Principles of

Imaging Science and Protection

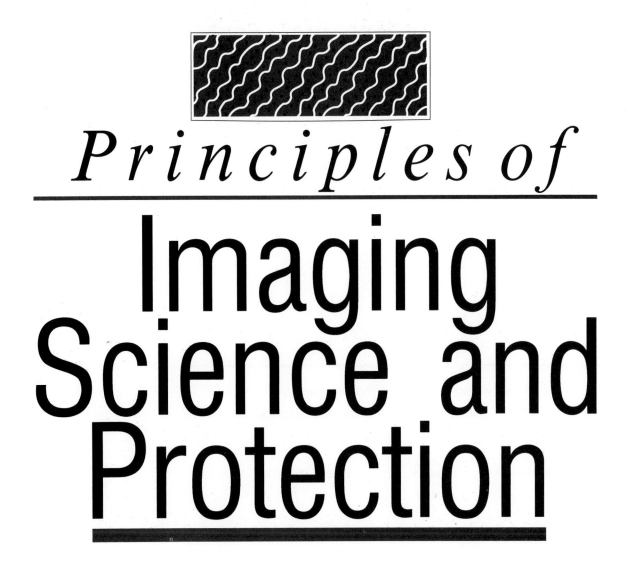

Principles of Imaging Science and Protection

Michael A. Thompson, M.S.
Professor, Medical Physics
Division of Medical Imaging and Therapy
The University of Alabama at Birmingham
Birmingham, Alabama

Janice D. Hall, M.A.Ed., R.T.(R.)
Assistant Professor and Director
Advanced Imaging Program
The University of Alabama at Birmingham
Birmingham, Alabama

Marian P. Hattaway, B.S., R.T.(R.)
Associate Professor
Radiography Program
The University of Alabama at Birmingham
Birmingham, Alabama

Steven B. Dowd, Ed.D., R.T.(R.)
Program Director
Assistant Professor
Radiography Program
The University of Alabama at Birmingham
Birmingham, Alabama

W.B. Saunders Company
A Division of Harcourt Brace & Company
Philadelphia   London   Toronto   Montreal   Sydney   Tokyo

W.B. SAUNDERS COMPANY
A Division of Harcourt Brace & Company
The Curtis Center
Independence Square West
Philadelphia, Pennsylvania 19106

Library of Congress Cataloging-in-Publication Data

Principles of imaging science and protection/Michael A. Thompson . . . [et al.].—1st ed.
    p.   cm.
ISBN 0-7216-3428-1
1. Diagnostic imaging.   2. Radiography, Medical.   3. Radiation-Safety measures.
4. Medical physics.   I. Thompson, Michael A.   II. Title.
    [DNLM: 1. Radiography.   2. Health Physics.   3. Radiation Protection.   WN 200
P957 1994]
RC78.7.D53P76   1994
616.07′54—dc20
DNLM/DLC   93-12638

PRINCIPLES OF IMAGING SCIENCE AND PROTECTION   0-7216-3428-1

Last digit is the print number: 9   8   7   6   5   4   3   2   1

To my parents, Elizabeth and Alfred, who recognized the importance of education. To all the parents who, like my own, sacrifice to provide a quality education for their children.

Contributors

Duane Akroyd, Ph.D., R.T.(R.)
Associate Professor and Director, Health Occupations Education, North Carolina State University, Raleigh, North Carolina

Charles Burns, M.S.P.H., R.T.(R.)
Associate Professor, Division of Radiologic Science, University of North Carolina School of Medicine; University of North Carolina Hospitals, Chapel Hill, North Carolina

LaVerne T. Gurley, Ph.D., FASRT
Professor Emeritus, Shelby State Community College, Memphis, Tennessee

Alfred J. Lawson, Ph.D.
Administrative Director, Radiation Oncology Center of East Memphis; Clinical Assistant Professor, Department of Radiology, University of Tennessee, Center for the Health Sciences, Memphis, Tennessee

Preface

Principles of Imaging Science and Protection is a text written by eight radiography educators and edited by four, each of whom has had at least 10 years experience in the clinic and the classroom. When W.B. Saunders Company first contacted me several years ago to oversee this project, I knew that I wanted to involve experienced individuals, professionally recognized in their area of expertise, who have the ability to convey this information to students. It is hoped that the readers of this text will agree that we have been very successful in this respect.

Our introductory chapter, written by Duane Akroyd of North Carolina State University, provides a brief overview of radiography and introduces the student to a typical radiology department, the types of personnel employed within a department, and the types of equipment within such a department.

Chapters 2 through 5 provide the student with a basic background information in mathematics, physics, electricity, and magnetism needed to understand radiography equipment, radiation production, and radiation interaction in matter.

Many instructors have indicated that they would like to minimize mathematics and physics content. We all must recognize, however, that in doing so we weaken the professional preparation of radiographers and minimize their chances of advancing in the field of medical imaging. As a result, we do not apologize for the level of mathematics and physics in this text. We do recognize that all students entering radiography programs do not have exactly the same educational background. We have, therefore, sought to strike a balance between the theoretical and the practical application of physics to the clinical practice of radiographers. This is the purpose of these basic review chapters.

I personally believe that a radiographer should know about other types of radiation in medicine. Radiographers and radiation therapists need to be aware of all types of radiation sources for the safety of patients, staff, and members of the public, as well as for themselves—this basic information is included in Chapter 3.

Chapters 6 and 7 concentrate on the x-ray tube and the circuitry of the x-ray machine. Chapters 8 and 9 summarize the basic methods by which photons interact with matter and the characteristics of the radiation produced by the x-ray machine.

Chapters 10 through 14 describe image production. LaVerne Gurley, a highly respected radiography educator, has produced an excellent chapter on film. Mar-

ian P. (Pat) Hattaway, associate professor in the radiography program at the University of Alabama at Birmingham, wrote Chapters 11 and 13. They describe, in detail, general radiographic image production, effects of technical factors, and mechanical devices that are used to improve radiographic image quality. Janice D. Hall, assistant professor and director of the advanced imaging program at the University of Alabama at Birmingham wrote Chapters 12 and 14, which describe the effects of geometrical factors and patient status on the radiographic image. These chapters are very thorough and provide numerous radiographic images to illustrate specific points.

Chapter 15 on fluoroscopy was written by Steven B. Dowd, author, educator, and director of the radiography program at University of Alabama at Birmingham. The chapter provides the student with a generalized view of fluoroscopic units and image generation.

Chapters 16 and 17 are relatively unique to introductory radiography texts. Chapter 16 describes common equipment problems that affect the radiographic image and practical solutions to these problem. This chapter stresses the critical thinking skills needed by a professional radiographer confronted with equipment problems. Chapter 17 addresses the topic of quality control from a practical approach. Both chapters were written by Charles Burns of the University of North Carolina School of Medicine, with contributions from Dr. Dowd.

Chapters 18 through 21 concentrate on radiation biology—the application of its principles to clinical situations and the resulting concepts developed for radiation protection purposes. Chapter 18, which provides a summary of radiation biology concepts, was written by Alfred J. Lawson, a respected radiation biologist and educator, with contributions from Dr. Dowd. Chapter 19, written by Dr. Dowd, attempts to answer the student's question of why one must learn radiobiology by relating radiobiology to clinical practice.

Chapter 20 approaches the topic of health physics (radiation protection) from the viewpoint of a medical physicist, and Chapter 21 approaches the topic from the standpoint of the radiographer.

Chapter 22 concludes the text with an overview of other imaging modalities in just enough detail to provide the student with a working knowledge of these other modalities.

Each chapter concludes with a summary, important terminology, and review questions in both multiple choice and short answer formats. When numerical calculations are performed, exercises to test the student's problem-solving abilities are included in the review questions. Additional review questions, exercises, and practical laboratory exercises are provided in the workbook/laboratory manual that is available with this text. The text and its supplements continually stress the professional, critical thinking skills needed by today's radiographer to operate a variety of types of complicated imaging equipment.

I would like to extend personal thanks to Ms. Uvarta Coleman who prepared the manuscript and in the midst of chaos found time to give birth to a beautiful daughter. Her patience and determination to produce flawless work is greatly appreciated. Another individual on whom I depended was Ms. Lisa Morgan who did an excellent job preparing the camera-ready workbook/laboratory manual. It was a pleasure working with two such professional women.

For technical assistance, I would like to extend my appreciation to Varian-EIMAC, Philips Medical Systems, P and S X-Ray, Siemens, Picker International, American College of Radiology Institute, Eastman-Kodak, Liebel-Flarsheim, and OEC-Diasonics and to Dr. Robert Ford. A special thanks to both Mr. Dewey Narkates, chief service engineer for the University of Alabama Hospitals Radiology Department, for several afternoons of enlightening discussions in regard to x-ray equipment and to Mr. Bob Nelson, quality assurance supervisor for the University of Alabama at Birmingham radiology department. Our thanks is also extended to Ms. Donna Burr for her assistance in the duplicating of images and locating of materials.

I would also like to extend my appreciation to Lisa Biello and Peg Waltner of the W.B. Saunders Company for their patience and understanding when unavoidable problems arose—and to my co-authors, contributors, and colleagues for their encouragement and support. Most of all I extend appreciation to our students who keep their instructors mentally and professionally challenged in the classroom and in the clinic. Lest we forget, our students are the future of medical imaging.

MICHAEL A. THOMPSON

Contents

These variations can result in technical difficulties for the radiographer if not taken into consideration. This chapter describes the variations in patient size and anatomy and their effects on the final radiographic image. Included are the effects as a result of variations in tissue composition, pathological condition, age, and sex, and the presence of contrast media.

C H A P T E R   1 5

Fluoroscopy: Viewing Motion with X-ray 361
Steven B. Dowd, Ed.D., R.T.(R.)

The fluoroscopic unit is described. General descriptions of applications of fluoroscopy are also provided. Special attention is devoted to the equipment—x-ray tube, image intensification tube, fluoroscopic generator, viewing system, and means of recording the image. Mobile fluoroscopy is also briefly described.

C H A P T E R   1 6

Equipment and Accessory Malfunctions or Misapplications 379
Charles Burns, M.S.P.H., R.T.(R.)
Steven B. Dowd, Ed.D., R.T.(R.)

Reducing repeat exposures is a critical task of the technologist. Not all suboptimal images are due to poor technique. Being able to recognize common equipment- or accessory-related malfunctions or errors minimizes the number of exposures. This knowledge helps eliminate "chasing" a good image when the problem is equipment- or accessory-related rather than technique. This chapter reviews a number of such problems that may occur.

C H A P T E R   1 7

Quality Control 395
Charles Burns, M.S.P.H., R.T.(R.)
Steven B. Dowd, Ed.D., R.T.(R.)

This chapter describes quality control and the relationship between quality assurance and quality control. The focus of this chapter is on first- and second-level quality control tests performed by radiologic technologists. More complex tests are also presented briefly, as is a short discussion of repeat analysis.

C H A P T E R   1 8

General Radiation Biology 415
Alfred J. Lawson, Ph.D.
Steven B. Dowd, Ed.D., R.T.(R.)

Radiation biology is the study of how radiation may affect the function of living tissue from the subcellular level to the organism. The basic principles of radiation biology represent the collective attempt to explain how the known interactions of radiation within matter result in the diverse responses evident following that energy transfer. The results of radiation energy transfer within the cellular environment are dependent upon a variety of factors. These include radiation type, energy of the radiation employed, dose and dose rate, volume irradiated, specific molecules affected by the energy transfer, and secondary effects on adjacent neighboring molecules.

C H A P T E R   1 9

Applying Radiation Biology to Clinical Practice 439
Steven B. Dowd, Ed.D., R.T.(R.)

This chapter refines the theory presented in Chapter 18 in terms of risk/benefit considerations. This discussion provides a foundation for the following chapters in which maximum permissible doses and radiation protection are discussed. Means of expressing risk, risk-benefit continuums, dose-response curves, stochastic and nonstochastic effects, and specific risks of radiation are presented.

C H A P T E R   2 0

Radiological Health Physics....................453
Michael A. Thompson, M.S.

Health physics is the name given to the science of radiation protection. It encompasses the techniques of radiation measurement, the determination of radiation dose, and the assessment of potential biological effects as a result of radiation exposure. From these assessments, the development and implementation of radiation protection regulations are based. This chapter defines basic radiation protection units, discusses current radiation protection philosophy, identifies agencies that establish radiation protection standards, and summarizes current and proposed changes in those standards. Methods of occupational dose assessment are also discussed.

C H A P T E R   2 1

Radiation Protection 475
Steven B. Dowd, Ed.D., R.T.(R.)

The foundations of the profession of radiography are the production of a diagnostic image and radiation protection of the patient. The radiographer must also practice personal radiation protection. This chapter describes means by which the radiographer can practice sound protection principles. The general radiation protection principles of time, distance, and shielding as well as specific action strategies, such as patient communication, immobilization techniques, and film critique, are presented. Special topics include protection during mobile radiography and angiography and protection of the pregnant and potentially pregnant worker and employee.

CHAPTER 22

Michael A. Thompson, M.S.

The past two decades have seen significant advances in medical imaging. With significant numbers of technologists training in more than one imaging modality, it is important for new technologists to become familiar with these other types of medical imaging. A brief description is provided of other imaging modalities. The principles by which each operates and a brief description of the equipment used are also presented.

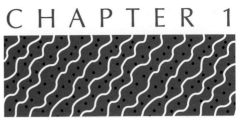

CHAPTER 1

An Introduction to Radiography — Principles, Equipment, and Departmental Operation

Duane Akroyd, Ph.D., R.T. (R)
Michael A. Thompson, M.S.

Chapter Outline

Chapter Objectives

On completion of this chapter, you should be able to

- Define basic radiography terms discussed in the chapter and summarized at the end.
- Describe the general design and operation of an x-ray tube.
- Describe in general the method by which x-rays are used in conventional radiography to produce images on radiographic film.
- Explain what is meant by "technical factors" and how each factor affects the x-rays produced and the resulting radiograph.
- Briefly describe what is meant by the ALARA concept and tell how it can be implemented in the radiology department.
- Indicate techniques used to monitor the radiographer's occupational radiation exposure and how they work; tell why monitoring one's radiation exposure is important.
- Specify the three primary planes of the body.
- Explain each of the following terms and describe their effects on the resulting radiograph:
  - *scatter radiation*
  - *grids*
  - *screens*
- Explain the term *artifact;* and indicate the effect of artifacts on diagnostic usefulness of radiographs.
- Briefly describe the principle of image production for each of the following imaging modalities usually associated with diagnostic radiology departments:
  - *ultrasound*
  - *nuclear medicine*
  - *magnetic resonance imaging*

HISTORICAL BEGINNINGS

Medical radiography had its beginnings on November 8, 1895, in Würzburg, Germany, in the laboratory of Wilhelm Conrad Röntgen. Röntgen, a mechanical engineer and physicist, was conducting ongoing investigations on the passage of electricity through high-vacuum discharge tubes known as Crookes tubes. These tubes were simple in design and basically consisted of a positive and a negative electrode within a sealed glass tube, as illustrated in Figure 1–1. Air was removed from

1

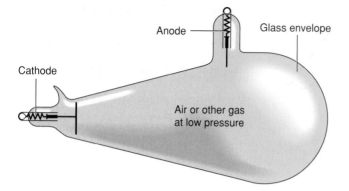

FIGURE 1–1. Diagram of a Crookes tube, the forerunner of the modern x-ray tube. (Courtesy of Arnold Feldman, Ph.D.)

the tube, using a vacuum pump, and trace amounts of elemental gases (such as hydrogen; mercury, sodium, or neon vapor) could then be introduced into the tube to test their electrical conductive properties. When a current (now recognized to be a flow of *electrons*) passed through the gas within the tube, the gas would glow with a characteristic color, depending on the type of gas within the tube. This color is known as the emission spectrum of the element (e.g., yellow light is emitted from sodium and bluish-purple light from mercury) and is unique for each element.

As higher vacuum conditions were established within the tube (i.e., more and more of the gas was removed from the tube), the tube became completely dark with the exception that its glass walls now began to give off a faint light. Further investigation and experimentation identified the origin of this emitted light (known as *fluorescence*) from the glass walls to be streams of particles that appeared to originate from the negative electrode or cathode of the tube. At the time, these particles, which today we know to be electrons were designated *cathode rays*. During investigations into the nature of cathode rays, it had also been observed that when certain materials known as *phosphors* were struck by these cathode rays, light would be emitted. One such material used by Röntgen in his studies of cathode rays was barium platinocyanide.

Thus with the use of a suitable phosphor such as barium platinocyanide, one could detect the passage of cathode rays (i.e., electrons) from the *cathode* (negative terminal) to the *anode* (positive terminal) of the tube when an appropriate voltage was applied. The voltage, from a high-voltage power supply, is necessary to pull the electrons across the tube to the anode.

Röntgen's discovery of x-rays came about by accident. In an effort to better see the fluorescence produced by the cathode rays striking the glass walls of the tube, Röntgen had enclosed the tube with a cardboard shield. Upon closer inspection when the room lights were lowered, he noticed that when a current was passed through the tube, no light leaked through the makeshift cover. However, a phosphor-coated sheet lying near the enclosed tube began to glow dimly.

■ FLUORESCENCE, PHOSPHORS, AND PHOSPHORESCENCE

A metal wire, such as the filament of a light bulb, can be heated to a point at which it gives off visible light. When a material is heated to such a temperature that visible light is emitted, the process is referred to as incandescence.

There are substances, known as phosphors, that can be made to emit visible light without the use of heat. Some of these materials need only be exposed to invisible electromagnetic radiation (e.g., x-rays or ultraviolet radiation) in order to emit visible light. If the visible light is emitted immediately after the material is exposed and ceases to be emitted when the exposure is terminated, the material is said to be fluorescent as in the case of fluorescent lights. In the fluorescent light tube, an electric current is passed through a gas mixture containing mercury vapor. The mercury atoms absorb energy from the electric current and emit ultraviolet (UV) radiation. A fluorescent powder coating the inner walls of the tube absorbs the UV radiation and then emits visible light. When the source of energy (i.e., the electric current) is removed by switching off the current, no additional light is emitted from the tube.

Other substances may absorb energy, but it may be emitted slowly over an extended period of time ranging from minutes to hours rather than immediately. Such materials are said to be *phosphorescent*. An example is the luminous numbers on the face of a clock that absorb visible light during daylight hours and re-emit visible light in the dark.

Use of such phenomena has played an important role in the study of radiation, for it allowed early investigators such as Röntgen to detect the presence of the otherwise unseen. Phosphors have been an important part of the investigation into the nature of radiation and continue to be used in radiation detection instruments, x-ray image production, and television and computer display screens.

Röntgen reasoned that some type of radiation originating from the tube was passing through the cardboard shield, striking the phosphor-coated screen and causing it to fluoresce. This new radiation was designated as *x-rays—x* meaning *unknown*. This terminology has remained intact, even though today the properties of this radiation are well known.

Although Röntgen's discovery occurred in November 1895, he chose not to announce his discovery until January 1896. After further investigations, Röntgen published his findings at the end of December 1895. In this initial publication, Röntgen listed his

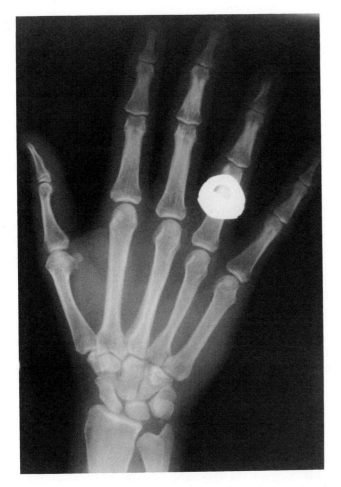

FIGURE 1-2. Radiograph of the hand similar to the first radiograph made by Röntgen, December 22, 1895.

findings regarding the properties of the new rays, which included the following:

- the degree to which a material is penetrated by x-rays depends on its thickness and density
- many materials can be penetrated by x-rays to varying degrees

- a phosphor can be made to fluoresce when exposed to x-rays
- photographic plates darken as a result of exposure to x-rays
- x-rays do not exhibit measurable reflection from surfaces they encounter
- x-rays are not deflected by magnetic fields

The ability of the new rays to penetrate matter held great potential for their usefulness. On December 22, 1895, Röntgen made the first reported medical radiograph—his wife's hand—similar in appearance to the radiograph in Figure 1-2. Then on January 23, 1896, Röntgen made a second, similar radiograph of an individual's hand during a public lecture (Fig. 1-3). The image produced showed the bones of the hand clearly, since bones tend to stop x-rays. Soft tissue structures stop x-rays to varying degrees but not to the extent as do bones. Therefore, on the radiographic image, bones show up as light areas (or areas of low radiographic density) against a background of shades of gray. On such a radiograph, the degree of darkening of the film is determined by the degree of x-ray penetration. The field of medicine immediately recognized the potential usefulness of this new type of radiation in medical diagnosis.

At about the same time in the United States, a physics instructor, Frank E. Austin, is reported to have performed amazing demonstrations with similar rays in his laboratory at Dartmouth College in New Hampshire. It is not clear, however, whether Austin's work with x-rays occurred before, concurrently with, or after Röntgen's discovery. Regardless of the timing, it is possible that Austin's radiographs were the first made in the United States. Austin had tried to interest persons in the medical profession, but found little enthusiasm in those he approached—at least until Röntgen's first publication began to circulate through the American medical community.

On February 3, 1896, Dr. Gilman Frost of the Mary Hitchcock Memorial Hospital, with the assistance of his brother, who was a physicist, employed x-rays to

FIGURE 1-3. Röntgen's first public demonstration of x-rays in Würzburg in January 1896. (Courtesy of Parke-Davis, a division of Warner Lambert Company.)

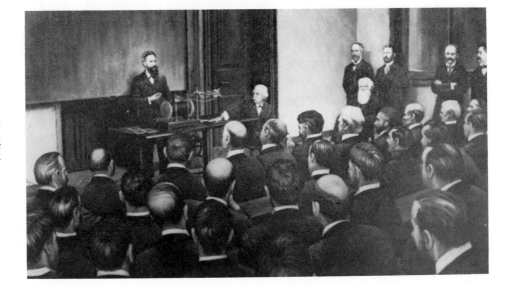

diagnose the extent of injuries of a young boy who had fallen while skating on the Connecticut River. The x-ray was made in the physics laboratory at Dartmouth College (Fig. 1–4). This became the first case in which x-rays were used for medical diagnosis in the United States.

In the years that have passed since these beginnings, the diagnostic radiology department has become one of the most important diagnostic departments within modern health care facilities. Beyond making standard x-ray films, a wide variety of radiographic procedures is usually conducted within these departments. Also within many radiology departments are found the other modes of medical imaging:

Diagnostic Ultrasonography. Utilizes sound waves to view internal structures of the body

Nuclear Medicine. Utilizes chemical compounds tagged with trace amounts of radioactive material (i.e., unstable form of an element that emits radiation) to obtain images indicating whether or not an organ is functioning properly

Magnetic Resonance Imaging (MRI). Utilizes radiowaves and strong magnetic fields to generate images of internal body structures; these images yield complex information about body structures and the chemical changes that occur as a result of the onset of disease

Computed Tomography (CT). A specialized form of radiography using an x-ray tube that rotates around the patient's body and a sophisticated computer system to generate "slice," or *tomographic,* images through a plane of the body; this type of radiography requires the use of a computer to reconstruct the final image

Each of these imaging modalities, including conventional radiography, has its own individual advantages and disadvantages in diagnosing various health problems. The making of an accurate diagnosis is dependent on the knowledge of the patient's referring physician (i.e., the physician who orders the particular imaging study) and the *radiologist* (i.e., the physician who reviews and interprets radiographic studies) in choosing the most appropriate imaging modality to provide the information desired.

As a future *radiographer,* you will become an integral part of a team of modern health care professionals dedicated to providing quality care to each patient. Whether you become a member of a small department in a rural hospital, a staff technologist in an outpatient diagnostic center, or a technologist in a large medical center, the first steps in making an accurate diagnosis begin with you and your ability to obtain a quality radiograph. Your radiologist depends on your ability to work with patients and your knowledge of the equipment that you use to obtain the sharpest and most detailed images technically possible.

At the conclusion of your studies and clinical instruction, you will become a member of a proud profession with a rich history and perhaps unmatched in the rate of its technical advancement over the past two decades. As a medical imaging specialist, your career opportunities will be limited only by your own desires to learn and to become more technically proficient in your clinical skills.

THE X-RAY TUBE: AN OVERVIEW

The x-rays that are used to produce a medical x-ray image (known as a *radiograph*) are generated by an x-ray tube, the basic components of which are illus-

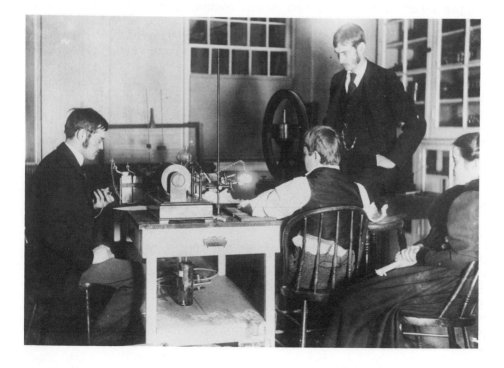

FIGURE 1–4. The first medical radiograph in the United States, performed by Dr. Gilman D. Frost in the physics laboratory at Dartmouth College on February 3, 1896. (Reprinted with permission of the Dartmouth-Hitchcock Medical Center, Hanover, New Hampshire.)

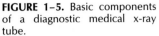
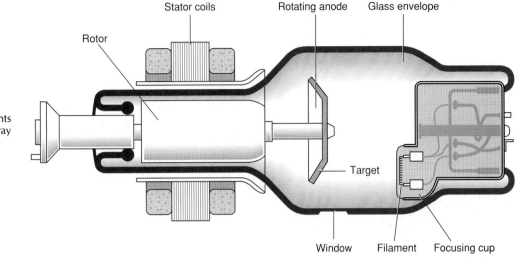

FIGURE 1–5. Basic components of a diagnostic medical x-ray tube.

trated in Figure 1–5. These basic components consist of a positive electrode (or anode), a negative electrode (or cathode), a *filament,* and a *target.* The primary technique used to generate x-rays in conventional x-ray tubes is to accelerate charged particles (electrons) to very high speeds then to let them strike a high Z number (i.e., *atomic number*) target. As the electrons are accelerated and slam into the target, their kinetic energy (energy of motion) is converted into two other types of energy—heat and x-rays. Slightly more than 99% of the electrons' kinetic energy is converted into heat, whereas less than 1% is converted into x-rays. This fact becomes more important in later chapters when we more closely consider the specifics of x-ray tube design.

In the x-ray tube, the filament is the source of electrons. The filament itself is a long, thin coil of tungsten wire that, when heated by an electric current, releases electrons from its surface (a process referred to as *thermionic emission*). Once the electrons are released from the filament surface, a force must then be provided that will pull the electrons at great speed into the anode target. This force is provided by a high-voltage generator that greatly amplifies the incoming line voltage, from hundreds of volts to tens of thousands of volts. The higher the voltage across the x-ray tube electrodes, the faster the electrons move and the more energetic or penetrating the x-rays produced. Therefore the radiographer has the ability to change the penetrating power of the x-rays simply by adjusting the voltage across the tube.

The target into which the electrons from the filament are drawn is also conventionally made of the element tungsten. Tungsten is used as the target material because of its high Z number (Z = 74) and its extremely high melting point (~ 3300°C). Most x-ray tubes in modern x-ray departments use rotating anodes to assist in the dissipation of the large quantities of heat generated at the target. Special motors allow anode targets to rotate at speeds up to 10,000 revolu-

tions per minute (expressed as 10,000 rpm). Most x-ray machines do not allow x-rays to be produced by the tube until the anode target rotates at its designated speed, in order to minimize the chance of heat damage to the target.

The components of the x-ray tube are enclosed within a protective *glass envelope* that serves several purposes. First, it is necessary that the tube electrodes be enclosed within a *vacuum* (i.e., a region from which all air has been removed) for proper tube operation. If air is present between the electrodes during the tube operation, collisions between the fast-moving electrons from the filament and the air molecules will result in x-ray production that can be controlled neither in terms of number of x-rays produced (related to what is termed x-ray intensity) nor in their energy (related to their penetrating ability). Thus the glass envelope serves to maintain vacuum conditions within the tube. Second, it provides mechanical support for the tube components and the high-voltage cables that provide the electrical energy for the tube. The glass envelope is commonly made of Pyrex to withstand the high levels of heat generated during tube operation.

When one first sees an x-ray unit in an imaging room, the actual x-ray tube is not visible, since it is enclosed within the *tube housing* as shown in Figure 1–6. The tube is surrounded by oil, also within the tube housing, that aids in the removal of heat. Fans circulating air are also used to assist in cooling of the tube and its housing. X-rays leave the tube through the exit window, proceeding through a series of *filters* (used to remove low-energy x-rays from the beam) and lead *collimators* (lead strips used to restrict the size of the beam) before striking the patient. Both filtration and collimation of the emerging x-rays are for the purpose of reducing patient radiation dose. Also occupying the same compartment as the collimators is a small light source that allows the radiographer a visible method to approximate the size of the x-ray beam before energizing the tube (Fig. 1–7).

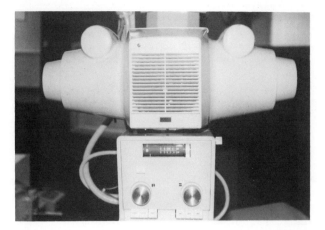

FIGURE 1–6. An x-ray tube as it would normally appear in its tube housing.

PRODUCTION OF THE RADIOGRAPH: AN OVERVIEW

The production of medical radiographs is based on the fact that x-rays of appropriate energy will pass through structures within the body to varying degrees. If a piece of radiographic film is placed behind the body structure exposed to the x-ray beam, the x-rays

striking the film will darken areas on it when it is processed. Areas on the film that appear dark represent those areas of the body easily penetrated by the x-rays. Those dark regions are said to be regions of high *radiographic density.* Soft tissue, muscle, and organs produce regions of varying degrees of darkness or shades of gray on the radiographic image. Bone is effective at stopping x-rays, not allowing them to interact with the film; it appears as light areas (i.e., areas of low radiographic density) on the film. This is illustrated in Figure 1–8 along with the radiographic image that would be obtained.

When the patient enters the imaging room, the radiographer first confirms his or her identity and the type of x-ray image that has been ordered by the patient's own physician, the department radiologist, or both. Body thickness measurements should be made by the radiographer in order to determine the appropriate x-ray energy that will produce the best possible image. After body thickness measurements have been made and recorded, the radiographer chooses the proper size film, which has been previously loaded into a *cassette.* (During the exposure of the film to the x-ray beam, the cassette provides mechanical support; it also contains flexible sheets known as *screens* that serve to intensify the image produced on the film. Screens are discussed further in later chapters.) The radiographer then loads the film cassette into a cassette-holding device that may be located under the x-ray table top (this type of holder is known as the

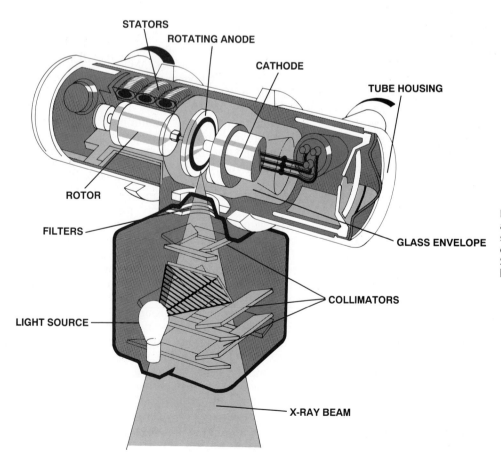

FIGURE 1–7. Schematic drawing of a medical x-ray tube and associated structures within the metal housing of a radiographic unit. (Courtesy of Siemens Medical Systems, Inc., Iselin, NJ.)

STATORS
ROTATING ANODE
CATHODE
TUBE HOUSING
ROTOR
FILTERS
GLASS ENVELOPE
LIGHT SOURCE
COLLIMATORS
X-RAY BEAM

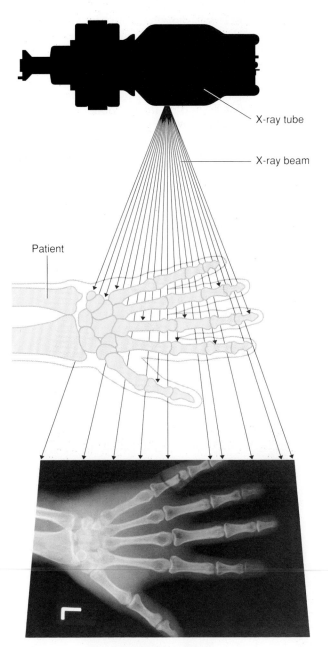

X-ray tube

X-ray beam

Patient

Image receptor (film)

Photons penetrating tissue cause film to darken.
Photons absorbed by bone result in light areas on the radiograph.

FIGURE 1–8. Relative positions of x-ray tube, patient, and film necessary to make the radiograph shown. Bones tend to stop diagnostic x-rays, but soft tissue does not. This results in the light and dark regions that form the image.

Bucky tray) or mounted vertically on a wall. Both types of cassette-holding devices are shown (Figs. 1–9 and 1–10). Films are also properly labeled with patient information and markers to designate his or her particular position shown on the radiograph.

Prior to actually making the radiographic exposure, the *radiological technologist* should briefly discuss the procedure and carefully inform the patient of any special breathing instructions that will be used. The nor-

mal motion that occurs during breathing can reduce image clarity for certain radiographs. Therefore the patient may be asked to take a deep breath and hold it or to expel the air in the lungs and stop breathing momentarily prior to the exposure. Since unnecessary motion affects image clarity, restraining devices (e.g., straps or positioning blocks) may on occasion need to be used for immobilization.

The technologist must also make sure that the patient does not have any jewelry, buttons, watches, earrings, hairpins, and so forth on the area of the body to be radiographed. If any article such as those mentioned is not removed, its image will be superimposed on the radiograph. This was illustrated earlier in Figure 1–2, in which a ring is shown on a radiograph of a hand. When an object such as this creates a feature on a medical image that does not represent an actual body structure, it is referred to as an *artifact*. Artifacts are not desirable in medical imaging, since they can obscure body structures and possible pathologies and in certain cases, can even mimic pathologies, which could result in a misdiagnosis. Finally, the patient is correctly positioned in relation to the x-ray machine and the film cassette.

Using the body thickness measurements obtained earlier, the technologist then refers to what is known as a technique chart, which will provide the proper *technical factors* to produce the best image quality possible. The technical factors are those imaging parameters that the technologist can vary and that have profound effects on the image produced. These technical factors include the following:

- Peak kilovoltage (kVp) refers to the voltage sent across the x-ray tube electrodes; it affects the number of x-rays produced and determines their energy or penetrating ability*
- Milliamperes (mA) refers to the magnitude of the electric current (i.e., the number of electrons) that flows between the tube electrodes when an exposure is made; this is also known as the tube current and is used to regulate the number of x-rays produced
- Exposure time is normally measured in seconds or fractions of a second; refers to the length of time that the x-ray tube produces x-rays during a radiographic exposure

The technique chart provides numerical values for these technical factors for a body part (e.g., hand, chest, abdomen, etc.) of specific thickness that will produce the best diagnostic-quality radiograph. Care must always be taken to utilize only the technique chart specifically formulated for the x-ray equipment being used.

After the proper technical factors are determined from the technique chart, their numerical values are entered into the equipment at the console, or control

*The abbreviations kV and kVp are often used interchangeably; kVp more correctly indicates that the voltage across the tube electrodes typically varies in magnitude. And kVp indicates the peak value of voltage, which determines the maximum energy of the x-rays produced.

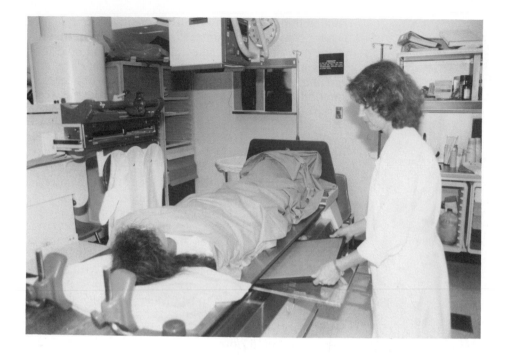

FIGURE 1-9. A radiographic film cassette being loaded into a Bucky tray in a radiographic imaging table.

panel, which is usually located behind a physical barrier (e.g., a lead-lined wall, lead shield, or other protective structure) designed to protect the radiographer from *scatter radiation* (e.g., x-rays that scatter in many directions as a result of their initial interaction with the patient's body, the imaging table and so forth). The technologist should always stand behind protective barriers when the x-ray tube is energized. Final instructions are given to the patient, the rotating anode is brought up to speed, and the exposure is made. The patient is told to relax while the technologist prepares to process the film.

The radiographer then removes the film cassette from the cassette holder and carries it into the *darkroom*—a room having greatly reduced light intensity that is the storage area for unexposed film and the place where film cassettes are loaded and unloaded. The door to the darkroom must always remain closed when it is in use. The only light allowed within the room during film loading and unloading is that provided by the *safe light* located inside the darkroom. It produces sufficient light to aid the radiographer in darkroom work but of low enough intensity not to affect the film. In the darkroom, the technologist removes the film from the cassette and carefully feeds it into the *automatic film processor.*

The film processor contains tanks of chemical solutions and rinses through which the film automatically moves by a system of rollers. As the film passes through these solutions, the *latent image* (i.e., the hidden image) caused by the radiographic exposure now becomes visible on the film. This hard copy film image is retrieved from the exit tray of the film processor,

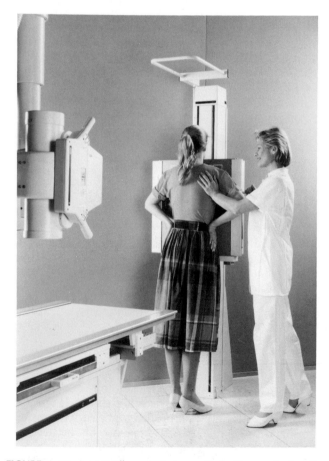

FIGURE 1-10. A vertically mounted cassette holder used primarily in making chest radiographs. (Courtesy of Medica Mundi–Philips Medical Systems, Best, the Netherlands.)

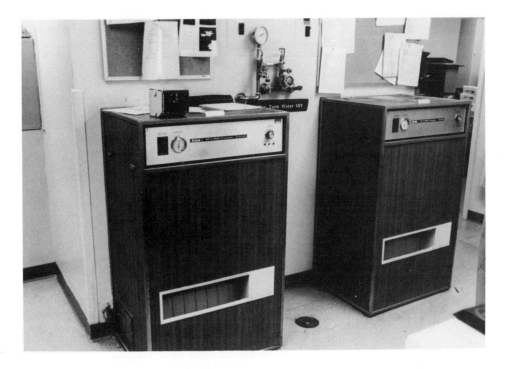

FIGURE 1–11. Automatic film processors positioned outside a radiology department darkroom.

which is normally located in a room adjacent to the darkroom. Two such automatic film processors located just outside a radiology darkroom are shown in Figure 1–11. In many departments, radiographers make the radiographs and process their own film. In larger departments, when workloads warrant, darkroom technicians may perform all darkroom work for the radiographers.

After the radiographer obtains the final x-ray images and approves the image quality, the patient is released, and the images are placed in the patient's folder and forwarded to the department radiologist who reads, or interprets, the radiograph. The radiologist's findings are contained in a written report, which is forwarded to the patient's personal physician or to the referring physician who originally ordered the test. The referring physician and the patient discuss the findings, and a course of treatment is planned if test results warrant. The patient's radiographic images are placed in his or her file, which is stored in the radiology department file room in the event that they are needed for reference at a later time. A typical radiology file room is shown in Figure 1–12.

THE TYPICAL RADIOLOGY DEPARTMENT

X-ray departments vary widely in size, depending on the type of facility. X-ray units are found in large medical facilities, clinics, outpatient diagnostic centers, dental offices, and even private physicians' offices. The purpose of the next part of the chapter is to familiarize you with the various sections of a large hospital radiology department, the personnel who work in the department, the various types of equipment, and the work of radiographers.

Perhaps the first person one meets when entering a radiology department is the department's receptionist. She or he usually has the responsibility of greeting patients, obtaining and recording general patient information, assisting with patient scheduling, and informing the technologist when patients arrive for their imaging studies. Patients usually sit in the patients'

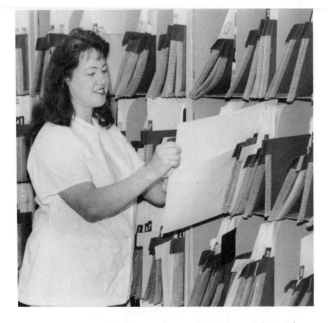

FIGURE 1–12. On completion of a study, patient radiographs are stored in the department file room for future reference.

waiting area until they are escorted to the imaging room by the technologist who will perform the study.

Most large radiology departments have several imaging rooms, containing various types of radiographic equipment. Some of the more general types of equipment design and imaging areas found in larger radiology departments are described in the following paragraphs.

General Purpose X-ray Units

General purpose x-ray units are perhaps the most common type of equipment found in an x-ray department regardless of size. This type of unit consists of a radiographic table and an x-ray tube positioned above the table (Fig. 1–13). The tables used with the units may be stationary or of a design that allows the patient to be moved in a number of directions. Many tables also allow the patient to be tilted through various angles to obtain different projections. Most of these radiographic tables contain a device known as a Bucky assembly. This device contains a grid and a cassette tray in which the loaded film cassette is placed prior to radiographic exposure. The grid is composed of a large number of thin lead strips separated by a material through which x-rays can pass. The purpose of this device is to decrease the amount of scatter radiation that strikes the film, since scatter radiation degrades the image quality of the radiograph (see the boxed material on grids and screens). X-ray tubes associated with this type of unit can be positioned so that the x-ray beam is either perpendicular or parallel to the tabletop. This allows the technologist to use the radiographic table in image production or to use a wall-mounted cassette holder such as that for making chest films (see Fig. 1–10). Typical studies conducted with this equipment include imaging of bones and joints, the chest, skull, abdomen, spine, and pelvis.

Radiographic and Fluoroscopic (R/F) Equipment

More versatile than the general purpose radiographic unit is an R/F unit. A modern unit of this type is equipped with two x-ray tubes—one mounted above the imaging table for general purpose radiography and the other under the imaging table for fluoroscopic studies. Each unit is used independently of the other, depending on the study to be performed. The radiographic unit is used in conjunction with standard film cassettes and is employed for conventional radiographic imaging. When imaging involving motion are required, the radiographic unit is swung out of position and replaced by the fluoroscopic unit. Modern fluoroscopic units utilize a device known as an *image intensifier,* located above the imaging table, to convert x-rays emerging from the patient into a visible image that can be viewed on a TV monitor and recorded on videotape for later study. Since these studies result in higher radiation doses to the patient and commonly employ the use of *contrast media* (gases, barium, or iodinated compounds introduced into the patient's body to enhance the radiographic image), the studies are performed by a radiologist assisted by the radiographer.

The fluoroscopic unit is also equipped with either a special film cassette holder or a roll of 105 mm radiographic film that allows the radiologist to record a particular image displayed on the TV monitor. Such an image is referred to as a *spot film.* Thus in addition to conventional radiographic studies, the fluoroscopic component allows the R/F unit to be used in fluoroscopic studies such as those of the upper and lower gastrointestinal (GI) tract, small bowel, esophagus, spinal cord, and joints. All personnel involved with fluoroscopic procedures are required to wear *lead aprons* for radiation protection purposes. A typical R/F unit is shown in Figure 1–14.

Portable Units (Mobile Radiography)

In the event of serious illness or injury, a patient may be unable to be transported to the radiology department. In these cases, most routine radiographic studies can be conducted at the patient's bedside with the use of mobile x-ray units. These are motorized, battery-powered, self-contained units that allow radiographs to be made of patients hospital rooms, intensive care units (ICUs), the emergency room (ER), or the operating room (OR). Portable fluoroscopic units may also be found in larger departments. A typical portable unit is shown in Figure 1–15.

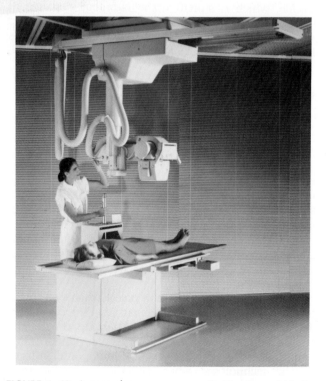

FIGURE 1–13. A general purpose x-ray unit. (Courtesy of Medica Mundi–Philips Medical Systems, Best, the Netherlands.)

■ GRIDS AND SCREENS

When x-rays pass through matter such as a patient's body, the x-ray may interact in one of three primary ways:

The x-ray may be transmitted. If this occurs, the x-ray passes through the patient's body and interacts with the radiographic film to produce a dark area on the film or an area of increased radiographic density.

The x-ray may be absorbed. If this occurs, the x-ray is absorbed within the denser soft tissue or bone structures. Since fewer x-rays penetrate these regions of the body and strike the radiographic film, these areas on the film appear light.

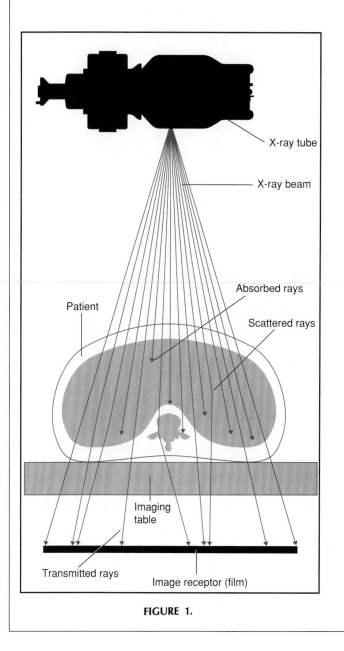

FIGURE 1.

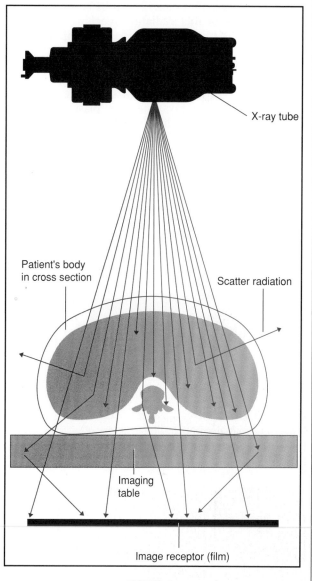

FIGURE 2.

The x-rays may be scattered. When an x-ray is scattered, the direction in which it was originally traveling is changed.

Scatter radiation results in a darkening of the radiographic film in areas where the film would have remained light had the direction of the x-ray not been changed. Each of these types of tissue interactions are shown in Figure 1.

Transmission and absorption provide specific diagnostic information about the tissue directly in front of each area on the radiographic film. Scatter radiation does not contain useful information, since it originated at random locations within the body, as illustrated (Fig. 2).

Scatter radiation lessens the sharpness and clarity of a radiographic image. It also produces a general

(continued)

darkening (known as *film fog*) over the entire radiograph. Radiographic images can thus be improved if the amount of scatter radiation reaching the radiographic film is minimized. This is accomplished by the use of a device known as a *grid,* which is placed between the patient and the film cassette. A grid consists of a series of regularly spaced lead (Pb) strips separated by a radiolucent substance (i.e., easily penetrated by x-rays) such as plastic or other synthetic materials. Such a typical arrangement and its placement in relationship to the patient and film cassette is shown in Figure 3.

Since scatter radiation originates from many sites within the irradiated volume of the patient's body (Fig. 3) as well as from the top of the imaging table if one is used, a great portion of this radiation is absorbed by the Pb strips. Scatter radiation cannot

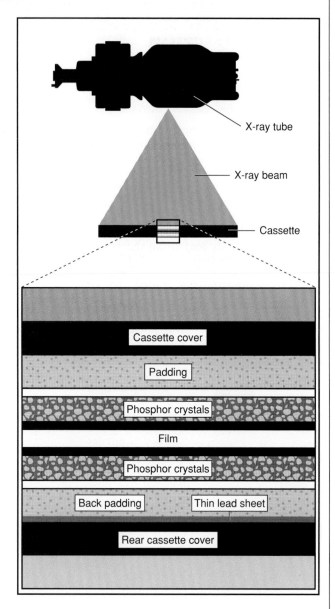

FIGURE 4.

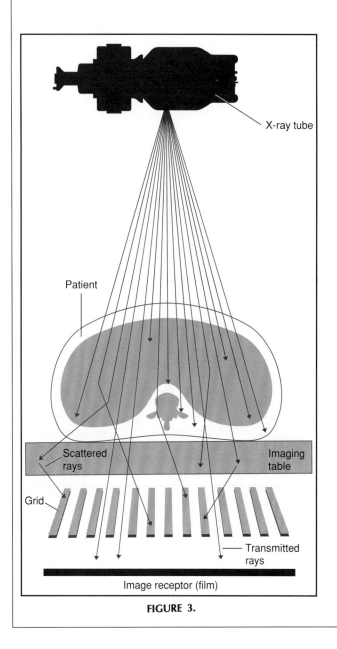

FIGURE 3.

be totally eliminated, but the use of grids produces radiographs of greatly improved diagnostic quality.

Another technical device used to affect the diagnostic quality of the resulting radiograph is the *intensifying screen.* An intensifying screen is a specially designed plastic or cardboard sheet that is coated with phosphor crystals. These crystals are compounds (e.g., cesium iodide, zinc cadmium sulfide, barium strontium sulfate) that when struck by x-rays, emit visible light. Since radiographic film is relatively insensitive to direct interaction with x-rays, radiographic images can be produced much more effectively by "sandwiching" the film in the film cassette between two such screens (Fig. 4).

In this way, x-rays that pass through the patient's body interact with the screens. The screens emit visible light to produce the image on the film. This technique greatly improves radiographic image quality. From a practical standpoint, when screens are used, much less radiation is required for image production, which in turn reduces patient radiation dose. The use of screens also allows the use of shorter exposure times, thereby reducing the chances of patient motion during the procedure.

More information on grids and screens is provided in later chapters.

Special Procedures

Many types of advanced radiological examinations involve the introduction of contrast media into the body through a catheter or puncture. These procedures must be performed by a physician or radiologist under sterile conditions to assure patient safety. These studies are referred to as *special procedures;* they normally involve the use of more complex radiographic and fluoroscopic equipment (Fig. 1–16). Tests conducted in these special imaging areas include procedures such as cardiac catheterization (to visualize blockages in coronary arteries), renal arteriography (to view the renal arterial system), cerebral arteriography (to demonstrate the blood vessels supplying the brain), and therapeutic catheterization techniques (to diagnose and treat diseases in the blood vessels). Therapeutic catheterization methods may include such techniques as infusion therapy (injection of specific drugs into a blood vessel to increase or decrease blood flow) and percutaneous transluminal angioplasty (PTA), designed to dilate or reopen occluded areas within a vessel by compressing plaque against the vessel wall with a balloon catheter. Special procedure imaging areas are usually located in restricted access sections of the department.

Tomographic Imaging

Many times a radiograph contains obscured information as a result of the superimposed images of tissues and organ structures lying above and below a region of diagnostic interest. An imaging technique that is often employed in these instances is known as *tomography* (from the Greek *tomos,* meaning *cut* or *slice*). Conventional tomographic imaging equipment is used to produce a radiograph of a selected body plane of predetermined thickness. Tomographic imaging is performed to minimize any additional image information coming from regions outside the specific area of interest. This particular type of imaging is most important, since a lesion (i.e., a site of disease or disease structure) may be masked or hidden by overlying structures. One technique used to obtain this type of image in radiography is known as conventional (or linear) tomography. With conventional tomographic equipment (Fig. 1–17), a special mechanism allows the x-ray tube and film to be moved in opposite directions simultaneously (Fig. 1–18). As the tube and film are moved during a radiographic exposure, only structures located in the focal plane remain in focus. Structures above and below this focal plane are blurred by the

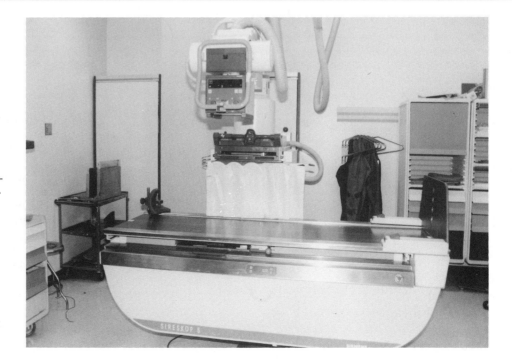

FIGURE 1–14. A typical radiographic and fluoroscopic (R/F) unit.

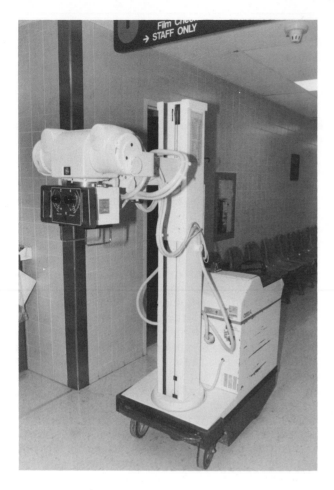

FIGURE 1-15. Mobile x-ray units allow radiographs to be made at locations outside the radiology department.

FIGURE 1-16. Special procedures are conducted under sterile conditions by a radiologist with the assistance of a radiographer.

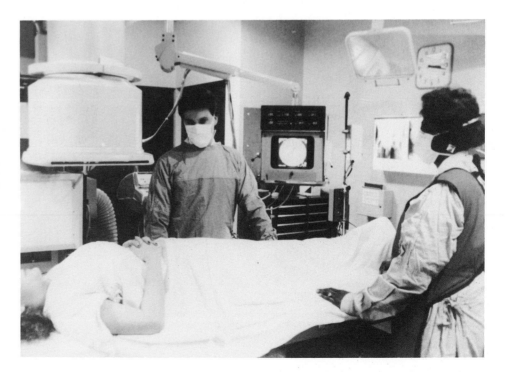

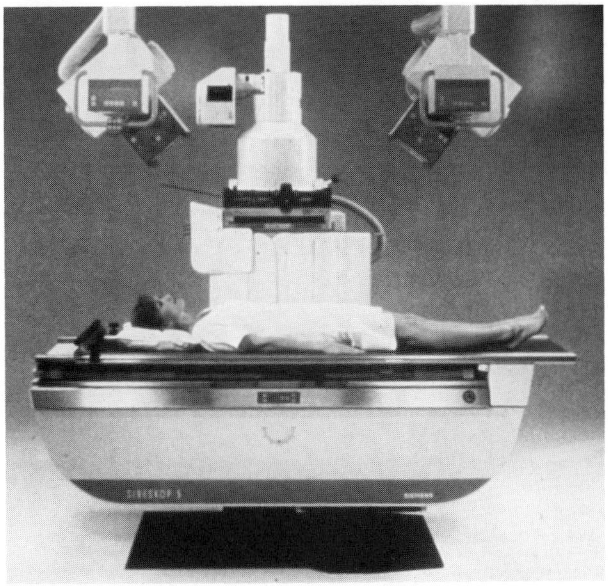

FIGURE 1–17. A linear tomographic x-ray unit used to obtain radiographic images at specific depths within the patient's body. (Courtesy of Siemens Medical Systems, Inc., Iselin, NJ.)

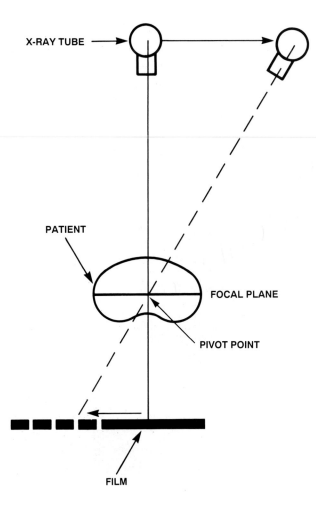

X-RAY TUBE →

PATIENT

FOCAL PLANE

PIVOT POINT

FILM

FIGURE 1–18. In conventional tomography, the film and x-ray tube are moved horizontally in opposite directions during the exposure. The plane through the pivot point remains in focus, whereas structures above and below this plane are blurred by the motion. (Courtesy of Eastman-Kodak Company.)

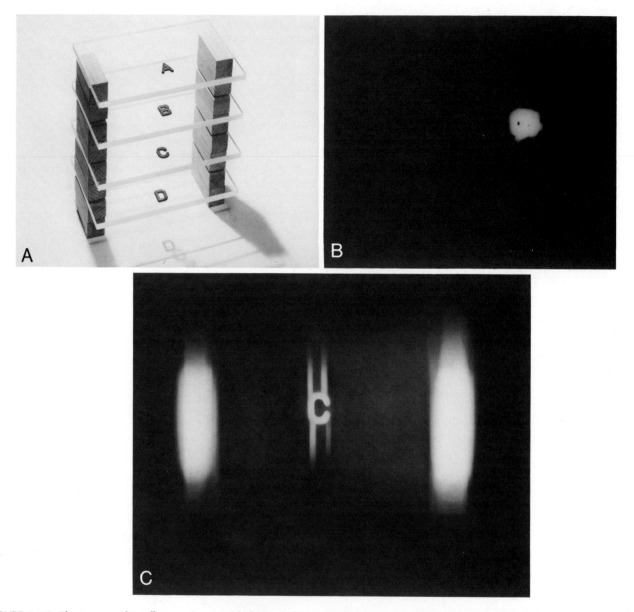

FIGURE 1–19. The tomographic effect: *A*, A series of plastic shelves, each holding a lead letter, is used as a test object. *B*, A radiograph made with conventional equipment. The x-ray beam passed vertically through the test object, and all letters are superimposed. C, A radiograph made with conventional tomographic equipment. The fulcrum plane was located at the level of the letter C, which shows quite clearly. The other letters are blurred by motion. Notice the streaking effect associated with tomography of linear objects. (Courtesy of Eastman-Kodak Company.)

made radiographic examinations of the breast a routine procedure in many departments, outpatient diagnostic centers, and women's clinics. Mammography units (Fig. 1–22) are designed for the specific purpose of performing soft tissue radiography and are thus considered *dedicated units* (i.e., x-ray units only for specific types of study). Unlike conventional x-ray tubes, which use only tungsten targets, mammography tubes may use tungsten or, perhaps more commonly, molybdenum targets. Molybdenum targets produce a greater number of low-energy x-rays at low kVp settings. It is these lower-energy x-rays that are needed in imaging soft tissue structures to maximize the ability to detect structural and pathological changes.

Image Processing

After a radiographic film has been exposed to x-rays in any radiographic procedure, it must be processed to convert the latent radiographic image in the film into a visible image. Since the film used in radiography is

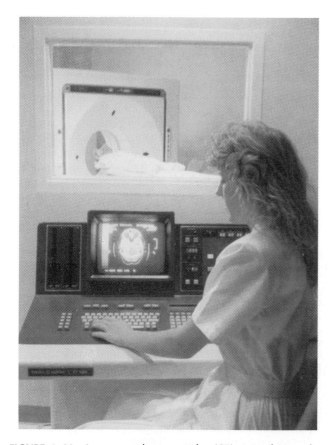

FIGURE 1–20. A computed tomography (CT) unit obtains slice images using an x-ray tube that moves around the patient and a computer that generates the final images. (Reprinted from ''Your Career Opportunities in Radiologic Technology,'' American Healthcare Radiology Administrators, Sudbury, MA.)

motion (Fig. 1–19). Typically, conventional tomographic units find great use in the performance of intravenous pyleograms (IVPs) used to visualize renal structures.

A more complex method of obtaining tomographic images is *computed tomography (CT)*. CT units (Fig. 1–20) have a very different appearance from previously discussed radiographic equipment. These units are usually square with a circular opening at the center within which the patient is positioned. The tomographic images are produced by an x-ray tube that is rotated around the patient's body on a mechanized track (Fig. 1–21). The number of x-rays that pass through the body at the different angles is recorded by a series of detectors opposite the tube. In CT, rather than recording the image directly on radiographic film, the information is fed into a computer, from which an image is generated. CT imaging is an advanced mode of radiographic imaging and is not considered a routine study because of its complexity and the higher radiation dose to the patient. It is used however when more detailed images are required for a diagnosis.

Mammography Units

The relatively high incidence of breast cancer in the United States and the emphasis on early detection has

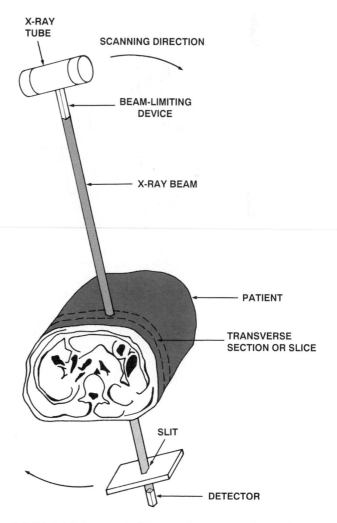

FIGURE 1–21. In computed tomography, a narrow beam of x-rays is passed through the patient's body to detectors that remain aligned with the x-ray tube as it rotates about the patient. From the information obtained at the different positions, a computer-generated image is constructed. (Courtesy of Eastman-Kodak Company.)

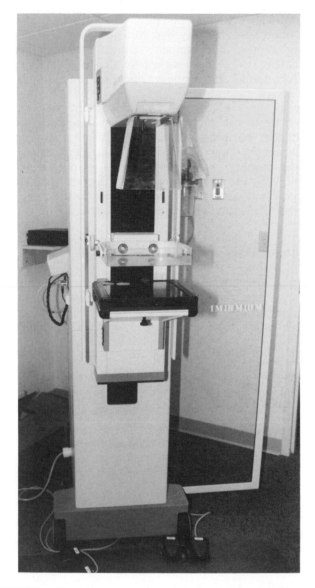

FIGURE 1–22. A mammography unit most commonly utilizes a molybdenum target to improve soft tissue images of the breast.

Some processing systems reduce or eliminate the need for a darkroom. These are known as *daylight systems* because cassettes can be loaded and unloaded and film can be processed without the use of a darkroom.

Images are carefully reviewed by the radiologist in the *reading room.* After detailed examination of the images, the radiologist writes a report of his or her findings, which is returned to the patient's referring physician for final action. The actual radiographs produced during the study and a copy of the radiographic findings are placed in the patient's files, which are maintained in the department's file room in the event that they are needed for future reference.

TYPES OF RADIOGRAPHIC IMAGES AND RECORDING DEVICES

Depending on the exact type of radiographic study being conducted, the radiologist requests certain projections (radiographic images with the patient's body or the x-ray machine in specific positions). These positions allow the radiologist to obtain the best visualization of body structures and pathologies that might otherwise be obscured or overlooked if only one projection was taken. In radiography the specific positions can also be referred to as projections. A projection indicates the path taken by the x-rays as they emerge from the x-ray tube and travel through the patient's body to the image receptor. Some of the more common projections include the following:

Anteroposterior (AP). With this projection, if an imaging table is used, the patient is supine (face

sensitive to visible light (e.g., room light) as well as x-rays, the loading of unexposed film into film cassettes and its removal for processing must take place in near-total darkness. In the radiology department, the loading and unloading of film cassettes occurs in the departmental darkroom.

The darkroom is usually centrally located to all imaging areas to maximize work flow efficiency. Since the door to the darkroom should never be opened when it is in use, all darkrooms are equipped with a device known as a *passbox* (Fig. 1–23). This device allows film cassettes to be passed into the darkroom and back again without permitting light to enter the darkroom work area. The darkroom also serves as a storage area for unexposed film. Here it is stored in light-tight *film bins* until it is used to reload film cassettes. Film bins are usually located under the darkroom countertops and contain separate compartments for film of different sizes.

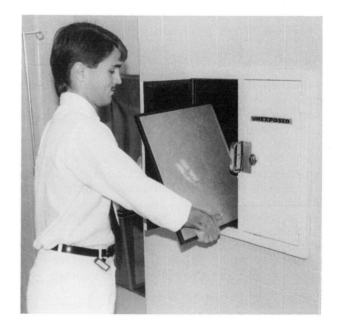

FIGURE 1–23. The passbox allows exposed and unexposed film cassettes to be transferred into and out of the darkroom without light entering.

up) with his or her back against the radiographic table. If a vertically mounted chest chamber is used, the patient's back is placed against this device. In either imaging technique, the x-ray beam enters the front or anterior surface of the body and exits the back or posterior side before striking the image receptor (Fig. 1–24A).

Posteroanterior (PA). If an imaging table is used with this projection, the patient is placed in a prone (face down) position on the radiographic table. If a chest chamber is used, the patient is erect, facing the vertically mounted device. With either technique, the x-ray beam enters the patient's back, or posterior surface, and exits the front, or anterior, surface before striking the image receptor (Fig. 1–24B).

Lateral. A lateral view implies a side view. Patient may be positioned on the right or left side on a radiographic table or with either side against a vertical chest chamber (Fig. 1–24C). Whether a particular projection is termed a right lateral or left lateral is determined by which side of the body is nearest the radiographic film.

Oblique. An oblique projection implies a projection made at an angle. The body part being imaged is rotated so that neither a frontal (AP or PA) nor a lateral view is produced. Oblique projections are illustrated in Figure 1–24D.

It is common to hear the term *view* used to describe various radiographic projections. Technically, a view represents the radiographic image as seen from the vantage of the film or image receptor. A view is the exact opposite of a projection.

In addition to specific projections commonly used in conventional radiography, the more widespread application of tomographic techniques to produce slice images in all modes of medical imaging makes recognition of body planes extremely important. With the body erect, feet together, and arms at the sides (Fig. 1–25), the three fundamental body planes are defined as follows:

Coronal. This plane divides the body into an anterior (front) and posterior (back) portion

Sagittal. This plane divides the body into a right side and a left side

Transverse (Axial). This plane produces cross-sectional slices and divides the body into superior (upper) and inferior (lower) portions

To illustrate the use of these body planes in medical imaging, Figure 1–26 shows tomographic images pro-

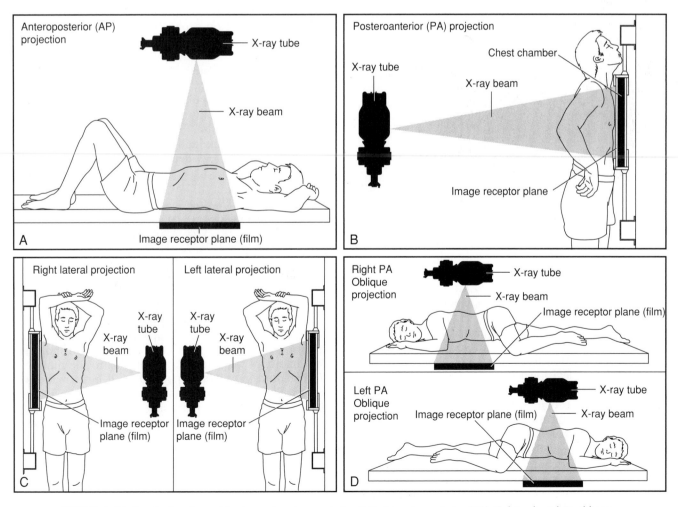

FIGURE 1–24. Standard radiographic views: *A,* anteroposterior (AP), *B,* posteroanterior (PA), *C,* lateral, and *D,* oblique.

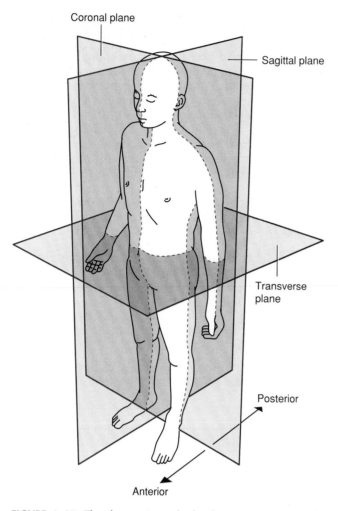

Coronal plane

Sagittal plane

Transverse plane

Posterior

Anterior

FIGURE 1–25. The three primary body planes: transverse (axial), coronal, and sagittal.

duced by a magnetic resonance imaging (MRI) unit in each of these three body planes.

The images produced in modern radiology departments vary in complexity and methods used to record them. Conventional radiographs that do not contain motion information (known as *static images*) are recorded and stored on various sizes of radiographic film. This is one of the oldest and most commonly used methods of image production and storage. Fluoroscopy gave the radiologist the ability to visualize anatomical motion but these images were produced on a fluorescent screen. The images originally produced were of poor quality and disappeared when the x-ray machine was turned off. Today these radiographic motion pictures (referred to as *cine* from the term *cinema*) are viewed on television monitors, and the images are recorded on motion picture film, videotape, or magnetic disc. Fluoroscopic images may in the near future be recorded on optical discs, which have greater information storage capability.

The development of newer imaging techniques such as CT, which uses computers to generate images, produces the images on a computer screen at the operator console. These images can then be stored on magnetic discs or tapes, and if needed, hard copies can be pro-

duced on radiographic film. The use of computers in the production of medical images has also led to further advancements, such as *digital radiography.* In this specialized mode of radiography, the information contained in a medical radiography (e.g., the various shades of gray on a radiographic image that represent the degree of x-ray penetration through the tissues) is depicted by the computer in an image *matrix,* which consists of a fixed number of rows and columns (Fig. 1–27). Each row and column consists of individual picture elements or *pixels.* In generating its images, the computer assigns each pixel a numerical value representing a specific shade of gray. These computer-generated images are known as *digital images* and can be mathematically manipulated to enhance their diagnostic quality.

Many radiology departments today are overburdened by space-consuming film files. However, the use of computers offers the alternative of storing large volumes of information on magnetic discs, magnetic tapes, or floppy discs. Many departments today are utilizing combinations of image storage devices to minimize space storage problems.

More recent developments in image-recording devices have seen the introduction of filmless cassettes. These specially designed cassettes are similar in appearance to standard cassettes, the major difference being that they do not contain radiographic film. With this type of cassette, the image generated by the x-ray exposure is stored on a phosphor-coated screen within the cassette. The exposed cassette is then loaded into a filmless cassette unit that uses a laser light beam to read the stored image. The image information obtained is then digitized and stored. The digital information can be manipulated within limits to produce somewhat higher-quality images prior to their transfer onto radiographic film. Such units could reduce the need for repeat films and perhaps even the need for darkrooms in radiology departments of the future.

SUPPORT AND ADMINISTRATIVE DEPARTMENTAL PERSONNEL

Almost every radiology department has one radiographer who has been designated chief technologist. It is this individual's responsibility to supervise the daily scheduling of radiographic examinations and to make the most efficient use of equipment and personnel in performing imaging procedures. The chief technologist also maintains departmental records as to the numbers of procedures conducted, patients, and films made per patient. Such information is most important in issuing charges to patients, proposing future budget allotments, reviewing efficiency of equipment use, and evaluating personnel.

A number of technical tests are conducted on a regular schedule (many are performed daily) on x-ray units and film-processing equipment to assure their proper operation. These tests may be performed by an experienced technologist or a quality assurance super-

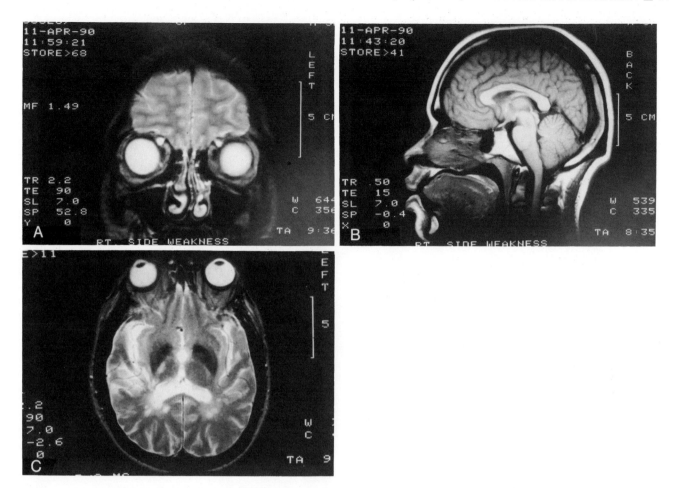

FIGURE 1–26. Medical images of the head obtained in each of the three primary body planes using a magnetic resonance imaging (MRI) unit. A, coronal, B, sagittal, and C, transverse (axial).

visor. This individual typically runs and inspects appropriate test films on each film processor at specified times during each workday. This technologist is also usually trained in minor repair and in replenishment of film-processing chemicals whenever these are required. In addition to these duties, this person may perform or assist with acceptance testing of new x-ray units and routine testing of existing units as required by regulating agencies.

With the increased complexity of radiographic equipment and the heavy patient load of most radiology departments, many larger departments may find it cost-effective to have an equipment service engineer as a permanent staff member. The service engineer is responsible for keeping all radiographic units in peak operational condition and performing any necessary repairs and new equipment acceptance testing.

RADIATION PROTECTION

Radiographers use penetrating x-rays to produce medical radiographs. X-rays are a form of *electromagnetic radiation*, like light, but much more penetrating.

X-rays are classified as *ionizing radiation*, which indicates that they have sufficient energy to remove electrons from neutral atoms (i.e., create ions) that make up the materials (e.g., air and tissue) through which they pass. This ability of x-rays to produce ionization events can also potentially produce biological harm. As a radiation worker, otherwise known as an *occupationally exposed individual,* the radiographer works under radiation protection rules established by state and federal regulating agencies.

In order not to exceed recommended radiation exposure limits, the radiographer wears a film badge to monitor whole-body radiation doses. Several types of film badges are shown in Figure 1–28. The film in the badge is processed and replaced at the beginning of each month. The degree of darkening of the film is an indication of the amount of radiation encountered in performing clinical studies during the month it was worn. A ring badge is also assigned to each radiographer to monitor radiation dose to the hands. Ring badges usually contain a small crystal that absorbs radiation energy and re-emits this as light when the crystal is heated. This type of radiation monitor is known as a thermoluminescent dosimeter (TLD). Both devices are known as *personnel dosimeters,* or devices used to measure radiation dose.

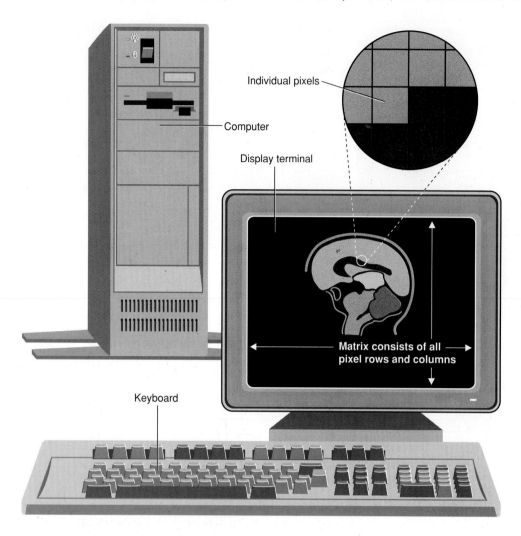

Individual pixels

Computer

Display terminal

Keyboard

Matrix consists of all
pixel rows and columns

FIGURE 1–27. A computer-generated image is formed by a matrix consisting of rows and columns of individual picture elements (pixels).

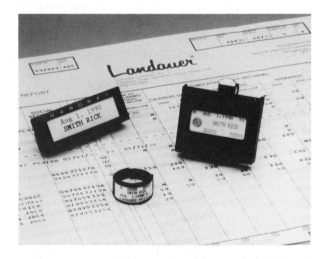

FIGURE 1–28. Film badges are worn to monitor whole-body radiation dose, and finger rings monitor radiation dosage to the hands. Monthly reports are posted in a designated location within the department for review by the radiographer. (Courtesy of Landauer, Inc., Glenwood, IL.)

In order for these devices to provide accurate estimates of your radiation exposure, care must be taken to always observe the following precautions:

● Film badges and finger rings must always be worn when conducting radiographic procedures
● Personnel dosimeters must never be stored near radiation sources
● Personnel dosimeters should never be exposed to extreme heat

In most radiographic procedures, the radiographer energizes the x-ray unit from behind a lead-lined barrier, greatly reducing the radiographer's exposure to scatter radiation. Some procedures may require the radiographer to be present in the room near the patient when the x-ray tube is energized (e.g., certain fluoroscopic examinations). For those procedures in which the use of protective barriers may be inappropriate, lead aprons must always be worn to protect the radiographer from scatter radiation. The film badge must also be worn at the collar level outside the lead apron to monitor exposure to unprotected areas of the body not covered by the apron.

When working with any source of radiation there are three basic techniques to reduce one's radiation exposure:

- Time: Reduce time spent near the radiation source
- Distance: Increase your distance from the radiation source
- Shielding: Use appropriate shielding (e.g., barriers and lead aprons) when available

Each of these methods of reducing your own radiation exposure should be committed to memory and practiced daily in the clinical setting.

Protecting oneself from unnecessary radiation exposure must not be the only concern of the medical radiographer. The current philosophy in radiation protection is that radiation exposure should be kept as low as reasonably achievable (known as the *ALARA* concept). This principle applies not only to all radiation workers but also to patients.

How can radiation exposure to the patient be reduced when it is the patient at whom the x-ray beam is directed? The radiographer can reduce patient radiation exposure by a combination of methods:

- Proper beam collimation: Conventional radiographic equipment has beam restriction devices known as collimators (see Fig. 1–7); by opening and closing the collimators, one can effectively restrict the size of the x-ray beam so that it covers only the area of the body to be imaged on the radiograph
- Use of gonadal shielding: Since the reproductive organs are most sensitive to the effects of radiation, every effort should be made to protect this region of the body during radiographic procedures; this may involve draping a lead apron over the pelvic region or the use of specially designed gonadal shields
- Use of proper technical factors: As mentioned earlier in this chapter, the selection of the proper technical factors of mA, kVp, and exposure time (seconds) determines whether a diagnostic quality radiograph is obtained; the choice of the proper technical factors is determined by the type of study and thickness of the body part. When improper technical factors are chosen, repeat radiographs must be taken, and repeat studies increase the radiation dose to the patient

As a medical radiographer, it is vitally important to use appropriate radiation protection practices for both yourself and your patients. Medical radiation is one of the greatest contributors of radiation exposure to the general population. Therefore the medical radiographer and other medical professionals who utilize radiation play a major role in determining the amount of radiation to which the general population is exposed. Further coverage of radiation protection and associated practices is discussed in later chapters.

BECOMING A PROFESSIONAL MEDICAL RADIOGRAPHER

Thus far this introductory chapter has attempted to present an overview of radiographic equipment, the method of producing x-rays, practical methods of radiation protection, and general organization of a radiology department. However, no radiology department regardless of its size can operate without its skilled technologists. Becoming a skilled and valued radiological technologist is not always an easy task regardless of the type of educational program in which you are enrolled. Educational programs for medical radiographers may be administered by hospitals, technical schools, colleges, or universities. These programs are regularly reviewed and evaluated. If the review is favorable and meets established criteria, accreditation is granted by an appropriate accrediting agency. The classroom education provided by these programs provides future radiographers with the information necessary to understand the equipment with which they will work and the reasoning behind the ways in which radiographic studies are conducted. It is necessary to master this information, for it is required in making sound clinical decisions.

A second component of the radiographer's education is the clinical component. Experienced clinical instructors who are also certified radiological technologists supervise the clinical education of future radiographers. Under the watchful supervision of the clinical instructor, student radiographers learn the practical aspects of radiography—patient positioning, operation of equipment, image processing, and so forth. Students are directly involved with actual patient studies under the guidance of the clinical instructor.

On completion of appropriate course work and satisfactory performance in clinical education courses, a student radiographer is eligible to take the national certification examination administered by the *American Registry of Radiologic Technologists (ARRT)*. After passing this examination, covering all aspects of medical radiography, the student becomes a certified radiologic technologist. Certification leads to professional recognition and increased job opportunities.

In addition to mastery of skills and classroom information, many personal qualities such as the following contribute to making you a valued employee of any radiology department:

- Pride in your work: Your department's radiologists depend on your use of technical skills to produce the best diagnostic quality images
- Consideration of your patients: Most patients are frightened of diagnostic studies when they don't know what to expect. Treat patients the way you would like to be treated if you were in their condition
- Going beyond what is minimally expected of you: Whenever possible, assist your co-workers and physicians, especially during times of heavy workloads
- Punctuality: Make every effort to be on time; delays can cause major problems in patient scheduling
- Willingness to learn: Take advantage of opportunities to learn new techniques, new equipment, and new modes of medical imaging

Medical imaging is perhaps one of the most rapidly changing and technologically advanced areas of medicine. Each specific imaging modality—radiography, ultrasound, nuclear medicine, and MRI—has seen rapid advancements over the past decade. Each of these various "windows to the body" continues to be perfected in order to obtain the most accurate diagnostic information possible. As a medical radiographer, you join a select number of health care professionals who utilize their scientific knowledge and technical skills to assist the physician in the diagnosis and treatment of disease.

Medical radiography has made almost unbelievable advancements in its technical capabilities during the first century of its existence. It is a proud profession, steeped in rich, scientific history, and by all indications, it possesses an equally bright future. On becoming a medical radiographer, you will have an important role in its second century of application in the ever-continuing battle against disease.

Chapter Summary/ Important Concepts

X-rays are a penetrating form of electromagnetic radiation that travel in the form of photons (i.e., small packets of pure energy)

X-rays were discovered by Wilhelm Conrad Röntgen in November 1895 and were first used on a human subject in December 1895 to produce the first radiograph

X-rays are produced in an x-ray tube when fast moving electrons strike a target with a high atomic number such as tungsten

Primary components within an x-ray tube include a negative electrode (i.e., cathode), a filament (source of electrons), a target with which the electrons collide, and a positive electrode (i.e., anode)

The number of x-rays produced by the x-ray tube is primarily determined by the tube current (i.e., the number of electrons that flow between cathode and anode); the tube current is designated by the mA

The energy, or penetrating ability, of the x-rays produced is controlled by the kV placed across the tube electrodes

The production of medical radiographs is based on the fact that exposure of radiographic film to x-rays will turn the film dark when it is processed; therefore dark areas on a radiograph indicate tissue that is radiolucent (i.e., easily penetrated by x-rays),

whereas light areas represent structures or materials that are radiopaque (i.e., tend to reduce x-ray penetration)

Less than 1% of the total energy used to produce x-rays is actually converted into diagnostically useful x-rays; the greater percentage of the energy is transformed into heat

Other important components of a complete radiographic system include the following:
  a. Filters screen out low-energy x-rays and thereby reduce radiation dose to the patient
  b. Collimators reduce the size of the x-ray beam that strikes the patient
  c. Grids reduce the amount of scatter radiation that strikes the film
  d. Intensifying screens increase the effect of the x-ray beam on the film while reducing radiation dose to the patient

The technical factors used by the radiographer to vary the appearance of the medical radiograph are the kVp, mA, and exposure time

Tomographic imaging (e.g., CT and conventional tomographic x-ray units) allows production of "slice" images through the body

Fluoroscopy allows the visualization of motion

In addition to the use of conventional radiographic film, radiographic images can also be generated using the computer to produce digital images, which allow image manipulation to enhance their diagnostic quality

Exposure to x-rays and any other form of ionizing radiation has the potential for biological harm

Radiation-monitoring devices (i.e., film badges and finger rings) to measure the radiation exposure must always be worn by the radiographer during any occupational procedure involving radiation.

Radiation exposure can be minimized by using appropriate shielding, minimizing time spent near any radiation source, and increasing the distance between the individual and any source of radiation

X-ray machines produce radiation only when the x-ray tube is energized

Radiation dose to patients can be reduced by the radiographer's proper use of beam restriction devices, gonadal shielding, and proper selection of technical factors to avoid repeat films

Important Terminology

ALARA. Current philosophy of radiation protection, which proposes that a person's radiation exposure should be kept as low as reasonably achievable.

American Registry of Radiologic Technologists (ARRT). The agency that offers certification examinations for eligible candidates in radiography, nuclear medicine, and radiation therapy

Anode. The positive electrode

Artifact. An image feature that does not represent an actual body structure

Atomic Number (Z number). The number of protons in the nucleus of an atom

Automatic Film Processor. A piece of equipment that will automatically perform all the appropriate processing requirements when an exposed x-ray film is fed into it

Bucky Tray. A device, located under the x-ray table top, that holds the film cassette

Cassette. A device that holds the radiographic film during a radiographic exposure; this device also usually contains two intensifying screens, one positioned on either side of the radiographic film

Cathode. The negative electrode

Cathode Rays. The early name given to the stream of electrons that flows from the cathode to the anode of a Crookes tube when a high voltage is placed across these electrodes

Cine Image. An image that allows the visualization of motion

Collimator. A device attached to the x-ray tube housing that enables automatic or manual control of the extent of the area to be irradiated

Computed Tomography (CT). A specialized mode of medical imaging that utilizes a rotating x-ray machine and detectors in conjunction with computer systems to obtain "slice" images through a plane of the patient's body

Contrast Medium. A material introduced into the body or body cavity to assist with the radiological visualization of body structures that otherwise could not be seen

Coronal Plane. A plane that divides the body into anterior (front) and posterior (back) portions

Darkroom. A room that excludes outside light and is used for the handling of exposed and unexposed x-ray film

Daylight System. A system that enables the radiographer to unload and load cassettes and to process film without using a darkroom

Dedicated Unit. An x-ray machine used for one specific purpose

Digital Image. A computer-generated image, consisting of numbers of individual pixels; the color or shade of gray assigned to each pixel is determined by the numerical value assigned to it, based on some image parameter such as x-ray transmission

Digital Radiography. An advanced radiographic technique using computers to generate digital radiographic images that in many cases can be electronically manipulated to produce higher quality diagnostic images

Electromagnetic Radiation. Photon radiation having neither mass nor electric charge; "packets" of electromagnetic energy such as x-rays, visible light, ultraviolet, infrared, and radiowaves

Electron. The smallest known unit of negative electric charge

Filament. The long, thin tungsten wire that when heated becomes the source of electrons in the x-ray tube

Film Bin. A bin in the darkroom in which unexposed x-ray film is placed for transfer into empty cassettes

Film Fog. An overall darkening of exposed radiographic film, resulting primarily from scatter radiation; film fog decreases the diagnostic quality of a radiograph

Filter. A thin sheet of specific metal such as aluminum or copper used to remove or reduce the number of low-energy x-rays in an x-ray beam in order to diminish radiation dose to the patient

Fluorescence. The emission of visible light by a substance when it is exposed to an activating source such as x-rays, fast-moving charged particles, light, or chemical reactions; the visible light is emitted less than 10^{-8} seconds after exposure to the activating source

Fluoroscopy. A procedure that utilizes x-rays to image "real time" movement and motion; it is generally associated with higher radiation doses

Glass Envelope. The glass tube in which the primary components of the x-ray tube are sealed

Grid. A device whose purpose is to absorb scatter radiation; both cassettes and grids are located between the x-ray table top and the Bucky tray

Image Intensifier. A device associated with fluoroscopic units that converts x-rays to a visible image during fluoroscopy

Intensifying Screen. A phosphor-coated sheet that gives off visible light when struck by x-rays; a screen helps produce the image on the x-ray film

Ionizing Radiation. Either photon or particle radiation having sufficient energy to produce ionization events in materials through which it passes; diagnostic x-rays are one form of ionizing radiation

Kilovoltage (kV). The voltage, or potential difference, placed across the electrodes of an x-ray tube; the higher the kV, the more penetrating the x-rays produced

Latent Image. The image produced in the chemical emulsion of x-ray film on radiographic exposure; this "hidden" image is converted into a visible image when the film is chemically processed

Lateral. A side projection or view

Lead Apron. An apron made of an approximately 0.5-mm thickness of lead or its equivalent that should be worn during fluoroscopy or any radiographic procedure in which more substantial shielding is either unavailable or inappropriate

Magnetic Resonance Imaging (MRI). A mode of medical imaging that uses strong magnetic fields and radiowaves to obtain detailed images of the body

Mammography. Radiographic examination of the breast

Matrix. The sum of all rows and columns of pixels used to represent a computer image

Milliamperage (mA). A measure of the tube current that flows between the electrodes of the x-ray tube; the higher the mA, the more x-rays are produced

Nuclear Medicine. A mode of medical imaging that uses trace amounts of radioactive materials attached to a wide variety of chemical compounds to obtain functional information about organs and organ systems

Oblique. A projection or view taken at an angle other than 0° or 90°

Occupationally Exposed Individual. A person whose occupation will likely result in his or her exposure to ionizing radiation

Passbox. A device that allows cassettes to be passed to and from the darkroom without light entering

Personnel Dosimeter. A device such as a film badge or finger ring that monitors radiation exposure; it must be worn by personnel working with radiation

Phosphor. In radiology, crystals of specific inorganic salts that emit visible light when exposed to an activating source

Phosphorescence. The emission of visible light by a substance when it is exposed to an activating source; in this case, the visible light emissions are delayed beyond 10^{-8} seconds

Photon. A packet of electromagnetic radiation from x-rays, gamma rays, radiowaves, visible light, and so forth; photons are pure energy and carry neither mass nor electric charge

Pixel. A picture element; one individual component of a digital image

Portable X-ray Machine. A compact mobile x-ray unit that can be moved to various locations when a patient cannot come to the radiology department

Radiograph. A film that contains an image of a body structure created by the passage of x-rays through a patient's body

Radiographic Density. The degree of darkening on a radiographic film; high density implies dark areas, low density implies light areas on the film

Radiological Technologist (Radiographer). An individual who uses x-ray equipment to obtain radiographs of a variety of anatomical structures

Radiological Technology. The profession associated with the use of radiation for the diagnosis or treatment of disease or injury

Radiologist. A physician specializing in the use of radiant energy in the diagnosis or treatment of disease or injury

Radiology Department. The department within a medical facility that offers a variety of radiological services for patients

Radiolucent. A material easily penetrated by x-rays (e.g., plastic or soft tissue)

Radiopaque. A material not easily penetrated by x-rays (e.g., lead or bone)

Reading Room. A room in which radiographs are read or interpreted by the radiologist

R/F Unit. A room that has both a conventional x-ray machine and a fluoroscope

Safe Light. A type of lighting found in the darkroom that does not affect exposed or unexposed x-ray film

Sagittal Plane. A plane that divides the body into right and left sides

Scatter Radiation. Radiation that has been deflected from the direction in which it was originally traveling; it is of lower energy and is likely to be absorbed in the next medium through which it travels

Screen. Sheet coated with a selected phosphor that emits visible light when struck by x-rays; the visible light emitted by the screen interacts with the radiographic film to produce an intensified image, minimizing the need for high radiation doses in the patient

Special Procedure. A more complex radiographic procedure that usually involves the introduction of contrast media into the body by catheter or puncture; it must be performed by a radiologist under sterile conditions

Spot Film. A radiograph that can be produced during fluoroscopy using a cassette and x-ray film

Spot Film Camera. A device attached to a fluoroscopic unit, containing a roll of x-ray film that can be used to produce radiographic images

Static Image. An image that does not allow the visualization of motion

Target. On the x-ray tube anode, the tungsten plate, which when struck by fast-moving electrons, generates x-rays

Technical Factors. The combination of mA, kVp, and exposure time (seconds) for a set distance between the x-ray tube anode and film

Thermionic Emission. The process of using heat energy to release electrons from the tungsten filament of the x-ray tube

Tomography. A specialized form of medical imaging (e.g., CT, MRI, ultrasound) in which the images produced represent "slices" through the patient's body

Transverse Plane. A plane that produces cross-sectional (or axial) slices and divides the body into superior (upper) and inferior (lower) portions

Tube Housing. The metal shield that contains the x-ray tube

Ultrasonography. A mode of diagnostic medical imaging that uses sound waves of ultra-high frequencies to obtain images of internal body structures

Vacuum. A region from which air or gas has been removed

X-ray Energy. Relates to the penetrating ability of the x-rays

X-ray Intensity. Relates to the number of x-rays, or total energy, passing through a specified area per second

X-rays. Penetrating electromagnetic radiation traveling in the form of photons having neither mass nor electrical charge; discovered by Wilhelm Conrad Röntgen in 1895

▨▨▨ Review Questions

1. X-rays travel in the form of photons. Indicate properties of these photons in regard to their mass, electric charge, and penetrating ability.
2. Briefly, explain in a general way how x-rays are produced in an x-ray tube.
3. Indicate the purpose of each of the following components of an x-ray tube: filament, cathode, target, anode, glass envelope, high-voltage generator.
4. What relationship exists between
   a. the number of electrons flowing between the x-ray tube cathode and anode and the number of x-rays produced?
   b. the voltage (kVp) across the tube electrodes and the energy (or penetrating ability) of the x-rays produced?
5. When an x-ray beam strikes a patient's body, each photon within the beam may interact in any of three primary methods. Briefly, explain what occurs in each interaction and how each type of interaction affects the degree of darkening that appears on the radiograph.
6. What can be said about the effect of scatter radiation on the diagnostic quality of medical radiographs?
7. Considering the location of the film cassette as it is placed in the Bucky tray of a radiographic imaging table, indicate briefly two sources of scatter radiation.
8. Indicate three basic ways to reduce one's own radiation exposure when working with any radiation source.
9. Indicate three ways the radiographer can reduce radiation dose to the patient.
10. Indicate why your film badge should never be stored in areas where it could be exposed to radiation.

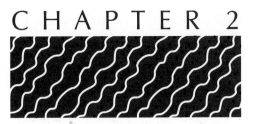

C H A P T E R   2

Mathematics and Physics Review

Michael A. Thompson, M.S.

Chapter Outline

Chapter Objectives

Upon completion of this chapter, you should be able to

- Perform simple computations involving fractions, decimals, and percentages.
- Set up and solve a simple proportion, given sufficient information.
- Explain and identify direct, inverse, and inverse square relationships.
- Explain the relationship between an exponent and a logarithm.
- Explain the difference between a "common" and a "natural" logarithm.
- Solve a simple exponential or logarithmic equation with the aid of a pocket calculator.
- Interpret and extract data from a linear or semilog graph.
- Identify, sketch, or identify and sketch, the graph of a positive or negative exponential.
- Express any number in proper form using scientific notation.
- Perform calculations using the rules of scientific notation.
- Perform unit conversions using the technique of dimensional analysis.
- Define and perform simple calculations, indicating proper units, involving any of the following physical quantities:
  - *velocity (or speed)*
  - *acceleration*
  - *linear momentum*
  - *kinetic energy*
  - *rest energy*
  - *power*
  - *temperature*
- Indicate the relationship between the joule and the electron volt, and perform simple conversions between the two energy units.
- Specify the speed of light *(c)* in vacuum or air, indicating appropriate units.
- Define the following quantities:
  - *force*
  - *potential energy*
  - *temperature*
  - *electron volt*
  - *heat*
  - *conduction*
  - *convection*
  - *radiation*
- Explain what is meant by
  - *conservation of energy*
  - *the direction of heat flow*

THE NEED FOR PHYSICS AND MATHEMATICS IN RADIOGRAPHY

As a future radiologic technologist, you will become an important component of a highly skilled medical team whose primary objective is the accurate diagnosis of a patient's health problems so that appropriate medical treatment can be provided. As a medical radiographer, you have become a part of one of the most rapidly expanding and technologically advanced areas of medicine, specifically known as diagnostic medical imaging. In the medical imaging departments of most modern hospitals, your professional associates will be individuals like yourself who work in areas such as ultrasound (utilizes sound waves to produce images of the body), nuclear medicine (utilizes small amounts of radioactive tracers to determine if organs are functioning properly), and magnetic resonance imaging (MRI) (uses magnetic fields and radiowaves to obtain chemical and structural information about the body).

The field of radiography, although the oldest of these imaging modalities, has advanced rapidly in its capabilities. As a result, qualified radiographers can enhance their skills to work in areas such as fluoroscopy, computed tomography (CT), and digital subtraction radiography. Many radiographers also "cross-train" to become competent in more than one imaging speciality. A good imaging technologist skilled in more than one imaging modality can be of great value to a health care facility.

As an imaging specialist, you will use some of the most scientifically and technologically advanced equipment found in medicine today. It is therefore important to possess not only a firm understanding of the scientific principles but also the necessary technical skills to use the equipment safely and correctly. Your radiologist will greatly depend on you to use your knowledge and technical abilities to obtain the best images possible to assure an accurate diagnosis.

In order to understand the physical principles behind the production and use of x-rays in medical imaging, this chapter reviews the more important mathematical rules and physical concepts that find use in radiography. This does not imply that an extensive knowledge of mathematics and physics is required to be a good radiographer, but a sound understanding of certain fundamental concepts is necessary.

This chapter begins with a review of mathematical rules and relationships that you will find useful in your study of radiography. Mathematics is the language of science, and we often need to make measurements and quantitative determinations in discussions of radiation and the equipment used to produce it. The following material provides you with a review of the concepts on which this exciting field of study is based.

MATHEMATICS REVIEW

Fractions and Decimals

A fraction is the quotient of two numbers. The number above the dividing line is known as the numerator, and the number below the line is known as the denominator, as indicated below:

$$\frac{3}{4} \longleftarrow \text{numerator} \atop \longleftarrow \text{denominator}$$

Fractions may exist in several forms:

- Proper fractions are those fractions which, when the numerator is divided by the denominator, the quotient is less than one

))))) EXAMPLES

$$\frac{1}{3}, \frac{2}{3}, \frac{3}{4}, \frac{2}{5}$$

- Improper fractions are those fractions, which when the numerator is divided by the denominator, the quotient is greater than one

))))) EXAMPLES

$$\frac{4}{3}, \frac{6}{5}, \frac{7}{2}, \frac{9}{4}$$

- Decimal form: Any fraction can be expressed in decimal form by simply dividing its numerator by its denominator

))))) EXAMPLES

$$\frac{3}{4} = 0.75, \frac{5}{2} = 2.5, \frac{5}{4} = 1.25$$

Addition and Subtraction

Fractions can be added or subtracted by either of two methods:

Method I: Conversion to Decimal Form

All fractions can initially be converted to decimal form and then added or subtracted, using the standard rules for decimals.

))))) EXAMPLES

a) $\frac{1}{4} + \frac{1}{2} + \frac{9}{8}$

$= 0.25 + 0.5 + 1.125$

$= 1.875$

b) $\dfrac{5}{4} + \dfrac{3}{2} - \dfrac{3}{8}$

$= 1.25 + 1.5 - 0.375$

$= 2.750 - 0.375$

$= 2.375$

Method II: Determination of Least Common Denominator

Fractions may be added or subtracted also by first finding the least common denominator (LCD) (i.e., the smallest number into which all denominators will divide evenly). Each fraction is placed over the LCD; then the mathematical operation is performed.

)))))) EXAMPLES

a) $\dfrac{1}{4} + \dfrac{1}{2} + \dfrac{9}{8}$

$= \dfrac{2}{8} + \dfrac{4}{8} + \dfrac{9}{8}$

$= \dfrac{15}{8}$

Note. If the preceding example is converted to decimal form, it should be seen that the earlier result is reached again. That is,

$$\frac{15}{8} = 1.875$$

b) $1\dfrac{2}{3} - \dfrac{4}{5} - \dfrac{1}{4}$

$= \dfrac{5}{3} - \dfrac{4}{5} - \dfrac{1}{4}$

$= \dfrac{100}{60} - \dfrac{48}{60} - \dfrac{15}{60}$

$= \dfrac{100}{60} - \dfrac{63}{60}$

$= \dfrac{37}{60}$

Multiplication

Multiplication of fractions is accomplished simply by multiplying the numerators and the denominators of the individual fractions.

)))))) EXAMPLES

a) $\dfrac{2}{3} \times \dfrac{1}{4}$

$= \dfrac{2 \times 1}{3 \times 4}$

$= \dfrac{2}{12}$ or $\dfrac{1}{6}$

b) $\dfrac{3}{4} \times \dfrac{1}{2} \times \dfrac{2}{3}$

$= \dfrac{3 \times 1 \times 2}{4 \times 2 \times 3}$

$= \dfrac{6}{24}$ or $\dfrac{1}{4}$

Division

Division by a fraction is accomplished by inverting the number or fraction in the denominator and then multiplying.

)))))) EXAMPLES

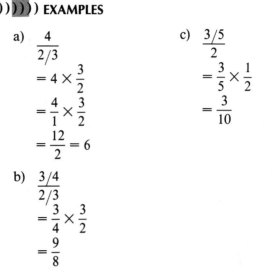

a) $\dfrac{4}{2/3}$

$= 4 \times \dfrac{3}{2}$

$= \dfrac{4}{1} \times \dfrac{3}{2}$

$= \dfrac{12}{2} = 6$

b) $\dfrac{3/4}{2/3}$

$= \dfrac{3}{4} \times \dfrac{3}{2}$

$= \dfrac{9}{8}$

c) $\dfrac{3/5}{2}$

$= \dfrac{3}{5} \times \dfrac{1}{2}$

$= \dfrac{3}{10}$

Ratios and Proportions

Fractions can be used to express the relationship that exists between like quantities. When fractions are used to express these relationships, they are known as ratios. Ratios are specifically used in radiography in establishing relationships between units of measurement, solving particular problems in x-ray circuitry, and relating various radiation exposure factors to other imaging parameters.

Ratios may be expressed in any of several forms. These include primarily fractional form or ratio notation form.

)))))) EXAMPLE

As an example of a ratio, consider the relationship between inches and feet. Since 12 inches = 1 foot, we can express this as a ratio in fractional form as

$$\frac{12 \text{ inches}}{1 \text{ foot}}$$

or using ratio notation, this is written as 12:1 and is read as "a 12 to 1" ratio.

Ratios find their greatest usefulness in radiography when used to establish a proportion. By definition a proportion is an expressed equality between two ratios. Proportions can be used to solve a variety of problems in which specifically defined relationships between quantities exist. To illustrate this concept, we use the ratio defined in the previous example to solve a simple problem containing a proportion.

)))))) EXAMPLE

Determine the number of inches in 3.5 ft. Use the previously determined ratio to write the following proportion:

$$\frac{12 \text{ inches}}{1 \text{ foot}} = \frac{x \text{ inches}}{3.5 \text{ feet}}$$

To solve this for x, simply cross-multiply:

$$(x \text{ inches}) (1 \text{ foot}) = (12 \text{ inches}) (3.5 \text{ feet})$$
$$x = (12 \text{ inches}) (3.5 \text{ feet})/(1 \text{ foot}) = 42 \text{ inches}$$

Note. It should be observed that when the proportion is originally set up, "like quantities" are placed in the respective numerators (i.e., inches) and denominators (i.e., feet) prior to solving for the unknown quantity.

)))))) EXAMPLE

Use the relationship 1 kg = 2.2 lb to determine the weight of a 120-lb patient in kilograms. Based on the information provided, set up the following proportion:

$$\frac{1 \text{ kg}}{2.2 \text{ lb}} = \frac{x \text{ kg}}{120 \text{ lb}}$$

Now, cross-multiplying, the result is

$$(x \text{ kg}) (2.2 \text{ lb}) = (1 \text{ kg}) (120 \text{ lb})$$

$$x = \frac{(1 \text{ kg}) (120 \text{ lb})}{(2.2 \text{ lb})}$$

$$x = 54.5 \text{ kg}$$

Mathematical Relationships

In your study of radiography, you will find that many quantities are related. In order to use these parameters most effectively to produce quality radiographs, the radiographer must have an understanding of how these quantities are related. Formulas are simply the shorthand notation that science uses to indicate the relationships among quantities. Formulas should serve as helpful reminders demonstrating the relationships among quantities with which you deal.

Two quantities are said to vary directly or to have a *direct relationship* if as one quantity increases, the second quantity also increases, and vice versa. Such quantities—for example, x and y—when they vary directly with each other can have this relationship expressed in equation form as

$$\boxed{\frac{x}{y} = \text{constant}} \quad \text{Direct relationship}$$

Recall that a constant is any numerical value that does not change; therefore it can be shown that as x

increases in value, y must correspondingly increase so that the numerical value of $x/(y)$ remains constant.

)))))) EXAMPLE

Verify that x varies directly with y in the equation given by

$$\boxed{\frac{x}{y} = 5}$$

Developing a table of x and y values that will satisfy this equation, the result is

x	y
1	$\frac{1}{5}$
5	1
10	2
40	8
50	10

It can be seen that as x increases, y correspondingly increases verifying a direct relationship between x and y.

An *indirect*, or inverse, *relationship* exists between two quantities if as one quantity increases the other quantity decreases, and vice versa. Two quantities x and y, that vary in this manner may have this relationship expressed in equation form as

$$\boxed{xy = \text{constant}} \quad \text{Inverse relationship}$$

This equation indicates that the product of x and y remains constant. Thus as x increases, y must decrease so that their product remains constant.

)))))) EXAMPLE

Verify that x and y vary inversely in the equation given by

$$xy = 20$$

Again, this can be easily verified by producing a table with values for x and y that satisfy the above equation. This is shown as follows:

x	y
20	1
10	2
5	4
2	10

Again, it is easily seen that as x decreases, y correspondingly increases, verifying an indirect relationship between x and y.

As you continue the study of radiography, you will find that certain quantities may vary in a somewhat more complex way. These quantities may vary as squares. It is important to understand these types of relationships, since many quantities used in radiography vary as squares and perhaps even more important, as inverse squares.

Begin by considering a relationship in which one quantity, y, varies directly with the square of a second quantity, x. Write this first as a proportionality:

$$y \propto x^2$$

Note. This is read, "y is directly proportional to x squared."

This proportionality can be easily converted into an equation by including what is known as proportionality constant, k. This then becomes

$$\boxed{y = kx^2} \quad \text{Direct square relationship}$$

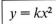 **EXAMPLE**

Verify that the equation given by

$$y = 2x^2$$

represents a direct relationship.

To verify this relationship, again substitute values for x and find the corresponding values for y. These values are shown in the following table:

x	y
1	2
2	8
3	18
4	32

Note that as x increases, y also increases, verifying that this is a direct relationship. It should however be seen that y increases in value much more rapidly, since it varies as the square of x. This is characteristic when quantities change in this manner. Also, and extremely important, a quantity may vary indirectly as the square of another quantity. This is known as an inverse square relationship. If y varies inversely as the square of quantity x, it may be expressed in the following form:

$$y \propto 1/x^2$$

Or, inserting a proportionality constant, k, we have the relationship expressed in the form of the equation

$$\boxed{y = k/x^2} \quad \text{Inverse square relationship}$$

 EXAMPLE

Verify that the equation given by

$$y = 1/x^2$$

represents an inverse relationship between x and y.

To verify this relationship, again generate data in a table of x values and corresponding values of y:

x	y
1	1
2	$\dfrac{1}{4}$
3	$\dfrac{1}{9}$
4	$\dfrac{1}{16}$

It should be noted here that not only does y decrease as x increases (verifying an indirect, or inverse, relationship) but y decreases quite rapidly with increases in x. The importance of this type of relationship is evident later in discussions of electrical forces, radiation exposure, and even radiation protection.

Exponents and Logarithms

An *exponent* is the *power* to which a number is raised. In the example show,

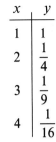

10 is the base number, which has been raised to the second power. Exponents may be whole numbers (as shown) or even fractions. Fractional exponents represent roots as indicated:

$$4^{1/2} = \sqrt{4} = 2$$
$$10^{1/3} = \sqrt[3]{10} \approx 2.15$$
$$2^{0.5} = 2^{1/2} = \sqrt{2} \approx 1.41$$

In contrast, a *logarithm* (log) is the power to which a number must be raised to give a specific numerical value. As an example, consider the following numerical equation:

$$10^2 = 100 \qquad \text{Exponential Equation} \qquad (1)$$

In terms of logarithms, we could write

$$\log_{10} 100 = 2 \qquad \text{Logarithmic equation} \qquad (2)$$

Essentially, both equations say the same thing. Equation (1) is known as an exponential equation, and (2) is a logarithmic equation. In equation (2), the 10 is known as the base number. Since the log in this equation equals 2, it simply indicates that 100 is obtained when the base number, 10, is raised to the second power. Similarly, if the equation

$$\log_{10} 45 = 1.653$$

is given, this simply indicates that

$$10^{1.653} = 45$$

Logs to the base 10 are known as common logs. Many natural occurrences, however, vary exponentially but to the base number 2.718 (represented in mathematics by the letter *e*). These are known as natural logs and are generally written as *ln* rather than *log*. Several examples follow.

)))))) **EXAMPLE**

$$ln\ 420 = \underline{\hspace{2cm}}$$

Using a standard scientific pocket calculator, on entering 420 then depressing the *ln* key, you find

$$ln\ 420 \approx 6.04$$

This means that

$$e^{6.04} \approx (2.718)^{6.04} \approx 420$$

Note. This can be easily verified by using the y^x key and entering 2.718 for *y* and 6.04 for *x*.

)))))) **EXAMPLE**

$$log\ 200 = \underline{\hspace{2cm}}$$

Again, using a pocket calculator, on entering 200 then depressing the log key, you find

$$log\ 200 \approx 2.301$$

This means that

$$10^{2.301} \approx 200$$

This again can be easily verified, using the y^x or 10^x key.

Thus a logarithm is a power to which a number known as the base number is raised to give a certain number. The base number may be 10, in which case the log is known as a common log, or it may be 2.718, in which case the log is known as a natural log.

Solving Logarithmic and Exponential Equations

There will be a need on occasion to determine exact information, such as the thickness of lead (Pb) required to safely shield radiography personnel from radiation or how much radiation will penetrate a given thickness of body tissue. At such times it is necessary to know how to solve simple logarithmic and exponential equations. These solutions are simple once the method is understood.

Begin with solving the logarithmic equation. A logarithmic equation is one in which the term *log* or *ln* appears. An example of such an equation would be

$$log\ x = 2.5$$

To solve such an equation, we need only recall from earlier discussions that a logarithm is a power to which a base number is raised to give a specific number. Thus when writing

$$log\ x = 2.5 \tag{3}$$

it actually means

$$10^{2.5} = x \tag{4}$$

or

$$x \approx 316.2$$

Note. The actual numerical value of $10^{2.5}$ (i.e., 316.2) is obtained by substituting the appropriate values and using the 10^x or y^x key on a pocket calculator.

Once the initial logarithmic equation (3) has been rewritten in its equivalent form (4), the equation is solved. Any logarithmic equation can be solved in this manner. Consider the following example, which involves natural logs.

)))))) **EXAMPLE**

Solve the following for *x*:

$$5\ ln\ x = 12$$

To solve this equation, start by getting the logarithm on one side of the equation by itself. Here, divide both sides by 5 to obtain

$$ln\ x = \tfrac{12}{5} = 2.4$$

Then rewrite the equation based on the definition of a logarithm, recalling that the base number for natural logs is *e*, or 2.718:

$$e^{2.4} = x$$

or

$$x = (2.718)^{2.4} \approx 11.02$$

Note. In this case, the base number is $e = 2.718$ since this was a natural log. The numerical value of $e^{2.4}$ is obtained by using either the e^x or y^x key on a pocket calculator.

Both of these examples were solved in exactly the same way, the only difference is that when common logs are involved, the base 10 is used, whereas the base $e = 2.718$ is used for natural logs.

The opposite of the logarithmic equation and perhaps more useful from the practical point of view is the exponential equation. Since an exponent is a power, the base number may be 10, *e*, or any other number. An example of each is considered to illustrate that the methods of solution are quite similar. In each case, the problem can be solved by applying the same general rules:

1. Isolate the term containing the unknown exponent.
2. If the base number is 10, take the common log of both sides of the equation. If the base number is *e*, take the natural log of both sides. If the base is neither 10 nor *e*, take either the common or natural log of both sides.
3. Use the general rule

$$log\ (a)^b = b\ log\ a$$

or

$$ln\ (a)^b = b\ ln\ a$$

4. Solve algebraically for the unknown quantity.

This method of solution is now used to solve each of the following exponential equations for x.

))))))) **EXAMPLE**

$$5\ (10^{2x}) = 200$$

Using the rules described, isolate the term containing the unknown by dividing both sides by 5 to get

$$10^{2x} = 40$$

Since the base number is 10, now take the common log of both sides. That is

$$\log(10)^{2x} = \log 40$$

Apply rule (3) to the left hand side and use the calculator to obtain the log of 40 and get

$$2x\ \log 10 = 1.6$$

But $\log 10 = 1$, so the above equation reduces to

$$2x\ (1) = 1.6$$

or

$$x = \frac{1.6}{2} = 0.8$$

))))))) **EXAMPLE**

$$4\ e^{x/2} = 18$$

First isolate the unknown by dividing both sides by 4:

$$e^{x/2} = \frac{18}{4} = 4.5$$

Since the base number here is e, take the natural log of both sides:

$$ln\ (e^{x/2}) = ln\ 4.5$$

Applying rule (3) to the left hand side and using the calculator to obtain $ln\ 4.5$ we get

$$(x/2)\ ln\ e = 1.5$$

But $ln\ e = 1$, so the above reduces to

$$x/2\ (1) = 1.5$$

Multiply both sides by 2 to obtain

$$x = 3.0$$

))))))) **EXAMPLE**

$$(0.5)^{5x} = 0.10$$

In this problem, the unknown term is already iso-

lated. In addition it is noted that the base number is 0.5. Since the base number is neither 10 nor e, it doesn't matter which log is used. Taking the natural log of both sides, we obtain

$$ln\ (0.5)^{5x} = ln\ 0.10$$

Applying rule (3) to the left hand side and using a calculator to obtain $ln\ 0.10$, we get

$$5x\ ln\ 0.5 = -2.30$$

Again use the calculator to find that $ln\ 0.5 = -0.693$, and make this substitution in the above equation to now obtain

$$5x(-0.693) = -2.30$$

$$5x = -2.30/-0.693 \approx 3.32$$

$$x = 3.32/5 \approx 0.66$$

Note. It is important to include all signs when working with equations of this type. It should also be noted that if the common log of both sides of the original equation had been taken, the same value of x would be obtained.

Although solving these equations may seem somewhat complex, it should be noted that each was solved using the same general rules (steps 1 to 4). Applying these simple rules to equations of this type permits solution of a wide variety of practical problems involving radiation.

Graphs and Graphical Interpretation

The old adage that states, "A picture is worth a thousand words," is also true when visualizing the relationships that exist between quantities. These relationships may be described in words, equations, or graphical representations. In previous discussions, we worked with the first two methods, now we concentrate our efforts on the third method.

Linear Graphs

The graph with which most of us are familiar is the *linear graph* (i.e., all squares appearing on the graph are of equal size), which is used to describe the relationship between two quantities—for example, x and y. Later, we replace x and y with actual physical quantities such as current and voltage, but for now, the general rules must be mastered, so use of x and y simplifies the discussion. The x (horizontal) and y (vertical) axes are drawn and labeled appropriately (Fig. 2–1). One may then obtain data, perhaps from a simple laboratory experiment, in which values of x are chosen and corresponding values of y are determined. Prior to plotting these values on a graph, an appropriate scale should be chosen for both the x and y axes. It should be noted that the axes need not use the same scale, but whatever scale is chosen, it must be used consistently along the full length of the axis. This is

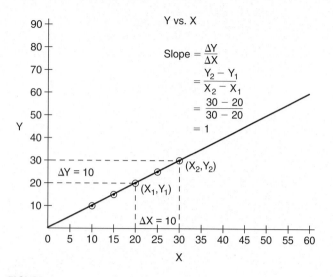

FIGURE 2-1. Direct linear relationship plotted on linear graph paper.

illustrated in Figure 2-1 in which each small square has a numerical value of 5 along the x axis and a numerical value of 10 along the y axis. Axes should be appropriately labeled, indicating units of measurement whenever units are used.

When data is plotted on the graph, a graph like that in Figure 2-1 may be obtained. On close inspection of Figure 2-1, the following information can be found:

- A linear relationship exists between x and y (since the graph is a straight line),
- Accurate data can be obtained even in the region beyond that in which there are data points (i.e., in the region beyond $x = 30$), since a constant relationship exists between x and y, and
- A direct relationship exists between x and y (since y increases as x increases).

In addition to these bits of information, all straight lines have a constant slant, or slope. The slope represents the "tilt" of the line, and its numerical value is determined by the formula

$$\text{Slope} = m = \frac{\Delta y}{\Delta x}$$

$$= \frac{y_2 - y_1}{x_2 - x_1}$$

Note. Δ is the Greek letter *delta*, which represents change; (x_1, y_1) and (x_2, y_2) represent coordinates of any two points that lie on that line.

Use the two points indicated on Figure 2-1 to determine the slope of this line.

$$m = \frac{y_2 - y_1}{x_2 - x_1}$$

$$= \frac{30 - 20}{30 - 20}$$

$$= \frac{10}{10} = 1$$

Also notice the following regarding slopes:

- Any straight line has a constant slope (i.e., a slant or tilt that does not change) and a numerical value of its slope that does not change regardless of which two points on the line are chosen
- The slope has a positive value when the line runs from the lower left to the upper right corner and a negative value when the line runs from the upper left to the lower right corner

Later, you will find that the slope of a graph can have important physical meanings when actual quantities are plotted instead of x and y.

Any straight line graph can be represented by an equation of the form

$$y = mx + b \qquad (5)$$

where

m = slope
b = y intercept (i.e., the point at which the straight line crosses the y axis)

For the graph in Figure 2-1, the equation is

$$y = (1)x + (0)$$
$$y = x$$

Note. This equation is verified, since for each point that lies on this line, $x = y$.

Now, if a different set of data is plotted on a similar graph, the graph might resemble that in Figure 2-2. Again, on inspection of the second graph, the following information is evident:

- A linear relationship exists between x and y (since the graph is a straight line)
- Accurate data can be obtained in regions along the line from $x = 0$ to $x = 40$
- An inverse, or indirect relationship, exists between x and y, since y decreases as x increases)

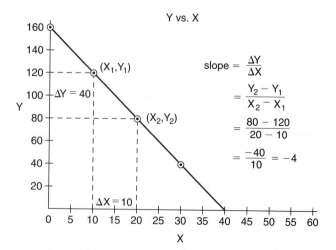

FIGURE 2-2. Indirect linear relationship plotted on linear graph paper.

From the two data points indicated on the graph, the slope of this graph is found to be

$$m = \frac{\Delta y}{\Delta x}$$

$$\frac{y_2 - y_1}{x_2 - x_1} = \frac{80 - 120}{20 - 10}$$

$$= -\frac{40}{10} = -4$$

Note. The negative value of the slope indicates that the line graph is oriented from upper left to lower right as shown.

Once again, the graph in Figure 2–2 can be represented in equation form by using equation (5), which applies to any straight line graph:

$$y = mx + b$$
$$y = (-4)x + 160$$
$$y = -4x + 160$$

It should be noted that if $x = 20$, the value of y can be found as follows:

$$y = -4(20) + 160$$
$$= -80 + 160$$
$$= 80$$

Thus when $x = 20$, $y = 80$, which is verified by the graph. This simple example serves to illustrate the reason for developing equations that express the relationships between quantities—the power of prediction. One of the true strengths of science is its ability to predict accurately how quantities will vary under given sets of conditions. It is this ability that allows prediction of the energy of x-rays needed to produce a quality radiograph, the amount of radiation that will penetrate a known thickness of lead shielding, or the radiation dose a patient will receive during a diagnostic procedure. The answer to these and many other important questions can be determined by applying the equations demonstrating such relationships.

Exponentials and Semilogarithmic Graphs

When relationships between quantities are represented in graphic form, a linear, or straight-line, graph is not always obtained. Many relationships in radiation science vary exponentially (recall from earlier discussions that an exponent is a power). Two basic types of commonly encountered exponential relationships are quantities that vary as positive or negative exponentials. It therefore is important to recognize these types of relationships in graphic form.

First, consider the positive exponential. Two quantities that are related in a positive exponential manner can be described by equations of the following form:

$$y = 10^x \text{ or } y = e^x$$

When values are given to x and corresponding

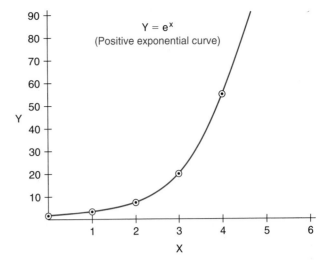

FIGURE 2–3. A positive exponential plotted on linear graph paper.

values for y are found and plotted, a typical positive exponential relationship looks like that in Figure 2–3.

The positive exponential curve characteristically begins slowly to increase numerical values of y for small values of x, then rises rapidly as x continues to increase.

Closely related to the positive exponential curve and definitely more important in the study of radiation is the negative exponential curve. Typically, negative exponential curves are described by equations of the form

$$y = 10^{-x} \text{ or } y = e^{-x}$$

Again, if values are assigned to x and corresponding values for y are found and plotted, a typical negative exponential curve like that in Figure 2–4 is obtained.

The negative exponential curve characteristically starts high on the y axis and falls rapidly toward the x axis but never crosses the axis. This indicates that as the quantity plotted on the x axis gets larger, y contin-

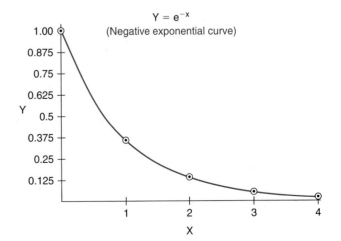

FIGURE 2–4. A negative exponential plotted on linear graph paper.

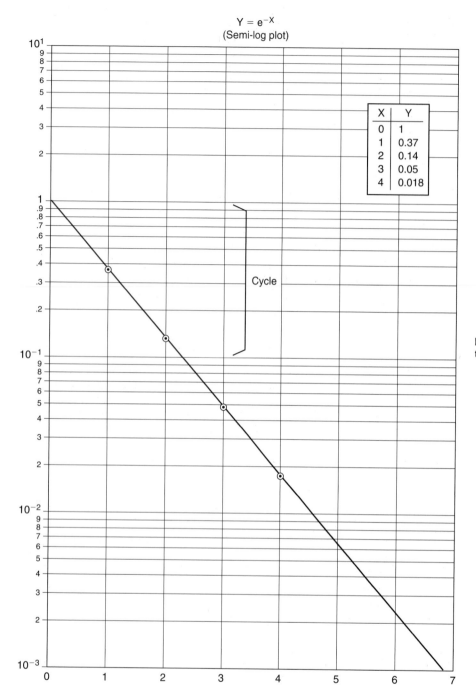

$$Y = e^{-X}$$
(Semi-log plot)

X	Y
0	1
1	0.37
2	0.14
3	0.05
4	0.018

Cycle

FIGURE 2-5. Negative exponential plotted on semilog graph paper.

ues to decrease but never theoretically reaches zero. This is another characteristic of exponential relationships. The negative exponential curve is an important mathematical relationship in radiation science, since it is used to describe such phenomena as radioactive decay and the transmission of radiation through matter.

Since exponential relationships are extremely common when working with radiation, their graphic representations would be considerably easier to work with if they could be represented by lines rather than curves such as those in Figures 2-3 and 2-4. The complex exponential relationships can easily be converted into linear form if the data is plotted on *semilogarithmic*

(semilog) graph paper rather than conventional linear graph paper. Semilog paper has a logarithmic scale along the y axis but a linear scale along the x axis. This is easily seen in Figure 2-5, in which the data used to plot Figure 2-4 is now plotted on semilog paper.

Note that the individual squares on the y axis vary in size, and each individual horizontal segment or grouping of squares (known as a cycle) represents a power of 10. This is in contrast to the x axis (the linear scale), where all squares are the same size. When data is plotted on this type of graph paper, the paper automatically takes the logarithm of the data plotted along the y axis.

Information important to radiographers is often plotted on semilog graphs, and it therefore is most important to be able to read these graphs and extract information from them correctly. It should carefully be noted that, unlike linear graphs, the squares on the logarithmic axis vary in numerical value, and one must pay attention to the power of 10 indicated in each cycle in order to determine the value of the individual squares.

Scientific Notation

To begin discussion of radiation and its use in diagnostic imaging, we need to use numbers that range from the large to the very small. The easiest way to work with numbers that vary in size over a wide range is to use *scientific notation*. To use this technique, first recall that powers of 10 can be written in the forms indicated:

Positive powers of ten
$$
\begin{cases}
10^4 = 10,000. \\
10^3 = 1,000. \\
10^2 = 100. \\
10^1 = 10. \\
10^0 = 1.
\end{cases}
$$

Negative powers of ten
$$
\begin{cases}
10^{-1} = \dfrac{1}{10} = 0.1 \\
10^{-2} = \dfrac{1}{100} = 0.01 \\
10^{-3} = \dfrac{1}{1000} = 0.001 \\
10^{-4} = \dfrac{1}{10,000} = 0.0001
\end{cases}
$$

From these examples, it can be seen that a positive exponent of ten moves the decimal point that same number of places to the right. That is

$10^0 = 1.0$

$10^1 = 10$ (1 place to the right)

$10^2 = 10 \times 10 = 100$ (2 places to the right)

$10^3 = 10 \times 10 \times 10 = 1000$ (3 places to the right)

and so on. On the other hand, a negative exponent of ten moves the decimal point that same number of places to the left. That is,

$10^0 = 1.0$

$10^{-1} = \dfrac{1}{10^1} = \dfrac{1}{10} = 0.1$ (1 place to the left)

$10^{-2} = \dfrac{1}{10^2} = \dfrac{1}{100} = 0.01$ (2 places to the left)

$10^{-3} = \dfrac{1}{10^3} = \dfrac{1}{1000} = 0.001$ (3 places to the left)

Therefore powers of ten can be used to move decimal points either to the right or left depending on the sign of the exponent. It also follows that any number, regardless of how large or how small, can be written in terms of a number between 1 and 10 times an appropriate power of ten. This is known as putting the number in the proper form. The following examples illustrate this point.

))))) EXAMPLES

Place each of the following numbers in proper form.

a) 480
   $480 = 4.8 \times 10^2$

b) 73100
   $73100 = 7.31 \times 10^4$

c) 0.0531
   $0.0531 = 5.31 \times 10^{-2}$

d) 0.000062
   $0.000062 = 6.2 \times 10^{-5}$

The fact that any number can be expressed as a number between 1 and 10 times an appropriate power of ten, allows complex mathematical computations to be performed rather easily. To review the simple rules that govern calculations using scientific notation

Multiplication

Rule: $10^a \times 10^b = 10^{a+b}$
That is, when multiplying powers of ten, simply add the exponents

))))) EXAMPLES

Perform the following calculations using scientific notation. Express the final answer in proper form.

a) 6200×1000
$$
\begin{aligned}
6200 \times 1000 &= (6.2 \times 10^3) \times (1 \times 10^3) \\
&= (6.2 \times 1) \times (10^3 \times 10^3) \\
&= 6.2 \times 10^6
\end{aligned}
$$

b) 420×0.0005
$$
\begin{aligned}
420 \times 0.0005 &= (4.2 \times 10^2) \times (5 \times 10^{-4}) \\
&= (4.2 \times 5) \times (10^2 \times 10^{-4}) \\
&= 21.0 \times 10^{-2} \\
&= 2.1 \times 10^1 \times 10^{-2} \\
&= 2.1 \times 10^{-1}
\end{aligned}
$$

c) 0.0051×0.002
$$
\begin{aligned}
0.0051 \times 0.002 &= (5.1 \times 10^{-3}) \times (2 \times 10^{-3}) \\
&= (5.1 \times 2) \times (10^{-3} \times 10^{-3}) \\
&= 10.2 \times 10^{-6} \\
&= 1.02 \times 10^1 \times 10^{-6} \\
&= 1.02 \times 10^{-5}
\end{aligned}
$$

Division

> Rule: $\dfrac{10^a}{10^b} = 10^{a-b}$
>
> That is, when dividing powers of ten, subtract the exponent of the denominator from the exponent of the numerator

))))) EXAMPLES

Solve each of the following, using scientific notation. Place the final answer in proper form.

a) $\dfrac{10{,}840}{200}$

$$\dfrac{10{,}840}{200} = \dfrac{1.084 \times 10^4}{2 \times 10^2}$$
$$= \dfrac{1.084}{2} \times \dfrac{10^4}{10^2}$$
$$= 0.542 \times 10^2$$
$$= 5.42 \times 10^{-1} \times 10^2$$
$$= 5.42 \times 10^1$$

b) $\dfrac{255}{0.005}$

$$\dfrac{255}{0.005} = \dfrac{2.55 \times 10^2}{5 \times 10^{-3}}$$
$$= \dfrac{2.55}{5} \times \dfrac{10^2}{10^{-3}}$$
$$= 0.51 \times 10^{2-(-3)}$$
$$= 5.1 \times 10^{-1} \times 10^5$$
$$= 5.1 \times 10^4$$

c) $\dfrac{0.082}{0.02} = \dfrac{8.2 \times 10^{-2}}{2 \times 10^{-2}}$

$$= \dfrac{8.2}{2} \times \dfrac{10^{-2}}{2 \times 10^{-2}}$$
$$= 4.1 \times 10^{-2-(-2)}$$
$$= 4.1$$

Raising to a Power

> Rule: $(10^a)^b = 10^{ab}$
>
> That is, when raising a power of ten to a power, multiply the exponents

))))) EXAMPLES

Perform the following computations using scientific notation. Express the answer in proper form.

a) $(3 \times 10^3)^2$
$$(3 \times 10^3)^2 = (3)^2 \times (10^3)^2$$
$$= 9 \times 10^6$$

b) $(2 \times 10^{-2})^3 = (2)^3 \times (10^{-2})^3$
$$= 8 \times 10^{-6}$$

c) $(2 \times 10^2)^{-2} = (2)^{-2} \times (10^2)^{-2}$
$$= 1/(2)^2 \times 10^{-4}$$
$$= 1/4 \times 10^{-4}$$
$$= 0.25 \times 10^{-4}$$
$$= 2.5 \times 10^{-1} \times 10^{-4}$$
$$= 2.5 \times 10^{-5}$$

Addition and Subtraction

> Rule: When adding or subtracting numbers expressed in scientific notation, convert all numbers to the same power of ten, then add or subtract in the normal manner

))))) EXAMPLES

Perform the following computations. Express the final answer in proper form.

a) $(5 \times 10^2) + (0.2 \times 10^1) + (0.002 \times 10^1)$
$$= (50 \times 10^1) + (0.2 \times 10^1) + (0.002 \times 10^1)$$
$$= (50 + 0.2 + 0.002) \times 10^1$$
$$= 50.202 \times 10^1$$
$$= 5.0202 \times 10^2$$

b) $(50.05 \times 10^{-2}) - (1.5 \times 10^{-3})$
$$= (50.05 \times 10^{-2}) - (0.15 \times 10^{-2})$$
$$= (50.05 - 0.15) \times 10^{-2}$$
$$= 49.9 \times 10^{-2}$$
$$= 4.99 \times 10^{-1}$$

Metric Units and Conversions

To begin the study of radiation, the principles developed in physics help to explain how x-ray machines work, the nature of radiation, and how to predict its behavior in matter. Physics relies heavily on precise and accurate measurement. In order for any measurement to have meaning it must not only have some numerical value (magnitude), it must also have units.

Units of measurement are arbitrary. Over the centuries some units have been defined but later have faded into nonexistence. Others have however stood the test of time. The most widely used of the devised systems of units is known as the metric system. First introduced in France some 200 years ago, the metric system has become the system of choice in science and engineering. The simplicity of the system lies in the fact that it is based on units of 10. This means that in making unit conversions within the metric system, in most cases, one need only move a decimal point to the right or left.

The current version of the metric system is referred to as the *SI system of units* (Systeme International d' Unites) and employs the units indicated in Table 2–1 for the basic units of length, mass, time, electric current, and *temperature*. However, the sizes of these

Table 2–1: SI UNITS FOR BASIC PHYSICAL QUANTITIES

Quantity	Unit	Unit Abbreviation
Length	Meter	m
Mass	Kilogram	kg
Time	Second	sec
Electric current	Ampere	A
Temperature	Kelvin	K

units are not always appropriate, and in those cases, multiples and submultiples are used. These are identified by the use of Greek prefixes. Some of the most commonly used prefixes that should be committed to memory are indicated in Table 2–2.

Often, conversions must be made between metric and British units (Fig. 2–6). In order to do this, one need only remember two basic conversion factors:

$$1 \text{ inch} = 2.54 \text{ cm}$$
$$\text{and}$$
$$1 \text{ kg} \approx 2.2 \text{ lbs}$$

These can be used in conjunction with your knowledge of metric prefixes with a technique to make unit conversions known as dimensional analysis. The technique utilizes the concept of multiplication by a series of factors that have a numerical value of 1. When a quantity is multiplied by a series of such factors, its initial value remains unchanged, although the units in which it is measured will change. Individual factors are written so that unit cancellation occurs. When all units have been canceled except the one to which the initial quantity is being converted, simply multiply the individual terms to arrive at the final answer. The following examples illustrate this technique.

))))))) EXAMPLES

Use dimensional analysis to make the following conversions:

a) Convert 30 ft to mm
First write the quantity to be converted, then multiply by factors that have a numerical value of 1.

Table 2–2: COMMONLY USED METRIC PREFIXES

Prefix	Numerical Meaning	Symbol
mega-	$10^6 = 1,000,000$	M
kilo-	$10^3 = 1,000$	k
centi-	$10^{-2} = 1/100 = 0.01$	c
milli-	$10^{-3} = 1/1000 = 0.001$	m
micro-	$10^{-6} = 1/1,000,000 = 0.000001$	μ
nano-	$10^{-9} = 1/1,000,000,000 = 0.000000001$	n

$$30 \text{ ft} \times \frac{12 \text{ in}}{1 \text{ ft}} \times \frac{2.54 \text{ cm}}{1 \text{ in}} \times \frac{10 \text{ mm}}{1 \text{ cm}}$$
$$= (30 \times 12 \times 2.54 \times 10) \text{ mm}$$
$$= 9144 \text{ mm}$$

Note. Factors are determined and arranged in such a way that all units cancel except the one to which the initial quantity is being converted. This desired unit should always appear in the numerator of the final term.

b) Convert 10 lb to μgm

$$10 \text{ lbs} \times \frac{1 \text{ kg}}{2.2 \text{ lb}} \times \frac{10^3 \text{ gm}}{1 \text{ kg}} \times \frac{10^6 \text{ } \mu\text{gm}}{1 \text{ gm}}$$
$$= (10 \times 1/2.2 \times 10^3 \times 10^6) \text{ } \mu\text{gm}$$
$$= 1/2.2 \times 10^{10} \text{ } \mu\text{gm}$$
$$= 0.45 \times 10^{10} \text{ } \mu\text{gm}$$
$$= 4.5 \times 10^9 \text{ } \mu\text{gm}$$

c) Convert 10 min to ns

$$= 10 \text{ min} \times \frac{60 \text{ s}}{1 \text{ min}} \times \frac{10^9 \text{ns}}{1 \text{ s}}$$
$$= (10 \times 60 \times 10^9) \text{ ns}$$
$$= 6 \times 10^{11} \text{ ns}$$

As problems are worked, great care must always be taken to observe units and to assure proper cancellation of terms.

On occasion, there is a need to work with areas and volumes. For the most part, areas represent two-dimensional measurements and are measured in square units (e.g., m^2, cm^2, ft^2), whereas volumes are measured in three dimensions and are expressed in cubic units (e.g., m^3, cm^3, ft^3). Conversions of these units can also easily be made, using the technique of dimensional analysis. The following examples illustrate this point.

))))))) EXAMPLES

Make the following conversions using dimensional analysis.

a) Convert 10 ft² to m²

$$10 \text{ ft}^2 \times \left(\frac{12 \text{ in}}{1 \text{ ft}}\right)^2 \times \left(\frac{2.54 \text{ cm}}{1 \text{ in}}\right)^2 \times \left(\frac{1 \text{ m}}{10^2 \text{ cm}}\right)^2$$

Note. Here, each term must be squared so that units cancel out appropriately. Observe that both units and numerical values must be squared.

$$= 10 \text{ ft}^2 \times \frac{144 \text{ in}^2}{1 \text{ ft}^2} \times \frac{6.45 \text{ cm}^2}{1 \text{ in}^2} \times \frac{1 \text{ m}^2}{10^4 \text{ cm}^2}$$
$$= (10 \times 144 \times 6.45 \times 10^{-4}) \text{m}^2$$
$$= 0.93 \text{ m}^2$$

b) Convert 10 in³ to cc (Note: 1 cc = 1 cm³)

$$10 \text{ in}^3 \times \left(\frac{2.54 \text{ cm}}{1 \text{ in}}\right)^3$$

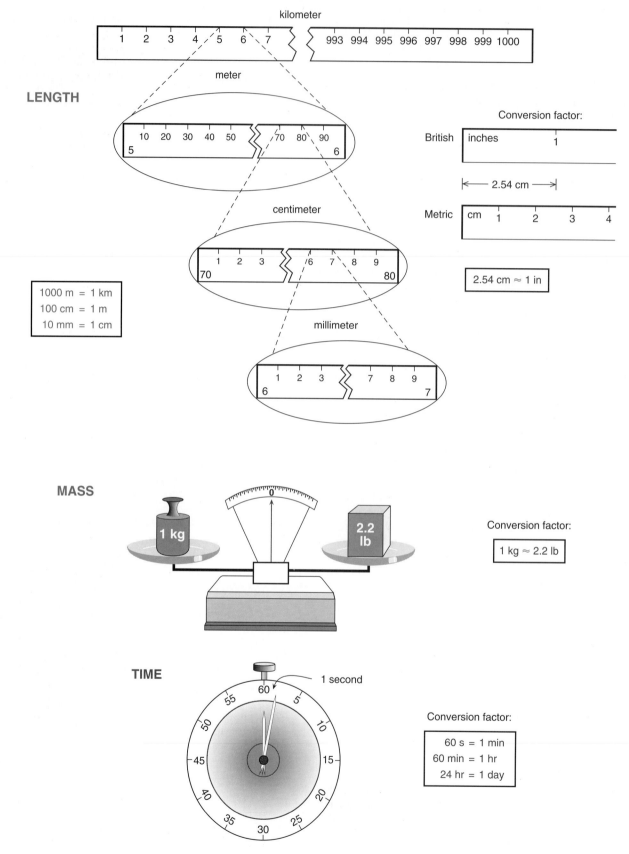

LENGTH

1000 m = 1 km
100 cm = 1 m
10 mm = 1 cm

Conversion factor:

2.54 cm ≈ 1 in

MASS

Conversion factor:

1 kg ≈ 2.2 lb

TIME

Conversion factor:

60 s = 1 min
60 min = 1 hr
24 hr = 1 day

FIGURE 2–6. SI units and conversion factors.

Here, factors must be cubed to assure cancellation of units.

$$= 10 \; \cancel{in^3} \times \frac{16.4 \; cm^3}{1 \; \cancel{in^3}}$$
$$= 164 \; cc$$

Care must always be taken in working with such problems, not only to raise the units but also the individual numerical values to the appropriate power.

PHYSICS REVIEW

Concepts of Motion

When an x-ray tube is activated, electrons move at tremendously high rates of speed from the negative to the positive terminals. The faster electrons move, the more penetrating are the x-rays produced. What factors are responsible for making these electrons move faster or slower? How fast are they moving? X-rays travel through air at the speed of light. What is the speed of light, and how is it measured?

In order to answer any of these questions, one must be familiar with the basic concepts used to describe motion. When an object moves through a distance, d, in a time period, t, the object is said to move with a *velocity* (or speed) given by the equation in units of m/sec, ft/sec, mm/sec, and so forth (Fig. 2–7).

$$\text{Velocity} = \frac{\text{distance traveled}}{\text{time required}}$$
$$\text{or}$$
$$v = d/t$$

Note. For our purpose, the terms *speed* and *velocity* are used interchangeably.

It should also be mentioned at this point that any formula used to define a specific quantity such as velocity can be treated as any algebraic equation and can therefore be solved for any quantity in the defining equation. This is illustrated in the following examples:

))))) EXAMPLES

a) An electron moves a distance of 80 cm in a time of 0.1 μsec. How fast is this electron moving? Express the final answer in m/sec.
Given: $d = 80$ cm and $t = 0.1$ μsec; $v = ?$ From the definition,

$$v = d/t$$
$$= \frac{80 \; cm}{0.1 \; \mu sec}$$
$$= \frac{0.8 \; m}{10^{-1} \times 10^{-6} \; sec}$$
$$= 8 \times 10^6 \; m/sec$$

b) How long would it take this same electron to move a distance of 10 m? Given: $v = 8 \times 10^6$ m/sec and $d = 10$ m; $t = ?$ To solve this problem, simply solve the defining equation for time, t:

$$v = d/t$$
$$vt = d$$
$$t = d/v$$
$$= \frac{10 \; m}{8 \times 10^6 \; m/sec}$$
$$t = 1.25 \times 10^{-6} \; sec \; or \; 1.25 \; \mu sec$$

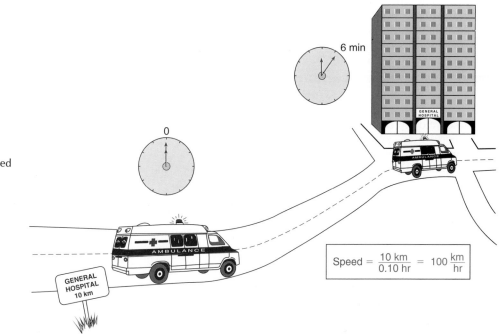

FIGURE 2–7. Concept of speed (velocity).

$$\text{Speed} = \frac{10 \; km}{0.10 \; hr} = 100 \; \frac{km}{hr}$$

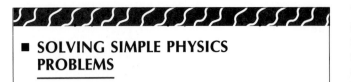

■ SOLVING SIMPLE PHYSICS PROBLEMS

It is at about this time, just after the first problem has been solved, that many students either begin to feel extremely depressed or give up altogether. Perhaps this is due to a lack of confidence in their own mathematical and problem-solving abilities. The availability of pocket calculators should eliminate the fear of mathematical computations. Solving problems does however require a degree of logic and organization that almost anyone can acquire with a little determination and practice.

Every physics problem that you encounter in this text can be solved by following several simple steps:

1. Read the problem carefully, and determine what quantity you are being asked to find.
2. Identify all the information you're given, and give each piece of information a symbol (e.g., t for time, v for velocity, and so on).
3. Choose the equation that contains all of these symbols with the exception of one unknown quantity.
4. Substitute numerical values given for the symbols, and solve for the unknown quantities.
5. Convert all multiple or submultiple units to basic units before performing mathematical calculations (e.g., convert mm, cm, km to meters; msec, μsec to seconds).
   Note. Care should always be taken to observe units of measurement. If unit conversions have been properly performed, unit cancellations will occur to provide proper units for the quantity desired.
6. Perform any necessary mathematical computations, and express your final answer with appropriate units. Watch carefully in all future example calculations how each step is performed. If you, too, follow each of these steps carefully, your problem solving will be greatly simplified.

Simple velocity calculations like those illustrated are easily performed and will become more important when energy concepts are discussed. It is easy to recognize velocity terms, since these are always expressed in units of distance/(time) (e.g., m/sec, cm/sec, ft/sec, miles/hr).

One extremely important speed with which you will frequently work is the speed of light (designated by the letter c). This value is

$$c = 3 \times 10^8 \text{ m/sec}$$ Speed of light in vacuum or air

The preceding value is the accepted speed of light in vacuum or in air (light tends to travel at lower speeds when it travels through matter such as water or glass).

This speed converts roughly to 186,000 miles/sec. It also serves as an upper limit of speeds for objects in the universe. That is, nothing is known to travel faster than the speed of light in vacuum. (Note: When an object approaches the speed of light, conventional physics relationships are no longer valid and must be replaced with equations developed by Einstein in his theory of relativity.)

When most objects move, they do not move at a constant speed. Realistically, objects may speed up, slow down, or change the direction in which they move. If an object does increase or decrease its speed or change its direction of motion, the object is said to undergo an *acceleration* (Fig. 2–8). This is easy to remember, since the accelerator in an automobile is used to change its speed. The faster the speed changes, the greater the acceleration. In our shorthand equation form, acceleration is defined as

$$\text{Acceleration} = \frac{\text{change in speed}}{\text{time required to make the change}}$$

or

$$a = \frac{\Delta v}{\Delta t}$$

Note. Δ is the Greek letter *delta* and is a symbol commonly used to represent *change.*

Acceleration terms are also easily recognized, because they always have two time units in the denominator and a distance unit in the numerator—for example, m/sec², ft/sec², cm/min-sec.

)))))) EXAMPLES

a) A particle moving initially at a speed of 10 m/sec increases its speed to 100 m/sec in a time of 10 msec. Determine the acceleration that this particle undergoes.

Given initial velocity $= v_i = 10$ m/sec
final velocity $= v_f = 100$ m/sec
$$\Delta t = 10 \text{ msec} = 10 \times 10^{-3} \text{ sec}$$
$$= 10^{-2} \text{ sec}$$
$$a = ?$$

Using the definition of acceleration,

$$a = \frac{\Delta v}{\Delta t}$$

We note that the change in velocity, or Δv, is just the difference between the final and initial velocities:

$$a = \frac{v_f - v_i}{\Delta t}$$
$$= \frac{100 \text{ m/sec} - 10 \text{ m/sec}}{10^{-2} \text{ sec}}$$
$$= \frac{90 \text{ m/sec}}{10^{-2} \text{ sec}}$$
$$= 90 \times 10^2 \text{ m/sec}^2$$
$$= 9 \times 10^3 \text{ m/sec}^2$$

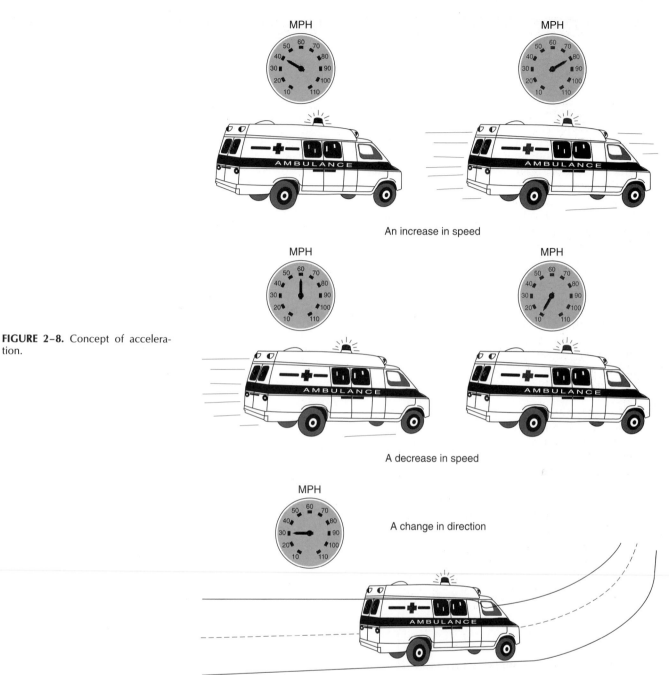

FIGURE 2–8. Concept of acceleration.

An increase in speed

A decrease in speed

A change in direction

Thus the particle undergoes an acceleration of 9000 m/sec².

b) Find the acceleration that the same particle undergoes if it initially moves at 10 m/sec but comes to rest in 2 sec.

Given $v_i = 10$ m/sec
$v_f = 0$ (i.e., it comes to rest)
$\Delta t = 2$ sec
$a = ?$

Again applying the definition of acceleration,

$$a = \frac{\Delta v}{\Delta t}$$
$$= \frac{v_f - v_f}{\Delta t}$$
$$= \frac{0 - 10 \text{ m/sec}}{2 \text{ sec}}$$
$$= -5 \text{ m/sec}^2$$

■ ACCELERATION DUE TO GRAVITY (g)

Another example of accelerated motion is the acceleration due to gravity, designated as *g*. If a box is dropped from rest from the top floor of your hospital (Fig. 1) and you were able to make some measurements to determine how fast it was moving 1 sec, 2 sec, and 3 sec after being dropped, you would obtain the information shown in the drawing. Using the definition of acceleration, you could determine the acceleration the box would experience:

$$a = \frac{\Delta v}{\Delta t}$$

$$= \frac{v_3 - v_1}{t_3 - t_1}$$

$$= \frac{96 \text{ ft/sec} - 32 \text{ ft/sec}}{3 \text{ sec} - 1 \text{ sec}}$$

$$= \frac{64 \text{ ft/sec}}{2 \text{ sec}}$$

$$= 32 \text{ ft/sec}^2$$

Since this acceleration comes about only as a result of the gravitational force of attraction between the box and the earth, it is known as *g*, the acceleration due to gravity.

$$g = 32 \text{ ft/sec}^2 = 9.8 \text{ m/sec}^2 = 980 \text{ cm/sec}^2$$

This means that theoretically a body at rest dropped from a high point increases its speed as it falls downward at a rate of 32 ft/sec each second until it hits the ground. Actually, it accelerates at a rate somewhat lower than this as a result of air resistance. Air resistance allows a freely falling body to reach a maximum speed of only ~544 m/sec (~120 miles/hr), which is known as terminal velocity.

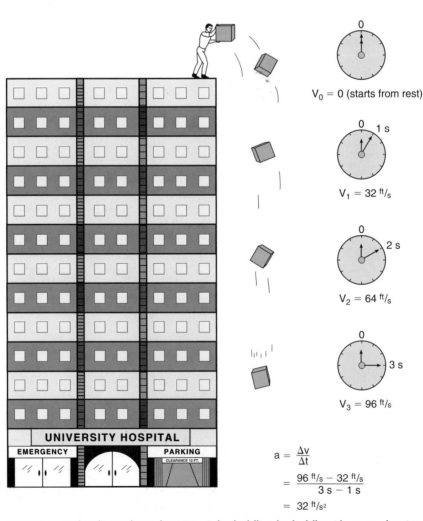

$V_0 = 0$ (starts from rest)

$V_1 = 32 \text{ }^{ft}/_s$

$V_2 = 64 \text{ }^{ft}/_s$

$V_3 = 96 \text{ }^{ft}/_s$

UNIVERSITY HOSPITAL

EMERGENCY   PARKING
CLEARANCE 12 FT.

$$a = \frac{\Delta v}{\Delta t}$$

$$= \frac{96 \text{ }^{ft}/_s - 32 \text{ }^{ft}/_s}{3 \text{ s} - 1 \text{ s}}$$

$$= 32 \text{ }^{ft}/_{s^2}$$

FIGURE 1. Uniformly accelerated motion. A freely falling body falls with an acceleration due to gravity, known as "g."

Note. The negative value that automatically arises here simply indicates that the particle is slowing down or decelerating.

Force and Momentum

A net *force* must be applied to a body in order for it to undergo an acceleration. That is, a net force must be applied in order for a body to increase its speed, decrease its speed, or cause the body to change its direction of motion. (By net force, we simply mean a force that is not counterbalanced by another.)

The idea of using forces to explain the motion of bodies comes from the great British physicist, Issac Newton (1642–1727). Two of Newton's three laws of motion are especially important in your present and future study of radiation science. Newton made the following observations:

1. An unbalanced (net) force is required to cause a body to increase its speed, decrease its speed, or change its direction of motion (Fig. 2–9).
2. The acceleration a body experiences is directly proportional to the size (or magnitude) of the net force applied to it. In our shorthand notation:

$$F_{net} \propto a$$

Note. Since this is a direct relationship, the larger the force applied, the greater the acceleration the body will undergo.

These laws of motion will have direct application when we investigate the factors that increase the speed of electrons moving between the electrodes of the x-ray machine. Here, the radiographer has the ability to change the magnitude of the applied force and thereby the resulting penetrating ability of the radiation produced. It is interesting to note that all forces existing in nature can at this moment in time be classified into four basic categories.

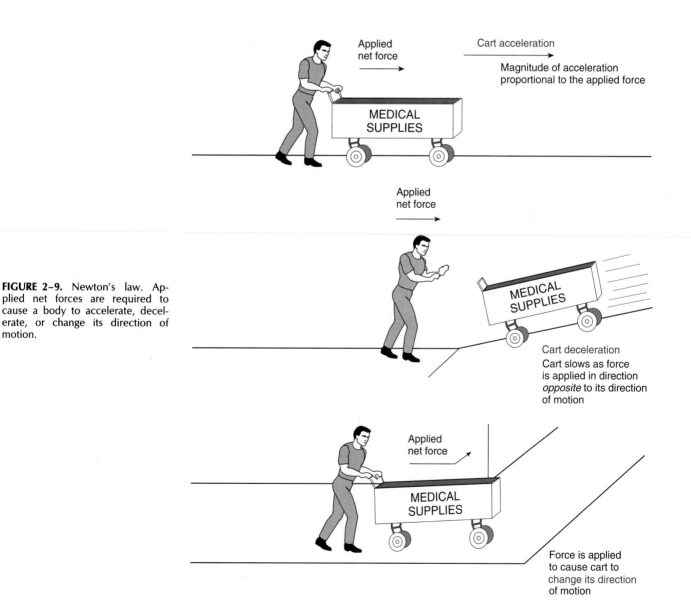

FIGURE 2–9. Newton's law. Applied net forces are required to cause a body to accelerate, decelerate, or change its direction of motion.

Force	*Relative Strength*
1. Strong force: The force that holds nuclei together; the strongest force known to exist in nature	1
2. Weak force: A nuclear force associated with the beta mode of radioactive decay; not well understood	10^{-13}
3. Electromagnetic force: The force that arises between electric charges or magnetic poles; may be attractive or repulsive	10^{-2}
4. Gravitational force: The force of attraction that arises between all objects having mass; the weakest of all the known forces in nature	10^{-40}

The primary force dealt with in radiography is the electromagnetic force.

Another term of importance is the concept of *linear momentum*. The linear momentum of a body is defined as follows:

> Linear momentum = mass × velocity
> or
> $$p = m \times v$$

Linear momentum

It is just the product of a body's mass and its speed. The larger this numerical quantity, the greater the tendency of the body to follow a straight-line path (Fig. 2–10).

))))) EXAMPLES

A truck that rolls down a small incline tends to move in a straight line because its large mass gives it a large linear momentum.

Similarly, a bullet fired from a gun tends to follow a straight line path because of its high velocity.

Both objects tend to travel in straight lines because the product of mass times velocity determines the magnitude of the linear momentum.

Energy

Perhaps one of the most important terms discussed here is the concept of *energy*. The energy of the radiation used determines its penetrating ability. If sufficiently penetrating radiation is not used, an image is not produced on the radiographic film. Physics defines energy as the ability to do work. Energy exists in many forms—heat, sound, light, solar, nuclear, mechanical, electrical, and magnetic—to name a few (Fig. 2–11). Today there are many devices and appliances whose primary purpose is to convert one form of energy to another, more useful form—an electric stove converts electrical energy into heat to cook food, the light bulb converts electrical energy into heat and light, and automobiles convert chemical energy (i.e., gasoline stored in the tank) into the mechanical energy of motion. Any device that converts one form of energy into another is termed a *transducer*.

The following are three important classifications of energy (Fig. 2–12).

1. *Kinetic energy:* Kinetic energy represents energy of motion. Any body that has mass and speed possesses kinetic energy. The amount of energy it carries is determined as follows:

> Kinetic energy = $\frac{1}{2}$ (mass) (velocity)^2
> or
> $$KE = \frac{1}{2} mv^2$$

2. *Potential energy:* Potential energy is energy that is stored. Stored energy can take many forms—the energy stored in a battery, in an electrical or mag-

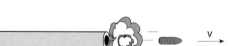

Linear momentum, p = m × v

Small mass × *high* velocity = large linear momentum

FIGURE 2–10. Linear momentum. Two conditions that require a large applied force to alter straight line (linear) motion owing to large values of linear momentum.

HOSPITAL SUPPLIES

Large mass × low velocity = large linear momentum

Forms of Energy

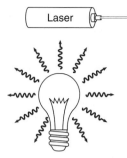

Light
(Electromagnetic Energy)

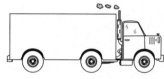

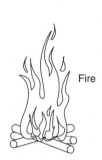

Fire

Heat Energy

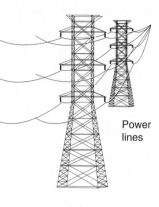

Power
lines

Electrical energy

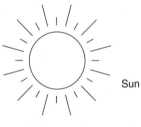

Sun

Solar energy

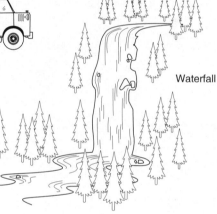

Mechanical energy
of motion

Waterfall

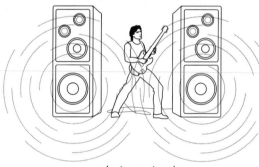

Instrument and
sound system

Sound energy

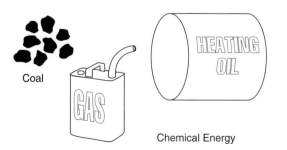

Coal

Chemical Energy

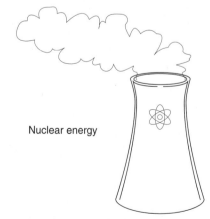

Nuclear energy

Cooling tower

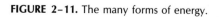

FIGURE 2–11. The many forms of energy.

Kinetic Energy
(Energy of motion)

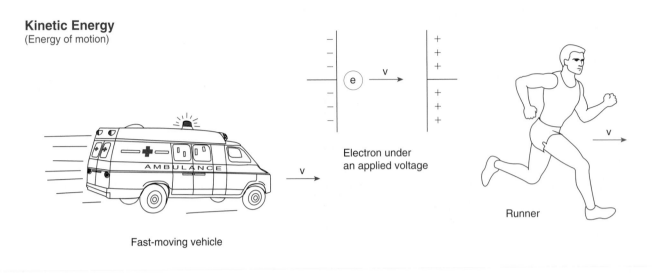

Electron under an applied voltage

Fast-moving vehicle

Runner

Potential Energy
(Stored energy)

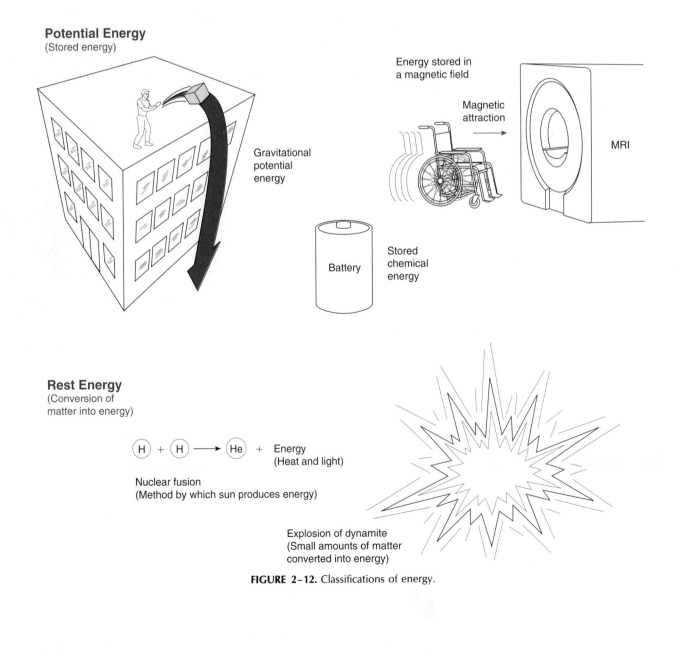

Gravitational potential energy

Energy stored in a magnetic field

Magnetic attraction

MRI

Battery

Stored chemical energy

Rest Energy
(Conversion of matter into energy)

$$H + H \longrightarrow He + \text{Energy (Heat and light)}$$

Nuclear fusion
(Method by which sun produces energy)

Explosion of dynamite
(Small amounts of matter converted into energy)

FIGURE 2-12. Classifications of energy.

netic field, or in the food we eat. Because of the variety of forms of stored energy, there is no single formula for potential energy, but it can be measured.

3. *Rest energy:* Rest energy is the energy a body possesses by virtue of the fact that it has mass. Einstein expressed this fact in his universally recognized equation:

> Rest energy = (mass) (speed of light)^2
> or
> $E = mc^2$

This equation simply indicates that matter can be converted into energy, which has been verified on numerous occasions. It is recognized as the source of energy generated by the sun. In the sun, atoms of hydrogen are "fused" together to form the next heavier element, helium. Each time this occurs, a small amount of matter is converted into energy in the form of heat and light.

In the SI system of units, energy, regardless of its form, is measured in *joules* (J). From the previously stated formula for kinetic energy, a joule would be the approximate energy carried by a 4.5-lb ($\approx$ 2-kg) stone moving at a speed of approximately 2.2 miles per hour ($\approx$ 1 m/s). That is,

$$KE = \frac{1}{2} mv^2$$

$$= \frac{1}{2} (2 \text{ kg}) (1 \text{ m/sec})^2$$

$$= 1 \frac{\text{kg} - m^2}{\text{sec}^2}$$

$$= 1 \text{ joule}$$

The joule, although an appropriate unit of energy when working with objects having masses measured in kilograms, is not convenient for use with smaller bodies such as atomic particles. A smaller unit of energy is the *electron volt* (eV). Since both the electron volt and the joule are units of energy, they must be related in some manner. This relationship is shown here:

> $1 \text{ eV} = 1.6 \times 10^{-19} \text{ J}$

This relationship can be used as a conversion factor whenever needed. The following simple energy calculations illustrate concepts of energy and the units in which it is measured.

))))) EXAMPLES

a) A 120-lb (54.5-kg) student runs to class at a speed of 6 miles/hr ($\approx$ 2.7 m/sec). What is this student's kinetic energy in joules? Since the joule is an SI unit of energy, all units used in the equation for KE must also be SI units, for example.

$$KE = \frac{1}{2} mv^2$$

$$= \frac{1}{2} (54.5 \text{ kg}) (2.7 \text{ m/sec})^2$$

$$= \frac{1}{2} (54.5 \text{ kg}) (7.29 \text{ m}^2/\text{sec}^2)$$

$$\approx 198.7 \text{ J}$$

b) An electron having a mass of 9.1×10^{-31} kg moves along a path at a velocity of 2×10^6 m/sec. Determine its energy in joules and electron volts. Since the electron is moving, it has kinetic energy. Therefore

$$KE = \frac{1}{2} mv^2$$

$$= \frac{1}{2} (9.1 \times 10^{-31} \text{ kg}) (2 \times 10^6 \text{ m/sec})^2$$

$$= \frac{1}{2} (9.1 \times 10^{-31} \text{ kg}) (4 \times 10^{12} \text{ m}^2/\text{sec}^2)$$

$$\approx 1.8 \times 10^{-18} \text{ J}$$

Now, to convert this energy in joules to electron volts use dimension analysis and the conversion factor:

$$KE = 1.8 \times 10^{-18} \text{ J} \times \frac{1 \text{ eV}}{1.6 \times 10^{-19} \text{ J}}$$

$$= 11.25 \text{ eV}$$

From this example, it is easily seen that the energy of the electron was a very small fraction of a joule (i.e., 1.8×10^{-18} J) but was a larger number in smaller electron volt units (i.e., 11.25 eV).

c) The head of a pin is weighed and is determined to have a mass of 1 mg. If all of this matter is converted into energy, how much energy would be produced?

If matter is to be converted into energy, use the rest energy equation:

$$E = mc^2$$
$$= (1 \text{ mg}) (3 \times 10^8 \text{ m/sec})^2$$
$$= (1 \times 10^{-6} \text{ kg}) (9 \times 10^{16} \text{ m}^2/\text{sec}^2)$$
$$= 9 \times 10^{10} \text{ J}$$

Note. When 1 kg ($\approx$ 2.2 lb) of dynamite explodes, approximately 5.4×10^6 J of energy are released. The energy in the head of a pin would be approximately 17,000 times this amount!

One of the most important laws in nature is the law of conservation of energy. This law simply states:

> Energy can be neither created nor destroyed but can be changed in form.   Conservation of energy

The law states that energy can be converted from one form to another without any loss of energy in the conversion process. Another way of saying this is that total energy before an interaction occurs must equal the total energy after the interaction.

Power

As indicated previously, in most cases energy is not available in its most useful form and must be converted into a form in which it can be utilized. As an example, electrical energy is of little use until a lamp is plugged into a wall outlet, and the electrical energy is converted into light. The rate at which energy is converted or used is known as *power* (P). In shorthand formula notation,

$$\text{Power} = \frac{\text{energy}}{\text{time}}$$

or   Power

$$P = \frac{E}{t}$$

In the SI system of units, in which energy is measured in joules and time in seconds, power is measured in a unit known as the *watt* (W) where

$$\text{watt} = \text{joules/second}$$

The watt is a commonly recognized unit, since the power of light bulbs, ovens, hair dryers, and other appliances is measured in terms of their wattage. The higher the wattage of a device, the more quickly it uses energy.

))))) EXAMPLE

The heating element on an electric stove converts 750,000 J of electrical energy into heat energy over a 10-minute time period. What is the power rating of this heating unit?

Given: $E = 750,000$ J

$t = 10 \text{ minutes} = 600 \text{ sec}$

$P = ?$

Using our definition for power,

$$P = \frac{E}{t}$$

$$= \frac{7.5 \times 10^5 \text{ J}}{6 \times 10^2 \text{ sec}}$$

$$= 1.25 \times 10^3 \text{ W}$$

$$= 1250 \text{ W}$$

Thus the power rating of the heating unit is 1250 watts.

))))) EXAMPLE

How long would it take this same heating unit to generate 200 kJ of heat energy?

Given: $E = 200 \text{ kJ} = 200 \times 10^3 \text{ J} = 2 \times 10^5 \text{ J}$

$P = 1250 \text{ W}$

$t = ?$

Again, use the same definition of power, but now solve for the time, *t*:

$$t = \frac{E}{P}$$

$$= \frac{2 \times 10^5 \text{ J}}{1250 \text{ W}}$$

$$= \frac{2 \times 10^5 \text{ J}}{1.25 \times 10^3 \frac{\text{J}}{\text{sec}}}$$

$$= 1.6 \times 10^2 \text{ sec}$$

$$= 160 \text{ sec or} \approx 2.7 \text{ min}$$

Heat and Methods of Heat Transfer

Heat is a form of energy. Normally, heat manifests in the form of an increase in the kinetic energy of the molecules of a substance. That is, as heat energy is added to matter, we see an increase in the motion of the atoms and molecules making up that substance. This can be visualized in the turbulence generated in a pot of boiling water on the heating unit of a stove.

The physical quantity or parameter used as an indicator of the amount of heat that has been added to or removed from a body is its *temperature* (T). Temperature can be measured in either Fahrenheit (°F) units or Celsius (°C) units (also known as centigrade units). Formulas have been derived that allow conversions from one temperature scale to another. These are given with examples of their use.

$$T_C = \tfrac{5}{9} (T_F - 32°)$$
and
$$T_F = \tfrac{9}{5} T_C + 32°$$

Temperature conversions

))))) EXAMPLES

a) On a cold winter day, the temperature reaches a high of 22°F. Express this temperature in °C.

Given: $T_F = 22°F$

$T_C = ?$

Using the equation for T_C,

$$T_C = \tfrac{5}{9} (T_F - 32°)$$
$$= \tfrac{5}{9} (22° - 32°)$$
$$= \tfrac{5}{9} (- 10°)$$
$$= -5.6°C$$

b) The temperature of a room is 23°C. What is this temperature in °F?

Given: $T_C = 23°C$

$T_F = ?$

Using the equation now for T_F,

$$T_F = \tfrac{9}{5} T_C + 32°$$
$$= \tfrac{9}{5} (23°) + 32°$$
$$= 41.4° + 32°$$
$$= 73.4°F$$

Heat energy can be transferred from one point to another. When two objects at different temperatures are placed in contact with one another, heat energy will flow from the warmer object to the cooler object. This indicates that there is a preferred direction of heat flow:

> When two objects at different temperatures are placed in contact, heat will flow from the higher temperature body to the lower temperature body.

Direction of heat flow

METHODS OF HEAT TRANSFER

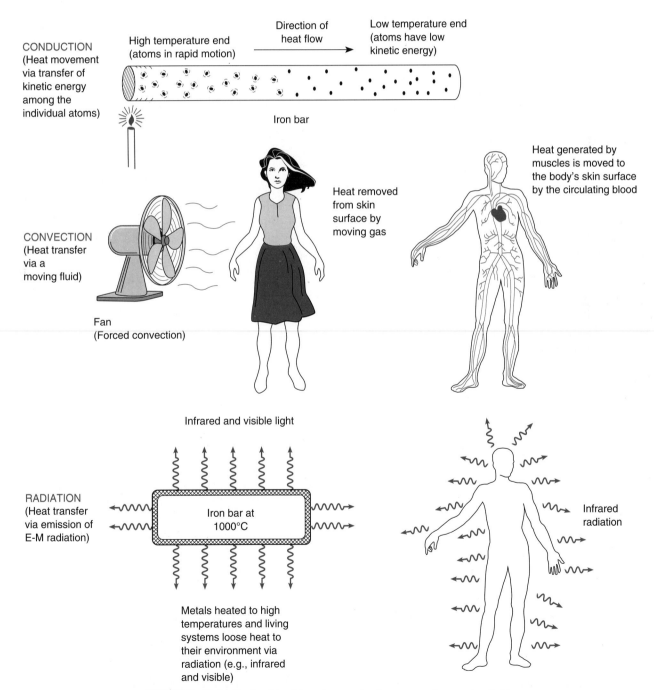

FIGURE 2–13. Methods of heat transfer: conduction, convection, and radiation.

There are three recognized methods by which heat can be transferred (Fig 2–13):

1. *Conduction:* The transfer of heat energy by the random collision of fast-moving molecules (i.e., high-temperature region) with slower moving molecules (i.e., lower-temperature region) in a body; this is typically the method of heat transfer in metals
2. *Convection:* The transfer of heat energy by a moving fluid (Note: a "fluid" may be either a liquid or a gas); as the fluid absorbs heat, it expands, becomes less dense, and rises; the warmer fluid is replaced by cooler, more dense fluid, and the cycle repeats itself, producing convection currents, which are responsible for "wind chill factors" and convection winds at seashores; it is also the reason that we use fans in the summer to keep cool
3. *Radiation:* The transfer of heat energy from a body by electromagnetic waves; although for the most part this radiation is classified as infrared radiation (i.e., heat radiation) but if heated to a high enough temperature, the radiation may fall into the visible portion of the spectrum; this method, unlike the first two, requires no material medium for the heat energy transfer to occur. Evidence of this is the transfer of heat energy from the sun through the vacuum of space

Each of these methods of heat transfer finds application in the design of the conventional x-ray machine, in which large amounts of heat are generated and must be dissipated effectively to avoid equipment damage.

Chapter Summary/ Important Equations, Constants, Relationships

Rules of scientific notation
  Multiplication: $10^a \times 10^b = 10^{a+b}$
  Division: $\dfrac{10^a}{10^b} = 10^{a-b}$
  Raising to a power: $(10^a)^b = 10^{ab}$

Metric conversions
  1 inch = 2.54 cm
  1 kg ≈ 2.2 lb

Velocity (or Speed): $v = \dfrac{d}{t}$

Speed of light: $c = 3 \times 10^8$ m/sec

Acceleration: $a = \dfrac{\Delta v}{\Delta t} = \dfrac{v_f - v_i}{t}$

Linear momentum: $p = mv$

Kinetic energy: $KE = 1/2\ mv^2$

Rest energy: $E = mc^2$

Electron volt: $1\ eV = 1.6 \times 10^{-19}$ joules

Power: $P = E/t$

Temperature conversions: $T_C = 5/9\ (T_F - 32°)$
$T_F = 9/5\ T_C + 32°$

Important Terminology

Acceleration. A measure of how quickly a body changes its speed or direction of motion

Conduction. A method of heat transfer in which heat energy is moved from one point to another by the collision of fast-moving molecules with slower-moving molecules; the primary method of heat transfer in metals

Convection. A method of heat transfer in which heat energy is moved from one point to another by a moving fluid

Direct Relationship. A mathematical relationship between two quantities in which an increase in one produces a corresponding increase in the other and vice versa

Electron Volt (eV). A small unit of energy equivalent to 1.6×10^{-19} joules

Energy. The ability to do work

Exponent. The power to which a quantity or number is raised

Force. Any influence that causes a body to increase or decrease its speed or change its direction of motion

Heat. A form of energy that manifests itself as a change in the kinetic energy of the molecules or atoms that make up a substance

Indirect (or Inverse) Relationship. A mathematical relationship between two quantities in which an increase in one produces a corresponding decrease in the other and vice versa

Joule. SI unit of energy

Kinetic Energy. Energy possessed by any body in motion

Law of Conservation of Energy. A fundamental natural law stating that energy can be neither created nor destroyed but can be changed in form

Linear Graph Paper. A graph paper that has equally sized squares on both the horizontal and vertical axes

Linear Momentum. A measure of the tendency of a body to maintain straight line motion; the greater its numerical value, the more difficult it is to alter its direction of motion

Logarithm. The power to which a base number (10, or e) must be raised to give a specific number

Potential Energy. Stored energy

Power. The rate at which energy is used or converted to another form

Rest Energy. The energy a body possesses by virtue of its mass

Scientific Notation. A technique to simplify mathematical calculations in which numbers are expressed as a number between 1 and 10 times an appropriate power of 10

Semilogarithmic (Semilog) Graph Paper. Graph paper that is usually characterized by a linear scale on the horizontal axis and a logarithmic scale on the vertical axis

SI System of Units. The metric system of measurement of which fundamental units are the kilogram, meter, and second; the accepted system of measurement of the international scientific and medical communities

Temperature. The physical quantity used to describe the amount of heat energy added or removed from a body

Transducer. Any device used to convert energy from one form to another

Radiation. A method of heat transfer by way of electromagnetic waves

Velocity (or Speed). The rate of movement of a body from one point to another

Watt. SI unit of power equivalent to 1 joule/second

Bibliography

Beiser, A. Modern Technical Physics, 5th ed. Reading, MA: Addison-Wesley, 1987.

Urone, P.P. Physics with Health Science Applications. New York: Harper & Row, 1986.

Waterhouse, M. Practical Mathematics in Allied Health. Baltimore-Munich: Urban & Schwarzenberg, 1979.

Wilson, J.D. Physics: A Practical and Conceptual Approach, 2nd ed. Philadelphia: W.B. Saunders, 1989.

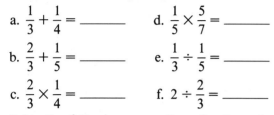 **Review Questions**

1. Perform the following computations:

   a. $\dfrac{1}{3} + \dfrac{1}{4} = $ _____

   b. $\dfrac{2}{3} + \dfrac{1}{5} = $ _____

   c. $\dfrac{2}{3} \times \dfrac{1}{4} = $ _____

   d. $\dfrac{1}{5} \times \dfrac{5}{7} = $ _____

   e. $\dfrac{1}{3} \div \dfrac{1}{5} = $ _____

   f. $2 \div \dfrac{2}{3} = $ _____

2. Solve the following proportions for the unknown quantity:

   a. $\dfrac{3}{5} = \dfrac{x}{6}$

   b. $\dfrac{1}{4} = \dfrac{2}{x}$

   c. $\dfrac{5}{6} = \dfrac{x}{4}$

   d. $\dfrac{x}{3} = \dfrac{8}{7}$

3. Convert each of the following fractions to their decimal equivalents:

   a. $\dfrac{1}{4}$ b. $\dfrac{2}{3}$ c. $\dfrac{2}{5}$ d. $\dfrac{1}{10}$

4. Convert each of the following decimal representations to their fractional equivalents:

   a. 0.25   b. 0.60   c. 0.125   d. 0.20

5. Use your pocket calculator to determine each of the following:

   a. $2^5 = $ _____

   b. $e^3 = $ _____ (Recall that $e = 2.718$)

   c. $\log 150 = $ _____

   d. $ln\ 28 = $ _____

   e. $\log 1 = $ _____

6. For the graphs shown below, identify the type of relationship (e.g., linear, positive or negative exponential, direct or indirect)

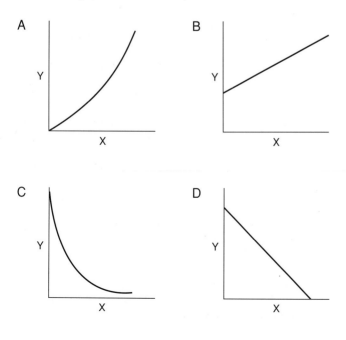

7. Express each of the following in proper form, using scientific notation:

   a. 25600   d. 0.000012

   b. 1.00   e. 4153

   c. 0.00323

8. Perform the following computations without the use of a calculator, using the rules of scientific notation. Express your final answer in proper form:

   a. $2400 \times 0.0002 = $ _____

   b. $0.0006 \times 0.002 \times 0.00005 = $ _____

   c. $25 \times 2000 \times 0.002 = $ _____

   d. $(2 \times 10^3)^2 = $ _____

   e. $80000/0.004 = $ _____

   f. $0.0006/400 = $ _____

9. Using a pocket calculator and the technique of dimensional analysis, make the following conversions. Express your final answer, with appropriate units, in proper form.

   a. Convert 10 cm to inches

   b. Convert 120 lb to kg

   c. Convert 10 inches to mm

   d. Convert 2 hours to msec

   e. Convert 50 kg to lb

   f. Convert 5 m to μm

   g. Convert 10 km to cm

Velocity and Acceleration

10. A particle moves a distance of 15 m in a time of 0.5 sec. What is its speed in m/sec?

11. A gas molecule moves a distance of 40 m in 10 msec. What is its speed in m/sec?

12. A particle changes its speed from 10 m/sec to 50 m/sec in a time of 0.1 sec. What is its acceleration?

13. How can a body experience an acceleration without changing its speed?

14. What is necessary for a body to experience an acceleration?

Force and Momentum

15. What is meant by the term *net force*?

16. When a net force is applied to an object, how does it affect its motion?

17. What type of relationship exists between a body's linear momentum and its mass? its speed?

18. Is it more or less difficult to change the direction of motion of a body that has a large linear momentum?

19. A 10-kg body moves at a speed of 20 m/sec. What is its linear momentum?

Energy

20. A body that has a mass of 5 kg moves at a speed of 10 m/sec. What is its kinetic energy?
21. A body having a mass of 100 gm moves at a speed of 4 m/sec. What is its kinetic energy?
22. What type of relationship exists between a body's kinetic energy and its mass? its velocity?
23. The energy of a diagnostic x-ray is 1.6×10^{-14} J. What is the energy of this x-ray in eV? in keV?
24. If 1 gm of matter is converted into pure energy, what is the energy produced in joules?
25. Explain why each of the following devices can be termed a transducer:
    a. an electric heater
    b. a stereo system
    c. an electric light
    d. a remote control device (e.g., for a TV or VCR)
    e. a radio

Power

26. A light bulb converts electrical energy into light at the rate of 50 J every 0.5 sec. What is the power rating of this bulb?
27. A 2000-W burner on an electric stove uses how many joules of energy in 1 min?
28. A sound system generates 100 J of sound energy in 0.25 sec. What is the power rating of this system?

Heat and Temperature

29. Although heat is normally measured in a unit known as the Calorie, why can it also be measured in joules?
30. Indicate which method of heat transfer is exemplified by each of the following:
    a. the transfer of heat generated within the body by the blood
    b. the transfer of heat along a metal rod when one end is placed in a flame
    c. the transfer of heat from the body by cool, moving air
    d. the loss of heat from a piece of metal which is glowing "red hot"
31. Use the temperature conversion formulas to perform the following:
    a. Convert 10°F to °C
    b. Convert 50°C to °F
    c. Convert -100°C to °F
    d. Convert 0°F to °C

Exercises

1. Perform the following computations, using pocket calculator and the techniques of scientific notation, and express your final answer in proper form:
    a. $(3 \times 10^{-2})^2 (2 \times 10^4)^3 =$ _____
    b. $(100)° (2 \times 10^6)^3 =$ _____
    c. $(2 \times 10^5) (5 \times 10^1)/(200)^3 =$ _____
    d. $(\sqrt{400}) (10^6)^{-2} =$ _____
2. Solve each of the following for the unknown quantity:
    a. $1/x = 1/3 + 1/4$
    b. $1/2 = 1/x + 1/5$
    c. $10 \text{ in}/x = 1 \text{ in}/2.54 \text{ cm}$
    d. $20 \text{ kg}/x = 1 \text{ kg}/2.2 \text{ lb}$
    e. $x/5 \text{ min} = 6 \times 10^4 \text{ msec}/1 \text{ min}$
3. Use your pocket calculator and the technique of dimensional analysis to make the following conversions. Express your final answer, with appropriate units, in proper form:
    a. Convert 10 oz to mg
    b. Convert 1/4 lb to μgm
    c. Convert 10 m² to ft²
    d. Convert 100 cc to in³
    e. Convert 10^{20} μsec to days
    f. Convert 10 ft³ to mm³
4. Solve each of the following for the unknown quantity using your pocket calculator:
    a. $\log 250 =$ _____   g. $5 e^x = 25$
    b. $ln\ 250 =$ _____   h. $10 e^x = 45$
    c. $ln\ 1 =$ _____   i. $\log x = 1.8$
    d. $\log 1 =$ _____   j. $ln\ x = 2.1$
    e. $x = e^{2.5}$ k. $10(0.5)^x = 2$
    f. $x = 10^{2.5}$ l. $4(0.5)^x = 0.6$
5. Interpretation of graphics:
    a. From Figure 2–1, what is the value of y when $x = 45$?
    b. From Figure 2–2, what is the value of x when $y = 64$?
    c. From Figure 2–3, what is the value of y when $x = 3.5$?
    d. From Figure 2–3, what is the value of y when $x = 0$? Is this verified by the equation of the curve?
    e. From Figure 2–4, what is the value of y when $x = 0$?
    f. In Figure 2–4, does y vary directly or indirectly with x?
    g. In Figure 2–5, what is the value of y when $x = 0.5$?
       when $x = 2.5$?
       when $x = 5.8$?
       when $x = 6.5$?
    h. In Figure 2–5, how many powers of 10 are indicated on the y axis?

6. If an electron moves at a speed of 10^3 m/sec, how far will it travel in 1 minute? How far is this in miles?

7. If an electron moves at a speed of 10^3 m/sec, how long will it take to travel a distance of 2 inches?

8. A particle changes its speed from 10 m/sec to 150 m/sec in a time period of 0.5 minute. What is its acceleration in m/sec^2?

9. What can be said about the acceleration a body experiences as the net force applied to it increases?

10. What does it mean to say that a body experiences a "negative acceleration"?

11. The kinetic energy of a body is 10 J. If the body's mass is 5 kg, how fast is it moving?

12. The mass of an electron is 9.1×10^{-31} kg. If this entire mass is converted into energy, how much energy is produced? Express your answer in joules, electron volts, and kiloelectron volts.

13. How much energy is used in 1 hour by a device that has a power rating of 1200 W?

14. If 12,000 J of energy are needed to heat a container of water, how long will it take a 2000 W heating unit to provide the necessary energy?

15. On your electric power bills, you are charged for the number of kilowatt hours you use each month. What type of physical quantity does a kilowatt hour represent?

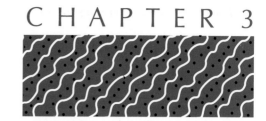

CHAPTER 3

Radiation: Its Atomic and Nuclear Origins

Michael A. Thompson, M.S.

Chapter Outline

Chapter Objectives

Upon completion of this chapter, you should be able to

■ Distinguish between particulate and electromagnetic radiation.
■ Identify the following on a transverse wave.
  • *crest*
  • *trough*
  • *wavelength*
  • *amplitude*
■ Define the following wave parameters:
  • *wavelength*
  • *frequency*
  • *wave velocity*
■ Indicate the relationships which exist between
  • *wavelength and frequency*
  • *energy and wavelength*
  • *energy and frequency*
■ Identify various types of electromagnetic radiation (e.g., x-rays, visible light, infrared, and ultraviolet) and their relative positions in the electromagnetic energy spectrum.
■ Use the general wave equation (i.e., $v = f\lambda$) to perform simple computations.
■ Identify units of measurement of wavelength, frequency, and wave velocity.
■ Use the equation $E(keV) = 12.4/[\lambda(\text{Å})]$ to perform simple photon computations.
■ Identify the following and explain the relation of each to general atomic structure:
  • *proton*
  • *neutron*
  • *electron*
  • *nucleus*
  • *mass (A) number*
  • *atomic (Z) number*
  • *electrical neutrality*
  • *electronic energy levels*
  • *electronic binding energy*
■ Locate the K, L, M, and N shells in relation to the nucleus of the atom and indicate how each relates to the others in terms of energy.
■ Explain what is meant by electronic transitions.
■ Determine the energy of photons emitted as a result of electronic transitions.
■ Explain the meaning of the following terms:
  • *ion*
  • *ionization event*
  • *ion pair*
  • *ionizing radiation*
■ Explain what is meant by a characteristic x-ray and how it is identified using K_α notation.
■ Explain the term *fluorescence* and tell how it differs from *phosphorescence*.
■ Define these terms:
  • *isotope*
  • *radioisotope*

(continued)

Chapter Objectives

- *radionuclide*
- *neutron to proton ratio*
- *nuclear binding energy*

■ Identify each of the following types of nuclear radiation in respect to origin and general characteristics.
  - *gamma rays*
  - *alpha particles*
  - *beta particles (or negatrons)*
  - *positrons*

■ Indicate the difference between x-rays and gamma rays.

■ Define the term *activity,* give the units in which it is measured, and explain how it relates to the intensity of radiation emitted from a radioactive source.

■ Define the term *physical half-life.*

■ Perform simple activity computations.

■ Draw a general "activity versus time" graph on semilog graph paper, and use the graph to determine the activity remaining after a specified time has passed.

ELECTROMAGNETIC RADIATION: A NEW WAY OF LOOKING AT LIGHT

Wave Parameters and Relationships

As mentioned initially, *radiation* is a general term used to describe a wide variety of emissions that may originate from a radiation source. One of the most useful forms of radiation is light, otherwise known as *electromagnetic* (EM) *radiation.* For many years physicists sought to discover the true nature of light—does it travel as a particle or as a wave? Particles have specific properties (e.g., mass and their existence as individual, discrete units) as do waves (see box). Prior to 1900 experiments seeming to indicate that light travels as a wave had been conducted by scientists. However, in 1887, an experiment now known as the photoelectric effect could not be explained on the assumption that light behaved as a wave. In 1905 a German physicist, Albert Einstein, refined a theory proposed some years earlier by another German physicist, Max Planck, to satisfactorily explain the experimental results. This new theory proposed that light has a "dual nature"—behaving as a wave in large-scale interactions but as a particle in interactions that occur at the atomic level. This is known as the wave-particle duality of light.

Einstein and Planck proposed in their theory that on the atomic level, light consists of individual, discrete packets of pure energy known as *photons* (thus light is also known as photon radiation). The energy (E) of these photons is directly related to the *frequency* (f). That is, in formula notation

$$E \propto f \qquad \text{Energy of a photon is directly related to its frequency}$$

From the general wave equation ($v = \lambda f$) applied to light traveling through air or vacuum where $v = c$ (i.e., c = speed of light in vacuum or air), a general wave equation for light emerges:

$$c = \lambda f \qquad \text{General wave equation for light}$$

Since c is assumed to be constant, note that λ and f vary inversely. That is, as λ increases, f decreases, and vice versa. This is an important relationship to remember. Since this inverse relationship exists between f and λ, then

$$E \propto 1/\lambda \qquad \text{Energy of a photon is inversely related to its wavelength}$$

From these relationships it can be said that as the frequency of light increases, its energy increases. But as the *wavelength* of the light gets longer, the energy of the light decreases. Normally, it is more common to discuss light in terms of its wavelength than in terms of its frequency. The reason is that when white light is passed through a prism, it is split into its component wavelengths, which we see as the individual colors of the visible spectrum (Fig. 3–1).

The colors of the visible spectrum range from the longest wavelength of 7000 Å (700 nm), which corresponds to red light, to the shortest wavelength of 4000 Å (400 nm), which corresponds to violet light. All the other colors in the visible spectrum fall between these wavelength limits.

The Electromagnetic Energy Spectrum

Visible light represents only a small portion of the electromagnetic (EM) energy spectrum. The entire EM spectrum with its classifications is shown in Figure 3–2. Note where the various types of EM radiation fall in the spectrum in relation to wavelength, frequency, and especially energy. It is energy that is used to determine the ability of radiation to penetrate materials (e.g., tissue or protective shielding) and that can produce biological effects. The major classifications of EM radiation include the following:

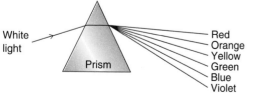

White light → Prism → Red / Orange / Yellow / Green / Blue / Violet

$\lambda = 7000$ Å (longest visible wavelength)

$\lambda = 4000$ Å (shortest visible wavelength)

FIGURE 3–1. The visible spectrum as seen when white light passes through a prism.

■ WAVE PROPERTIES

Many forms of energy travel in the form of waves—light and sound being two primary examples. Several parameters that are used to describe any type of wave motion are discussed here. Light travels in the form of a transverse wave such as those that move through the ocean. These waves have high points *(crests)* and low points *(troughs)* as shown in Figure 1. The maximum height of the wave, as measured from the equilibrium position, is known as the *amplitude* of the wave.

The distance between any two consecutive crests, any two consecutive troughs, or the distance covered by one full crest and one full trough is known as the *wavelength* (Fig. 2). Wavelength is indicated by the Greek letter lambda (λ). Wavelength can be measured in any unit of length (e.g., m, cm, ft, etc.). One older unit of wavelength is the angstrom (Å), where

$$1 \text{ Å} = 10^{-10} \text{ m}$$

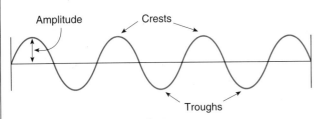

FIGURE 1. The transverse wave.

Another parameter important in wave discussions is wave *frequency (f)*. The frequency of a wave represents the number of waves that pass a given point per second. Frequency is measured in units of second^{-1}, also known as the hertz (Hz). Frequency is determined by counting the number of waves passing per second. Examples of a high- and low-frequency wave are shown in Figure 3.

$$\text{Frequency} = \frac{\text{number of waves}}{\text{seconds}}$$

The speed at which a wave travels through a medium is known as the *wave speed,* or *wave velocity (v)*. Wave speed is measured in conventional velocity units (e.g., m/sec). These last three parameters (i.e., wave speed, frequency, and wavelength) are related through one extremely important relationship known as the general wave equation:

$$\text{Wave speed} = \text{wavelength} \times \text{frequency}$$
or
$$v = \lambda f$$

General wave equation

This relationship is valid for light, sound, ocean waves, waves in a string, and so forth. It is an extremely important relationship that will also be of significance in discussions of electromagnetic radiation.

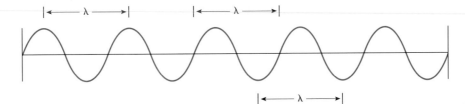

FIGURE 2. Wavelength measurement of a transverse wave ($\lambda =$ lambda).

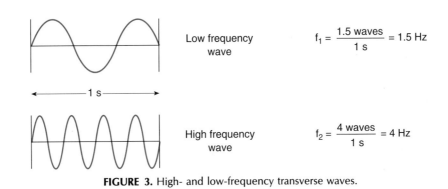

Low frequency wave $\quad f_1 = \dfrac{1.5 \text{ waves}}{1 \text{ s}} = 1.5 \text{ Hz}$

High frequency wave $\quad f_2 = \dfrac{4 \text{ waves}}{1 \text{ s}} = 4 \text{ Hz}$

FIGURE 3. High- and low-frequency transverse waves.

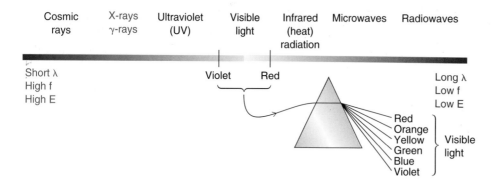

FIGURE 3-2. The electromagnetic spectrum.

Radiowaves. Radiowaves comprise a broad band of frequencies (~20 kHz to 1 GHz) within the spectrum and refer to those frequencies used in aircraft and marine navigation, short-wave radio signals, AM and FM radio transmissions, and television broadcasts. These frequencies are often referred to as RF (i.e., radiofrequency) radiation. Frequencies in the lower MHz (i.e., megahertz, or 10^6 Hz) range correspond to those currently used with magnetic resonance imaging (MRI) devices.

Wavelength range: ~1.5×10^4 m to 3×10^{-1} m

Frequency range: ~2×10^4 Hz to 1×10^9 Hz

Energy range: ~10^{-10} eV to 10^{-6} eV

Microwaves. The microwave region of the spectrum consists of those EM waves within the approximate frequency range of 1 to 30 GHz. In the past, microwaves have been used primarily in radar and satellite communications. In addition to these applications, microwave ovens make use of specific microwave frequencies, readily absorbed by the water molecules in food, that in turn generate heat. Microwaves are also used in long distance telephone transmission and in speed determination by law enforcement agencies (i.e., "radar guns"). In medicine, microwaves (~2450 MHz) are used for deep tissue heating and show promise in the treatment of certain types of cancer in conjunction with other modes of therapy. The use of microwave radiation in medical therapy is referred to as microwave diathermy. Microwaves are also used in devices known as linear accelerators in radiation therapy departments to produce high-energy beams of electrons and high-energy x-rays in the treatment of both superficial and deep-seated tumors.

Wavelength range: ~0.3 m to 0.01 m

Frequency range: ~10^9 Hz to 3×10^{10} Hz

Energy range: ~10^{-6} eV to 10^{-4} eV

Infrared Radiation. Also referred to as *IR radiation,* these EM waves occupy the region of the spectrum in which wavelengths are just longer than the longest portion of the visible spectrum. *Infra* indicates that the corresponding *frequencies* are just "below" the red (i.e., long wavelength) portion of the visible spectrum. IR radiation is commonly associated with radiation emitted from "heat lamps" and other warm bodies that are not at temperatures high enough to make the body glow (i.e., not hot enough to emit light in the visible portion of the spectrum). The human body emits radiation having wavelengths in the approximate range of 6000 nm to 15,000 nm (i.e., 60,000 Å to 150,000 Å), which falls in the infrared region. Devices sensitive to this radiation can be used to detect small temperature variations over the surface of the body as a means of locating sites of inflammation, areas of impaired blood flow, and certain types of tumors and to diagnose and evaluate wound healing, arthritis, burns, and frostbite. This technique of medical diagnosis is known as medical thermography.

Wavelength range: ~3×10^{-3} m to 8×10^{-7} m

Frequency range: ~10^{11} Hz to 3.8×10^{14} Hz

Energy range: ~4×10^{-4} eV to 1.55 eV

Visible Light. That portion of the electromagnetic energy spectrum to which our eyes respond is visible light. Wavelengths, which correspond to the various colors of visible light (i.e., red, orange, yellow, green, blue, and violet) range in wavelength from 700 nm to 400 nm (i.e., 7000 Å to 4000 Å). Other than stimulating our sense of vision, visible light, which occupies only a very narrow region within the EM spectrum, is used in a wide range of applications in medicine. A process known as transillumination utilizes visible light passed through body structures to obtain specific types of information. This method has been used on structures such as the breast to locate and determine the nature of lumps. The amount of light transmitted can indicate if the lump is solid or cystic (i.e., fluid-filled). This technique has also been used on infants to detect such conditions as water on the brain (hydrocephalus) and collapsed lungs.

Use of lasers, extremely intense and pure wavelength light sources, has also become common in medicine over the past several years. Lasers have become the "bloodless scalpels" of many of today's surgical procedures, since the heat generated by the absorption of this emitted light actually cauterizes small blood vessels as tissue is vaporized by the laser beam. Lasers find application in surgery of the eye, plaque removal from arteries, and surgery to remove skin lesions and certain types of cancer.

Wavelength range: ~7 × 10^{-7} m to 4 × 10^{-7} m

Frequency range: ~4.3 × 10^{14} Hz to 7.5 × 10^{14} Hz

Energy range: ~1.8 eV to 3.1 eV

Ultraviolet Radiation. *Ultraviolet (UV) radiation* extends just beyond the violet portion of the visible spectrum. UV radiation has more energy than visible light and has the capability of destroying certain types of organic materials. As a result UV radiation produced by special UV lamps can be used to kill certain microorganisms on the surfaces of food and even on surgical instruments. By far one of the largest sources of UV radiation is the sun. Most of the sun's UV light, however, is absorbed by the earth's atmosphere. The UV light that does penetrate the atmosphere is responsible for stimulation to produce the skin pigment melanin, which results in the "tanning" of the skin as a defense mechanism against UV radiation.

Overexposure of the skin to UV radiation can produce skin cancer. All exposure to UV is not harmful, in that it is a necessary component for the body's production of vitamin D, required for healthy bones and teeth and the proper absorption and utilization of phosphorous and calcium. For this reason, controlled exposure to UV radiation is used to treat a variety of skin conditions.

Wavelength range: ~4 × 10^{-7} m to 1.8 × 10^{-9} m

Frequency range: ~7.5 × 10^{14} Hz to 1.7 × 10^{17} Hz

Energy range: ~3.1 eV to 0.7 keV

X-Rays and Gamma Rays. Both *x-rays* and *gamma (γ) rays* occupy the same portion of the EM spectrum. The only difference between the two is their origin — x-rays originate from outside the nucleus of the atom and gamma rays originate from within the nucleus. This portion of the spectrum represents high-energy, penetrating radiation. At high intensities, x-rays can produce skin burns and can lead to more serious biological complications. At lower intensities, these rays can be used to visualize the body's internal structures by the techniques of radiography. The x-radiation on the patient's body is transmitted to varying degrees (i.e., transmitted by soft tissue but stopped, or attenuated, by more dense structures such as bone), producing a "shadow" image on a sheet of photographic film. The image produced is known as a radiograph.

Gamma rays originate from the nucleus of an unstable (i.e., radioactive) atom. Radioactive materials that emit this type of penetrating radiation find use in nuclear medicine departments, where they are used to diagnose a wide variety of diseases and medical conditions. Radiation therapy departments use both x-rays (from x-ray machines and accelerators) and gamma rays (from radioactive materials) to treat tumors and various types of cancer. Gamma radiation also finds extensive applications in medical research in an effort to understand and develop better methods to treat disease.

Wavelength range: ~1 × 10^{-7} m to 1.8 × 10^{-17} m

Frequency range: ~3 × 10^{15} Hz to 1.7 × 10^{25} Hz

Energy range: ~12.4 eV to 6.8 × 10^{7} keV

Note. It should be mentioned that in an effort to classify these various types of EM radiation, the wavelength, frequency, and energy ranges given may seem to indicate that there are sharp divisions between each classification, but this is not so. There is overlap in these various regions, and therefore numerical ranges given for each do not represent strict absolutes.

Thus EM radiation represents many specific types of photon radiation — visible light, microwaves, UV, RF, and so forth. Each differs in its interaction with matter and in individual characteristics, but each is fundamentally a photon of pure energy having no mass (as far as we currently know) and no electric charge but possessing a specific quantity of energy.

Several features should be evident as you read the properties of each of these types of EM radiation:

- Recall the inverse relationship that exists between wavelength (λ) and frequency (f); that is,

$$\lambda \propto 1/f$$

Observe in each case that as the frequency increases, the wavelength decreases.
- There exists a direct relationship between energy (E) and frequency (f); that is,

$$E \propto f$$

In each case, as the frequency of the photon increases, its energy also increases.
- An indirect relationship exists between energy and wavelength; that is,

$$E \propto 1/\lambda$$

and in each case, as the wavelength decreases, the energy of the photon increases.

These relationships exist only for photons, since we are using Einstein's and Planck's theory, which ascribes wave characteristics (i.e., wavelength and frequency) to particles of pure energy known as photons. It is essential to remember these general relationships, for they will become more important when there is further discussion of the nature of the x-rays produced by the x-ray machine.

■ PHOTON CALCULATIONS

The relationships developed initially were general proportionalities. Recall that a proportionality can be converted into an equation by the inclusion of an appropriate constant. For the photon relationships we have

a) $E \propto f$

which becomes

Energy of a photon in terms of frequency (1)

$$\boxed{E = hf}$$

where

h = Planck's constant
= 6.63×10^{-34} joule-seconds (J-sec)

f = frequency (Hz or sec^{-1})

E = energy (J)

b) $E \propto 1/\lambda$

which becomes

$$\boxed{E = \frac{hc}{\lambda}}$$
Energy of a photon in terms of wavelength (2)

where

h = Planck's constant
= 6.63×10^{-34} J-sec

c = speed of light in vacuum
= 3×10^8 m/sec

λ = wavelengths (m)

E = energy (J)

A more usable and more meaningful relationship is

$$\boxed{E\ (keV) = \frac{12.4}{\lambda(\text{Å})}}$$
Energy of photon in terms of wavelength (modified form) (3)

where

E = energy (in keV)

λ = wavelength (in Å where 1 Å = 10^{-10} m)

c) $\boxed{\lambda f = c}$ General wave equation for photons (4)

which is the general wave equation for light where

λ = wavelength (m)

f = frequency (Hz or sec^{-1})

c = speed of light in vacuum (3×10^8 m/sec)

Each of these equations can be used to determine specific numerical values for any of the individual parameters. The following examples are provided to illustrate their use:

))))))) EXAMPLE

a) Determine the energy in keV of a photon has a frequency of 2×10^{20} Hz.
Using equation (1),

$E = hf$
$\quad = (6.63 \times 10^{-34}$ J-sec$)\ (2 \times 10^{20}$ sec$^{-1})$
$\quad = 13.26 \times 10^{-14}$ J

Then using appropriate conversion factors, we have:

$$E = 13.26 \times 10^{-14}\ \cancel{J} \times \frac{1\ \cancel{eV}}{1.6 \times 10^{-19}\ \cancel{J}} \times \frac{1\ keV}{10^3\ \cancel{eV}}$$

$$= 828.8\ keV$$

b) What is the wavelength in angstroms of the same photon, which has a frequency of 2×10^{20} Hz?
This can be determined by either of two methods.

Method I
The result of part (a) can be used in equation (3):

$$E(keV) = \frac{12.4}{\lambda(\text{Å})}$$

or

$$\lambda(\text{Å}) = \frac{12.4}{E(keV)}$$

$$= \frac{12.4}{828.8\ keV}$$

$$= 0.015\ \text{Å}$$

Method II
The general wave equation for photons (4) can be used:

$$\lambda f = c$$

$$\lambda = c/f$$

$$= \frac{3 \times 10^8\ \text{m/sec}}{2 \times 10^{20}\ \text{1/sec}}$$

$$= 1.5 \times 10^{-12}\ \text{m}$$

Then using appropriate conversion factors the following is obtained:

$$\lambda = 1.5 \times 10^{-12} \ \cancel{m} \times \frac{1 \ \text{Å}}{10^{-10} \ \cancel{m}}$$

$$= 1.5 \times 10^{-12} \times 10^{10} \ \text{Å}$$

$$= 0.015 \ \text{Å}$$

the same result, as it should be, obtained by Method I.

c) Determine the energy in keV of a photon that has a wavelength of 4×10^{-7} m (violet light).

Method I

Equation (2) can be used with appropriate conversion factors:

$$E = \frac{hc}{\lambda}$$

$$= \frac{(6.63 \times 10^{-34} \ \text{J-sec}) \ (3 \times 10^{8} \text{m/sec})}{4 \times 10^{-7} \ \text{m}}$$

$$= 4.97 \times 10^{-19} \ \text{J}$$

$$E = 4.97 \times 10^{-19} \ \cancel{J} \times \frac{1 \ \text{eV}}{1.6 \times 10^{-19} \ \cancel{J}} \times \frac{1 \ \text{keV}}{10^{3} \ \cancel{eV}}$$

$$= 0.003 \ \text{keV}$$

Method II

$$\lambda = 4 \times 10^{-7} \ \cancel{m} \times \frac{1 \ \text{Å}}{10^{-10} \ \cancel{m}}$$

$$= 4 \times 10^{3} \ \text{Å}$$

Then using equation (3)

$$E(\text{keV}) = \frac{12.4}{\lambda(\text{Å})}$$

$$= \frac{12.4}{4 \times 10^{3} \ \text{Å}}$$

$$= 3.1 \times 10^{-3} \ \text{Å}$$

$$= 0.0031 \ \text{Å}$$

which agrees with the result obtained in Method I.

GENERAL ATOMIC STRUCTURE AND THE ORIGIN OF CHARACTERISTIC X-RAYS

Atomic Components

The *atom* is the smallest unit of matter that has the identifiable properties of a particular element. Thus from specific physical and chemical properties (e.g., melting point, freezing point, density) atoms of hydrogen, helium, oxygen, nitrogen, and each of the other 88 naturally occurring elements can be identified. Each atom, regardless of its identity, is composed of three basic particles—*electrons, protons,* and *neutrons.* It is the number of protons within the tiny, dense core of the atom, known as the *nucleus* that determines the identity of an atom.

A comparison of various physical characteristics of these three primary particles is summarized in Table 3–1. These properties should be reviewed carefully.

Table 3–1: SELECTED PHYSICAL PROPERTIES OF ATOMIC PARTICLES

Particle	Symbol	Relative Mass (in Terms of Proton Mass, m_p)	Electric Charge
Proton	p	1 m_p	$+1.6 \times 10^{-19}$ coulombs
Neutron	n	~1 m_p	0
Electron	e	~1/2000 m_p	-1.6×10^{-19} coulombs

From the table it can be seen that protons and neutrons have about the same mass (actually, the neutron is a little heavier than the proton), but in comparison the electron's mass is about 1/2000 the mass of the proton. So protons and neutrons are massive particles, like "atomic bowling balls," compared with the lighter mass electron, which is like an "atomic pea" in comparison. In addition, the proton and electron carry the same magnitude of electric charge (which also happens to be the smallest charge known currently to exist in nature) but opposite signs.

Only protons and neutrons are found in the nucleus of an atom. Since these are the two massive particles that constitute more than approximately 99% of the total mass of an atom, the sum of the protons and neutrons of an atom is known as the *mass number,* or *A number.* Since the number of protons within the nucleus of an atom determines the identity of an atom (i.e., identifies the atom as carbon, nitrogen, oxygen, lead, etc.), the number of protons is known as the *atomic number,* or *Z number.* Together these two numbers, A and Z, are used to identify specific atoms or different forms of the same atom. These atoms are easily identified by using their chemical symbol along with their A and Z numbers. The general, commonly used, form is

Mass number $\longrightarrow$ A
Atomic number $\longrightarrow$ Z   X $\longleftarrow$ chemical symbol

For our purposes, this is designated as atomic notation. In almost all cases, the Z number is omitted, since the chemical symbol automatically indicates the number of protons in the nucleus.

It should also be noted that under normal conditions, all atoms are also electrically neutral, which simply means that an atom has the same number of positive and negative charges.

))))))) EXAMPLE

A carbon (C) atom has 6 protons and 8 neutrons in its nucleus.

a) How many electrons does this atom have?
This atom has 6 electrons to balance the 6 protons, so the atom is electrically neutral.
b) What are this atom's A and Z numbers?
Z = number of protons = 6
A = number of protons + neutrons
= 6 + 8 = 14
c) How would this atom be represented using atomic notation?

$$^{14}_{6}C \quad \text{or} \quad ^{14}C$$

The electrons in an atom are arranged in shells or energy levels around the nucleus. To move away from the nucleus is to move in the direction of increasing energy. These shells are designated by the letters K, L, M, N, and so forth, the K shell, nearest to the nucleus, representing the lowest energy state. This is shown schematically in Figure 3–3.

Only a specified number of electrons can exist in each energy level, and when a shell has its maximum number of electrons, it is said to be filled. Another important concept to remember is that an electron always tends to seek the lowest energy level in which it can exist. Electrons are held in their respective shells by the electrostatic force of attraction between the negatively charged electron and the positively charged nucleus. This force of attraction drops off rapidly the farther the electron is from the nucleus. (In reality this force drops off as an inverse square with distance as discussed in more detail in the next chapter.) This is verified by observing the binding energies (E_1, E_2, E_3, etc.) indicated in Figure 3–3. The binding energies represent the energy that is required to remove an electron from a particular shell. The negative signs on

these energies simply indicate that this energy does not come from the atom and must be supplied. From the diagram, 1 keV of energy is required to remove the electron from the K shell. Note that only 40 eV of energy is needed to remove an electron from the M shell. The reason for this difference is that an electron in the M shell is much less tightly bound to the atom, since the electron is farther away from the nucleus. Therefore, it takes less energy to remove an M-shell electron than a K-shell electron.

(Note: An electron in the M shell is said to exist in a "higher energy state" than an electron in the K or L shells. One way to think of this is that in terms of binding energies, −40 eV is larger, or "higher," than −1000 eV or −850 eV. That is, the last two values are "more negative" than −40 eV. Therefore, as an electron moves away from the nucleus, it is moving to higher energy levels.)

If sufficient energy is provided, an electron may be removed from an atom. What remains of the atom, which now is no longer electrically neutral, is known as an *ion*. The ejected electron and the ion are known as an *ion pair*. The creation of an ion pair is known as an ionization event. It generally requires approximately 33 to 35 electron volts of energy to produce an ionization event in the gases of the air. We use this then as a numerical marker and say that radiation having energy greater than 33 to 35 eV is classified as *ionizing radiation*. Diagnostic x-rays, which have energies within the approximate range of 60 keV to 100 keV, definitely are ionizing radiation.

Electronic Transitions

Electronic transitions refer to the movements of electrons within the shell structures of the atom. Again, consider an electron located in its lowest energy level (i.e., the K shell) as shown in Figure 3–3. Energy (in the form of heat, light, or electric current) must be supplied in the exact proper amount to raise an electron from a low energy state to a higher energy state. For example, 960 eV of energy must be supplied to raise the electron in Figure 3–3 from the K to the M shell. The amount of energy that must be supplied is just the difference between the two energy levels. This is shown in Figure 3–4.

Almost immediately on being raised to the higher energy level, the electron drops back to the lower energy level. When this occurs, energy is given off in the form of a photon, known as a *characteristic x-ray,* as shown in Figure 3–5. The energy of the emitted photon is determined simply by determining the difference in the binding energies of the two energy levels. As in this case,

$$\begin{aligned} E_{x\text{-ray}} &= E_3 - E_1 \\ &= -40 \text{ eV} - (-1000 \text{ eV}) \\ &= -40 \text{ eV} + 1000 \text{ eV} \\ &= 960 \text{ eV} \end{aligned}$$

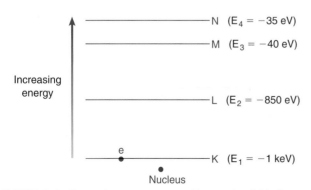

FIGURE 3–3. Electronic energy states with associated binding energies. An electron is shown in the lowest energy state.

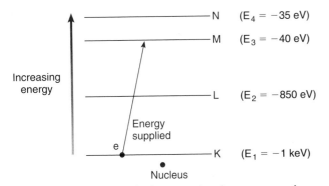

FIGURE 3–4. Having absorbed energy, the electron moves from a low to a higher energy state.

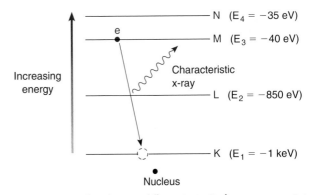

FIGURE 3–5. As the electron falls again to its lower energy state, energy is released in the form of a characteristic x-ray.

The photons emitted during these electronic transitions are called characteristic x-rays, since the binding energies for the respective shells are characteristic of the atoms of each element. This idea is demonstrated in Figure 3–6, in which there are atoms of three different elements, A, B, and C. An electron makes a transition from the M shell to the K shell in each case. It is noted, however, that a characteristic x-ray of different energy is emitted from each element even though exactly the same transition occurred in each case. Thus the photon energy is characteristic of the element.

Characteristic x-rays are designated according to the shell to which the electron falls and the specific shell from which the electron originated. In the examples shown in Figure 3–7, the characteristic x-ray designated as L_β indicates that the electron fell to the L shell, and the subscript β indicates that the electron originated from two shells away. When the electron falls to the K shell from one shell away, the characteristic x-ray is designated as K_α. K_γ indicates that the electron is from three shells away, so the subscript is γ (gamma).

Characteristic x-rays become important components of the total spectrum of x-rays produced by the conventional x-ray machine. They also are important in mammographic x-ray equipment in which x-ray tube target materials are made from different elements to capitalize on specific energies of the characteristic x-

rays produced. This is discussed in greater detail when the design and components of the x-ray machine are considered.

Another important process is the absorption of a light photon by a material that subsequently emits a lower-energy photon. This process, which occurs almost instantaneously, is known as *fluorescence*. If there is significant time delay between absorption and subsequent re-emission of the light, this is known as *phosphorescence*. A common example of fluorescence is the fluorescent light, in which an electric current is run through a tube containing a small amount of mercury vapor. The current provides the necessary energy to push electrons within the mercury atom up to higher energy levels. Almost immediately, these electrons fall to lower energy levels, resulting in the emission of ultraviolet (UV) radiation. This UV radiation is absorbed by a material (e.g., zinc sulfide) that coats the inner walls of the glass tube and re-emits light that falls into the visible portion of the EM spectrum. When the source of energy (i.e., the electric current) is removed, no more light is emitted. Phosphorescent paints are often used on the numbers of a clock. During the daylight hours, energy is absorbed in the form of visible light and re-emitted slowly in the form of visible light at night. This allows the numbers to be seen even in a totally darkened room.

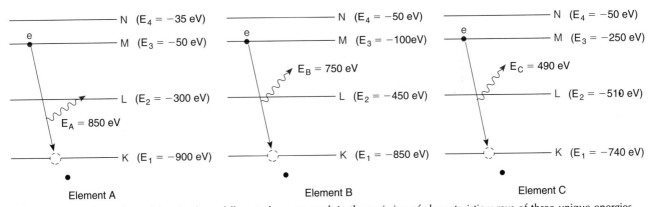

FIGURE 3–6. Identical transitions in three different elements result in the emission of characteristic x-rays of three unique energies.

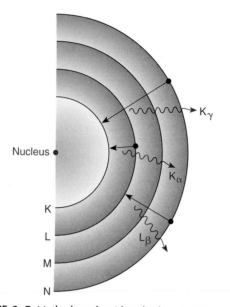

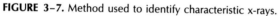

FIGURE 3-7. Method used to identify characteristic x-rays.

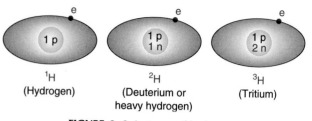

FIGURE 3-8. Isotopes of hydrogen.

RADIONUCLIDES AND NUCLEAR RADIATION

Factors Affecting Nuclear Stability

Estimates indicate that a typical atom has a diameter on the order of 10^{-10} meters, whereas a typical nuclear diameter is on the order of 10^{-15} meters. This indicates that a nucleus is roughly 100,000 times smaller (i.e., 10^5) than the atom itself. To get an idea of what this means in terms of relative sizes, if a nucleus expanded to the size of a baseball, its circling electron would be roughly three miles away. This example implies that an atom contains a considerable amount of empty space. This fact becomes important later when we consider the relative chance of photon radiation interacting with an atomic electron or even a nucleus. With all this empty space, it might be expected that the chances of a photon striking a shell electron or a nucleus are rather small, and we later find that this is true.

It has already been indicated that the nucleus contains only protons and neutrons (together known as *nucleons*) and that as the number of protons within the nucleus is changed so is the identity of the element. An atom may exist in several forms yet maintain its chemical identity by keeping the same number of protons but varying the number of neutrons. Different forms of the same element that vary only in the number of neutrons within their nuclei are known as *isotopes*. Three isotopes of the element hydrogen are shown in Figure 3–8.

As elements are produced by increasing the number of protons within the exceedingly small dimensions of the nucleus, there would seem to be a natural tendency for the nucleus to blow itself apart, since all protons

are electrically positive and like charges repel. This does not occur, however, since we know that atoms such as iron (Z = 26), gold (Z = 76), and lead (Z = 82) do exist in nature. Therefore something must hold all these protons together in a stable configuration.

Two factors appear to lend stability to these nuclei with higher Z numbers.

1. Neutron-to-Proton ("N to P") Ratio: As higher Z-number atoms are built, it is found that more and more neutrons must also be added to produce a stable atom (i.e., one that does not spontaneously emit radiation). This can be seen in Figure 3–9 in what is known as the stability line. This line simply shows that for elements with low Z numbers, approximately the same number of protons as neutrons are needed for stability. However, the higher the Z number, the greater is the number of neutrons needed for stability.

2. Nuclear Binding Energy: Just as electrons are bound, or held, to their respective shells by an *electronic binding energy,* nucleons are also bound to the nucleus by a nuclear binding energy. The source of this energy comes from the fact that an assembled atom has a total mass that is less than the total of the masses of the individual particles composing the atom. That is, a small amount of mass has been converted into energy (i.e., $E = mc^2$), and this en-

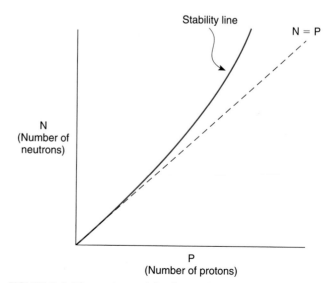

FIGURE 3-9. The nuclear stability line (solid line). As nuclei having more protons are formed, it is seen that more neutrons are required to provide nuclear stability.

ergy binds the particles within the nucleus together. It should be mentioned that although it takes energy of the order of eV to remove an electron from an atom, it takes energy of the order of MeV to remove a nucleon from the nucleus—approximately a million times more energy!

These two factors together determine whether a particular nuclear configuration of protons and neutrons is stable or unstable (i.e., radioactive). Those nuclei whose proton-to-neutron ratio does not fall on the stability line, that is, those having too many protons, too many neutrons, or too many of both, are radioactive and emit radiation spontaneously. The type of radiation emitted depends on whether the unstable nucleus, known as a *radioisotope,* or *radionuclide,* needs to rid itself of protons, neutrons, or both. The types of nuclear radiation, discussed next in more detail, are a result of the attempts by unstable nuclei to achieve a stable neutron-to-proton ratio.

Alpha (α) Radiation

When an unstable nucleus has too many protons and too many neutrons, it tends to emit alpha (α) radiation. *Alpha particles* consist of 2 protons and 2 neutrons, equivalent to a doubly ionized helium atom, which is identical to a helium nucleus. This is shown in Figure 3–10.

This type of radiation is characteristic of heavy (Z > 82), unstable nuclei such as the unstable forms of uranium, thorium, radium, and plutonium. When an alpha particle is emitted from an unstable nucleus, it provides a means for that nucleus to rid itself of 2 protons and 2 neutrons, thus altering its neutron-to-proton ratio. Because of its strong positive charge resulting from its two protons, the alpha particle is considered to be heavily ionizing radiation. An alpha particle does not have to hit an atomic electron directly to ionize an atom but can simply pass by an atom and by electrical attraction pull off loosely bound outer shell electrons. Therefore an alpha particle's primary mode of interaction with matter through which it passes is electrical. Highly ionizing radiation, such as alpha radiation, is said to have a high *specific ionization (SI),* which indicates the number of ion pairs created by the radiation per unit of *path length* traveled. SI is indicated in units, such as ion pairs per

centimeter. For alpha particles traveling through air, the SI may be as high as 70,000 ion pairs/cm. Since the ionizing capabilities of the various types of radiation are directly linked to their potential for biological harm, the SI is an important quantity in evaluating biological interactions.

Alpha particles also tend to expend their energy rapidly as they pass through materials. The average amount of energy lost per unit of path length traveled by the radiation is known as its *linear energy transfer (LET).* LET is analogous to gasoline mileage on an automobile. Gasoline mileage indicates how far a car will travel on a gallon of gasoline. LET indicates how much energy is used or expended per unit of distance traveled. Alpha particles have high LET, which indicates that they tend to lose their energy rather quickly and do not travel far in matter. In air, the approximate LET of alpha radiation is 1 MeV/cm. The maximum distance traveled, or *range,* in air by alpha particles is approximately only 4 to 10 cm, depending on the energy of the individual particles.

Alpha particles are also single-energied. That is, all alpha particles coming from a specific radionuclide have the same energy. In addition, alpha radiation tends to travel in straight lines as a result of high linear momentum.

When an alpha particle is ejected from an unstable nucleus, the nucleus loses 2 protons along with 2 neutrons. Recall that when the nucleus changes its number of protons, it changes its chemical identity. Therefore each nucleus that emits an alpha particle changes its identity, decreasing its Z number by 2 and its A number by 4. This is indicated by the general alpha decay equation shown here with an example of how this general equation is applied:

$$\underset{\text{Parent}}{_{Z}^{A}X} \xrightarrow{\alpha\text{-decay}} \underset{\text{Daughter}}{_{Z-2}^{A-4}Y} + \underset{\substack{\text{Alpha}\\\text{particle}}}{_{2}^{4}\alpha} \quad \substack{\text{General}\\\text{alpha decay}\\\text{equation}}$$

)))))) EXAMPLE

$$_{94}^{239}Pu \xrightarrow{\alpha\text{-decay}} {_{92}^{235}U} + {_{2}^{4}\alpha}$$

In the above example, plutonium 239 (^{239}Pu) is termed the parent nucleus, and the uranium 235 (^{235}U) is known as the daughter, or decay product. It should be noted that in "balancing" a nuclear equation such as that shown, the sum of the superscripts on the right hand side must equal the sum of the superscripts on the left hand side (i.e., 239 = 235 + 4). This must also always be true of the subscripts (i.e., 94 = 92 + 2).

Because of the heavy ionizing capability of alpha radiation and its minimal penetrating capabilities, alpha radiation essentially has no current applications in medicine. Alpha particles cannot penetrate the skin of the body and would therefore not result in a radiation dose to internal organs as long as the alpha radiation source remained outside the body. If taken into

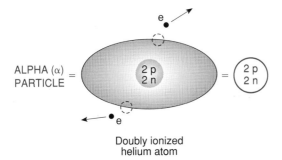

FIGURE 3–10. The alpha particle is identical to a doubly ionized helium atom, leaving only its nucleus—2 protons and 2 neutrons.

the body through inhalation, ingestion, or open wounds, then an alpha source can become extremely hazardous. This can be a problem with patients involved in radiation accidents at nuclear power facilities, weapons production facilities, or nuclear fuel fabrication plants. However, accidents such as this occur rarely.

Although this type of radiation is rarely if ever used, its characteristics (i.e., high SI, high LET, straight-line paths, range, etc.) are used in comparisons with other types of radiation.

Negative Beta, or Negatron, Radiation

If a nucleus is unstable as a result of having too many neutrons (a condition known as being neutron-rich), it will need to rid itself of one or more excess neutrons. However, no nucleus spontaneously emits neutron radiation. Therefore some alternative method to reduce the number of neutrons must exist. What occurs is the nuclear transformation of a neutron into the following particles:

$$\underset{\substack{\text{Nuclear}\\\text{neu-}\\\text{tron}}}{{}^1_0\text{n}} \xrightarrow{\text{transforms into}} \underset{\text{Proton}}{{}^1_1\text{p}} + \underset{\text{Electron}}{{}^0_{-1}\text{e}} + \underset{\substack{\text{Anti-}\\\text{neutrino}}}{{}^0_0\bar{\nu}}$$

This indicates that within the nucleus, one of the excess neutrons converts into a proton (which remains within the nucleus), an electron (which is ejected from the nucleus and is known as a *negative beta (β^-) particle, or negatron*), and an elementary particle known as an antineutrino, which is also ejected from the nucleus. When this conversion process occurs within an unstable nucleus, the nucleus loses a neutron and gains a proton, which alters its neutron-to-proton ratio toward a more stable nuclear configuration. Since a proton is gained, the daughter product has a different chemical identity from that of the parent. The general nuclear equation, indicating what occurs in negative beta decay, is shown here with an example:

$$\underset{\substack{\text{Parent}\\\text{nucleus}}}{{}^A_Z\text{X}} \xrightarrow{\beta^- \text{ decay}} \underset{\substack{\text{Daughter}\\\text{nucleus}}}{{}^A_{Z+1}\text{Y}} + \underset{\substack{\text{Beta}\\\text{particle}}}{{}^0_{-1}\beta} + \underset{\substack{\text{Anti-}\\\text{neutrino}}}{{}^0_0\bar{\nu}}$$

)))))) EXAMPLE

$$\underset{15}{{}^{32}_{15}\text{P}} \xrightarrow{\beta^- \text{ decay}} {}^{32}_{16}\text{S} + {}^0_{-1}\beta + {}^0_0\bar{\nu}$$

This general equation indicates that the unstable parent nucleus, which decays by the emission of a negative beta particle, or negatron, produces a daughter nucleus whose Z number is increased by one. In addition, a negatron, equivalent to a nuclear electron (Z = −1, A = 0), is also emitted along with the antineutrino, a highly penetrating particle having no charge and essentially no mass. This last particle, the antineutrino, is not considered a radiation hazard because it is so penetrating. Antineu-

trinos are thought to be able to penetrate light-years (one light-year is the distance light travels in a year, which is about 5.86×10^{12} miles) of pure iron without interacting with any of the iron atoms. The antineutrinos cannot be detected with conventional radiation detectors, because they are too penetrating and do not interact with the detectors. Thus from a practical standpoint, we are not concerned with the antineutrino radiation that accompanies each negatron emission.

However, the negatron is the important radiation of this decay process. This particle is an electron that is emitted from an unstable, neutron-rich nucleus. It is in every way identical to an electron in an atomic shell. It has the same mass ($m_e = 9.1 \times 10^{-31}$ kg), the same electrical charge ($e^- = -1.6 \times 10^{-19}$ coulomb) and the same physical dimensions. When emitted from a nucleus, beta particles travel at speeds approaching that of light. As they pass through air, these negatrons, or negative beta particles, tend to lose their energy through electrical interactions and scattering events. These interactions result in the production of ion pairs and the redirection of the negatrons from their original direction of motion. Recall that a change in direction of motion is known as an acceleration. When a charged particle such as an electron undergoes an acceleration, it loses energy in the form of photon radiation, namely *x-rays*. This is also known as *bremsstrahlung*, which means *braking radiation* in German, denoting the braking, or slowing down, of the negatrons as they are deflected.

The production of bremsstrahlung, or x-rays, is especially important to radiographers in that inadvertently, in discussing charged particle interactions in matter, we have found the way to artificially produce x-rays. Bremsstrahlung production can occur with any charged particle, but the number of x-ray photons produced, related to what is referred to as the intensity of the radiation, depends on such factors as

- The magnitude (or size) of the charge on the particle
- The number of charged particles
- The mass of the charged particles
- The Z number of the material with which the charged particle interacts
- The energy of the charged particles

Bremsstrahlung intensity is greatest for low-mass, charged particles (e.g., negatrons and electrons), which interact with high Z number materials. Considering the other factors indicated, more x-rays are also produced when there are more electrons and the electrons are moving faster (i.e., when they have more energy). It is for this reason that lead (Pb), which has a high Z number (Z = 82), is not used to provide protective shielding against high-energy negative beta radiation. That is, in protecting against exposure to the negatron radiation, it is not desirable to produce bremsstrahlung (x-rays) that present a different type of radiation hazard. Therefore when shielding against negative beta radiation, low Z number material (e.g., plastic, wood, cardboard, plexiglas) is commonly used. Bremsstrahlung radiation is discussed in much more detail in later chapters.

Compared with alpha particles, negatron radiation produces considerably fewer ion pairs per unit of path length traveled. The negative beta particle traveling through air may produce on the order of hundreds of ion pairs per centimeter compared with thousands per centimeter created by alpha radiation. Therefore, it can be said that negative beta particles have a lower SI than alpha particles. Negatrons also have lower LETs, meaning that they tend to lose less energy per unit of distance traveled than does alpha radiation. As a result, beta particles tend to travel farther or penetrate deeper into matter. As an indication of this, the range (i.e., the farthest distance traveled from the starting point) of negative beta particles in air is approximately 12 ft/MeV.

Whereas alpha particles are *monoenergetic* (i.e., all alphas emitted from the same radionuclide have the same energy), negatrons are *polyenergetic*. This means that negatrons are emitted from a radionuclide with energies ranging from zero to some maximum energy (E_{max}) determined by the particular radionuclide. The reason for this range of energies is that the total energy available to the decay process is divided between the negatron and the antineutrino. In the decay of one nucleus, the negatron may take 90% of the energy and the antineutrino the remaining 10%. In the decay of another nucleus, the negatron may take 20% of the energy, whereas the antineutrino takes 80%, and so on. When the emissions of many nuclei are analyzed, an entire spectrum of beta energies ranging from zero to E_{max} can be observed. As an example, the radioactive form of the element phosphorus, identified as ^{32}P, emits beta particles with E_{max} of 1.71 MeV. This implies that from a sample containing many ^{32}P nuclei, one might expect to obtain betas ranging in energy from zero to 1.71 MeV. The average beta energy ($\bar{E}$) is approximately 1/3 E_{max}, which for ^{32}P would be

$$\bar{E} \approx \frac{1}{3}\, E_{max}$$

$$\approx \frac{1}{3}\,(1.71\ \text{MeV})$$

$$\approx 0.57\ \text{MeV or } 570\ \text{keV}$$

Generally, very few of the beta particles emitted would have the maximum energy of 1.71 MeV, but

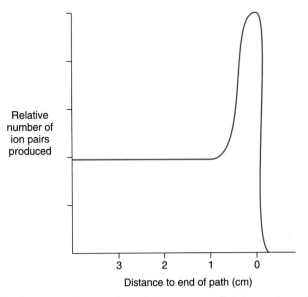

FIGURE 3–11. The number of ion pairs created by a charged particle as it travels through matter greatly increases as it loses energy and comes to the end of its path.

E_{max} is a useful concept, especially in radiation protection. That is, to shield sufficiently against the most energetic (and therefore the most penetrating) of the radiation, is also to have shielded effectively against all the lower energy beta radiation.

As a charged particle such as the negatron moves through matter, the number of ion pairs created per unit of distance does not remain constant (as indicated in Fig. 3–11). This graphical representation indicates that as the particle starts out, SI is relatively constant. However, as the particle approaches the end of its path, now having lower energy and moving more slowly a significant increase in the SI is noted. This comes about because as the charged particles lose energy, they spend more time in the vicinity of atoms of the media through which they are passing and therefore have more time to interact with loosely bound, outer shell electrons. This results in the creation of more ion pairs.

Since ionization events in a biological system have the potential to produce biological harm, this characteristic of charged *particle radiation* is used advantageously in radiation therapy. In treating certain types of superficial tumors, it is most effective to use elec-

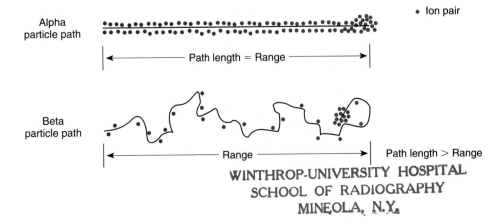

FIGURE 3–12. Comparison of the paths followed by alpha and beta particles as they travel through matter.

tron beam radiation in which the appropriate energy of the particles can be chosen, usually within the 4 to 15 MeV range; thus the particles penetrate to the depth of the tumor (usually less than 5 cm) and deliver their increased radiation dose at that point (as a result of the increased SI) with minimal dose to surrounding healthy tissue.

Another dissimilarity between negative beta and alpha radiation is the type of path followed by each as it travels into matter. Recall that alpha particles tend to follow rather straight line paths because of their relatively high linear momentum resulting from their large mass (~8000 times the mass of an electron). Beta particles, being extremely light in mass, do not possess enough linear momentum to produce straight line paths and as a result follow more erratic and tortuous paths as indicated schematically in Figure 3–12.

In the case of negatrons, there must now be a clearer distinction between terms used to describe how far the particle travels in matter. Whereas range indicates the farthest distance traveled by the particle from its starting point, the term *path length* is now introduced as representing the total distance traveled by the particle. In the case of alpha particles, range is essentially equivalent to path length, but for beta particles, the path length is usually considerably greater than the range.

Although the range of beta particles in air is approximately 12 ft/MeV, it is considerably less in more dense materials such as tissue (as is true for most types of radiation). Negative beta emitters in the form of radioactive ^{131}I (iodine 131) find use in nuclear medicine in the destruction of cancerous and hyperactive thyroid tissue. The negatrons emitted from radioactive ^{32}P (phosphorus 32) also have numerous therapeutic uses, from treatment of ovarian cancer to palliative treatment for recurring bone pain.

Positive Beta (β^+), or Positron, Radiation

When an unstable nucleus has an excess number of protons (a condition known as being proton-rich), there is a need to reduce the number of protons and to increase the number of neutrons. Since there are no radioactive nuclei that spontaneously emit protons, there must be an alternative method for a nucleus to reduce its number of protons. If sufficient energy is available within the nucleus, a proton may undergo the following nuclear conversion:

$$\underset{\text{Proton}}{^{1}_{1}p} \longrightarrow \underset{\text{Neutron}}{^{1}_{0}n} + \underset{\text{Positron}}{^{0}_{1}e^{+}} + \underset{\text{Neutrino}}{^{0}_{0}v}$$

In this process, one of the protons within the unstable nucleus converts into a neutron (which remains within the nucleus), a *positron* (also known as a *positive beta particle*), and an elementary particle known as a neutrino. The positron and the neutrino are ejected from the nucleus during a decay process. The original unstable nucleus has now changed its chemical identity, since it has decreased its proton number by one. This

process is indicated in the general decay equation for positron emission shown below with an example:

$$\underset{\substack{\text{Parent} \\ \text{nucleus}}}{^{A}_{Z}X} \xrightarrow{\beta^{+} \text{ Decay}} \underset{\substack{\text{Daughter} \\ \text{nucleus}}}{^{A}_{Z-1}Y} + \underset{\text{Positron}}{^{0}_{+1}\beta^{+}} + \underset{\text{Neutrino}}{^{0}_{0}v}$$

)))))) EXAMPLE

$$\underset{\substack{\text{Carbon} \\ \text{(parent)}}}{^{11}_{6}C} \xrightarrow{\beta^{+} \text{ Decay}} \underset{\substack{\text{Boron} \\ \text{(daughter)}}}{^{11}_{5}B} + \underset{\text{Positron}}{^{0}_{+1}\beta^{+}} + \underset{\text{Neutrino}}{^{0}_{0}v}$$

It should be noted in the above nuclear equations that all of our former rules still apply (i.e., sum of superscripts on the right must equal the sum of the superscripts on the left and the same must be true for the subscripts).

The neutrino ($^{0}_{0}v$) that is emitted has properties similar to the antineutrino in that it essentially has zero mass and zero electric charge and is extremely penetrating—again, so penetrating that it is of little concern.

The positron (positive beta particle) on the other hand, is unlike any radiation previously encountered. The positron is identified as a positive electron, and for this reason, the symbol often used for this particle is either ($^{0}_{+1}\beta$) or ($^{0}_{+1}e^{+}$). In addition, it is a positive electron that is ejected from the nucleus. Perhaps, however, its most unusual property is that it is what is termed antimatter. Whenever a positron encounters an electron, its "real" matter counterpart, the two particles undergo annihilation as indicated in Figure 3–13. When this process occurs, the mass of the two particles is converted into pure energy through the Einstein relationship, $E = mc^2$. If the mass of an electron ($m_e = 9.1 \times 10^{-31}$ kg) is placed in this equation and the energy produced is converted to keV, the result would be

$$E = mc^2$$
$$= (9.1 \times 10^{-31} \text{ kg})(3 \times 10^8 \text{ m/sec})^2$$
$$\approx 511 \text{ keV}$$

Verification of this result occurs when the positron enters matter containing electrons. Almost immedi-

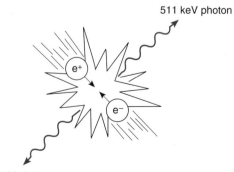

FIGURE 3–13. Annihilation radiation: Two 511-keV photons emitted in opposite directions result when a positron encounters an electron.

ately on encountering an electron, the electron and positron disappear, and in their place appear two 511-keV photons that travel outward in totally opposite directions (i.e., ~180° from each other).

The two 511-keV photons are known as annihilation radiation, and the production of these penetrating photons is characteristic of positron emitters. It is important to remember that the two 511-keV photons do not originate from within the nucleus but result from the interaction of the positron with an electron within the medium through which the positron passes after emission from the unstable nucleus.

On emission from a nucleus, the positron may travel a distance up to a few millimeters within a time of only about 10^{-9} sec to 10^{-6} sec before encountering an electron and undergoing annihilation. Prior to this occurrence, the positron loses energy in the creation of ion pairs. Since it, too, is an electron, but a positive one, prior to annihilation, it tends to interact with matter like its matter counterpart, the electron. Thus approximately the same values of LET and SI as with negatrons can be expected.

Like the negative beta particle, the positron is emitted with a spectrum of energies, since the positron shares with the neutrino the total energy available to the decay process. The positrons are emitted with energies ranging from zero to some E_{max}, determined by the identity of the nuclei. As an example, ^{15}O (oxygen 15) emits positrons with a maximum energy of 1.74 MeV. Therefore when an ^{15}O nucleus decays, a positron with energy somewhere between 0 and 1.74 MeV is emitted.

Positron emitters have not been used widely in medicine until relatively recent years when there has been a revival of interest in the highly specialized imaging modality known as positron emission tomography, or PET. Part of the interest lies in the fact that many positron emitters are radioactive forms of elements such as carbon, oxygen, nitrogen, and fluorine, which can be readily incorporated into biologically active substances such as carbon dioxide, ammonia, oxygen, water, and fluorodeoxyglucose. When inside the body, their utilization can be monitored using radiation detectors placed outside the body. These specialized detectors are designed to detect the annihilation radiation of the positron emitter. The imaging possibilities provided by PET techniques currently include research into areas such as definitive diagnosis of Alzheimer disease, effects of drug addiction, and early diagnosis of coronary artery disease. As the ability of clinical sites to obtain positron-emitting radionuclides increases, it is anticipated that PET imaging sites will experience continued growth.

Gamma Radiation

In a majority of cases, the emission of particle radiation from an unstable nucleus does not bring the nucleus to its lowest energy state. In these cases, the nucleus is said to be in an "excited" state and needs to rid itself only of excess energy. When this condition exists, the nucleus spontaneously emits photon radiation known as *gamma (γ) rays*. These photons are identical in nature to x-rays in every way except their origin—gamma-rays originate in the nucleus, and x-rays originate outside the nucleus of the atom. Gamma photons, like x-ray photons, have no mass and no electrical charge but are discrete in the energy that they carry. The energy carried by these photons is unique to the individual *radionuclide*. Several radionuclides commonly used in medicine are indicated here, together with the energy of the gamma photons emitted by each:

Radionuclide	Gamma Photon Energy	Medical Uses
Iodine 125 (^{125}I)	35 keV	Medical research: determination of hormone and drug levels
Iodine 131 (^{131}I)	364 keV	Treatment for certain types of thyroid conditions and thyroid cancer
Cesium 137 (^{137}Cs)	663 keV	Cancer treatment
Cobalt 60 (^{60}Co)	1.17 MeV, 1.33 MeV	Cancer treatment

Many radionuclides emit more than one type of radiation simultaneously. There are alpha-gamma emitters, beta-gamma emitters, and positron-gamma emitters. Also some radionuclides emit only one type of radiation; for example, ^{32}P is a pure beta emitter. Thus in evaluating the potential hazard associated with any type of radionuclide, one must consider all the types of radiation emitted by the specific radioactive substance. A good example of this is ^{131}I, used in nuclear medicine to treat thyroid cancer. ^{131}I is a beta-gamma emitter, and although it is the beta component that delivers the primary radiation dose to the cancerous thyroid tissue, producing no radiation exposure hazard to other individuals, radiation protection precautions must be taken to protect nursing staff, visitors, family members, and patients in adjacent rooms from the 364-keV gamma radiation that is also emitted.

Several important radionuclides do not emit their gamma photon radiation simultaneously with particle emission. The emission of the gamma radiation may follow within minutes to hours after a particle emission. This delay places the daughter product in what is termed a *metastable* state (i.e., an almost stable state). When this occurs, a metastable state is designated by the letter *m* (meaning metastable) in the superscript of the radionuclidic designation. An example of this is the metastable state of technetium (Tc), which is the most commonly used radionuclide in nuclear medicine, known as technetium 99m (i.e., ^{99m}Tc). ^{99m}Tc decays to ^{99}Tc by the emission of a 140-keV gamma photon. It is the 140-keV photon radiation that is detected by sensitive radiation detectors (known as scintillation cameras) outside the patient's body that allows compounds (known as radiopharmaceuticals) to be monitored in nuclear medicine studies. These types of studies are used to determine if specific organs are functioning properly and are often referred to as physiological imaging studies.

When an unstable nucleus emits a gamma photon, it loses only energy. The photon, whether it is a gamma- or an x-ray, carries no mass and zero electrical charge. As a result, the parent and daughter have the same chemical identity. The only difference between the two is that the daughter is in a lower energy state than the parent. In some instances, a nucleus that needs to release only energy is said to be in an excited state and may be indicated by an asterisk (*) on the superscript of the parent. A general decay equation for gamma emission is as follows:

$$\underset{\substack{\text{Parent} \\ \text{nucleus}}}{{}^{A}_{Z}X^*} \xrightarrow{\gamma\text{-decay}} \underset{\substack{\text{Daughter} \\ \text{nucleus}}}{{}^{A}_{Z}X} + \underset{\substack{\text{Gamma} \\ \text{photon}}}{{}^{0}_{0}\gamma}$$

))))))) **EXAMPLE**

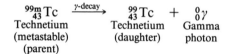

$$\underset{\substack{\text{Technetium} \\ \text{(metastable)} \\ \text{(parent)}}}{{}^{99m}_{43}Tc} \xrightarrow{\gamma\text{-decay}} \underset{\substack{\text{Technetium} \\ \text{(daughter)}}}{{}^{99}_{43}Tc} + \underset{\substack{\text{Gamma} \\ \text{photon}}}{{}^{0}_{0}\gamma}$$

Activity: The Amount of Radioactivity in a Radioactive Source

Radioactive sources used in medicine vary widely in strength, depending on whether the radioactivity is used to measure hormone levels in a patient's blood, diagnose a physical problem, or destroy a cancerous lesion. The greater the amount of radioactive material present in a sample, the greater the intensity of radiation emitted. The amount of radioactive material in a radiation source is designated by the *activity* of the source. Whenever a radioactive nucleus decays and emits its radiation, the decay process is known as a disintegration. Activity indicates the number of disintegrations that occur per second, abbreviated dps. Activity is measured in a unit known as the *curie* (Ci) where

$$\boxed{1 \text{ Ci} = 3.7 \times 10^{10} \text{ dps}}$$ The curie

A curie represents a large amount of radioactive material and is rarely found in the hospital environment except in radiation therapy departments in which curie-level quantities of ^{60}Co (cobalt 60) are used in teletherapy (radiation from a distance). It is more common to find lower activity sources in the millicurie (mCi) and microcurie (μCi) activity range in both radiation therapy and nuclear medicine departments as well as in medical research laboratories. These smaller activity units are defined as:

$$1 \text{ mCi} = 3.7 \times 10^7 \text{ dps}$$

and

$$1 \text{ } \mu\text{Ci} = 3.7 \times 10^4 \text{ dps}$$

The SI unit of activity is the *becquerel* (Bq) where

$$\boxed{1 \text{ Bq} = 1 \text{ dps}}$$ The becquerel

The following are relationships between the curie and its submultiples and the becquerel:

$$1 \text{ mCi} = 37 \text{ MBq (i.e., } 37 \times 10^6 \text{ Bq)}$$

and

$$1 \text{ } \mu\text{Ci} = 37 \text{ kBq (i.e., } 37 \times 10^3 \text{ Bq)}$$

The more disintegrations of nuclei that occur per second, the more radiation emitted from the source. Therefore the greater the activity of a radiation source, the more precautions should be taken in terms of radiation protection. Some commonly used medical radiation sources and their approximate activity levels are indicated in Table 3–2.

The sources listed represent only a small fraction of the many types of radiation sources used today in medicine. Continued new applications of radionuclides in the diagnosis and treatment of disease guarantee a bright future for their use for many years to come.

Physical Half-Life ($T_{1/2}$)

The activity of a radioactive sample does not remain constant but decays as time passes. As a result of this decay, the radioactive source becomes weaker and emits less radiation. Radionuclides decay with characteristic times known as their *physical half-life* ($T_{1/2}$). If

Table 3–2: REPRESENTATIVE ACTIVITIES OF COMMONLY USED MEDICAL RADIATION SOURCES

Medical Source	Radionuclide	Type of Radiation Emitted	Approximate Activity	Uses
Teletherapy sources	^{60}Co	γ	~6000 Ci	Cancer therapy and whole body irradiation
Cell irradiators	^{137}Cs	γ	~2000 Ci	Irradiation of blood products and medical research
Brachytherapy implants	^{137}Cs	γ	~25–75 mCi	Temporary implants used in cancer therapy
Nuclear medicine sources	^{99m}Tc	γ	~3–20 mCi	Diagnostic studies
Medical laboratory sources	^{125}I	γ	<10 μCi	Determination of drug and hormone levels in blood specimens

a radioactive source has an initial activity of 100 mCi and its physical half-life is 5 years, its activity after 5 years will be 50 mCi. After another 5 years have passed, the activity will be 25 mCi. Thus the activity of a radioactive source decreases in value by 50% for each physical half-life that passes.

The activity of any radioactive source can be determined by utilizing the concept of the physical half-life and a simple mathematical representation. If A is the activity of the radioactive source after time t has passed and A_0 is the initial activity of the source having a physical half-life, $T_{1/2}$, then

$$A = A_0 (0.5)^N \qquad (1)$$

where

A = source activity

A_0 = initial activity

N = number of half-lives that have passed

$$= \frac{t}{T_{1/2}}$$

)))))) EXAMPLE

Determine the activity of a ^{60}Co teletherapy source that when installed in January 1986, had an initial activity of 6000 Ci. ^{60}Co has a physical half-life of 5.3 years, and we wish to know its activity as of January 1990.

$$\text{Given:} \quad T_{1/2} = 5.3 \text{ years}$$

$$t = 4 \text{ years}$$

$$A_0 = 6000 \text{ Ci}$$

$$A = A_0 (0.5)^N$$
$$= (6000 \text{ Ci}) (0.5)^{4 \text{ yr}/5.3 \text{ yr}}$$
$$= (6000 \text{ Ci}) (0.5)^{0.75}$$
$$= (6000 \text{ Ci}) (0.59)$$
$$= 3540 \text{ Ci}$$

Note. When using the preceding equation to determine the activity of a source, it is necessary to express both t and $T_{1/2}$ in the same time units. This is essential for N to be a dimensionless quantity.

Physical half-lives vary widely among some 900 known radionuclides, ranging from seconds to millions of years. Physical half-lives of some of the more important radionuclides in both medicine and technology are indicated in the Table 3–3.

Radioactive decay is normally described mathematically by a negative exponential function of the form

$$A = A_0 e^{-\lambda t} \qquad (2)$$

where

A = activity of source

A_0 = initial activity

Table 3–3: TYPICAL PHYSICAL HALF-LIVES OF COMMONLY USED RADIONUCLIDES

Radionuclide	Physical Half-Life	Uses
^{11}C	20.4 min	Metabolic studies
^{3}H	12.3 yr	Medical and biologic research
^{137}Cs	30 yr	Cancer therapy
^{99m}Tc	6 hours	Nuclear medicine studies
^{131}I	8 days	Cancer therapy; thyroid and kidney studies
^{125}I	60 days	Drug and hormone level determinations
^{241}Am	432 yr	Smoke detectors
^{239}Pu	2.4×10^4 yr	Fuel source for nuclear reactors

λ = decay constant = $0.693/T_{1/2}$

t = length of time that has passed (in same unit as $T_{1/2}$)

Note, however, that since both equations (1) and (2) are used to determine the source activity, both will provide the same result. It is important to realize this, since equation (1) may be somewhat simpler to work with mathematically.

The activity of a radiation source can also be determined graphically, again using the concept of the physical half-life. If the percentage of activity remaining (i.e., 0% to 100%) is plotted on linear graph paper as a function of time expressed in half-life units (i.e., 1 $T_{1/2}$, 2 $T_{1/2}$, etc.), a curve typical of a negative exponential function is obtained (Fig. 3–14). It should be noted that this curve is obtained simply by using the fact that 100% of the activity occurs at time zero, 50% at one $T_{1/2}$, 25% at two $T_{1/2}$, and so forth. This graph can be used to determine the percentage of activity remaining, but it would be easier and more accurate if the graph were a straight line rather than a curve. This can easily be accomplished by recalling that plotting an

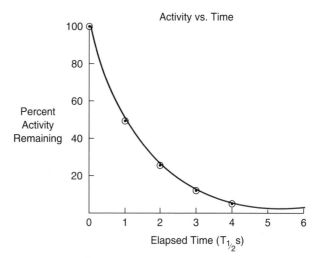

FIGURE 3–14. A linear plot of the activity of a radioactive sample that remains as a function of elapsed time. Plotting this information on linear graph paper verifies its negative exponential nature.

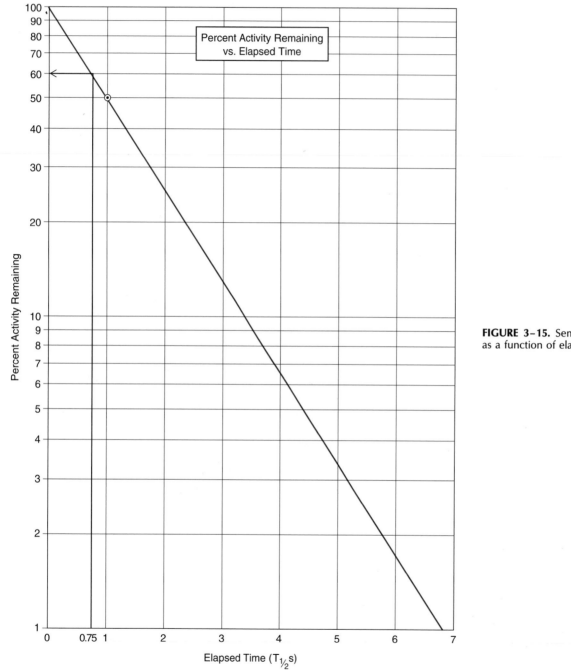

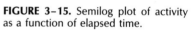

FIGURE 3–15. Semilog plot of activity as a function of elapsed time.

exponential function on semilog graph paper will yield a straight-line graph. The same data plotted in Figure 3–14 can then be plotted on semilog graph paper to obtain the graph shown in Figure 3–15. A review of this graphing technique is found in Chapter 2.

Recall that each cycle on the vertical axis represents a power of 10; then the top of the scale is chosen to represent 100% (i.e., 10^2 %); the next lower cycle 10% (i.e., 10^1 %); the next, 1% (i.e., 10^0 %); and so on. Usually, 2- to 3-cycle semilog paper is sufficient for most practical applications. The horizontal time axis is linear and again is chosen to be expressed in half-life units. When drawn with this method, the graph can be used for any radioactive source. The graph is used in the following example to determine the activity of the same source discussed in the previous example.

)))))) EXAMPLE

Use the semilog plot of Activity Remaining vs. Time shown in Figure 3–15 to determine the activity of a 6000-Ci ^{60}Co teletherapy source after 4 years of radioactive decay. Since this graph is plotted in terms of elapsed time in half-life units, first determine how many half-lives have passed. This is done by simply dividing the time that has passed by the physical half-life, $T_{1/2}$:

$$N = \frac{t}{T_{1/2}}$$
$$= \frac{4 \text{ yr}}{5.3 \text{ yr}}$$
$$= 0.75 \ T_{1/2}$$

This value is found on the time axis, and moving vertically from that point, it is determined that 60% of the initial activity remains. This corresponds to

$$A = (60\%) \ (6000 \text{ Ci})$$
$$= (0.60) \ (6000 \text{ Ci})$$
$$= 3600 \text{ Ci}$$

Note. This is approximately the same result obtained using decay equation (1). The slight difference between the two results comes only from approximations made in interpretations of graphical data.

Either of these methods, mathematical or graphical, can be used with confidence in determining the activity of a radioactive source, provided the initial activity (A_0), the physical half-life ($T_{1/2}$), and the elapsed time (t) are known.

▨▨◢ Chapter Summary/ Important Equations, Constants, and Relationships

General wave equation:

$$v = \lambda f$$

Wave units:

$$1 \text{ Å} = 10^{-10} \text{m}$$
$$1 \text{ Hz} = 1 \text{ sec}^{-1}$$

Photon energy relationships:

$$E \propto 1/\lambda$$
$$E \propto f$$

Photon energy:

$$E(\text{keV}) = 12.4/\lambda(\text{Å})$$

Visible light wavelength range:

$$4000 \text{ Å to } 7000 \text{ Å (400 nm to 700 nm)}$$

Charge on electron:

$$-1.6 \times 10^{-19} \text{ coulomb (C)}$$

Charge on proton:

$$+1.6 \times 10^{-19} \text{ C}$$

Activity equation:

$$A = A_0 \ (0.5)^N$$

Types of radiation summary (Table 3–4):

Table 3-4: SUMMARY OF THE VARIOUS TYPES OF RADIATION AND THEIR PHYSICAL CHARACTERISTICS

Type	Symbol	Origin	Identity	Charge	Mass	Range in Air	Penetrating or Nonpenetrating	Comments
Alpha particles	α	Heavy, unstable nuclei	2 protons, 2 neutrons (i.e., a helium nucleus)	+2	Massive ($\sim 8000 \times$ electron mass)	~ 1 cm/MeV	Nonpenetrating	Hazardous if taken internally; monoenergetic
Beta particles (negatron)	β^-	Unstable, neutron-rich nuclei	A nuclear electron	-1	Light (1 electron mass)	Up to 12 ft/MeV (~ 3.7 m/MeV)	Generally considered nonpenetrating	Can cause "skin burns" if radiation energy and intensity are sufficiently high
Positron	β^+	Unstable, proton-rich nuclei	A positive electron (antimatter)	+1	Light (1 electron mass)	A few mm	Nonpenetrating	The antimatter particle counterpart of the electron; when an electron is encountered, annihilation radiation, consisting of two penetrating 511-keV photons, emitted in opposite directions, is produced
X-ray	x	Produced as a result of electronic transitions or deceleration of a charged particle	Photon (EM energy)	0	0	Up to meters, depending on energy	Low to high penetration	Characteristic x-rays are monoenergetic and unique to a specific atom; bremsstrahlung, as produced by an x-ray machine, is polyenergetic
Gamma ray	γ	Emitted from an unstable nucleus that needs to rid itself only of excess energy	Photon (EM energy)	0	0	Up to meters, depending on energy	Low to high penetration	γ-rays are monoenergetic and are useful in identifying radionuclides from which emitted

EM = electromagnetic.

Important Terminology

Activity. A measure of the amount of radioactive material present in a radiation source

Alpha (α) Particle. Particulate radiation consisting of 2 protons and 2 neutrons; identical to helium nucleus; highly ionizing but not very penetrating

Amplitude. The maximum height of a wave as measured from its equilibrium position

Atom. The smallest unit of matter that retains the identity of a specific element

Atomic Number (Z Number). The number of protons in the nucleus of an atom; if this number changes, the chemical identity of the atom also changes

Becquerel (Bq). SI unit of activity equivalent to 1 dps

Beta (β⁻) Particle, or Negatron. Particulate radiation ejected from an unstable, neutron-rich nucleus; identical to an electron

Bremsstrahlung. X-rays produced when a charged particle undergoes a deceleration; known as "braking radiation"

Characteristic X-ray. X-ray photons emitted as a result of an electronic transition from a higher to a lower energy state within an atom; the energy of these photons is characteristic of the element from which they are emitted

Crest. The high point of a wave

Curie (Ci). A unit of activity equivalent to 3.7×10^{10} disintegrations per second (dps)

Electromagnetic Radiation. Photons or packets of pure energy having zero mass and no electrical charge

Electron. The smallest mobile unit of electric charge presently known to exist; the magnitude of the charge carried by this particle is -1.6×10^{-19} coulomb

Electronic Binding Energy. The energy with which an electron is bound to an atom

Electronic Transition. The movement of electrons among the energy shells of an atom; movement to higher energy levels requires that energy be supplied, whereas movement to lower energy states results in energy being released, usually in the form of photons

Fluorescence. The absorption of energy by an atom, resulting in the subsequent emission of photon radiation, commonly in the form of x-rays or visible light

Frequency (f). The number of waves passing a given point per second; measured in units of hertz, where 1 hertz (Hz) = 1 sec⁻¹

Gamma (γ) Rays. Penetrating photon radiation that originates from within the nucleus of an unstable atom; identical to x-ray except for origin

Infrared (IR) Radiation. Photon radiation having wavelengths just above the red portion of the visible spectrum, generally associated with heat radiation

Ion. An atom that by the loss or addition of an electron is no longer electrically neutral

Ion Pair. When an electron is ejected from a neutral atom, the ion pair consists of the ejected electron and the now positive ion created by its ejection

Ionizing Radiation. Radiation having energy greater than 33 to 35 eV, sufficient to produce an ionization event in air; any radiation that has sufficient energy to produce ion pairs in the medium through which it travels

Isotope. Form of an atom having the same number of protons but a different number of neutrons

Linear Energy Transfer (LET). The amount of energy lost per unit of distance traveled by a form of radiation

Mass (A) Number. The number of protons plus neutrons in the nucleus of an atom

Monoenergetic. Consisting of a single energy

Neutron. Particle having a mass approximately equal to that of the proton but carrying no electric charge

Nucleons. Protons and neutrons

Nucleus. The dense central core of the atom, containing only protons and neutrons and constituting approximately 99⁺ % of the entire mass of the atom

Particulate Radiation. Particles emitted from unstable nuclei

Path Length. Actual total distance traveled by a form of radiation from starting point to final stopping point

Phosphorescence. The absorption of energy by an atom resulting in the delayed emission of photon radiation

Photon. "Packet" of electromagnetic radiation having neither mass nor electrical charge

Physical Half-Life (T₁/₂). Characteristic time required for a radionuclide's activity to decay to half its original value

Polyenergetic. Consisting of many different energies

Positron, or Positive Beta (β⁺) Radiation. Particulate radiation emitted from an unstable proton-rich nucleus; a positive electron, the antimatter counterpart of the electron; when this particle encounters an electron, the particles are converted into two 511-keV photons (known as annihilation radiation)

Proton. Particle having a mass approximately 2000 times the mass of the electron and an electric charge of $+1.6 \times 10^{-19}$ coulombs

Radiation. Particles or photons emitted from an atom

Radioisotope, or Radionuclide. Isotope that is radioactive and spontaneously emits radiation

Range. Farthest distance traveled by a form of radiation

Specific Ionization (SI). The number of ion pairs created per unit of distance traveled by a form of radiation

Trough. The low point of a wave

Ultraviolet (UV) Radiation. Photon radiation having wavelengths just below the violet portion of the visible spectrum

Wavelength (λ). The distance between two successive crests or two successive troughs of a wave; also the distance spanned by one full crest and one full trough of a wave

Wave Speed, or Wave Velocity (v). The speed at which a wave travels in a particular medium

X-ray. Penetrating photon radiation that originates outside the nucleus of an atom as a result of electronic transitions or a deceleration of charged particles

Bibliography

Hendee, W.R. Medical Radiation Physics: Roentgenology, Nuclear Medicine, and Ultrasound, 2nd ed. Chicago: Year Book Medical Publishers, 1979.

Khan, F.M. The Physics of Radiation Therapy. Baltimore: Williams & Wilkins, 1984.

Rollo, F.D. Nuclear Medicine Physics, Instrumentation, and Agents. St. Louis: C.V. Mosby, 1977.

Sorenson, J.A.; Phelps, M.E. Physics in Nuclear Medicine, 3rd ed. New York: Grune & Stratton, 1987.

Review Questions

Wave Properties

1. Distinguish between particulate and photon radiation.
2. Explain what is meant by the "wave-particle duality" of light.
3. Indicate the number of wavelengths shown in each of the drawings below:

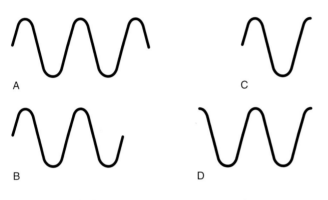

A

C

B

D

4. Use the information shown on the diagram below to answer the following questions:

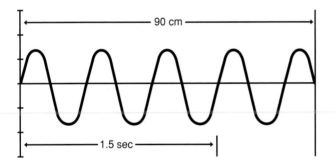

a. What type of wave is this?
b. What is the amplitude of the wave?
c. What is the wavelength?
d. What is the frequency of the wave?
e. How fast does the wave travel through this medium?

5. Use dimensional analysis to convert.
a. a wavelength of 1 mm to Å.
b. a wavelength of 1 Å to mm.

6. Determine the frequency (f) for each of the transverse waves shown below:

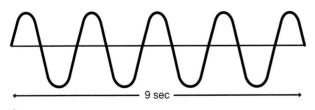

9 sec

A

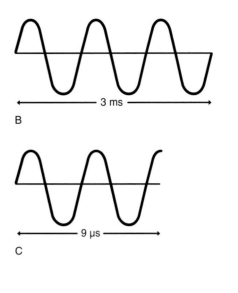

3 ms

B

9 µs

C

Photon Computations

7. Determine the following:
a. What is the frequency of photons of blue light having a wavelength of 400 nm? Recall that the speed of light in air is 3×10^8 m/sec.
b. What is the wavelength of an x-ray photon whose frequency is 3×10^{19} Hz?
8. Determine the energy in keV in the following, and explain your answers.
a. an x-ray photon having a wavelength (λ) equal to 0.177 Å
b. a red photon having $\lambda = 7000$ Å
c. an ultraviolet photon having $\lambda = 24.8$ Å
d. a gamma photon having $\lambda = 0.05$ Å
e. Which of the above photons would be classified as "ionizing"?

Atoms and Electronic Transitions

9. Use a periodic chart of the elements to identify the element and indicate the number of protons, neutrons, and electrons for each of the following atoms:

a. Z = 6, A = 12   c. Z = 42, A = 98
b. Z = 74, A = 182   d. Z = 1, A = 3

10. Use the energy level diagram, representing electronic energy states, to answer the following questions regarding electronic transitions and the resulting emitted photons:

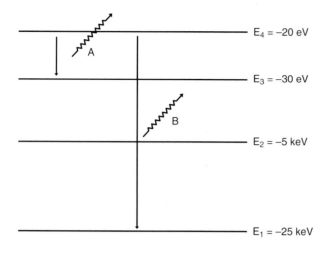

$E_4 = -20$ eV

$E_3 = -30$ eV

$E_2 = -5$ keV

$E_1 = -25$ keV

● Nucleus

a. Identify the individual shells (i.e., K, L, M, N) in the drawing.
b. Why are the binding energies indicated as negative quantities?
c. How much energy is required to completely remove an electron from the K shell? the N shell? Why is there such a large difference?
d. What is the energy of photon A, which results from an electronic transition from E_4 to E_3? Is it ionizing? Explain.
e. What is the energy of photon B, which results from an electronic transition from E_4 to E_1? Is it ionizing? Explain.

11. Use the energy level diagram shown here to identify the emitted x-ray photons, using the K_α notation.

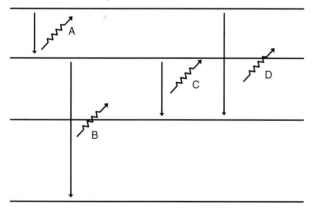

● Nucleus

12. For each of the isotopes indicated below, indicate (1) the number of nucleons, (2) the numbers of protons, (3) the number of electrons, (4) the number of neutrons, and (5) the name of the element
   a. $^{12}_{7}N$ d. $^{127}_{53}I$
   b. $^{60}_{27}Co$ e. $^{186}_{74}W$
   c. $^{96}_{42}Mo$

13. In reviewing the various types of radiation, which type(s) of radiation
   a. can use a few cm of air as shield?
   b. is identical to x-rays except for its origin?
   c. has a path length longer than its range?
   d. produces two 511-keV photons when it encounters an electron?
   e. is identical to an electron?
   f. is identical to a helium nucleus?
   g. would be classified as particulate radiation?
   h. would be classified as electromagnetic radiation?
   i. results from electronic transitions?
   j. is emitted from a nucleus that has excess energy?

Physical Half-Life

14. ^{60}Co has a physical half-life of 5.3 years. Use the activity equation to determine the activity remaining 13.25 years later. The initial activity of the source was stated as 5000 Ci.
15. How many half-lives would a radioactive source need to go through before its activity drops to 6.25% of its original activity?
16. Use the graph "Per Cent Activity Remaining vs. Elapsed Time" (Fig. 3–15) to answer the following questions:
   a. How many half-lives must pass before the activity drops to 30% of its initial activity?
   b. Determine the percentage of activity remaining after 6 half-lives have passed.
   c. If a certain radioactive source has a physical half-life of 20 days, how much time must pass before its initial activity drops to 80% of its initial value?

Exercises

1. For the waves shown below, find the wavelengths, frequencies, and corresponding wave velocities.

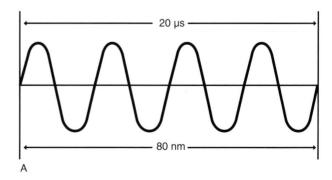

A

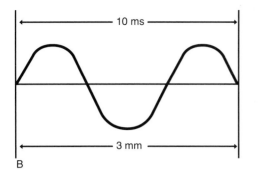

B

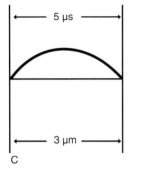

C

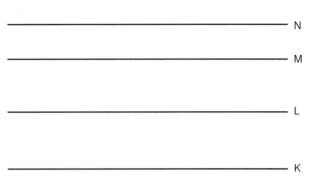

N

M

L

K

Nucleus

2. Determine the frequency and energy of each of the following photons:
   a. a yellow-green photon of 5500 Å wavelength
   b. a microwave photon of 1 cm wavelength
   c. a radiowave used in magnetic resonance imaging having a wavelength of 7 m
   d. a diagnostic x-ray photon having a wavelength of 1.77×10^{-2} nm

3. Use the energy level diagram shown here to answer the following questions regarding the electronic transitions shown.

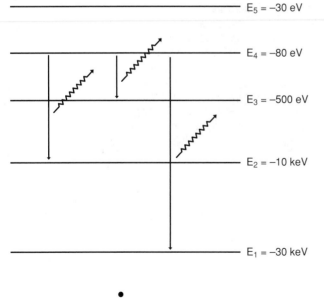

$E_5 = -30$ eV

$E_4 = -80$ eV

$E_3 = -500$ eV

$E_2 = -10$ keV

$E_1 = -30$ keV

Nucleus

a. How much energy is required to completely remove an electron from the K shell of this atom? from the M shell?
b. What is the energy of the characteristic x-ray A? How would it be designated?
c. What is the energy of x-ray B? How would it be designated?
d. What is the energy of x-ray C?
e. Are each of these x-rays ionizing? Briefly explain why or why not.

4. For a nuclear study, a patient is administered 10 mCi of a radioactive substance having a physical half-life of 6 hours. Owing to a scheduling delay, the patient is not scanned until 4 hours later.
   If 4 mCi has been excreted in the urine, how much activity is in the patient at the time of the scan?

5. Use the activity equation to determine the lengths of time for a radioactive sample to decay to 10% and 1% of its initial activity.
   Express your answer in units of physical half-life $(T_{1/2})$.

6. ^{131}I has a physical half-life of 8 days. How long will it take for a 200 mCi sample to decay to 50 μCi? Express your answer in days. (Note: You may need to refer to Chapter 2 to review solving exponential equations.)

7. It is often stated that a radioactive source that has decayed through 10 physical half-lives can be considered no longer radioactive. What percentage of the initial activity remains after 10 $T_{1/2}$ s? If the initial activity of a source is 10 Ci, what activity remains? Is this a valid rule of thumb?

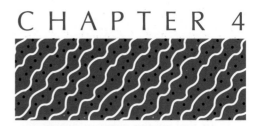

C H A P T E R 4

Electricity

Michael A. Thompson, M.S.

Chapter Outline

Chapter Objectives

Upon completion of this chapter, you should be able to

- Identify the electron as the smallest known mobile charge carrier.
- Specify signs and magnitudes of charge of both the electron and the proton.
- Explain what is meant by the statement that an object is electrically neutral.
- Explain or define the following terms: ion pair, positive ion, negative ion, Coulomb force, grounding, static electricity, current, voltage, resistance, Ohm's law, rheostat, series and parallel circuits, conductors, insulators, semiconductors, electric field, capacitor, AC current, DC current, sinusoidal wave, and power.
- Perform simple computations involving Coulomb's law when given sufficient information.
- Explain the need for electrical grounding and ways it is accomplished.
- Explain how humidity level affects static charge build-up in terms of the concept of electrical dipoles.
- Explain the charging of an electroscope in terms of the movement of electrons (charging by both conduction and induction).
- Explain the basic operation of a pocket dosimeter.
- Explain what is meant by an electric field and how its direction and magnitude are determined.
- Sketch the electric field lines of a single positive or negative charge or a combination of these.
- Perform simple computations using definitions of current, voltage, and resistance.
- Perform simple computations involving Ohm's law.
- Indicate the physical factors that affect the electrical resistance of a wire.
- Define the term *superconductor.*
- Explain the meaning of the term *60-cycle AC.*
- Perform simple computations involving capacitance and the RC time constant.
- Perform simple computations involving electrical power.

ELECTRICAL CHARGE AND COULOMB'S LAW

Current scientific investigations into the nature of electricity still indicate that the smallest unit of electrical charge is that carried by the *electron.* In the SI system of units, charge (*q*) is measured in *coulombs* (C). The coulomb represents a rather large quantity of electrical charge compared with the charge on a single electron, which has been determined to be

$$e^- = -1.6 \times 10^{-19}\ C \qquad \text{Charge on electron}$$

These important points should be emphasized in regard to the electron:

- In addition to carrying the smallest known unit of electrical charge, -1.6×10^{-19} C,
- The electron is a mobile charge carrier (i.e., the electron can move from one point to another).

The charge on the *proton* (p) is identical in magnitude to that of the electron except that it is positive, that is,

$$p^+ = +1.6 \times 10^{-19} \text{ C} \qquad \text{Charge on proton}$$

Unlike the electron, the proton is bound within the nucleus of the atom and is not free to move from one location to another. When an object is described as being *electrically neutral,* it means that the object contains equal numbers of positive and negative charges. An atom is electrically neutral, containing the same number of electrons in its shells as it has protons in its nucleus. When an electron is removed from an atom, what is left of the atom is known as a positive ion. The positive ion and the electron that has been removed together are known as an ion pair (Fig. 4–1). It is the formation of these ion pairs, produced as radiation passes through matter, that potentially results in biological harm when produced in living tissue.

When any two charges are brought together, a force is exerted between them. This is known as an *electrostatic,* or *Coulomb, force.* The electrical force may be either attractive or repulsive, depending on the signs of the two charges; unlike charges attract, and like charges repel each other. The magnitude of the electrical force (F_E) between two charges, q_1 and q_2, separated by some known distance (d) is given by Coulomb's law:

$$F_E = k \frac{q_1 \, q_2}{d^2} \qquad \text{Coulomb's law}$$

where

$$k = \text{coulomb constant}$$
$$= 9 \times 10^9 \frac{N\text{-}m^2}{C^2}$$

$$q_1, q_2 = \text{charge in coulombs}$$
$$d = \text{separation distance in meters}$$

From the expression for the electrical force, it is seen that the magnitude of the electrical force is directly related to the magnitude of the two charges and inversely related to the square of the distance between them (an inverse square relationship with distance). The inverse square relationship with distance explains why those electrons farthest from the positively charged nucleus are held less tightly to the atom.

)))))) EXAMPLE

a) Two charges of magnitude $+2 \times 10^{-5}$ C and -5×10^{-4} C are separated by a distance of 1 m. What is the magnitude of the electric force between them?

$$F_E = k \frac{q_1 \, q_2}{d^2}$$
$$= \left(9 \times 10^9 \frac{N\text{-}m^2}{C^2} \right)$$
$$\frac{(+2 \times 10^{-5} \text{ C})(-5 \times 10^{-4} \text{ C})}{(1 \text{ m})^2}$$
$$= (9 \times 10^9 \text{ N}) \, (-10 \times 10^{-9})$$
$$= -90 \text{ N} \qquad \text{(attractive)}$$

Note. The negative sign indicates only that this force is attractive. Positive values for F_E indicate that the force is a repulsive force.

b) What would be the magnitude of the electric force between the same two charges if the distance between them was doubled?

$$F_E = k \frac{q_2 \, q_2}{d^2}$$
$$= \left(9 \times 10^9 \frac{N\text{-}m^2}{C^2} \right)$$
$$\frac{(+2 \times 10^{-5} \text{ C})(-5 \times 10^{-4} \text{ C})}{(2 \text{ m})^2}$$
$$= \frac{-90 \text{ N}}{4} = -22.5 \text{ N} \qquad \text{(attractive)}$$

Thus doubling the distance between the two charges reduces the original force to one fourth of the initial strength. Tripling the distance would have brought it to $(1/3)^2$, or $(1/9)$, of its original value and so on, indicating the effect of an inverse square law.

The electric force represents one of the fundamental forces in nature and is most important in the production of x-rays used in medical diagnosis. It is used to control both the direction and speed at which charges move in the x-ray machine when producing x-ray photons of the appropriate energy for quality radiographs.

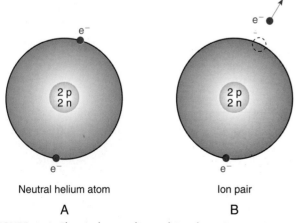

FIGURE 4–1. Electrical neutrality and ion formation. *A,* A neutral helium atom containing equal numbers of protons and electrons. *B,* A positive ion created by the removal of a shell electron.

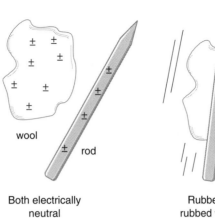
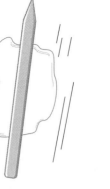
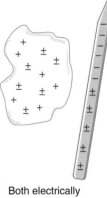

FIGURE 4-2. Generation of static electric charge on an insulator by frictional motion. Electrons are transferred from the wool to the rod, causing the wool to become positively charged and the rod negatively charged.

wool

rod

Both electrically
neutral

Rubber rod is
rubbed with wool

Both electrically
charged

STATIC ELECTRICITY

Matter is generally divided into one of three general classifications:

Insulator (also known as a dielectric or nonconductor). Material that does not allow an electrical charge to move freely, either through it or on its surface; examples: plastic, glass, rubber, and wood

Conductor. Material that allows a charge to move freely through it or on its surface; examples: most metals, melted salt, saline solutions, and many liquids

Semiconductor. Material through which a charge can move more easily than through an insulator but not as easily as through a conductor; examples: silicone and germanium

Static electricity, or static charge, refers to a charge that does not move but remains localized. If one takes two common insulators such as a hard rubber rod and a piece of wool, both of which are electrically neutral, and rub the two together, the rod will become negatively charged and the wool positively charged. Loosely bound outer shell electrons in the wool are transferred (by the mechanical motion of rubbing the two materials together) to the rubber rod (Fig. 4-2). This transfer of electrons from the wool causes it to become positively charged and the rod to become negatively charged. Since both materials are insulators (i.e., nonconductors), the transferred charges tend to remain highly localized in the region where contact between the two materials was originally made. The charges, being of the same sign, do not spread over the surface of the rod (or the wool) as they would if charges of like sign were deposited on the surface of a conductor (Fig. 4-3). This process of the transfer of electrical charge to produce static electrical charge build-up is fairly common when two nonconducting materials are rubbed across each other.

Static electricity is especially noticeable when the surrounding air is dry (i.e., condition of low humidity). It is not as much a problem when there is considerable moisture in the air (i.e., condition of high humidity).

The reason for this lies in the electrical properties of the water molecule. The water molecule, consisting of two atoms of hydrogen and one atom of oxygen (H_2O), is said to be electrically polar because electrons shared among the constituent atoms are shared unequally (Fig. 4-4*A*). The shared electrons spend more time near the oxygen end of the molecule, giving that end of the molecule a negative charge. Similarly, the hydrogen end of the molecule is more electrically positive. This separation of charges makes the molecule behave as an *electric dipole* (Fig. 4-4*B*). When static electrical charge is placed on a surface, the water molecules are attracted to and subsequently neutralize the excess charge on the surface (Fig. 4-4*C*). It is for this reason that static electricity is especially noticeable in the dry heat of a clothes dryer but is almost nonexistent on summer days when there is high humidity.

One simple device used to demonstrate several fundamental concepts of electrical charge is the electroscope (Fig. 4-5). The electroscope consists of a metal (conductor) sphere attached to a metal (conductor) rod from which hang two thin metal (conductor) foil strips. The electroscope is first neutralized by grounding the device. *Grounding* means the provision of a path (e.g., a wire) by which any excess charge can leave the device. (Metal cabinets containing electrical

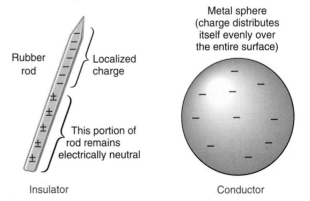

Rubber rod

Localized charge

This portion of rod remains electrically neutral

Insulator

Metal sphere (charge distributes itself evenly over the entire surface)

Conductor

FIGURE 4-3. Negative charge deposited on an insulator and on a conductor. When electric charge is deposited on an insulator, it remains localized. When charge is deposited on a conductor, it tends to spread out over the surface as a result of electrostatic repulsion.

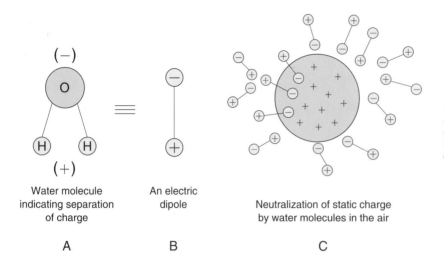

FIGURE 4–4. The electrical nature of water molecules. *A,* Polarity of the water molecule. *B,* An electric dipole, to which the water molecule can be likened. *C,* Electrical neutralization of static charge by water molecules in the air.

(−)

O

H   H

(+)

Water molecule
indicating separation
of charge

A

An electric
dipole

B

Neutralization of static charge
by water molecules in the air

C

motors or circuits are grounded as a safety measure to prevent electrical shock, which might occur when touched if electric charge has built up on the cabinet surface). The electroscope can be grounded by simply touching the sphere.

Recall that for an object to be electrically neutral, it must contain equal numbers of positive and negative charges. When a charged rod is brought near the sphere, a separation of the charge can be seen in the metal components. Because of electrostatic repulsive forces, the electrons within the metal are forced as far away as possible—that is, down to the thin metal leaves. Since both have the same electrical charge, they repel each other and spread apart. The more electrical charge on the leaves, the farther they spread apart.

If the metal sphere is touched by the charged rod, a negative charge (i.e., electrons) is conducted from the rod to the metal sphere, and the electroscope becomes negatively charged. (Recall that only the electron is mobile and capable of moving from one point to another.) This is known as charging by conduction (Fig. 4–6) (i.e., actual contact was made between the charged rod and the electroscope). When an electroscope is charged by conduction, the charge on the electroscope is the same as that on the charged rod.

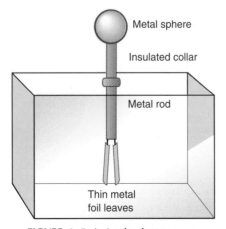

Metal sphere

Insulated collar

Metal rod

Thin metal
foil leaves

FIGURE 4–5. A simple electroscope.

The electroscope can also be charged positively with a negatively charged rod, using a second technique. Again, starting with a neutral electroscope (Fig. 4–7), the negatively charged rod is brought near the sphere but is not allowed to make contact. Again, observe that there is a separation of charge, as occurred initially. Recall that the electrons are repelled and move as far as possible from the charged rod (i.e., down to the metal foil strips). At this point, the electroscope is grounded, thus providing a path for the electrons on the metal strips to leave the device. This can be seen as the metal strips that once repelled each other now drop together. The ground is removed; then the rod is withdrawn, leaving the electroscope positively charged. This is known as charging by induction. With this technique, the electroscope is charged with the sign opposite that on the charged rod.

The electroscope demonstrates several important facts regarding electrical charge:

- Two types of electrical charge exist in nature—negative and positive.
- Like charges repel, and unlike charges attract. This force of repulsion and attraction is known as the electrostatic, or Coulomb, force.
- The electrostatic force that exists between charges becomes greater the closer charges are to each other. This force decreases rapidly as the distance between the charges increases. (Recall that this is a result of the inverse square relationship with distance.)
- Grounding refers to the process by which a path is provided for excess charge (e.g., excess charge build-up on a metal surface) to leave the surface. This is commonly done for the purpose of safety—to prevent electrical shock.
- When charge is deposited on an insulator (e.g., plastic, glass, wool), the charge remains localized and does not move.
- When charge is deposited on a conductor (e.g., a metal), the charge spreads over the surface as a result of electrostatic repulsion among the charges.

It is important to understand and master these basic concepts of electrical charge interaction, since these

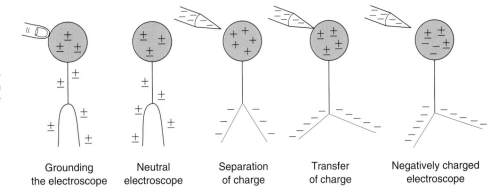

FIGURE 4–6. Charging an electroscope by conduction. Charge on the electroscope is the *same* as the charged rod.

Grounding the electroscope	Neutral electroscope	Separation of charge	Transfer of charge	Negatively charged electroscope

interactions are the basis of operation of many devices used in radiography and other medical imaging modalities. As is discussed later in this text, monitoring one's exposure to ionizing radiation is required by federal and state regulations because of its potential for biological harm. One device, based on the principles of the electroscope, that is used to measure radiation exposure is the pocket dosimeter (a dosimeter is a device used to measure radiation dose). The pocket dosimeter contains a thin quartz fiber (Fig. 4–8) and its mounting, which serve as the two central electrodes. When like charge is placed on both the quartz fiber and its mount (accomplished by using an accessory known as a charging base), the fiber moves away from the mounting as a result of electrostatic repulsion. When

viewed through the eyepiece, the quartz fiber casts a shadow on a scale within the dosimeter. As radiation enters the dosimeter and produces ion pairs within the air inside the device, the ions neutralize the charges on the fiber and mounting, allowing the fiber to move back toward the mounting. This in turn produces a reading on the scale that can be visualized when the dosimeter is held up to the light. The greater the amount of radiation to which the dosimeter is exposed, the more ion pairs created, the more charge neutralized, in turn resulting in a larger reading on the dosimeter scale. This type of direct-reading dosimeter is especially important in emergency situations in which an immediate estimate of one's radiation dose is needed.

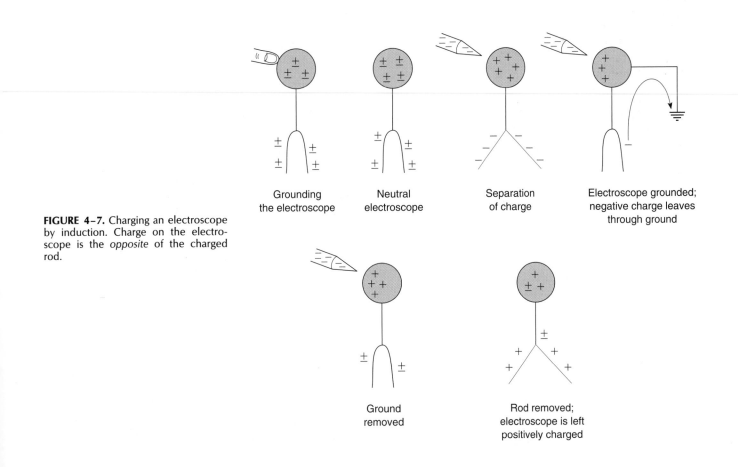

FIGURE 4–7. Charging an electroscope by induction. Charge on the electroscope is the *opposite* of the charged rod.

Grounding the electroscope

Neutral electroscope

Separation of charge

Electroscope grounded; negative charge leaves through ground

Ground removed

Rod removed; electroscope is left positively charged

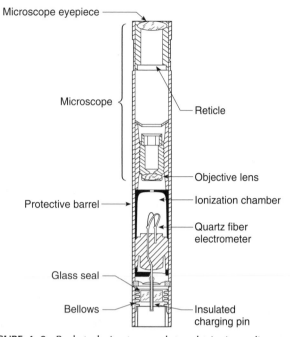

FIGURE 4–8. Pocket dosimeter used to obtain immediate estimates of radiation exposure. The operation of this device is based on the principle of the electroscope. (Courtesy of Dosimeter Corporation, Cincinnati, Ohio.)

ELECTRIC FIELDS: INVISIBLE FORCES SURROUNDING ELECTRICAL CHARGES

In almost all electrical devices there are, not one or two, but perhaps hundreds of thousands or more electrical charges. When working with large numbers of charges, it is much easier to use the concept of the *electric* (**E**) *field* in describing the behavior of electrical charges and predicting how they will behave under a specific set of conditions.

In physics a *field* is defined as a region of space in which a physical quantity has a definite value at every single point. To illustrate this idea, two types of fields are considered (Fig. 4–9). A room in which there is a fireplace or heater can represent a temperature field. That is, it represents a region of space (i.e., the space within the room) in which a physical quantity (i.e., temperature) has a definite value at every single point.

A gravitational field exists around the earth but in order to test the strength of this field, a "test mass" (m) must be used, since the earth only exerts its gravitational force of attraction on other masses. This field varies in strength, depending on the distance of the test mass from the earth as a result of the inverse square relationship, of the gravitational force with distance; recall that $F_G = G(m_1 \, m_2 / d^2)$. This variation in gravitational field strength with distance from the earth is indicated in the diagram by the spacing between the arrows. The gravitational field is strongest where the gravitation field lines (indicated by the arrows) are closest and weakest where the field lines are far apart. The field lines indicate not only the strength of the field but also the direction of the force exerted on the test mass. Thus from the diagram it is seen that the test mass (m) will be pulled to the earth as a result of the earth's gravitational attraction.

In much the same way as a gravitational field exists in the region of space around the earth, an **E** field exists around all electric charges. This indicates that charges exert forces on other charges around them— that is, through the Coulomb force, $F_E = k \, (q_1 q_2 / d^2)$. Like the gravitational field a test unit must be defined in order to measure the strength of the **E** field at various points and the direction in which it acts. By convention, we always use a small, positive test charge to determine electric field strength and the direction. The **E** field lines (arrows) for several charges and charge arrangements are shown in Figure 4–10. Recall that in each case

- The closer the field lines, the stronger the **E** field; the farther apart the field lines, the weaker the **E** field.
- A strong **E** field indicates that a strong electric force is exerted on any electrical charge in the region.
- The **E** field line direction indicates the direction of the electrical force exerted on a positive electrical charge.
- All electrical charges or charge distributions produce an **E** field in the region surrounding them.

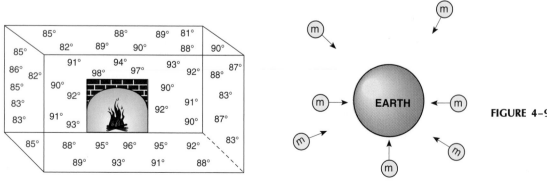

FIGURE 4–9. Types of fields.

A temperature field

The earth's gravitational field

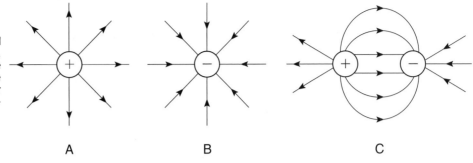

FIGURE 4-10. Electric fields for several charges and a charge distribution. *A,* An electric field for a single positive charge. *B,* Electrical field for a single negative charge. *C,* An electric field for a positive and negative charge configuration.

These concepts are demonstrated in the **E** fields shown in Figure 4-10. Figure 4-10*A* shows the **E** field of a single positive charge, and 4-10*B* indicates the **E** field surrounding a single negative charge. Figure 4-10*C* indicates the shape of the **E** field around a positive and negative charge combination. Note that the **E** field lines bend in the region between the two charges. The reason for this is that in the region between the charges, the positive test charge would simultaneously experience an attractive force from the negative charge and a repulsive force from the positive charge. The combined effect of the two forces produces field lines that curve as indicated. This specific field line pattern becomes particularly important when we later consider magnetic fields and the relationship that exists between electricity and magnetism.

E fields in themselves are important in that they provide one method of controlling the direction and speed of moving charges. Charged parallel metal plates can be used as shown in Figure 4-11 to direct the motion of a fast-moving electron. The **E** field between the plates exerts a force on the electron and produces a deflection in its motion. The strength of the field can be varied by increasing or decreasing the magnitude of the charge on the plates. Parallel charged plates are commonly used in controlling the motion of electric charges, since the **E** field between charged parallel plates is uniform in field strength.

ELECTRIC CURRENT: CHARGES IN MOTION

Current

When charges move, an *electric current* (I) is said to flow. In order for a current to flow, electrons must be available and free to move from one point to another. Conductors such as most common metals are characterized by having exceedingly large numbers of loosely bound outer shell electrons. These electrons are easily freed even by the heat energy available at room temperatures. These "free" electrons do not however flow in any one particular direction (Fig. 4-12) but in random directions. Thus there is no net flow of charge, and in order for a current to exist, there must be more charges moving in one direction than another. If one end of a metal wire is attached to the positive (+) terminal of a battery and the other end of the wire is attached to the negative (−) terminal, a current will flow, since now more electrons move from the negative to the positive terminal. Even though it is the electrons that are free to move, current flow is defined as the direction opposite that of electron flow (i.e., in the direction of flow of positive charge). These concepts are shown in Figure 4-12. Although direction of current flow is defined as opposite the direction of electron movement, current is nevertheless measured in terms of the amount of charge passing through a given area per unit of time. That is,

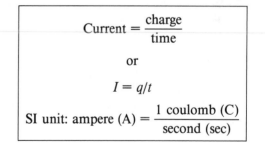

$$\text{Current} = \frac{\text{charge}}{\text{time}}$$

or

$$I = q/t$$

$$\text{SI unit: ampere (A)} = \frac{1 \text{ coulomb (C)}}{\text{second (sec)}}$$

When 1 C of electrical charge passes through a cross-sectional area of the conducting path per second, 1 A of current is said to flow.

The ampere is the SI unit of electric current and corresponds to a total charge of 1 C passing through a

FIGURE 4-11. Electric fields between parallel metal plates. *A,* Weak field between two lightly charged metal plates. *B,* Strong field between two heavily charged metal plates. *C,* Field between parallel charged metal plates used to redirect the motion of a moving electron.

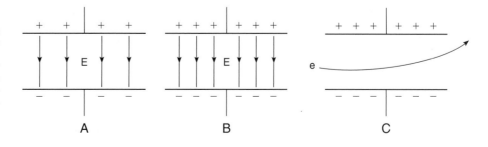

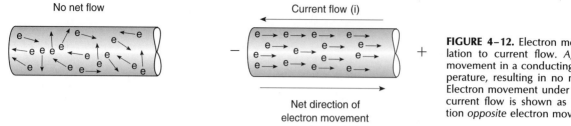

No net flow

Current flow (i)

Net direction of
electron movement

A   B

FIGURE 4–12. Electron movement and its relation to current flow. *A*, Random electron movement in a conducting wire at room temperature, resulting in no net current flow. *B*, Electron movement under an applied voltage; current flow is shown as being in the direction *opposite* electron movement.

cross-sectional area of the conducting path per second (Fig. 4–13). Recall that the electron is the mobile charge carrier and that each electron (e) carries a charge of -1.6×10^{-19} C; then a current of 1 A corresponds to

$$1 \text{ ampere (A)} = 1 \frac{\text{coulomb (C)}}{\text{second (sec)}}$$

$$= \frac{1 \text{ C}}{1.6 \times 10^{-19} \text{ (C/e}^-)/\text{sec}}$$

$$= 6.25 \times 10^{18} \frac{e}{\text{sec}}$$

6.25×10^{18} electrons flowing past any given point in the conducting path per second. From a practical point, an ampere generally represents a large amount of current, and as a result, currents of the order of milliamperes (mA) (i.e., 0.001 A) are encountered more commonly in radiographic procedures.

)))))) EXAMPLE

a) Determine the amount of charge that flows past a given point in a wire each second when a current of 100 mA flows through the wire.

$$I = 100 \text{ mA} = 10^2 \times 10^{-3} \text{ A} = 10^{-1} \text{ A}$$

$$10^{-1} \text{ A} = 10^{-1} \frac{\text{C}}{\text{sec}}$$

Thus 10^{-1} C of charge passes a given point within the wire each second.

Cross section of wire

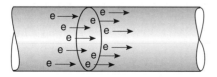

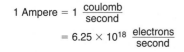

1 Ampere $= 1 \frac{\text{coulomb}}{\text{second}}$

$= 6.25 \times 10^{18} \frac{\text{electrons}}{\text{second}}$

FIGURE 4–13. A current of one ampere.

b) How many electrons (e) flowing past a given point within the wire each second does this correspond to?
10^{-1} C of charge flows. Since each electron carries 1.6×10^{-19} C of charge, then

$$\text{Number of electrons} = \frac{1 \times 10^{-1} \text{ C}}{1.6 \times 10^{-19} \text{ C/e}}$$

$$= 6.25 \times 10^{17} \text{ electrons}$$

Potential Difference, or Voltage

In order for a current to flow, charges must move. One will recall that bodies move from points of high potential (energy) to points of low potential (energy). A vase sitting on a tabletop (high potential energy) will naturally move to the ground (low potential energy) if it is tipped. Similarly, a metallic instrument held a short distance away from a powerful magnet (high potential) will move toward the magnet (low potential) when the instrument is released. And in the same manner, a charge must have a difference in potential, or potential difference, between points in the path (known as a *circuit*) through which it moves. (These concepts are demonstrated in Fig. 4–14). This potential difference may be provided by a battery or power supply.

Thus under normal operating conditions, two conditions must be satisfied in order for an electric current to flow:

1. The current must have a complete path through which to flow. (This means that there must be no breaks in the conducting path, a condition often referred to as an "open circuit." Most common electrical switches act to "open" or "close" conducting paths as a means of controlling the flow of an electric current.)
2. A potential difference *(voltage)* must exist between two points within the circuit or path through which the charge is to move. (This potential difference may be supplied by a battery, power supply, electrical outlet, and so forth.)

Potential difference is commonly referred to as voltage (V). When a charge is moved through the wires or conducting path of a circuit, energy must be used or expended. Voltage provides a measure of the amount of energy expended per unit of charge, that is, the amount of energy expended per coulomb. (Recall that

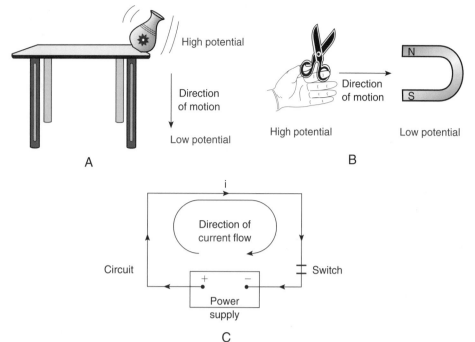

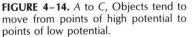

FIGURE 4–14. *A to C,* Objects tend to move from points of high potential to points of low potential.

the coulomb is the SI unit of electrical charge.) This can be written in equation form as

> $$\text{Voltage} = \frac{\text{energy expended}}{\text{charge}}$$
>
> or
>
> $$V = E/q$$
>
> SI units: volts (V) $= \dfrac{\text{joules (J)}}{\text{coulombs (C)}}$

))))))) EXAMPLE

Determine the energy used in moving a charge of 2 C through a circuit in which a power supply provides a potential difference of 100 V.

Given: $V = 100$ V

$q = 2$ C

$E = ?$

$V = E/q$

$E = Vq$

$E = (100 \text{ V})(2 \text{ C})$

$E = 200$ J

))))))) EXAMPLE

Determine the potential difference that exists within a circuit if 4.5 J of energy are expended per 0.01 C in moving charge through the circuit.

Given: $E = 4.5$ J

$q = 0.01$ C $= 10^{-2}$ C

$V = ?$

$V = E/q$

$= \dfrac{4.5 \text{ J}}{10^{-2} \text{ C}}$

$= 4.5 \times 10^2$ V or 450 V

In a conducting circuit, the voltage (or potential difference) provides the force that "pushes" charges through a conducting path such as a wire. The greater the voltage, the greater the force and the faster the charges move. As the charges move faster, the more charges move through the wire per second and thus the greater the current.

Resistance: Electrical Friction

Analogous to friction, which in a mechanical system always acts to oppose motion, *resistance* (R) in an electrical circuit acts to oppose current flow. Under normal conditions, resistance is present in all materials. Resistance is measured in a unit known as the *ohm,* represented by the Greek letter omega (Ω). In terms of electrical resistance, conductors (e.g., metals) are characterized as having low electrical resistance, whereas insulators (i.e., nonconductors such as wood, rubber, and plastics) are characterized as having high electrical resistance. In the case of wires used to conduct electric currents, resistance is determined not only by the material of which the wire is made but also by other physical factors such as the length (L) of the wire

Table 4-1: TYPICAL RESISTIVITIES OF COMMON MATERIALS

Material	ρ (Ohm-Meters)
Conductors*	
Copper	1.7×10^{-8}
Iron	1.2×10^{-8}
Platinum	11×10^{-8}
Silver	1.6×10^{-8}
Tungsten	5.6×10^{-8}
Insulators*	
Rubber	$\sim 1 \times 10^{15}$
Oil	$\sim 2 \times 10^{14}$
Glass	$\sim 1 \times 10^{12}$
Distilled water	5×10^{3}

* It should be noted that conductors typically have low resistivities (implying low resistance to the flow of current), whereas insulators have high resistivities (indicating high resistance to the flow of current).

and its cross-sectional area (A). This relationship is expressed as

$$R = \rho \frac{L}{A}$$

The symbol ρ (the Greek letter rho) represents resistivity, which is characteristic of the material from which the wire is made. L is the length of the wire in meters, and A is its cross-sectional area in meters squared. Typical values of resistivities of commonly used materials are shown in Table 4-1.

From this equation for electrical resistance (R), it is seen that as the length of the wire increases, resistance increases. Also, as the cross-sectional area of the wire decreases (i.e., as the wire becomes thinner or of smaller diameter), its resistance increases. When a current is pushed through a high-resistance wire, heat is generated. This principle is illustrated in the design of the filament of the common electrical light bulb. Here the purpose is to generate enough heat to cause the wire to glow and produce light. Thus a long, thin wire is used (i.e., to produce high electrical resistance) so that sufficient heat is generated as current is pushed through the wire. Most common filaments are made of tungsten, since tungsten has a high melting point (3370°C or 6098°F) and does not easily vaporize.

)))))) **EXAMPLE**

Determine the electrical resistance of a tungsten wire that is 80 cm long and has a radius of 0.1 mm.

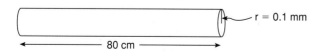

First, all units must be converted to SI units:

$$L = 80 \text{ cm} = 0.8 \text{ m} = 8 \times 10^{-1} \text{ m}$$

$$A = \pi r^2 = (3.14)(1 \times 10^{-4} \text{ m})^2$$
$$= (3.14)(1 \times 10^{-8} \text{ m}^2)$$
$$= 3.14 \times 10^{-8} \text{ m}^2$$

From Table 4-1, ρ for tungsten is 5.6×10^{-8} Ω-m. Therefore, using the relationship for resistance, R,

$$R = \rho \frac{L}{A}$$
$$= (5.6 \times 10^{-8} \text{ } \Omega\text{-m}) \frac{8 \times 10^{-1} \text{ m}}{3.14 \times 10^{-8} \text{ m}^2}$$
$$\approx 1.43 \text{ } \Omega$$

It should also be noted that electrical resistance for most materials also increases with increases in temperature. This comes about because as the temperature of a material increases, there is more random motion of the atoms that make up the material. When this occurs, the electron flow is hindered, and the material is said to have higher resistance.

Some materials, when cooled to extremely low temperatures, tend to lose all their electrical resistance. These materials are known as *superconductors*. Several materials and the temperatures (centigrade and kelvin) at which they become superconductors are listed below:

Aluminum (Al)	$-271.96°C$ (1.2 K)
Lead (Pb)	$-265.94°C$ (7.22 K)
Copper sulfide (CuS)	$-271.56°C$ (1.6 K)
Niobium titanium (Nb-Ti)	$-263.36°C$ (9.8 K)

When the temperatures of these materials are lowered below those indicated above, a current will flow through them indefinitely, provided a current is initially started and the temperature is maintained below the critical temperature. Currents have been made to flow in superconducting wires for several years without being connected to a battery, power supply, or electrical outlet. More will be said about superconductors in Chapter 22 in a discussion of magnetic resonance imaging; this technology has become most useful in the generation of strong magnetic fields.

OHM'S LAW: RELATING CURRENT, VOLTAGE, AND RESISTANCE

In general, as the voltage is increased in a conducting circuit (Fig. 4-15), if electrons are available (as they would be in a conducting wire), the electrons will move faster. As the electrons move faster, more of them pass through any cross-sectional area of the wire per second, and a larger current flows. This current is measured within a circuit by a type of measuring device known as an *ammeter*. Ammeters measure current flow in units of amperes or its subunits (e.g., milliamperes, microamperes).

The current flow is also affected, however, by the amount of resistance within the circuit. Any electrical

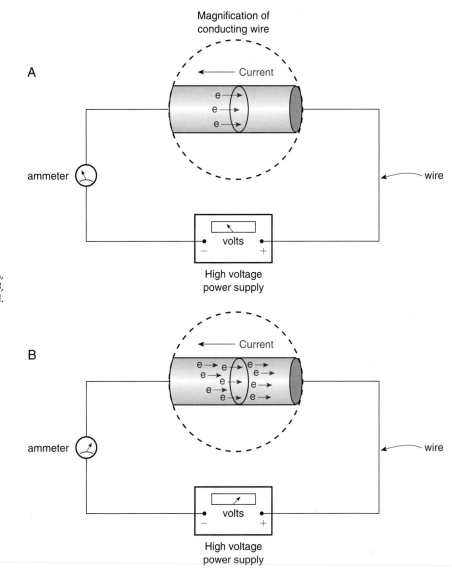

Magnification of
conducting wire

A

Current

ammeter

wire

volts

High voltage
power supply

B

Current

ammeter

wire

volts

High voltage
power supply

FIGURE 4–15. Simple electrical circuits. *A,* Low voltage results in low current flow. *B,* Current flow increases as voltage is increased.

device placed within an electrical circuit presents a certain amount of resistance to the flow of current. As mentioned earlier, certain devices such as incandescent lights (i.e., light bulbs), heaters, toaster ovens, electric irons, and the like act as pure high-resistance elements whose primary purpose is to generate heat. Resistances may also take the form of small circuit components whose primary purpose is not only to regulate the amount of current flowing but also to direct it through specific paths within a circuit. This is explained shortly when types of circuits are discussed.

The interrelationship between current (I), voltage (V), and resistance (R) for conductors is expressed by the formula known as Ohm's law:

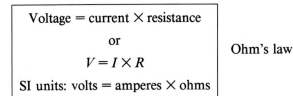

Voltage = current $\times$ resistance

or

$V = I \times R$

SI units: volts = amperes $\times$ ohms

Ohm's law

))$\rangle\rangle\rangle$) **EXAMPLE**

A 1.5-V battery produces a current of 300 milliamperes (mA). Determine the resistance of the circuit. Given

$$V = 1.5 \text{ V}$$
$$I = 300 \text{ mA} = 0.3 \text{ A}$$
$$R = ?$$

Using Ohm's law,

$$V = IR$$

or

$$R = V/I$$
$$= \frac{1.5 \text{ V}}{0.3 \text{ A}}$$
$$= 5 \text{ } \Omega$$

The circuit is found to have a resistance of 5 Ω.

FURTHER PRACTICE WITH OHM'S LAW: SERIES AND PARALLEL CIRCUITS

When placed in electrical circuits in specific physical arrangements, resistances can be used both to regulate the amount of current that flows in a circuit and to direct current to flow through specific paths. These specific arrangements of resistances are known as series circuits and parallel circuits. Each specific type of circuit has its own individual electrical rules so each is considered separately. As you read through each discussion and example, note how all the rules are applied and how Ohm's law is used to answer specific questions regarding the circuit.

Series Circuits

A circuit in which resistances are connected in a continuous line is known as a series circuit. Figure 4–16 shows three resistances—R_1, R_2, and R_3—connected in this type of arrangement. In addition to the individual resistances in the circuit shown there are four ammeters (I_T, I_1, I_2, and I_3) to measure the current flowing through the entire circuit and through

R_1, R_2, and R_3, respectively. Four voltmeters (V_T, V_1, V_2, and V_3) measuring the voltage (or potential difference) across the battery and each resistance are also shown. (Note: Voltmeters are connected across points in a circuit since they measure potential difference between two points. This method of connection is therefore different from that used with ammeters, which measure current flow through a circuit element).

When resistances are connected in a series arrangement within an electric circuit, several rules must be observed. These rules follow; they use the indicated quantities shown in Figure 4–16:

Rule #1
$I_T = I_1 = I_2 = I_3$. This simply indicates that the magnitude of the current that flows through each circuit component in a series circuit is constant.

Rule #2
$V_T = V_1 + V_2 + V_3$. The total voltage drop across the entire circuit (V_T) is the sum of the voltage drops across each individual resistance.

Rule #3
$R_T = R_1 + R_2 + R_3$. The total resistance of a circuit is the sum of the individual resistances.

These rules are now used to answer the following questions regarding the circuit shown in Figure 4–16.

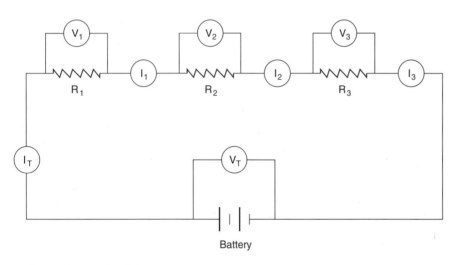

FIGURE 4–16. Resistances connected in a series circuit.

R_1 = resistance 1 = 8 Ω
R_2 = resistance 2 = 10 Ω
R_3 = resistance 3 = 6 Ω
I_T = ammeter measuring total current flow through circuit
V_T = voltmeter measuring voltage across battery = 12 volts
V_1, V_2, V_3: voltmeters (to measure voltage)
I_1, I_2, I_3: ammeters (to measure currents)

RULES FOR SERIES CIRCUITS:

1. $I_1 = I_2 = I_3 = I_T$
2. $V_T = V_1 + V_2 + V_3$
3. $R_T = R_1 + R_2 + R_3$

)))))) EXAMPLE

Three resistances are connected in series as shown in Figure 4–16. They have the following magnitudes:

$$R_1 = 8\ \Omega,\ R_2 = 10\ \Omega,\ R_3 = 6\ \Omega$$

Also,

$$V_T = 12\ \text{V}$$

a) What is the total current (I_T) that flows through the circuit?

To determine the magnitude of the current flowing through the entire circuit, first determine the total resistance (R_T) of the circuit. To find R_T, use

$$\begin{aligned} R_T &= R_1 + R_2 + R_3 \\ &= 8\ \Omega + 10\ \Omega + 6\ \Omega \\ R_T &= 24\ \Omega \end{aligned}$$

Now that the total resistance has been determined, use the total voltage (V_T) supplied here by a 12-V battery and Ohm's law to determine the total current, I_T:

$$V_T = I_T R_T \qquad \text{Ohm's law}$$

or

$$\begin{aligned} I_T &= \frac{V_T}{R_T} \\ &= \frac{12\ \text{V}}{24\ \Omega} \\ I_T &= 0.5\ \text{A} \end{aligned}$$

Thus 0.5 A flows through the entire circuit.

b) What is the magnitude of the current that flows through R_1, R_2, and R_3?

Rule #1 indicates that current is constant in a series circuit. Thus 0.5 A flows through each of the individual resistances as well as through the entire circuit.

c) Determine the voltage drop (or potential difference) across each resistance.

To find the voltage drop across each resistance, apply Ohm's law to each, keeping in mind that a constant current of 0.5 A flows through each:

$$\begin{aligned} V_1 &= I_1 R_1 \\ &= (0.5\ \text{A})\ (8\ \Omega) \\ &= 4\ \text{volts} \end{aligned}$$

$$\begin{aligned} V_2 &= I_2 R_2 \\ &= (0.5\ \text{A})\ (10\ \Omega) \\ &= 5\ \text{V} \end{aligned}$$

$$\begin{aligned} V_3 &= I_3 R_3 \\ &= (0.5\ \text{A})\ (6\ \Omega) \\ &= 3\ \text{V} \end{aligned}$$

As a check, by Rule #2 the total of these voltages should give the total voltage provided by the 12-V battery:

$$\begin{aligned} V_T &= V_1 + V_2 + V_3 \\ 12\ \text{V} &= 4\ \text{V} + 5\ \text{V} + 3\ \text{V} \\ 12\ \text{V} &= 12\ \text{V} \end{aligned}$$

Thus all rules for series circuit have been verified.

Note. With resistances connected in a series arrangement, it can be seen that if any individual resistance is so damaged that no current can flow through it, then no current will flow through the entire circuit. Strings of Christmas lights in which if one light burns out, all the lights in the string go out, are connected in a series arrangement.

Parallel Circuits

A circuit in which resistances are connected "side by side" is known as a parallel circuit. Figure 4–17 shows three resistances—R_1, R_2, and R_3—connected in a parallel arrangement. Ammeters (I_1, I_2, I_3, and I_T) are also connected in the circuit to measure the current flow through R_1, R_2, and R_3 as well as through the entire circuit. Voltmeters (V_1, V_2, V_3, and V_T) are again connected to measure the potential difference across each resistance. V_T is connected across the battery to measure the total potential difference across the entire circuit.

One major difference with the parallel circuit is that as the current travels through the circuit and arrives at the junction of the parallel branch, the current splits— a portion traveling through R_1, a second portion through R_2, and a third portion through R_3. It will always be true that the largest portion of the current travels through the branch having the least resistance. This is demonstrated in the example to follow. Unlike the series arrangement, if one resistance is damaged and the path through that resistance is broken, the current still has alternate paths through which it can travel. In a parallel circuit, any branch containing a broken path is seen by the current as having infinite resistance, and as a result, no current flows through that branch.

When resistances are connected in a parallel arrangement within an electrical circuit, again several rules must be observed. These rules are stated below using the indicated quantities shown in Figure 4–17:

Rule #1

$V_T = V_1 = V_2 = V_3$. In the parallel circuit, voltage is constant. That is, the potential difference across each resistance is the same as the potential difference across the battery.

Rule #2

$I_T = I_1 + I_2 + I_3$. This indicates that the total current flowing through the circuit will be the sum of the current that flows through each individual branch of the parallel circuit.

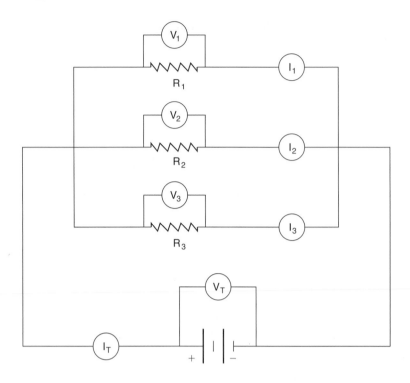

FIGURE 4–17. Resistances connected in a parallel circuit.

R_1 = resistance 1 = 4 Ω
R_2 = resistance 2 = 3 Ω
R_3 = resistance 3 = 12 Ω
I_T = ammeter measuring total current flow through circuit
V_T = voltmeter measuring voltage across the battery = 12 volts
V_1, V_2, V_3: voltmeters (to measure voltage)
I_1, I_2, I_3: ammeters (to measure current)

RULES FOR PARALLEL CIRCUITS:

1. $I_T = I_1 + I_2 + I_3$
2. $V_T = V_1 = V_2 = V_3$
3. $\dfrac{1}{R_T} = \dfrac{1}{R_1} + \dfrac{1}{R_2} + \dfrac{1}{R_3}$

Rule #3

$1/R_T = 1/R_1 + 1/R_2 + 1/R_3$. When resistances are connected in parallel, the reciprocal of the total resistance of the circuit is equal to the sum of the reciprocals of the individual resistance. R_T will always be less than the lowest individual resistance in the circuit.

The application of these rules is illustrated in the following example.

))⟫⟩) **EXAMPLE**

Three resistances are connected in parallel as shown in Figure 4–17 with the following information provided:

$$R_1 = 4\ \Omega,\ R_2 = 3\ \Omega,\ R_3 = 12\ \Omega$$

$$V_T = \text{voltage of battery} = 12\ V$$

a) What is the total current (I_T) that flows through the circuit? The total resistance determines the current that flows through the circuit. Using Rule #3 for the total resistance, R_T, we find

$$1/R_T = 1/R_1 + 1/R_2 + 1/R_3$$

$$= \frac{1}{4\ \Omega} + \frac{1}{3\ \Omega} + \frac{1}{12\ \Omega}$$

$$= \frac{3}{12\ \Omega} + \frac{4}{12\ \Omega} + \frac{1}{12\ \Omega}$$

$$1/R_T = \frac{8}{12\ \Omega}$$

$$R_T = \frac{12\ \Omega}{8} = 1.5\ \Omega$$

Note. R_T is less than the smallest individual resistance, which is 3 Ω.

Now, using Ohm's law,

$$V_T = I_T R_T$$

$$I_T = V_T/R_T$$

$$= \frac{12 \text{ V}}{1.5 \text{ Ω}}$$

$$I_T = 8 \text{ A}$$

b) What is the potential drop across each individual resistance?

$$V_T = V_1 = V_2 = V_3 = 12 \text{ V}$$

since voltage is constant in parallel circuits.

c) What current flows through R_1, R_2, and R_3? To determine the magnitude of the current that flows through each branch, we use Ohm's law once again, remembering that the voltage across each branch is constant.

The current that flows through R_1 is

$$V_1 = I_1 R_1$$

$$12 \text{ V} = (I_1) (4 \text{ Ω})$$

$$I_1 = \frac{12 \text{ V}}{4 \text{ Ω}}$$

$$I_1 = 3 \text{ A}$$

and the current through R_2 is

$$V_2 = I_2 R_2$$

$$12 \text{ V} = (I_2) (3 \text{ Ω})$$

$$I_2 = \frac{12 \text{ V}}{3 \text{ Ω}}$$

$$I_2 = 4 \text{ A}$$

and the current through R_3 is

$$V_3 = I_3 R_3$$

$$12 \text{ V} = (I_3) (12 \text{ Ω})$$

$$I_3 = \frac{12 \text{ V}}{12 \text{ Ω}}$$

$$I_3 = 1 \text{ A}$$

The largest current flows through the second branch (i.e., through R_2), since it is this branch that has the least resistance. In addition, if the three currents are added, the total current, I_T, should be obtained:

$$I_T = I_1 + I_2 + I_3$$

$$8 \text{ A} = 3 \text{ A} + 4 \text{ A} + 1 \text{ A}$$

$$8 \text{ A} = 8 \text{ A}$$

All rules for parallel circuits have now been verified.

CHARGE FLOW DIRECTION: AC VS. DC

Previously, a current was defined as charges in motion. If the charges move in only one direction, the current is said to be a direct current, abbreviated DC. A *DC current* is the type of current that is provided by a battery or DC power supply. Such a DC circuit is illustrated in Figure 4–18. In this circuit, it is seen that electrons move from the negative terminal to the positive terminal of the battery. Recall, however, that current flow is defined as being in the direction opposite that of electron flow; thus current flow is said to be from positive to negative terminals of the battery.

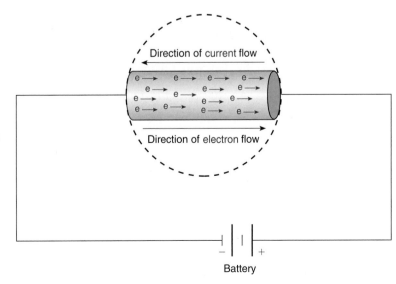

FIGURE 4–18. A DC circuit, indicating single direction of current flow.

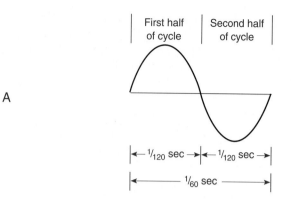

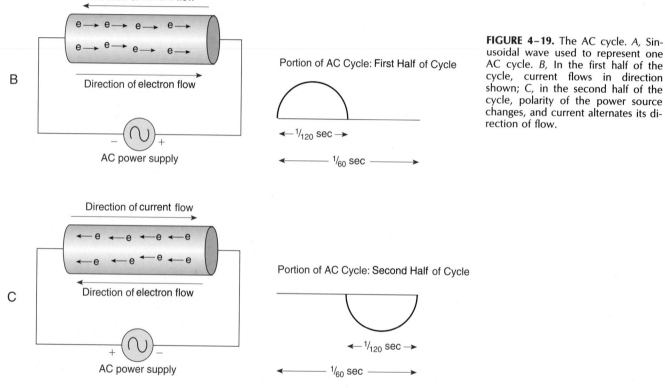

FIGURE 4-19. The AC cycle. *A,* Sinusoidal wave used to represent one AC cycle. *B,* In the first half of the cycle, current flows in direction shown; *C,* in the second half of the cycle, polarity of the power source changes, and current alternates its direction of flow.

A charge has only to be in motion to produce a current. From the practical standpoint, it is easier to generate a current that alternates its direction of motion. Such a current is known as an alternating current, abbreviated AC. An *AC current* is divided into cycles. During the first half of the cycle, the charge flows in one direction, and in the second half of the cycle, the charge flows in the opposite direction (Fig. 4–19). This cycle may be represented as a sinusoidal wave (Fig. 4–19*A*). In conventional AC current generated in the United States, 60 full cycles are produced each second. This is known as 60-cycle AC. Thus the time span of one cycle is 1/60 sec. Each half cycle occurs during half of this time period, or 1/120 sec. As shown in Figure 4–19*B*, the positive portion of the curve represents that half of the cycle in which the current flows to the left and the negative portion (Fig. 4–19*C*) of the curve represents the second half of the cycle, in which the current changes its direction and flows to the right.

OTHER USEFUL CIRCUIT COMPONENTS: CAPACITORS AND RHEOSTATS

Capacitors

Capacitors are devices that are used in an electrical circuit to store electric charge until a time that it is needed. A simple capacitor consists of two metal (conducting) plates separated by a space in which has been inserted some nonconducting material (e.g., oil, plastics, ceramics, glass). When a capacitor is placed in an electrical circuit in which there is a voltage source such as a battery, charge will flow to the conducting plates until the voltage across the plates is the same as the voltage produced by the battery. This "charging" of the capacitor does not occur instantaneously but requires a finite period of time that may range from seconds to minutes. The charging of a capacitor follows a typical charge build-up curve in which time is expressed in what is known as the *RC time constant.* (note that R × C = resistance × capacitance = ohms × farads = seconds). This is a characteristic time parameter for a particular circuit that includes a capacitor of known capacitance (C) and a known resistance (R). The capacitance, C, of a capacitor is defined as

$$\text{Capacitance} = \frac{\text{charge}}{\text{voltage}}$$

$$\text{SI units: farads} = \frac{\text{coulombs}}{\text{volts}}$$

Recall that changing the amount of charge on the plates changes the voltage across the plates. Capaci-

tance provides a measure of how much charge (of either sign) must be placed on a plate to produce a 1-V increase in potential difference across the capacitor plates. Capacitance in the SI system of units is measured in a unit known as the *farad (F)* in honor of the British physicist and chemist, Michael Faraday. A simple capacitor and its charging circuit is shown in Figure 4–20. Also shown is the charging curve for such a capacitor (Fig. 4–20C). It is noted that several RC time constants must pass before the capacitor approaches its maximum charge.

Table 4–2 indicates the general lengths of time required for a capacitor to reach a specific percentage of its full charge. From the table it is seen that during charging, after one RC time constant, the capacitor is achieving 63% of its full charge. After two RC time constants, it reaches 86% of full charge. Similarly, the discharge process also requires a finite period of time that again depends on the value of the RC time constant for the specific circuit. Table 4–2 also indicates general lengths of time required for a capacitor to discharge certain percentages of its full charge. It can be seen from the table that the capacitor can discharge rather rapidly, dropping to 37% of full charge after only one RC time constant has passed. Also note that

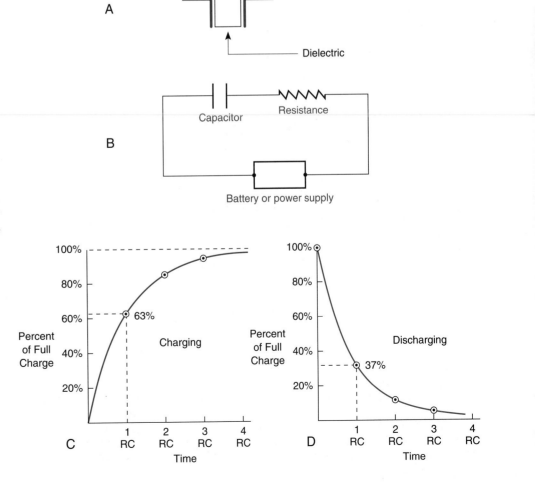

FIGURE 4–20. Design and characteristics of the simple capacitor. *A,* Basic design of a simple capacitor—parallel metal plates into which a dielectric (nonconductor) has been inserted. *B,* A simple circuit containing a capacitor and a resistance. *C,* Curve describing the time required to charge a simple capacitor in terms of the RC time constant. *D,* Curve describing the discharging of a simple capacitor in terms of the RC time constant.

Table 4-2: TIME CHARACTERISTICS ASSOCIATED WITH CHARGING AND DISCHARGING A CAPACITOR

Elapsed Time in RCs	Charging (% of Full Charge)	Discharging (% of Full Charge)
1	63	37
2	86	14
3	95	5
4	~98	~2
5	~99	~1

capacitors do not instantaneously discharge. When the charge that is stored in a capacitor is to be used, the charge does not leave the capacitor plates instantaneously but is discharged over a period of time determined by the RC time constant of the circuit as indicated in Table 4-2. It is also seen in Table 4-2 that during discharge, the charge drops to 37% of full charge after only 1 RC time constant has passed and to 14% of full charge after 2 RC time constants, and so on. This concept is also illustrated in the following example.

)))))) EXAMPLE

A 100-μF (microfarad) capacitor is used in a circuit that includes a 500-Ω resistance.

a) Determine the RC time constant for this circuit.

$$\text{RC time constant} = \text{resistance} \times \text{capacitance}$$
$$= R \times C$$
$$= (5 \times 10^2 \ \Omega)(10^2 \times 10^{-6} \ F)$$
$$= (5 \times 10^2 \times 10^{-4}) \ \text{sec}$$
$$= 5 \times 10^{-2} \ \text{sec or } 0.05 \ \text{sec}$$

b) When charging this capacitor within this circuit, how long does it take to charge the capacitor to approximately 98% of its full charge?

From Table 4-2, it takes a time period of 4 RC time constants to bring a capacitor to approximately 98% of full charge. Thus for this circuit, it will take

$$\text{Time to reach} \sim 98\% \text{ of full charge} = 4 \ RC$$
$$= 4 \ (0.05 \ \text{sec})$$
$$= 0.20 \ \text{sec}$$

c) If the capacitor is discharged, how long will it take to drop to 14% of its maximum charge?

From Table 4-2, it takes a time period of 2 RC time constants to drop to 14% of full charge. Therefore for this circuit this time will be

$$\text{Time to drop to 14\% of full charge} = 2 \ RC$$
$$= 2 \ (0.05 \ \text{sec})$$
$$= 0.10 \ \text{sec}$$

Note. In this problem, as with almost every physics problem, multiples and submultiples of quantities must be converted to basic SI units before performing calculations. Here, microfarads (μF) had to be converted to farads, the basic SI unit of capacitance, before arriving at the final numerical solution.

Capacitors come in many shapes and sizes, depending on their specific use within an electrical circuit. They are found in power supplies, electronic timing circuits, and many portable x-ray units. These particular applications are discussed in later chapters.

Rheostats

Up to this point, when using resistances in electrical circuits, they have been considered to have finite values. That is, a 10-Ω resistance in a circuit provides 10 Ω of resistance, no more and no less. You have seen that resistances can be used both to regulate the amount of current that flows in a circuit and to direct current flow through particular paths within a circuit (recall series and parallel circuits).

In many applications, there may be a need to vary the resistance in a circuit; this can be done by using a variable resistance known as a *rheostat*. In electric circuits, rheostats are used to produce gradual changes in voltage or current flow. In many electrical devices, rheostats may take the form of dials that are turned to adjust voltages or currents. A common household application of the rheostat is the light dimmer switch. By turning the dial in one direction one increases the electrical resistance, allowing less current to flow and resulting in a light that burns dimly. Turning the dial in the opposite direction decreases the resistance, allowing more current to flow, and the light burns brighter.

ELECTRICAL POWER

By definition, *power* is the rate at which work is done or the rate at which energy is used. In a DC electric circuit, the rate at which electrical energy can be converted into work is given by

> Power = voltage $\times$ current
>
> or
>
> $$P = V I$$
>
> SI units: watts = volts $\times$ amperes

When a current flows in a circuit in which there is electrical resistance, the stated relationship can be used to describe the power loss across the resistance. This power loss occurs in the form of heat generated as the current flows through the resistance. In order to see the effect of resistance on this rate of energy loss, Ohm's law can be solved for V,

$$V = IR \quad \text{Ohm's law}$$

and this result can be substituted in the preceding expression for power to obtain

$$P = VI$$
$$= (IR)I$$
$$\boxed{P = I^2 R}$$

SI units: watts = (amperes)² (ohms)

))))))) EXAMPLE

a) A DC current of 5 A flows through a circuit in which a potential difference of 120 V exists. What is the power generated in this circuit?

$$P = VI$$
$$= (120 \text{ V}) (5 \text{ A})$$
$$= 600 \text{ W}$$

b) A DC current of 10 A flows through a resistance of 20 Ω. What is the rate of energy loss from the resistance?

$$P = I^2 R$$
$$= (10 \text{ A})^2 (20 \text{ Ω})$$
$$= (100) (20) \text{ W}$$
$$= 2000 \text{ W (or 2000 J/sec)}$$

Note. Since a *watt* is the equivalent of 1 joule/sec, this latter form represents the rate of energy production or energy loss in the form of heat. Recall that heat energy may be measured in Calories or joules, since both are units of energy.

Chapter Summary/ Important Equations, Constants, and Relationships

Charge on the electron: $e^- = -1.6 \times 10^{-19}$ C

Charge on the proton: $p^+ = +1.6 \times 10^{-19}$ C

Coulomb's law: $F_E = k \dfrac{q_1 \, q_2}{d^2}$

where

$$k = \text{electric constant}$$
$$= 9 \times 10^9 \, \frac{\text{N–m}^2}{\text{C}^2}$$

Electric current: $I = q/t$

Voltage: $V = E/q$

Resistance: $R = \rho \dfrac{L}{A}$

Ohm's law: $V = IR$

Power: $P = VI$

Important Terminology

AC Current. Alternating current; current that constantly alternates its direction of flow

Ammeter. A meter placed in an electrical circuit to measure the magnitude of current flow; always connected in series

Ampere (A). SI unit of electrical current equivalent to 1 coulomb/sec

Capacitor. Device used in an electrical circuit to store electrical charge

Circuit. The physical path a charge follows in moving from one point to another

Conductor. Materials that allow electric currents to flow easily through them (e.g., copper, platinum, aluminum, saline solution, etc.)

Coulomb (C). The SI unit of electric charge

DC Current. Direct current; current that flows in only one direction (e.g., current produced by a battery or DC power supply)

Electric Current (I). Moving electric charge; direction of current flow is defined as opposite that of electron flow

Electrical Dipole. Two oppositely signed charges separated by a short distance

Electric Field (E). The force field that exists around every electric charge; its magnitude and direction are determined by using a small, positive test charge

Electrical Neutrality. Having equal numbers of positive and negative charges

Electron. The smallest known unit of electric charge capable of movement; the electron carries a charge of -1.6×10^{-19} coulombs

Electrostatic (Coulomb) force. The electrical force of attraction or repulsion that exists between two electrical charges

Farad (F). SI unit of capacitance equivalent to 1 coulomb/volt

Field. A region of space in which a physical quantity has a definite value at every single point

Grounding. Any process by which a path is provided for charges to leave a surface

Insulator (also known as **dielectric** or **nonconductor**). Materials that do not allow electric currents to flow through them (e.g., glass, rubber, plastic, wood, etc.)

Ohm (Ω). SI unit of electrical resistance

Power. The rate at which work is done or energy is converted to other forms

Proton. Atomic particle that carries a charge equal in magnitude to that of the electron but is positively charged

RC Time Constant. Time parameter used to describe the time required to charge and discharge a capacitor

Resistance. Opposes the flow of electric current in a circuit

Rheostat. A variable resistance

Semiconductor. Material that is neither a good conductor nor a good insulator

Static Electricity. A charge that does not move

Superconductor. Any material whose electrical resistance drops to zero when its temperature is lowered beyond a certain critical temperature

Volt (V). SI unit of electrical potential difference; equivalent to 1 joule/coulomb

Voltage (Potential Difference). The work done or energy expended in pushing a charge around a circuit; a measure of the difference in electrical potential between two points in a circuit

Voltmeter. A meter placed in an electrical circuit to measure the potential difference across two points in a circuit; always connected in parallel

Watt (W). SI unit of power equivalent to 1 joule/sec

Bibliography

Beiser, A. Modern Technical Physics, 6th ed. Reading, MA: Addison-Wesley, 1992.

Hazen, M.E. Experiencing Electricity and Electronics. Philadelphia: W.B. Saunders Company, 1989.

Thomas, S.R.; Dixon, R.L., eds. NMR in Medicine: The Instrumentation and Clinical Applications. New York: American Institute of Physics, 1986.

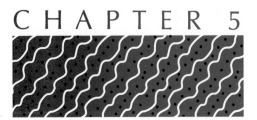

Magnetism and Its Relation to Electricity

Michael A. Thompson, M.S.

Chapter Outline

Chapter Objectives

Upon completion of this chapter, you should be able to

- Describe the interactions between like and unlike poles of a magnet.
- Describe and list the similarities and differences between electricity and magnetism.
- Indicate how magnets are produced (and weakened or destroyed) based on the concept of magnetic domains.
- Explain what is meant by a magnetic field, describe how its direction is determined, and give the SI unit in which it is measured.
- Sketch the magnetic field lines (both inside and outside) around a current-carrying wire and a permanent bar magnet.
- Describe the existence of electrical or magnetic fields or both in the vicinity of a stationary electric charge, a moving electric charge, stationary magnets, and changing magnetic fields across a conductor.
- Describe the magnetic properties of a current-carrying solenoid.
- Use Lenz's law to determine the magnetic polarity and the direction of the induced current in a solenoid produced by a bar magnet being thrust into or pulled out of the coil.
- Describe the method of operation of a generator and an electrical motor.
- Describe the process of rectification, and state the purpose of a rectifier.
- Describe what is meant by single-phase (1ϕ) and three-phase (3ϕ) rectification, how each is accomplished, and the resulting waveforms produced; explain the advantages and disadvantages of each.
- Describe what is meant by 60-cycle (or 60-Hz) AC, and state how this measurement is used to determine the time duration of voltage pulses produced by 1ϕ and 3ϕ generators.
- Using 60-cycle AC, determine the number of voltage pulses that occur per second, using single-phase, half-wave, and full-wave rectified voltage.
- Distinguish between DC and AC voltage by sketching voltage variation as a function of time for each.
- Explain what is meant by "six-pulse" and "twelve-pulse" generators, and describe the advantages of these units.
- Explain the term *ripple factor,* and give typical values for 1ϕ and 3ϕ generators.
- Explain the method of operation of the induction motor.
- Explain the principles of operation of the transformer and their use in x-ray circuitry.
- Use the transformer laws to perform simple calculations involving step-up and step-down transformers.
- Perform simple calculations involving transformer power ratings for both 1ϕ and 3ϕ units.

MAGNETS AND MAGNETIC FORCES

General Properties of Magnets

It has been proposed that as early as the sixth century B.C., it was known that certain types of stones, known as lodestones, had the ability to attract pieces of iron and other stones of this type. It is speculated that some of these first-known "natural magnets" were found in a region of Asia Minor known as Magnesia. From this name the term *magnet* is said to have been derived.

Around the first century A.D., the Chinese discovered that magnets could be artificially produced by simply stroking certain materials such as iron with a natural magnet. Perhaps the first technological application of magnets came with the development of the navigational compass. This instrument, also developed by the Chinese, consisted simply of suspending a magnetic needle on a point about which it could rotate freely. It was found that the magnetic compass needle would always tend to align itself in a north-south orientation. This behavior tended to indicate that the earth, too, behaved like a large magnet, exerting its magnetic force on the magnetic compass needle.

Each of these observations raised further questions regarding the nature and origin of magnetism. Experimentation continued and resulted in the following findings:

- A magnet consists of two types of magnetic poles—one designed north (N) and the other south (S).
- If a magnet is cut in two, each half will have a north and a south pole. This halving can continue, and in each case, each piece will have a north and a south pole. Even if the individual pieces consist of a single atom, it too will behave as if it has both magnetic poles. Thus a north pole cannot be isolated from a south pole.
- Like magnetic poles repel and unlike magnetic poles attract.
- The magnetic force (F_M) of attraction or repulsion between two magnetic poles (m_1 and m_2) is directly related to the strength of the individual magnets m_1 and m_2, respectively, and is inversely related to the square of the distance (d) between them. That is,

$$F_M \propto \frac{m_1 \, m_2}{d^2}$$

(Note: This takes the form of an inverse square law, seen previously with the electric force between charges.)

- The strength of a magnet can be adversely affected by heating or mechanically jarring (e.g., dropping or hammering) it
- Certain materials can be easily magnetized (e.g., iron, nickel, or cobalt), whereas other materials cannot.

(Note: Those metals that are most easily magnetized are said to be *ferromagnetic*.)

- Materials that are capable of being magnetized can be made so by leaving them for a period of time near a strong magnet or by stroking them with another magnet.
- Like electric charges, magnets have fields. That is, they have the ability to exert forces on other magnets or magnetic objects at a distance. (This is discussed more thoroughly in the next section.)

Many of these observations exposed important similarities between electricity and magnetism. Some of these similarities are indicated in Table 5–1, and it was these similarities that eventually led to the discovery of the intimate relationship between the two seemingly different phenomena.

Atoms—The Smallest Magnets

The type of magnet thus far referred to has been the common "bar magnet," usually consisting of a bar of iron or iron alloy that has been magnetized and has definite north and south magnetic poles. This type of magnet is also commonly referred to as a *permanent magnet* even though its magnetic properties are not "permanent" and can be altered by excessive heat or mechanical jarring. As previously mentioned, if a bar magnet is cut in two, each piece will behave as a separate bar magnet, each having a north and a south pole. This implies that each atom of the bar magnet material acts as a tiny magnet itself. This is illustrated in Figure 5–1.

Table 5–1: SIMILARITIES BETWEEN ELECTRICITY AND MAGNETISM

Properties of Electric Charge	Properties of Magnets
Two types of electric charge: positive and negative	Two types of magnetic poles: north and south
Like charges repel; unlike charges attract	Like magnetic poles repel; unlike magnetic poles attract
The electric force between charges depends on the magnitude of the charges and the distance between them	The magnetic force between magnets depends on the strength of the magnets and the distance between them
Some materials (conductors) conduct electric charges, and others (insulators) do not	Some materials (ferromagnetic) can be easily magnetized, whereas others cannot be
Electric fields exist around electric charges	Magnetic fields exists around magnets

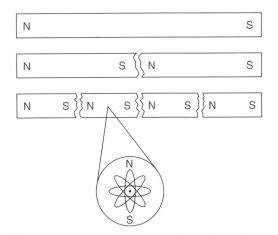

FIGURE 5–1. A permanent bar magnet. This figure demonstrates the nonexistence of an isolated north or south magnetic pole. Even an isolated atom from this metal will have north and south magnetic poles.

Since each atom behaves as a tiny magnet, it is thought that the behavior of a group of atoms, known as a magnetic domain, determines the overall magnetic properties of the bar as a whole. An unmagnetized bar has its magnetic domains (i.e., groupings of its magnetic atoms) randomly oriented, giving the bar no net or overall magnetic properties. That is, the random orientations would tend to "cancel out" any enhancement of magnetic properties of the bar. Conversely, if the magnetic domains are aligned or pulled into the same direction, the magnetic properties of the bar are enhanced, and the bar is then said to be magnetized (Fig. 5–2). These domains can be relatively easily aligned by taking a ferromagnetic material (e.g., iron or steel bar) and gently dragging a strong magnet across it many times. The magnetic force exerted by

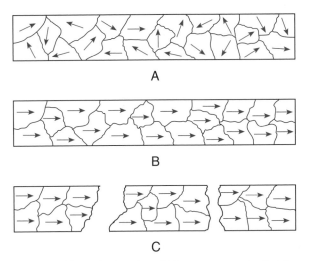

FIGURE 5–2. Magnetic domains within an unmagnetized and magnetized bar. In the unmagnetized bar (A), domains are randomly oriented, resulting in no net magnetic properties. If the bar is magnetized (B), the domains are aligned. When this occurs, even if the bar is cut into sections (C), each section behaves as an independent bar magnet, having a north and south pole.

the magnet pulls the domains into alignment, and now the bar too behaves like a magnet.

This also explains why heating and mechanical jarring can destroy a permanent magnet. Recall that when heat energy is added to a substance, its atoms increase their average kinetic energy by moving about. As more heat energy is added, the atoms and their magnetic domains become more randomly oriented, thereby decreasing the overall magnetic properties of the material. Mechanical jarring, such as hammering or dropping a magnet, would also tend to disturb the alignment of the domains and again would reduce the overall magnetic properties of the material. It should be pointed out that the source of the magnetic properties of an atom has yet to be explained. In addition, all atoms do not have magnetic properties. These ideas and observations are explained as you continue study of magnetism and magnetic effects.

MAGNETIC FIELDS

Magnets, like electric charges, have the ability to exert force over a distance. This implies that a *magnetic field* exists in the region of space surrounding the magnet, since the magnet can exert a force of attraction (or repulsion) on other magnets or magnetic materials brought into its vicinity. Also, like the electric field discussed in Chapter 4, magnetic fields have a direction associated with them. The electric field direction was defined as the direction of the force exerted on a small positive test charge. Recall, however, that unlike electric charges, magnetic poles cannot be separated. Therefore magnetic field lines are defined as being in the direction of force exerted on a small hypothetical north pole.

(Note: The term *hypothetical* means that a north magnetic pole does not actually exist by itself but its existence is assumed for purposes of definition.) Several sample magnetic fields are shown in Figure 5–3. Figure 5–3*A* shows the magnetic field of a permanent bar magnet. Since magnetic field lines represent the direction of force on a north magnetic pole, it is important to note that magnetic field lines are directed outward from the north pole of the magnet (since like poles repel) and are directed inward toward the south pole (since a north pole would feel a force of attraction from the south pole).

Magnetic field lines on the sides of the magnet bend since an individual north pole placed at these points feels both a force of repulsion from the magnet's north pole and a force of attraction to the south pole. Both of these forces acting simultaneously cause a north pole to curve as it travels from the north end of the magnet to the south end. From the illustration it can be said that outside a bar magnet, magnetic field lines travel from north to south. If we assume these magnetic field lines to be continuous, inside the bar magnet the magnetic field lines travel from south to north.

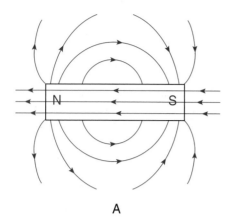

A

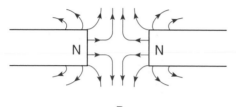

B

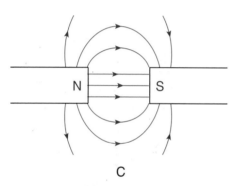

C

FIGURE 5–3. Magnetic field configurations. Magnetic field line directions are shown for a single permanent bar magnet *(A)*, two north poles of two bar magnets *(B)*, and a north and a south pole of two bar magnets *(C)*. These lines indicate the direction of the magnetic force that would be exerted on a hypothetical north pole.

This is important to remember for concepts discussed later in the chapter.

Also shown are magnetic field configurations for two magnetic north poles (Fig. 5–3*B*) and for a magnetic north and south pole (Fig. 5–3*C*). In your study of these patterns, recall that these field lines indicate the direction of the magnetic force exerted on a small north pole.

Magnetic field strength, indicating the magnitude of the magnetic force exerted on an object, is measured in the SI unit known as the *tesla (T)*. The strength of the earth's magnetic field at sea level is of the order of 3×10^{-5} T, whereas the magnetic field near a strong permanent magnet may be of the order of 0.1 T. Magnets now being commonly used in medical imaging (magnetic resonance imaging) have field strengths of 1.5 T, some 50,000 times stronger than the magnetic field of the earth at sea level. In illustrations and in text, as appropriate, the magnetic field is designated as **B**.

MAGNETIC FIELDS AND ELECTRICAL CURRENTS

Oersted's Experiment

The numerous similarities between electricity and magnetism (as outlined in Table 5–1) in addition to the almost identical field patterns produced by permanent magnets and certain electrical charge distributions (Fig. 5–4) led early investigators to suspect an even closer relationship between two seemingly different phenomena.

One of the early investigators who sought the missing link between electricity and magnetism was the Danish physicist Hans Oersted. Oersted's experimental approach was simple. He placed a compass needle (recall that it is just a small magnet) beneath a current-carrying wire. If the wire through which the current flowed produced any magnetic effects, the compass needle would be deflected. Unfortunately, Oersted originally oriented the compass needle perpendicular (i.e., at a 90° angle) to the wire that would carry the current (Fig. 5–5*A*). When the current was allowed to flow through the wire, no deflection of the needle was seen. Oersted had almost concluded that even though there were striking similarities between the two phenomena, there was no apparent connection between them. Then the story is told, one day Oersted was demonstrating his experimental apparatus. The equipment was accidentally jarred so that the compass needle was aligned parallel to the wire. To his amazement, when the current was switched on, the compass needle was deflected. Thus the compass needle had to be oriented parallel to the current-carrying wire for the effect to be seen (Fig. 5–5*B*). Two important concepts arise from this simple experiment:

1. A magnetic field is produced by electrical charges only when the charge is in motion. Note: This indicates that only electric currents produce magnetic fields. Stationary charges produce only electric fields but no magnetic fields.)
2. The **B** lines produced by a current-carrying wire encircle the wire in the form of concentric rings. The direction of the magnetic field lines is easily determined by the right-hand rule. (Note: Using only the right hand, position your thumb parallel to the wire and in the direction of current flow (I), i.e., in the direction opposite electron movement. Your remaining four fingers, wrapped around the insulated wire will indicate the direction of the wire's associated magnetic field. Application of this concept is shown in Figure 5–6.)

Thus the link between electricity and magnetism was established. Charges in motion produce not only electric fields but magnetic fields also. This physical principle allows magnets to be used to control the motion of fast-moving charged particles in many electronic devices.

Magnetic field lines   Electric field lines

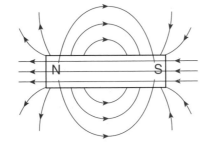

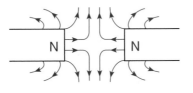
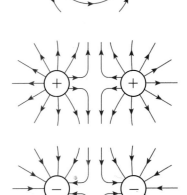

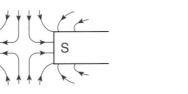

FIGURE 5–4. A comparison of magnetic and electric field line configurations for several magnetic pole and electric charge distributions. The similarities between the two indicate an apparent relationship between the two seemingly different phenomena.

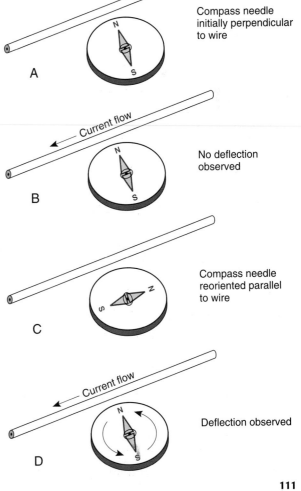

Compass needle initially perpendicular to wire

A

No deflection observed

B

Compass needle reoriented parallel to wire

C

Deflection observed

D

FIGURE 5–5. Oersted's experiment, which demonstrates that a current-carrying wire produces a magnetic field and also the importance of orientation in seeing the effect. In (A) the compass needle is oriented at a 90° angle to the wire, but no deflection is observed when a current is passed through the wire (B). If the needle is initially aligned along the wire (C), the needle is deflected when current flow is restored (D).

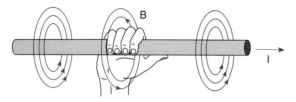

FIGURE 5–6. Use of the right hand rule to determine the magnetic field direction around a current-carrying wire. With the thumb of the right hand in the direction of current flow, the curled fingers indicate the direction of the associated magnetic field lines (B). I represents current flow. (Beiser, A. Modern Technical Physics, © 1992, Addison-Wesley Publishing co., Inc., Reading, Massachusetts. Reprinted with permission of the publisher.)

Magnetic Field of a Current-Carrying Solenoid

After Oersted's discovery that a current-carrying wire produced a magnetic field, it was found that if the wire was wound into a coil, known as a *solenoid* (Fig. 5–7A), one end of the coil would behave like a north magnetic pole, whereas the other end would behave like a south magnetic pole.

If the current (I) flow through the coil was reversed, the magnetic polarity of the coil would also reverse (Fig. 5–7B,C). The magnetic polarity of a current-carrying solenoid can easily be determined by again using the right-hand rule, remembering that such a device acts like a simple bar magnet.

In Figure 5–7B, current flow is shown flowing up the outside of the coil. Place the thumb of your right hand parallel to the direction of current flow on the outside of the coil as shown. When the remaining four fingers are curled into the center of the coil, these fingers (which represent the **B** lines), are directed from right to left. Thus the **B** lines travel within the coil

from right to left. Recall that a current-carrying solenoid behaves like a bar magnet and that magnetic field lines inside a bar magnet travel from south to north, then the right end of the coil behaves like a south magnetic pole and the left end behaves like a north magnetic pole. Determining which end of the coil behaves as the north and which as the south magnetic pole is known as determining the coil's *magnetic polarity*. If the direction of current flow through the coil is reversed, the right-hand rule can also be used to verify that the magnetic polarity also reverses. (Note: To apply the right-hand rule correctly, the palm of the right hand should always be directed toward you.)

The Search for Symmetry

Once it had been determined that an electric current could be used to generate a magnetic field, there began a search to determine if a magnetic field could be used

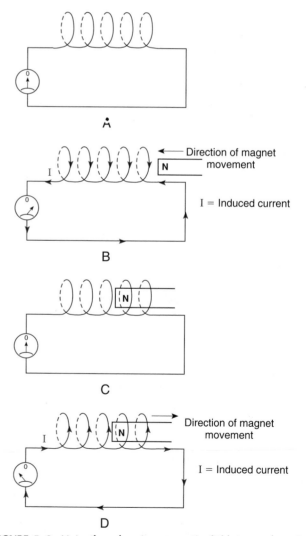

FIGURE 5–8. Use of a changing magnetic field to produce an electric current. A complete path is constructed containing a solenoid and galvanometer (A). When a magnet is thrust into the coil, a current is observed to flow (B). When there is no change in the magnetic field (i.e., the magnet is stationary), no current flows (C). If the magnet is withdrawn from the coil, a current is again induced in the wire, but it flows in the opposite direction (D).

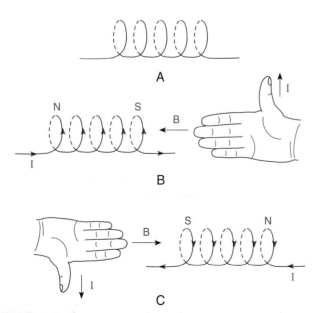

FIGURE 5–7. The magnetic polarity of a current-carrying solenoid. A solenoid (A) behaves like a bar magnet when a current is passed through the coils (B). If current direction is reversed, the magnetic polarity of the coil is also reversed (C).

to produce electricity—a search for symmetry. If a coil of wire (i.e., a solenoid) is placed in a simple circuit containing a device known as a *galvanometer* used to measure small amounts of current flow, as shown in Figure 5–8A, no current is observed to flow since the circuit does not contain a battery or power supply. However, when a bar magnet is thrust into the coil, the galvanometer needle deflects, indicating that a current momentarily flows in the wire. If the magnet remains still within the coil, no current flows. When the magnet is removed from the coil, the galvanometer needle is observed to deflect in the opposite direction, indicating again that a current momentarily flows in the circuit but in a direction opposite the original direction of flow. This is illustrated in Figure 5–8B to D.

Thus another important relationship was discovered. A magnetic field could be used to generate an electric current. However, in order to do this, the magnetic field had to be changing or there had to be relative motion between the wires and the magnetic field. (Note: Relative motion implies that it does not matter which is moving relative to the other—a magnetic field that changes across a stationary coil, a coil that moves through a stationary magnetic field, or a coil that moves through a changing magnetic field.)

Application to Radiography
Generators and electric motors (each is explained later in more detail)

■■■■

LENZ'S LAW: DETERMINING DIRECTION OF INDUCED CURRENT FLOW

When a magnetic field is moved across a coil of wire, a current (I) is induced or made to flow in the wires of the coil. The direction in which the induced current flows is determined by the use of a principle known as Lenz's law, which is stated as follows:

Lenz's Law: When a changing magnetic field is used to induce a current in a solenoid, the induced current flows in such a direction that its associated magnetic field opposes the change in the magnetic field that first induced the current to flow in the coil.

This principle is best understood by using a simple example. When the north pole of a bar magnet is pushed into a solenoid as shown in Figure 5–9A, the induced current must flow through the wires in such a direction that the magnetic field produced in the coil opposes the magnetic field of the magnet. The only way this can happen is if the right end of the coil takes on north pole characteristics (so as to oppose the north pole entering the coil) and the left end acquires south pole characteristics.

Lenz's law thus establishes the *magnetic polarity* of the coil, that is, which end is north and which south. Once this has been determined, one then needs only to apply the right-hand rule to determine the direction of current flow. Recalling that the coil behaves like a bar magnet and that **B** lines inside a bar magnet travel from south to north, the direction of induced current flow is determined by positioning the fingers of the right hand (which represents the direction of the magnetic field lines) in the coil in the direction from south to north. When this is done, the thumb is seen to be pointing downward on the outside of the coil as shown in Figure 5–9B. The thumb indicates the direction of the induced current flow.

In a similar manner, if the north pole is withdrawn from the coil, the right end of the coil must take on south pole characteristics so as to oppose the withdrawal of the magnet. This is shown in Figure 5–9C. Once the magnetic polarity of the coil has been determined, the right-hand rule can be used once again to determine the direction of the induced current as shown in Figure 5–9D. As seen in the figure, the di-

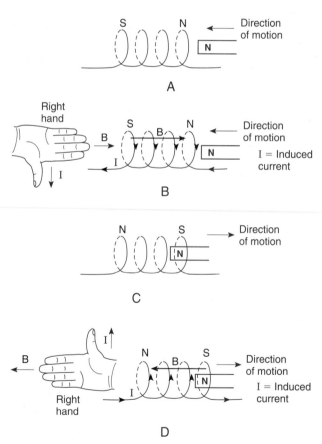

FIGURE 5–9. Application of Lenz's law to determine direction of induced current flow resulting from a changing magnetic field. *A,* North pole thrust into solenoid. *B,* By Lenz's law, a magnetic field of coil must oppose the north pole entering the coil. Since the coil acts as a bar magnet, the magnetic field inside is directed from south to north as indicated. Using the right hand with fingers directed inside the coil in the direction of B, the thumb indicates the direction of the induced current, i. *C,* The north pole is withdrawn from the coil. *D,* Coil polarity reverses, B field direction reverses, and induced current flow also reverses according to Lenz's law.

rection of the induced current flow is reversed when the magnet is withdrawn from the coil.

> **Application to Radiography Equipment**
> The principle of induction motors used to turn rotating anodes (this is explained later in more detail)

GENERATORS

A *generator* is a device designed to convert mechanical energy of motion into electrical energy. A generator utilizes the principle that a changing magnetic field can be used to produce a current. As previously mentioned, there need be only relative motion between a magnet and a coil in order to induce a current within the coil. "Relative motion" here implies that the coil can be moved through a stationary magnetic field, the magnetic field over the coil can be changed, or both can happen simultaneously with the same end result —namely, that a current is induced to flow through the wires of the coil. Therefore a simple device could be designed in which a coil of wire (solenoid) is made to rotate within a stationary magnetic field as shown in Figure 5–10. As the coil is rotated, an electrical current is generated in the wires of the coil. This device, which converts energy of motion (i.e., the rotation of the coil) into electrical energy (i.e., the electric current produced), is known as a generator. This type

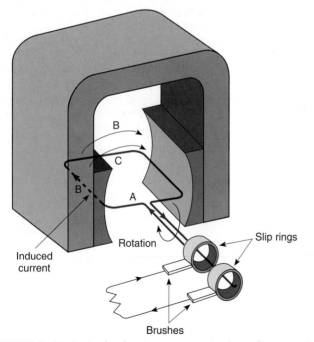

FIGURE 5–10. A simple electric generator. As the coil is rotated through the stationary magnetic field of the magnet, an electrical current is induced in the wire. (Beiser, A. *Modern Technical Physics*, © 1992, Addison-Wesley Publishing Co., Inc., Reading, Massachusetts. Reprinted with permission of the publisher.)

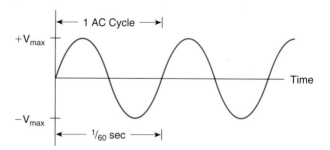

FIGURE 5–11. The sinusoidal variation of AC voltage. AC voltage (and current) fluctuates through maximum and minimum values in each AC cycle. The time required for one cycle of 60-Hz AC is 1/60 second.

of generator that utilizes a single coil is referred to as a single-phase generator.

The current produced by a generator in its simplest form is known as an *alternating current (AC)*. It is designated as such because the current produced within the coil alternates its direction of motion. Because there is a definite relationship between the position of the coil and the magnetic field lines through which the coil rotates, coil orientation within the magnetic field determines both the magnitude and the direction of the resulting induced current. As illustrated in Figure 5–11, as the coil is rotated through one full 360° revolution in the magnetic field (referred to as a cycle), a voltage is induced in the coil that varies in time in magnitude and sign. The resulting current also varies in time. This variation in time of the induced voltage and current is described most appropriately by a sinusoidal curve, also shown in Figure 5–11. (Note: This type of curve is designated as sinusoidal since it describes the variation of the trigonometric function known as the sine or cosine.)

To more completely describe an AC cycle by using the sinusoidal curve, refer to Figure 5–12. As the rotating coil turns through its first half turn (i.e., through 180°), the voltage induced in the wire of the coil increases from zero to the maximum voltage (designated V_{max}) then decreases back to zero. During the second half of the rotation, the voltage decreases from zero to a negative maximum voltage then returns to zero. The rotating coil returns to its original orientation, and as it continues to turn, a new AC cycle begins. In the United States, AC current is generated at a frequency (i.e., the number of cycles per unit time) of 60 cycles per second, or 60 Hertz. (Note: Hertz (Hz) is the SI unit of frequency and is equivalent to 1 cycle per second). This is referred to as *60-cycle AC*. In many portions of the world, AC current is generated at 50 cycles per second, or 50 Hz.

As the voltage fluctuates through each AC cycle, so does the induced current, similar to Figure 5–12. During the positive half of the voltage cycle, current increases from zero to some maximum value (I_{max}) then returns to zero. During the negative portion of the voltage cycle, the charges moving in the wire reverse and flow in the opposite direction. With 60-cycle AC, this reversal occurs 120 times each second. Thus the current stops 120 times each second, once at the be-

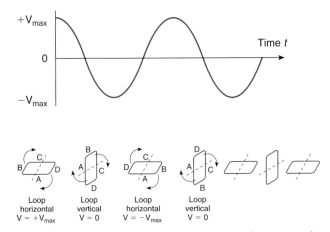

FIGURE 5–12. Generation of the AC voltage waveform as a coil in a stationary magnetic field. The sinusoidally varying voltage is produced as the coil makes a complete rotation in the magnetic field. Each rotation of the coil produces one AC cycle. (Beiser, A. *Modern Technical Physics,* © 1992, Addison-Wesley Publishing Co., Inc., Reading, Massachusetts. Reprinted with permission of the publishers).

ginning of the cycle and again at the midway point in the cycle. Several important points regarding AC current need to be emphasized:

- Electric charges moving in an AC current change their direction of flow 120 times each second (60-cycle AC). Recall that in order for a current to flow, charge must be in motion regardless of its direction of movement.
- An AC voltage fluctuates in a sinusoidal manner. During an AC cycle, voltage values range from zero to a maximum (V_{max}) then back to zero. Voltage then decreases to a minimum value ($-V_{max}$) and returns again to zero.
- As the AC voltage fluctuates, the resulting AC current also fluctuates sinusoidally. Recall that voltage provides the "push" that causes charges to move. The AC voltage variation in each AC cycle causes charges moving in the circuit to vary in speed and therefore in kinetic energy. The moving electrons have maximum kinetic energy at those points in the AC cycle at which voltage has maximum value, either positive or negative. Kinetic energy ranges from zero to these maximum values at all other points in the AC cycle.

Another important aspect of the AC cycle is the interpretation of the negative portion of the AC voltage curve shown in Figure 5–12. In a DC circuit, such as that including a battery as the voltage source, electrons only flow in one direction—from the negative to the positive terminal of the battery. With an AC voltage source, during the positive portion of the AC voltage cycle, electrons also flow from negative to positive. However, the negative portion of the AC voltage cycle has the same effect as reversing the electrical polarity of the voltage source. That is, the negative terminal becomes positive and the positive terminal becomes negative. As a result, electrons reverse their direction

of flow during this portion of the cycle—hence the name, alternating current.

The type of generator that has been discussed in this section involves a generator design consisting of a single coil of wire rotated in a stationary magnetic field and designated a single-phase (often abbreviated 1ϕ) AC generator. Single-phase generators are characterized by the production of single wave and sinusoidally varying voltages and currents. In later chapters on x-ray equipment, it is shown that single-phase generators are not the most efficient for the production of useful x-rays for medical diagnosis. As a result, a variation in this simple, single-coil design in order to produce a more efficient x-ray generator has been made. This more efficient generator is known as a three-phase (abbreviated 3ϕ) generator. This generator is discussed later in the chapter.

Application to Radiography Equipment
High-voltage generators are necessary for the production of x-rays in the x-ray tube

---

RECTIFICATION

The x-rays used in radiography are produced by an x-ray tube within the x-ray machine. The components and design of the tube are discussed in much greater detail in Chapter 6, but here is a basic description of how x-rays are generated. In general, an x-ray tube consists of a *glass envelope* which contains two basic *electrodes*—one positive (known as the *anode*) and the other negative (known as the *cathode*). Air is evacuated from the tube, and electrons are made to flow from the cathode to the anode by the application of high voltage provided by a high-voltage AC generator. The high voltage present across the electrodes provides the electrical force necessary to pull the electrons at high speeds to the positive anode. When these fast-moving electrons strike a small region on the anode

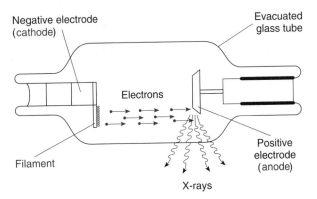

FIGURE 5–13. The standard x-ray tube produces x-rays only when fast-moving electrons flow from cathode to anode. Electrons emitted from the filament are accelerated from the cathode to the positively charged anode. Only when the electrons strike the anode are x-rays produced.

■ RECTIFIERS

Rectifiers are circuit components that allow current to flow in only one direction. These devices are needed in AC x-ray circuits, since in the conventional x-ray tube, x-rays are produced only when electrons flow from the cathode to the anode target. In past years, vacuum tubes containing two electrodes (i.e., a cathode and an anode) were used. These tubes were known as *diodes,* or valve tubes (Fig. 1). Similar in basic design to the x-ray tube, these tubes would allow electrons to move only from cathode to anode. This would certainly be true during the positive half of the AC voltage cycle when the cathode is negative and the anode positive. During the negative portion of the cycle, the anode is held at a relatively low voltage that prevents electron movement between the electrodes. Therefore electrons travel between the electrodes, and subsequent x-rays are produced only during the positive half of the AC cycle. Various numbers of these rectifiers could be arranged in an x-ray circuit to produce either half-wave or full-wave rectification.

It is more common today to find solid state rectifiers, specifically solid state silicon rectifiers (Figs. 2 and 3). These devices consist of a semiconductor (silicon) and an added substance known as an impurity (e.g., arsenic, antimony, indium, gallium, or aluminum). Depending on the impurity used, a semiconductor results that either has an excess number of electrons (known as donor) or a deficiency of electrons (known as acceptor). Junctions are formed between these two types of semiconducting materials within the solid state rectifier. Current will flow through these junctions only if the appropriate voltage polarity is applied. Thus the solid state device acts as a true rectifier—allowing current to flow in one direction during half of the AC voltage cycle but no current flow when the voltage polarity reverses.

Solid state rectifiers have several advantages over valve tubes in that they have longer life spans, produce more consistent x-ray output, and do not produce any radiation as a result of their use within the x-ray circuit.

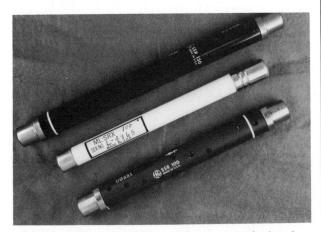

FIGURE 2. Solid-state silicon rectifiers commonly found in today's x-ray equipment.

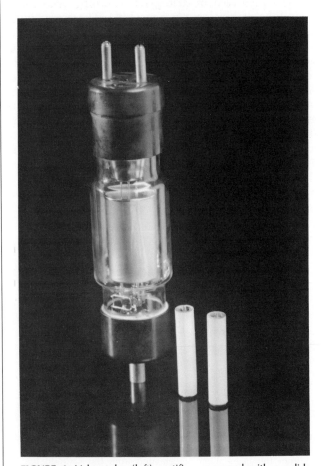

FIGURE 1. Valve tube (left) rectifier compared with a solid-state rectifier.

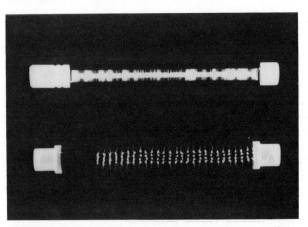

FIGURE 3. Radiograph of two solid-state silicon rectifiers, showing strings of diodes required to rectify kilovoltage levels of AC used in standard x-ray equipment.

known as the target, x-rays are produced. (In order for these x-rays to be produced, electrons must actually strike the target anode.) This is shown schematically in Figure 5–13.

A problem immediately arises, stemming from the fact that voltage across the electrodes is produced by an AC generator. Recall from the previous discussion that AC voltage fluctuates sinusoidally in every AC cycle. The first half of each cycle voltage is positive— that is, the anode is positive, the cathode is negative, electrons flow from cathode to anode, and x-rays are generated. During the second half of the cycle, however, voltage turns negative. When this occurs, electrical polarity of the electrodes is reversed—that is, the anode becomes negative, the cathode becomes positive, no electrons flow to the target anode with the result that there is no x-ray production.

Needless to say, this is an inefficient way to produce x-rays. X-rays would be produced only during the positive half of each AC cycle. With 60-cycle AC, there would be 60 "bursts" of x-rays each second, but only half of the electrical energy available for their production would be used. X-ray circuits that operate in this manner, producing x-rays during only half of an AC cycle, are said to be half-wave rectified. Circuit components known as rectifiers (see Rectifiers, in box) are used in x-ray circuits to perform specific functions with the sinusoidally varying AC voltage waveform. Rectifiers are circuit elements (designated in circuit diagrams by the symbol →|) that allow current to flow in only one direction. Depending on the number of rectifiers used within the circuit, these devices may be used in one of two ways: (1) to suppress the negative portion of the AC cycle (*half-wave rectification*) or (2) to make the negative portion of each AC cycle positive (*full-wave rectification*). (Recall that x-rays are produced only during positive portions of the AC cycle.)

Half-Wave Rectification

Half-wave rectification occurs when no rectifier or one or two rectifiers are used in the x-ray circuit. When no rectifier is used in the circuit, the x-ray tube itself acts as a rectifier, allowing electrons to flow only from cathode to anode. An x-ray circuit in which the x-ray tube is the only rectifier in the circuit is said to be *self-rectified*.

In half-wave rectified circuits, the rectifiers act to suppress the negative portion of the AC cycle (Fig. 5–14), resulting in 60 AC voltage pulses per second. Since x-rays are produced in the x-ray tube whenever there is a positive voltage pulse, an x-ray tube under 60-cycle, half-wave rectified voltage produces 60 "bursts" of x-rays each second. Each burst lasts one half of 1/60 second, or 1/120 second (Fig. 5–14).

Full-Wave Rectification

As previously pointed out, half-wave rectified voltage makes use of only half of the AC voltage waveform. If four rectifiers are used in the x-ray circuit, electrons

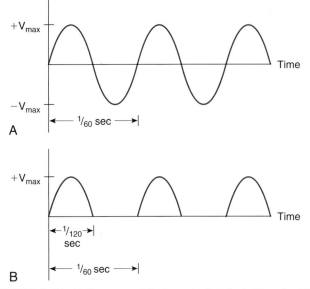

FIGURE 5–14. Half-wave rectification. *A,* Standard 60-cycle AC voltage waveform. *B,* Full-wave rectification inverts the negative portion of the AC cycle to produce 120-Hz pulsed DC.

are allowed to flow in only one direction, from cathode to anode, through both portions of the AC cycle. This has the effect of making the negative portion of each AC voltage waveform positive, which means that through each portion of the cycle, the tube cathode remains negative and its anode positive as indicated in Figure 5–15. As a result, electrons always flow from cathode to anode, resulting in x-ray production. When each portion of the AC voltage waveform is positive, 120 bursts of x-rays are produced each second (i.e., two bursts every 1/60 second), each burst lasting one half of 1/60 second, or 1/120 second. An obvious advantage of full-wave rectification is that the x-ray production approximately doubles compared with half-wave rectification.

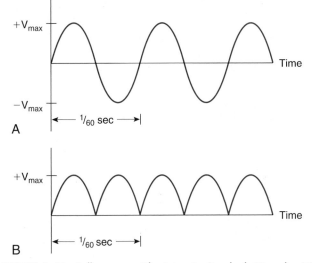

FIGURE 5–15. Full-wave rectification. *A,* Standard 60-cycle AC voltage waveform. *B,* Full-wave rectification inverts the negative portion of the AC cycle to produce 120-Hz pulsed DC.

THREE-PHASE GENERATORS

Single- vs. Three-Phase Generators

Earlier in this chapter, the simplest type of electric generator was discussed. This generator, known as a single-phase (1ϕ) generator, consists of a single coil of wire rotated within a stationary magnetic field. As the coil rotates, the coil experiences a changing magnetic field that "induces" or generates a voltage (and resulting current) within the wires of the coil. This AC voltage (current) generated by the rotating coil has been shown to vary in time as a sinusoidal wave with both positive and negative components (see Fig. 5–12). Since the direction of flow of electrons from cathode (−) to anode (+) cannot be reversed in the x-ray tube and still produce x-rays, rectifiers were introduced into the x-ray circuit to prevent this current flow reversal during the negative portion of the AC cycle. One problem, however, still remained. Using even half-wave or full-wave rectified circuits, the voltages across the electrodes of the x-ray tube drop to zero at times during each cycle. If the voltage across the electrodes is not at its maximum value, the x-rays generated are lower in energy and therefore not as penetrating. This generally results in a lower-quality image and increased radiation dose to the patient. In order to minimize these problems, three-phase (3ϕ) generators are more commonly used.

Before considering the differences in voltage outputs of 1ϕ and 3ϕ generators, let us first consider the meaning of *phase*. Phase refers to the relative position of the crests (high points) and troughs (low points) of one wave to the crests and troughs of a second wave (see Phase Relationships, in box).

Rather than utilizing a single coil of wire in a changing magnetic field to generate the standard AC waveform, the 3ϕ generator uses three wire coils, also known as *stator* windings, mechanically arranged 120° apart as shown in Figure 5–16. With these stator coils, each separated by 120° from the others, as each is exposed to a changing magnetic field, three AC sinusoidal waveforms are generated. The actual physical location of the three stators as described results in three AC waveforms that are 120° out of phase with each other.

The advantage of such an arrangement is seen in a comparison of the AC voltage waveforms produced by a 1ϕ generator and by a 3ϕ unit. As shown in Figure 5–15*A*, a 1ϕ generator produces a sinusoidal voltage waveform that when full-wave rectified, resembles the one shown in Figure 5–15*B*. Recall that this represents the voltage as it is applied across the x-ray tube electrodes, and it can be seen that the voltage fluctuates from zero to V_{max} (maximum voltage) then back to zero twice during each cycle. The primary problem

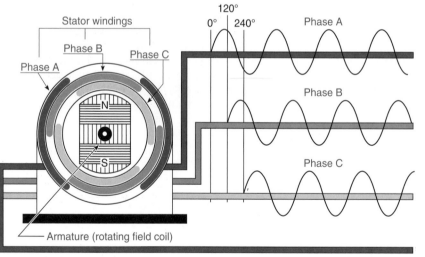

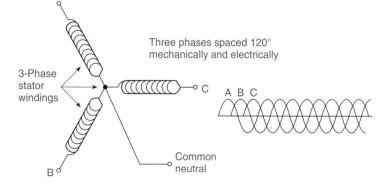

FIGURE 5–16. The three-phase AC generator. The three-phase generator produces three AC voltage waveforms which are each 120° out of phase with each other to produce a composite voltage waveform having minimal ripple. (From Hazen M., Experiencing Electricity & Electronics. Philadelphia: W.B. Saunders College Publishing, 1989.)

■ PHASE RELATIONSHIPS

Phase refers to the relative position of two or more waves in relation to each other. A sinusoidal wave consists of a repeating series of alternating crests (points of highest amplitude) and troughs (points of lowest amplitude) as shown here in Figure 4.

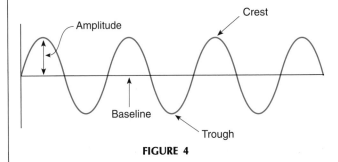

FIGURE 4

Waves can be added using a technique known as the principle of *superposition,* which consists of a point-by-point addition of the wave amplitudes. Amplitudes above the base line are considered to be positive and those below the base line, negative. The wave that results from this process of wave addition is known as a composite wave. The exact form and shape that the composite wave takes depends on the phase relationship existing between the two waves.

Two waves are totally *in phase* when "crests meet crests" and "troughs meet troughs" as shown in Figure 5. It should be noted that when waves A and B are added, the composite wave is a wave of increased amplitude.

Note: The composite wave shown above has an amplitude of 5 since the amplitudes of waves A and B are 2 and 3 respectively.

Two waves are totally *out of phase* (or what is commonly termed *180° out of phase*) when "crests meet troughs." When this occurs the composite wave is a wave of reduced amplitude as shown in Figure 6.

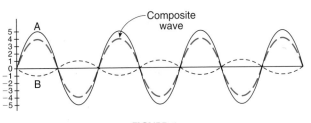

FIGURE 6

Note: The composite wave shown has an amplitude of 4 since the amplitude waves A and B are 5 and 1 respectively.

Composite waves of much greater complexity can be produced by using this method of adding waves having various phase relationships. The exact phase relationship between two waves is expressed by a phase angle that may range from 0° to 360°. Waves are then said to be in phase, 30° out of phase, 90° out of phase, 180° out of phase, and so forth. The final shape of the composite wave depends on the amplitudes and phases of the individual waves added as demonstrated in Figure 7.

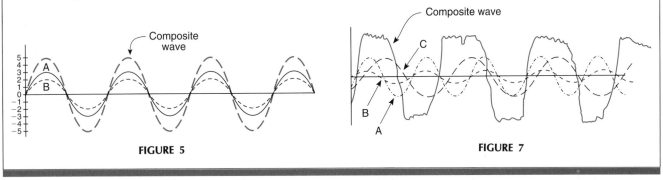

FIGURE 5

FIGURE 7

with this type of voltage variation is that no x-rays are produced when the voltage across the x-ray tube electrodes is zero. In addition, only lower-energy, less penetrating x-rays are produced when the voltage is lower than V_{max}. When full-wave rectification is used in conjunction with a 3ϕ generator, the resulting composite waveform (see Phase Relationships, in box) is one in which the voltage remains almost constant. This comes

about as a result of the addition of the three voltage waveforms generated 120° out of phase with each other. This resulting composite waveform is shown in Figure 5–17.

It can be observed that as the negative portion of each individual waveform is made positive through rectification, the result is six voltage "bumps," or pulses, each cycle (i.e., 1/60 second). These pulses in

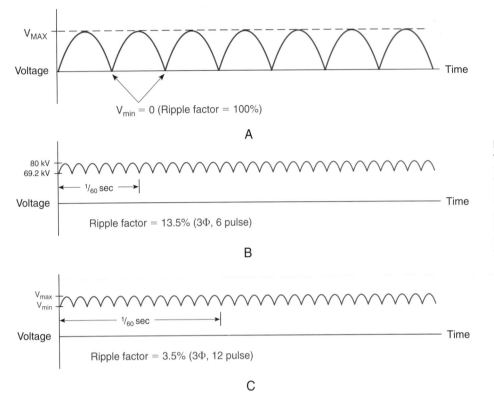

FIGURE 5–17. Typical voltage waveforms for single and three-phase generators. *A,* Voltage waveforms for a single-phase, full-wave rectified generator, demonstrating 100% ripple. *B,* Voltage waveform for a three-phase, six-pulse unit having a 13.5% ripple. *C,* A ripple factor of 3.5% obtained with a three-phase, 12-pulse generator.

the voltage waveform are referred to as voltage ripple. The *ripple factor* is the maximum drop in voltage expressed as a percentage of the V_{max}. This is demonstrated in Figure 5–17. Single-phase, full-wave rectified voltage has a 100% ripple factor (Fig. 5–17*A*), since the fluctuations in its voltage has a minimum value of zero (i.e., $V_{min} = V_{max} - 100\% \ V_{max} = 0$).

Three-phase generators in circuits producing six-pulse voltages exhibit ripple factors of 13.5%. As shown in Figure 5–17, in such a circuit, when the V_{max} is 80 kV (i.e., 80,000 volts), the lowest voltage across the x-ray tube electrodes should theoretically never drop below 80 kV − 13.5% (80 kV), or 69.2 kV. The ideal case would be to produce a constant, nonfluctuating voltage (i.e., 0% ripple). Modifications can be made in circuitry using 3ϕ generators to produce 12 pulses per AC cycle as shown in Figure 5–17*C*. The advantage of 3ϕ, 12-pulse voltage is that the ripple factor is theoretically reduced to 3.5%. Under actual working conditions, a ripple factor of approximately 5% is more realistic.

In the quest to obtain a near-constant voltage, 3ϕ generators have obvious advantages over 1ϕ units. Advantages include the following:

● Single-phase generators produce pulsating DC voltage (with the aid of appropriate rectifiers), whereas 3ϕ units (with proper rectification) produce DC voltage that more closely approximates a constant voltage source.
● Single-phase generators produce voltage pulses having a 100% ripple factor in comparison with 3ϕ units that with appropriate circuitry can produce voltages with ripple factors approaching 13.5% (6-pulse) and 3.5% (12-pulse).

● Three-phase generators produce more diagnostically useful x-rays per exposure, since the voltage supplied to the x-ray tube is nearer the maximum, or peak, voltage a greater percentage of the time in which the tube is activated. This results in the production of more x-rays of the desired energy.
● An x-ray unit utilizing a 3ϕ generator produces an x-ray beam of higher average energy than a beam produced by a 1ϕ unit as a result of the near-constant voltage provided by the 3ϕ system.
● Since the voltage across the x-ray tube electrodes is nearer the peak voltage a greater percentage of the time, more electrons can be pulled from the cathode to the anode of the tube per unit of time. This movement of charge between the tube electrodes is referred to as the *tube current.* This capability of 3ϕ units to produce high tube currents (1000 to 2000 mA for 3ϕ units compared with 300 to 500 mA for 1ϕ units) can greatly reduce the time required to produce a radiographic exposure (referred to as the *exposure time*). The ability to produce quality radiographs with extremely short exposure times along with the capability of making multiple exposures in rapid succession make 3ϕ units excellent for trauma radiography and fluoroscopic procedures.
● Patient radiation doses may be somewhat reduced with 3ϕ units, since higher-energy x-rays compose a larger portion of the x-ray beam. Higher-energy x-rays generally imply greater penetrating power and therefore less radiation energy deposited within the patient's body.

A comparison of 1ϕ and 3ϕ generators is summarized in Table 5–2.

Table 5–2: A COMPARISON OF TYPES OF X-RAY GENERATORS

	Generator Type			
Characteristics	**Single-Phase** (1ϕ)	**Three-Phase** (3ϕ) **6-Pulse**	**Three-Phase** (3ϕ) **12-Pulse**	**High-Frequency**
Waveform				
Method of producing waveform	Single 60-Hz AC voltage waveform	3 60-Hz AC voltage waveforms 120° out of phase with each other; also uses 3ϕ transformer with 6 or 12 rectifiers	3 60-Hz AC voltage waveforms 120° out of phase with each other; uses 3ϕ transformer having slight variation in coil design from 6 pulse units; also contains 12 rectifiers	1ϕ or 3ϕ 60-Hz AC voltage waveforms are rectified, then fed into a DC chopper where frequency is converted from 60 Hz to the kHz range
Ripple factor	100%	~13.5%	~3.5%	Less than 3.5%
Disadvantages to x-ray production	1. Voltage fluctuations result in nonefficient x-ray production 2. Voltage fluctuations result in x-rays of varying energies	1. Requires 3ϕ power 2. More expensive than 1ϕ units	1. Requires 3ϕ power 2. More expensive than 1ϕ units	1. More expensive units
Advantages to x-ray production	1. Usually less expensive than 3ϕ units 2. Can be made more efficient if full wave rectified	1. Voltage fluctuations minimized resulting in more efficient x-ray production 2. More efficient production of x-rays of appropriate energy	1. Even lower voltage variations result in higher x-ray production efficiency 2. More higher energy x-ray produced	1. Almost constant voltage results in perhaps highest x-ray production efficiency 2. More x-rays produced have the desired higher energies 3. Reduction in x-ray dose to patient 4. Smaller space requirements than other 3ϕ units

Other Types of X-ray Generator Units

Generators are designed to provide the voltage requirements necessary for proper x-ray tube operation. Without adequate voltage, diagnostic quality x-rays cannot be produced. The need for sufficiently high voltage could however pose serious problems when space is limited and in those cases in which radiographs must be made in locations other than the radiology department, such as the emergency room or intensive care units. The types of generators previously discussed, with their high-voltage transformers and associated circuitry, tend to be massive pieces of equipment not easily moved. Therefore other types of generators were designed to minimize these specific problems.

In the portable generator category, two specific types include the capacitor-discharge generator and now the more common battery-powered generator. Each of these generators lends itself to the portability required by mobile x-ray units but not without specific limitations. They are considered separately.

Capacitor-Discharge Generators

Recall from earlier discussions of circuit components that a capacitor is a device used to store electric charge. Therefore such a device could be designed that when charged, could provide the necessary kilovoltage to an x-ray tube to produce a diagnostic radiograph. Specifically, in this type of generator, standard incoming line voltage (110 or 220 V) is fed into the *primary* of the *step-up* (high-voltage) *transformer* (a device used to adjust voltage levels within the x-ray tube discussed later in this chapter). The *secondary* (output) voltage is rectified and is then used as the means of charging one or more capacitors. The voltage placed across the x-ray tube electrodes is controlled by the voltage across the capacitors. This is in turn governed by the output voltage of the high-voltage transformer, which is operator-controlled by adjustment of the kVp selector on the instrument control panel. This is schematically shown in Figure 5–18.

Capacitor-discharge units are usually compact and mobile. Most generators of this design have the capability of producing high tube currents with extremely short exposure times. Although tube currents produced with these units may be as high as 500 mA, limitations arise in the total amount of charge that can be supplied by the capacitors. The total charge that flows between the electrodes of the x-ray tube, which is equivalent to the tube current (in mA) multiplied by exposure time in seconds (s), referred to as mAs, is limited by the electrical characteristics of the capacitors used in the circuitry. (Note: mAs relates to the degree of darkening that occurs on an x-ray film as a result of exposure of the film to x-rays. Having an x-ray machine that can provide sufficient mAs, which varies with the portion of the body being radiographed as well as other factors, is fundamental in producing diagnostic quality radiographs. More will be said regarding mAs in later chapters.)

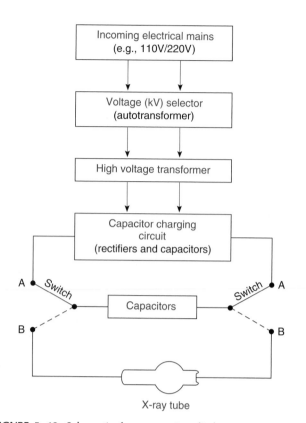

FIGURE 5–18. Schematic for a capacitor-discharge generator. Incoming line voltage is converted into the required high voltage through use of an autotransformer and a high-voltage transformer. When the switches are in the "A" position, this voltage is used to charge a capacitor or bank of capacitors. When the switches are in "B" position, the capacitors are discharged across the x-ray tube, allowing x-rays to be produced.

These units, as a result of their electrical design limitations, are commonly restricted to 30 to 50 mAs. As an example, 50 mAs could correspond to a tube current of 500 mA with an exposure time of 0.1 s (i.e., 500 mA × 0.1 s = 50 mAs). Short exposure times are most helpful in minimizing motion artifacts. Motion artifacts are image distortions caused by voluntary or involuntary body motion such as breathing, the motion of the heart, peristalsis, and so forth. However, for thicker body parts such as the abdomen, where higher mAs values are required, this type of generator system finds limited usefulness.

A drawback to this type of generator is that the kilovoltage across the x-ray tube falls with time. This occurs as a result of the characteristic method by which a capacitor discharges (see Chapter 4 of this text). Recall that as a capacitor discharges, the voltage across its plates drop exponentially with time. Thus for a capacitor-discharge unit, the kilovoltage across the tube would also drop exponentially with time, since it is dependent on the discharging of the capacitor. This factor can limit the use of this type of unit for radiographs requiring higher kilovoltage and longer exposure times.

Capacitor-discharge units must also be charged just prior to use (and after each exposure) by plugging the unit into an appropriate outlet. This occurs at the site where the radiograph is to be made.

Battery-Powered Generators

A more common design for today's mobile generators is the battery-powered generator. In this type of unit, a standard power supply (e.g., a standard AC wall outlet) is used to charge a bank of rechargeable nickel-cadmium batteries.

Recall that batteries provide DC current and that a high-voltage transformer (as any transformer) cannot operate on DC current since there is no constantly changing magnetic field. Therefore the current supplied by the batteries must first undergo modification. The modification is accomplished by passing the DC current from the batteries through a special circuit referred to as a DC chopper. This "chops" the otherwise constant current at regular intervals (typically 500 times each second, to produce 500-Hz pulsed DC current). This pulsed DC current is then directed to the primary side of the high-voltage transformer. The output voltage from this transformer is then rectified (since the output of a transformer is AC) and supplied to the x-ray tube in the form of a 1000-Hz, 1ϕ waveform. This waveform is then smoothed with appropriate circuitry to provide a near-constant voltage at the level required for quality diagnostic radiographs.

These units are usually larger and somewhat more difficult to maneuver. Batteries must routinely be charged, but the unit need not be connected to an electrical outlet to make x-ray exposures. Unlike the capacitor-discharge generator, in which kilovoltage and tube current drop through an exposure as a result of the method by which a capacitor becomes discharged, the battery-powered generator maintains constant voltage and tube current during an exposure.

As previously mentioned, x-ray generators are designed to provide as constant a voltage as possible to the x-ray tube. Maintaining an appropriate level of voltage that is constant and does not fluctuate is fundamental in producing sufficient numbers of x-rays and x-rays having sufficient energy (i.e., penetrating power). Single-phase generators having 100% ripple factors and subsequent improvements in design that led to the development of 3ϕ, 6- and 12-pulse generators in which ripple factors dropped significantly have been discussed previously. Still other generator designs were developed for specific radiographic applications, and their relative cost and size may greatly exceed those of designs previously discussed. Also, the determination must be made whether generators with a 1% or less ripple factor actually make better quality radiographs than those with a 3% ripple factor.

One major advancement in x-ray generator design has been the high-frequency generator. Use of high-frequency current has resulted in a generator having many advantages, such as more compact size, more efficient x-ray production, and voltage waveforms that may have less than a 3% ripple factor. As a result, high-frequency generators are becoming more commonplace in radiology departments.

The basic design of the high-frequency generator utilizes one of the basic physical principles of transformers:

> The magnitude of the voltage produced in the secondary coil of a transformer is directly proportional to how rapidly the current changes in the primary coil (a restatement of Faraday's law of induction).

Actually, the voltage output of the secondary coil is proportional to (1) how rapidly the magnetic field lines (or flux) change across the wires of the secondary coil, (2) the number of turns of wire on the secondary coil, and (3) the cross-sectional area of the coil. With this type generator, transformer output voltage is raised to the desired levels (40 kVp to 125 kVp) by increasing

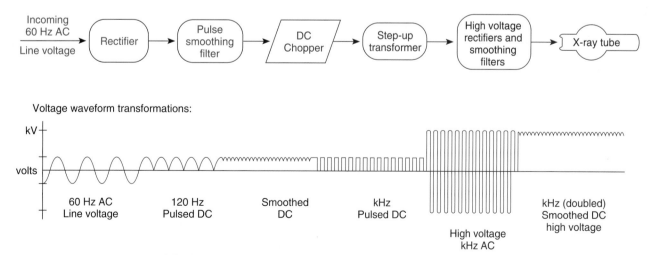

FIGURE 5–19. Basic components of the high-frequency generator and voltage waveform transformations as they occur in each component. Incoming 60-Hz AC line voltage is rectified, smoothed, and converted into high-frequency voltage that when rectified and further smoothed, results in almost constant DC high voltage as required for efficient x-ray production.

the frequency of the input current from 60-Hz AC to thousands of hertz, depending on generator design. Using higher-frequency current and with other circuitry modifications, the required increases in voltage can be obtained with simultaneous reductions in the number of turns of wire required on the secondary coil and reductions in the amount of iron on which the coil is wound. These modifications indicate that these generators are much smaller and more compact than conventional 1ϕ and 3ϕ units.

High-frequency generators take incoming 1ϕ, 60-Hz AC and pass this through rectification circuits to produce 120-Hz pulsed DC current. This current is smoothed and then put into a DC chopper in which its frequency is raised to thousands of hertz. This high-frequency, pulsed DC current is then directed into the primary of the high-voltage transformer. Since the output of the secondary is now AC, it is rectified once more, now doubling the output frequency. This high-frequency output waveform is smoothed again prior to being supplied to the x-ray tube. The voltage waveform supplied to the tube now has a ripple factor of less than the 3.5%, as is typical for 3ϕ, 12-pulse units that have greater space requirements. A general schematic outlay of a high-frequency unit is shown in Figure 5-19.

In summary, high-frequency units offer (1) a near-constant voltage to the x-ray tube; (2) more efficient production of diagnostic quality x-rays; (3) required kilovoltages produced by smaller, more efficient transformers, resulting in more compact design; and (4) extremely low ripple factors obtained using 1ϕ, 60-Hz AC line voltage. High-frequency generators are now found in both stationary and mobile x-ray equipment. More advantages of the high-frequency generator will be noted in later chapters.

ELECTRICAL MOTORS

Whereas electrical generators convert mechanical energy of motion (i.e., the motion of a coil of wire in a magnetic field or a stationary coil in a moving or changing magnetic field) into electrical energy, electrical motors do just the reverse. That is, an *electrical motor* is a device that converts electrical energy provided by an electrical current into mechanical energy of motion.

In a simple DC motor (i.e., one operating off a battery or DC power supply), one finds the same basic components as in the generator—specifically, coils of wire and a magnet (Fig. 5-20). The difference in this case is that an electrical current, produced by the battery or power supply, is sent through the wire coils.

As the current flows through the coils, a force is exerted on them as a result of the interactions of the two magnetic fields—that of the magnet and that generated around the current-carrying coils. To further enhance this effect, the coils are tightly wound around a ferromagnetic (e.g., iron) core. This assembly is then

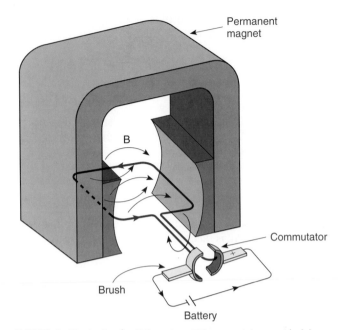

FIGURE 5–20. A simple DC motor. DC current is provided by a battery or DC power supply. Current flows through the wire coil, producing a magnetic field that interacts with the magnetic field of the magnet, producing rotation of the coil. The commutator acts to redirect the current flow in the coil to maintain a constant direction of coil rotation. (Beiser, A. Modern Technical Physics, © 1992, Addison-Wesley Publishing Co., Inc., Reading, Massachusetts. Reprinted with permission of the publisher).

mounted in such a way that it is free to rotate when an appropriate current is applied.

The force that causes the coil to rotate provides this "push" in one direction (e.g., clockwise) through only one half of a revolution of the coil. The direction of the force exerted on the coil reverses, however, during the second half of the turn of the coil as a result of the coil's new orientation within the magnetic field of the magnet. This can be prevented by reversing the direction of current flow in the coil during the second half of the rotation. In the DC motor, current flow reversal is accomplished every half revolution of the coil by the use of a split ring known as a commutator (also shown in Fig. 5-20). With this simple device, current flow in the coil is reversed every half rotation as the commutator makes contact with the brushes of reversed polarity. This action assures that the force applied to the coil always acts in the same direction to produce continuous rotation. As a result, the coil continues to rotate as long as current flow is maintained through it. The action of motors can be further improved with the use of (1) electromagnets rather than permanent magnets, (2) the use of more coils of wire, and (3) more turns of wire on each coil. In many motors, these multiple coils may be mounted on a slotted iron core (known as an *armature*) that is free to rotate when current flow begins. This basic design is illustrated in Figure 5-21.

An AC motor has the same basic design as the DC motor except that it does not need brushes or a commutator since the current flow naturally reverses its direction of flow 120 times per second (60-cycle AC).

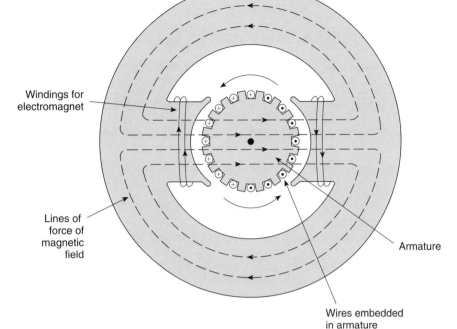

Windings for electromagnet

Lines of force of magnetic field

Armature

Wires embedded in armature

FIGURE 5–21. Armature of a simple electric motor. Multiple wire coils are wound through slots of the armature. The armature rotates as a result of the interacting magnetic fields of the electromagnet and the wires on the armature. (Beiser, A. Modern Technical Physics, © 1992. Addison-Wesley Publishing Co., Inc., Reading, Massachusetts. Reprinted with permission of the publisher).

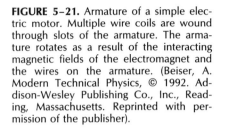

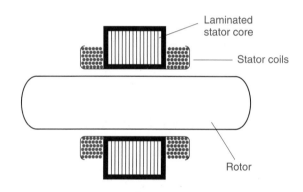

Laminated stator core

Stator coils

Rotor

A

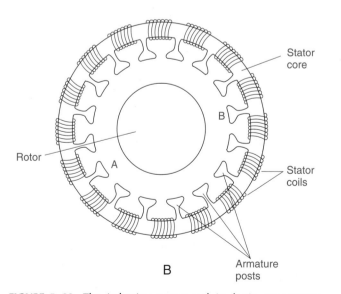

Stator core

B

Rotor

A

Stator coils

Armature posts

B

FIGURE 5–22. The induction motor and its basic components. A, Side view illustrating the relative locations of the stator coils and the rotor of an induction motor. B, End-on view of coil windings on a stator core surrounding the rotor.

These motors are designed to make the most effective use of the AC current supplied.

Two types of motors of special importance in radiography are synchronous and induction motors. A *synchronous motor* is designed to rotate at the same number of revolutions per minute (rpm) as the frequency of the current (such as 60-cycle AC) being supplied by the generator. Motors of this type are especially useful in timing devices such as clocks, since they can be made to make one revolution every 1/60 second or multiple thereof (e.g., 1/30 s, 1/20 s, 1/15 s).

The second type of motor extremely important in x-ray tube design is the *induction motor*. The basic components of this type of motor consist of a stator and a rotor. As shown in Figure 5–22, the stator is the outer, stationary portion of the motor, which normally consists of coils of copper wire wound on a ferromagnetic core. These are wound so as to form pairs of *electromagnets* that can be energized in sequence. The *rotor*, or part of the motor that is free to rotate, consists of a conducting copper cylinder (a metal cylinder on which a copper covering has been attached). The motor works on the principle of electromagnetic induction. During operation, the stator is supplied by a multiphase power source that activates each opposite pair (e.g., A and B, shown in Fig. 5–22B) of electromagnets. These electromagnetic pairs are powered in sequence in rapid succession. As a result, the conducting copper rotor is exposed to a changing magnetic field that in turn induces a current to flow in the copper. The interaction between the magnetic fields of the electromagnets of the stator and the magnetic fields induced in the copper results in a force being applied to the rotor that then causes it to rotate. Some induction motors can produce rotation rates as high as 10,000 rpm.

Application to Radiography Equipment
Synchronous motors are used in equipment timers and induction motors are used with rotating anodes

---

TRANSFORMERS

Principles of Operation

In the production of diagnostic energy x-rays it is necessary to increase or step-up incoming line voltage (i.e., the voltage supplied by your power company, usually 110 or 220 V) into the kilovoltage range. For other purposes, it may be necessary to reduce or step-down incoming line voltage to 5 to 10 V. The device that provides the capability to do either is the electric *transformer*.

Like generators and motors, transformers use the interactions between electricity and magnetism to accomplish their tasks. To understand the basic principles of operation, refer to Figure 5–23A. A standard transformer consists of two circuits—a primary and a secondary. The primary circuit is that portion of the circuit containing the power source, in this illustration circuit (1), which contains a battery (DC). In addition, a coil of wire, known as the primary coil, is also an integral part of this circuit. The secondary circuit, (2) in Figure 5–23A, consists of a coil known as the secondary coil and, in this illustration, a sensitive current-measuring device such as a galvanometer. Primary and secondary coils are in close proximity but do not make contact.

In Figure 5–23A, both primary and secondary circuits are shown. Initially, no current flows in either circuit. In *B*, the primary switch is closed, allowing a DC current to flow. As the current builds up to its maximum value, magnetic field lines also expand outward from the primary coil. As the **B** lines expand across the wires of the secondary, a current is induced to flow in it. As the current stabilizes in the primary, the **B** lines also stabilize and cease to expand. The secondary coil no longer discerns a changing magnetic field, and current ceases to flow in the secondary circuit (Fig. 5–23C).

If the switch in the primary circuit is opened, current flow in that circuit will cease. As the current flow begins to diminish, the **B** lines around the wire also begin to contract. As the diminishing **B** lines cut across the wires of the secondary circuit, a current is again induced to flow in this circuit (Fig. 5–23D).

As the current in the primary circuit diminishes to zero, so do the associated **B** lines. Magnetic field lines no longer cut across the coils of the secondary, and as a result, no current flow is detected in the secondary circuit. It is important to note that a current is induced in the secondary circuit only when there is a changing magnetic field in the primary circuit. With a DC power source, this occurs only when the primary circuit is either opened or closed. Instead of continuously opening and closing the switch to produce this effect, it is more efficient if the input current (i.e., that current produced in the primary circuit) is AC. The continuous reversal of current flow direction in the primary circuit assures that currents (and voltages) are induced in the secondary circuit.

The purpose of the transformer is to take incoming voltages (or currents) and increase or decrease them to appropriate levels to accomplish a particular task. Whether a transformer increases or decreases incoming voltages (or currents) depends on the ratio of the number of turns on the secondary coil (N_s) to the number of turns on the primary coil (N_p). This ratio, N_s/N_p, is known as the *turns ratio*. Transformers are classified as step-up or step-down according to what effect they have on incoming voltage. If incoming voltage is increased, the transformer is step-up. If incoming voltage is decreased, the transformer is step-down. In addition, *step-up transformers* have turns ratios greater than one, whereas ratios for *step-down transformers* are less than one.

Construction and Design

Transformers may take one of several forms depending on their specific use and circuit space requirements. Four specific types are of interest:

1. Air-core transformers. In its simplest form, an air-core transformer consists of insulated primary and secondary coils placed in close proximity to each other (Fig. 5–24A).
2. Open-core transformers. The open-core transformer design is similar to that of the air core with the exception that the primary and secondary wire coils are each wrapped around a ferromagnetic (e.g., iron) core. This serves to intensify the **B** lines in both primary and secondary coils when they become magnetized as current flows through each set of coils (Fig. 5–24B). A special type of open-core transformer is the autotransformer. The *autotransformer* consists of a single coil of insulated wire wrapped around a large ferromagnetic core (Fig. 5–24C). In this transformer, the single coil serves as both primary and secondary coils. Contacts are made on the primary side of the coil for incoming voltage and a variable moving contact is located on the secondary side of the coil as shown in the illustration. The movable contact can be positioned to vary the turns ratio on the autotransformer. Whereas the number of turns on most transformers are *fixed* and cannot be changed, the autotransformer is a *variable transformer*, since the turns ratio can be altered. Autotransformers are usually somewhat smaller than standard transformers and are used to produce only relatively small variations in incoming voltage. This concept of autotransformer is illustrated in Figure 5–25.

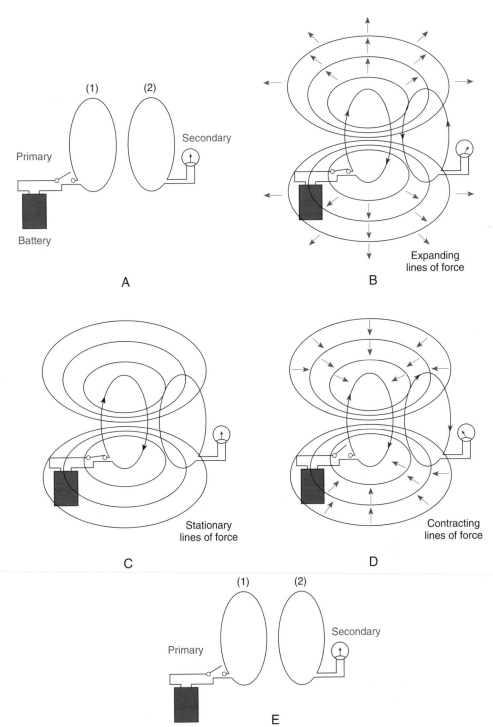

FIGURE 5–23. Principle of operation of the transformer. *A,* The primary and the secondary circuits. *B,* Current is induced in the secondary circuit as the magnetic field of the primary circuit expands outward when the switch is closed. *C,* No current is induced when there is no changing magnetic field. *D,* Current is once again induced in the secondary circuit when the switch is opened and the magnetic field decreases to zero. *E,* No current is induced when the magnetic field stabilizes to zero. (Beiser, A. Modern Technical Physics, © 1992, Addison-Wesley Publishing Co., Inc., Reading, Massachusetts. Reprinted with permission of the publisher).

Note: Standard transformers having separate primary and secondary coils operate on the principle of *mutual induction.* Autotransformers that utilize a single coil operate on the principle of self-induction. *Self-induction* refers to the induction of currents in a coil as a result of changing magnetic fields generated by an AC current flowing through the same coil.

3. Closed-core transformers. In a closed-core transformer, the insulated coils of the primary and secondary circuits are wrapped around a ferromagnetic core, usually iron or steel, in the shape of a circular or square ring (see Fig. 5–24D). Cores of this design tend to contain more of the **B** lines that are generated and in doing so make the transformer more efficient in its operation. The cores are normally composed of layers of metal plates rather than a solid core, in order to minimize energy loss in the form of heat produced by small opposing currents (known as eddy currents) generated within the metal core. A core that is composed of layers of metal plates is said to be laminated. The use of

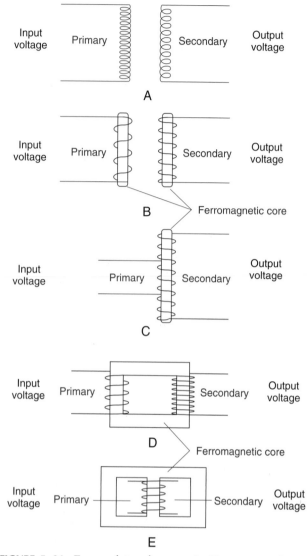

FIGURE 5-24. Types of transformers. *A,* Air core transformer. *B,* Open core design. *C,* Autotransformer. *D,* Closed core transformer. *E,* Shell type transformer.

laminated cores also tends to increase transformer efficiency.

4. Shell type of transformer. In the shell type of transformer (see Fig. 5–24*E*), the core once again consists of coated plates of iron or silicon steel. The design of the core plates is such that each contains two rectangular holes. Both primary and secondary coils are wrapped around the center post of the core. In this way the ferromagnetic core completely surrounds the coils. This traps more **B** lines generated in the coils and makes the transformer more efficient. Some of the largest power transformers are of this design.

In many high-voltage transformers both the core and coil assemblies are immersed in a special mineral oil that acts to provide both electrical insulation and a method by which heat is transferred from the coils.

Transformer Laws

The purpose of a transformer is to transfer energy from one circuit to another by means of electromagnetic induction. This electrical energy is transferred without a change in its frequency but with changes in voltage and current. The relationships that exist between incoming voltages and currents as registered at the primary coil and their output values as measured at the secondary coil are related to the actual number of turns of wire on each coil. These relationships are described by the following transformer laws.

Transformer Law #1: Voltage Related to Turns Ratio

A direct relationship exits between the voltages across the primary and secondary coils and the number of turns of wire on the respective coils. That is,

$$\frac{V_s}{V_p} = \frac{N_s}{N_p}$$
$$\left(\frac{N_s}{N_p} = \text{turns ratio}\right)$$

where

V_s = voltage across the secondary

V_p = voltage across the primary

N_s = number of turns on the secondary

N_p = number of turns on the primary

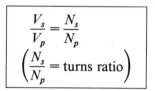 **EXAMPLE**

If an incoming line voltage of 220 V is placed across the primary of a transformer having 100 turns on the primary and 40,000 turns on the secondary coil,

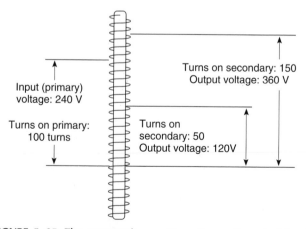

FIGURE 5-25. The autotransformer. Operating on the principle of self-induction, the autotransformer is used to produce only slight differences in incoming line voltage as shown. Depending on the relative number of turns on the primary and secondary circuits, output voltages may be halved or doubled.

what is the output (secondary) voltage of this transformer?

$$\frac{V_s}{V_p} = \frac{N_s}{N_p}$$

$$\frac{V_s}{220 \text{ V}} = \frac{40,000}{100}$$

$$V_s = (220 \text{ V}) (400)$$

$$V_s = 88,000 \text{ V or } 88 \text{ kV}$$

))))) EXAMPLE

What is the turns ratio for this transformer? Is this a step-up or step-down transformer?

$$\text{Turns ratio} = \frac{N_s}{N_p}$$

$$= \frac{40,000}{100}$$

$$= 400$$

Since the turns ratio is greater than 1, this is a step-up transformer.

Application to Radiography Equipment
  Step-up transformers are required to increase incoming line voltage to *the kilovolt* (kV) range to produce appropriate diagnostic energy x-rays.
  Step-down transformers are required to *lower* incoming line voltage to a voltage appropriate for generating electrons from the filament of the x-ray tube.
  The autotransformer may be used to slightly raise or lower incoming line voltage to obtain appropriate voltages across the x-ray tube.

Transformer Law #2: Current Related to Voltage
  In an ideal transformer, the power input into the primary coil equals the power output of the secondary coil (conservation of energy). Since electrical power (P) equals the product of voltage (V) times current (I), then

$$P_p = P_s$$

or

$$\boxed{V_p \, I_p = V_s \, I_s}$$

where

$$V_p = \text{voltage across the primary}$$

$$V_s = \text{voltage across the secondary}$$

$$I_p = \text{current in primary}$$

$$I_s = \text{current in secondary}$$

))))) EXAMPLE

The input voltage across the primary circuit of a transformer is 220 V, whereas the voltage output is 22 kV. If the current flow through the primary circuit is 20 A, what current flows through the secondary?
Given

$$V_p = 220 \text{ V}$$

$$V_s = 22 \text{ kV}$$

$$I_p = 20 \text{ A}$$

$$I_s = ?$$

$$V_p \, I_p = V_s \, I_s$$

$$(220 \text{ V}) (20 \text{ A}) = (22,000 \text{ V}) (I_s)$$

$$I_s = \frac{(220 \text{ V}) (20 \text{ A})}{22,000 \text{ V}}$$

$$I_s = \frac{(2.2 \times 10^2 \text{ V}) (2 \times 10^1 \text{ A})}{2.2 \times 10^4 \text{ V}}$$

$$= 2 \times 10^{-1} \text{ A, or } 0.2 \text{ A}$$

Note. As indicated in this problem, kilovolts must be converted into volts prior to performing any calculations. The conversion of multiples to basic units must be performed in working most problems, unless a special case is noted.
  As can be seen by this example, an inverse relationship exists between voltage and current in a transformer. As voltage increases, current must decrease and vice versa.

Transformer Law #3: Current Related to Turns Ratio
  From the first transformer law, it was found that

$$\frac{V_s}{.V_p} = \frac{N_s}{N_p}$$

and rearranging terms of the second transformer law produces

$$\frac{V_s}{V_p} = \frac{I_p}{I_s}$$

Since both of the preceding ratios for voltages are equivalent, then the following is also valid:

$$\boxed{\frac{I_p}{I_s} = \frac{N_s}{N_p}}$$

where

$$I_p = \text{current in primary coil}$$

$$I_s = \text{current in secondary coil}$$

$$N_s = \text{number of turns on the secondary coil}$$

$$N_p = \text{number of turns on the primary coil}$$

))))) **EXAMPLE**

The turns ratio of a certain transformer is 50. If the current that flows through the secondary coil is 5 A, what current flows through the primary coil?
Given

$$\text{Turns ratio} = \frac{N_s}{N_p} = 50$$

$$I_s = 5 \text{ A}$$

$$I_p = ?$$

$$\frac{I_p}{I_s} = \frac{N_s}{N_p}$$

$$\frac{I_p}{5 \text{ A}} = 50$$

$$I_p = (50)(5 \text{ A})$$

$$I_p = 250 \text{ A}$$

From the preceding example it is seen that an inverse relationship exists between the current flowing through the coils and the actual number of turns on the individual coils.

Transformer Power Ratings

Recalling that electrical power (P) is defined as the product of voltage (V) and current (I), that is,

$$P = VI$$

(Units: watts = voltage × amperes)

the maximum safe power output of a transformer secondary is generally expressed in this manner in units of kilowatts (kW). This *transformer power rating* is stated as a safety measure, for if it is exceeded, overheating that could result in heat damage to both the coil insulation and coil windings may occur.

The kilowatt power rating of a generator, of which the transformer is an integral part, is calculated in one of two ways, depending on whether the unit is 1ϕ or 3ϕ. With 3ϕ generators, in which there are only minor fluctuations in the supplied voltage, power ratings are calculated as follows:

$$\boxed{\text{Power rating}_{3\phi} \text{ (kW)} = \frac{\text{Kilovoltage (kV)} \times \text{current (mA)}}{1000}}$$

))))) **EXAMPLE**

A 3ϕ generator that operates at 70 kV and 300 mA would have a power rating of

$$\text{Power rating}_{3\phi} = \frac{(100 \text{ kV})(300 \text{ mA})}{1000}$$

$$= 30 \text{ kW}$$

In comparison, a 1ϕ generator supplies a voltage that fluctuates from zero to some maximum value referred to as the peak voltage. (Note: With x-ray units, this maximum voltage is referred to as the peak kilovoltage or simply the kVp). For this case, an effective voltage, known as the *root mean square (RMS) voltage* is used to determine an "average" or effective power rating, defined as

$$\text{Power Rating}_{1\phi} \text{ (kW)} = \frac{0.7 \times \text{kV} \times \text{mA}}{1000}$$

The factor of 0.7 that enters into this relationship results from the use of the RMS AC voltage. It is this effective value of the fluctuating AC voltage that has the same heating effect as a specific, nonfluctuating DC voltage or current. This effective, or RMS, voltage is related to the AC peak by the following:

$$V_{\text{RMS}} \sim 0.7 \text{ V}_{\text{peak}}$$

This factor is not used with 3ϕ units, since the kilovoltage is practically constant and does not fluctuate through maximum and minimum values.

))))) **EXAMPLE**

Determine the power rating of a 1ϕ generator operating at 100 kV and 200 mA.

$$\text{Power Rating}_{1\phi} \text{ (kW)} = \frac{(0.7)(100 \text{ kV})(200 \text{ mA})}{1000}$$

$$= 14 \text{ kW}$$

Since the power ratings are determined from the conditions of kilovoltage and milliamperage under which the generator can actually operate, these ratings can be used to determine if a particular generator is appropriate for specific needs. As an example, a 3ϕ generator having a power rating of 30 kW could possibly operate under the following combinations of voltage and current:

200 mA at 150 kVp (power = 30 kW)

400 mA at 75 kVp (power = 30 kW)

500 mA at 60 kVp (power = 30 kW)

This same generator would not be the one of choice if one must perform a significant number of studies requiring technical factors of 500 mA at 80 kVp, since this combination would exceed the power rating of the unit.

More is said later regarding power ratings and the practical limitations they place on radiographic procedures.

Chapter Summary/ Important Equations, Constants, Relationships, and Concepts

Two magnetic poles exist in nature: north and south

Like magnetic poles repel and unlike magnetic poles attract

Magnetic poles do not exist independently of each other in nature—that is, they cannot be separated

Magnetic forces of attraction or repulsion vary as an inverse square of the distance between them

Electric charges in motion (i.e., electric currents) produce magnetic fields

A current-carrying solenoid behaves like a bar magnet

Electrical motors convert electrical energy into mechanical energy of motion

Generators convert mechanical energy of motion into electrical energy.

With DC current, charge flows in only one direction. In AC current, charge continuously changes direction of motion

Rectification of AC voltage is required to obtain a current that flows in only one direction

Transformers are primarily used to increase or decrease incoming voltage by the process of mutual induction (standard transformer having separate primary and secondary coils) or self-induction (autotransformer having a single coil that acts as both primary and secondary)

Turns ratio for a transformer: N_s/N_p
$N_s/N_p > 1$, step-up transformer
$N_s/N_p < 1$, step-down transformer

Transformer laws:
a. $\dfrac{V_s}{V_p} = \dfrac{N_s}{N_p}$
b. $V_p I_p = V_s I_s$

c. $\dfrac{I_p}{I_s} = \dfrac{N_s}{N_p}$

Transformer power ratings:
$$P_{3\phi}\,(\text{kW}) = \frac{\text{kV} \times \text{mA}}{1000}$$
$$P_{1\phi}\,(\text{kW}) = \frac{0.7 \times \text{kV} \times \text{mA}}{1000}$$

Root mean square (RMS) voltage $\approx 0.707\ V_{\text{peak}}$

Important Terminology

Alternating current AC. Current that alternates or continuously changes its direction of motion

Anode. The positive terminal

Armature. That portion of an electrical motor or generator that rotates

Autotransformer. A variable transformer having a single coil that acts as both primary and secondary coils

Cathode. The negative terminal

Direct Current (DC). Current that flows in only one direction, such as that supplied by a battery or DC power supply

Diode. An electronic circuit component that allows current to flow in only one direction; in older x-ray units, a diode was a vacuum tube (known as a valve tube), but in more modern units, these have been replaced by solid state rectifiers, which are also diodes

Electrical Motor. A device used to convert electrical energy into mechanical energy of motion

Electrodes. Positive and negative terminals

Electromagnet. A type of magnet formed by wrapping a current-carrying wire around a ferromagnetic core; this type of magnet has magnetic properties only when an electric current flows through the wires

Exposure Time. The actual length of time that an x-ray machine generates x-rays to produce a radiographic exposure

Ferromagnetic Materials. Materials such as iron, nickel, or cobalt, which are easily magnetized

Fixed Transformer. A transformer whose turns ratio cannot be altered

Full-Wave Rectification. Rectification in which the negative portion of the AC cycle is made positive; this results in 120 voltage pulses being produced each second if 60-cycle AC voltage is used

Galvanometer. A sensitive current-reading device

Generator. A device used to convert mechanical energy of motion into electrical energy

Glass Envelope. The glass enclosure that contains the components of the x-ray tube

Half-Wave Rectification. Rectification in which the negative portion of the AC cycle is simply removed or negated; this results in 60 voltage pulses being produced each second if 60-cycle AC voltage is used

Induction Motor. A type of AC motor whose primary components are stators and a rotor; rotor rotation is produced by electromagnetic interaction between currents induced in the rotor by changing the magnetic fields in the surrounding stator windings

In-Phase. Term used to describe the phase relationship between two waves when "crests meet crests" and "troughs meet troughs"

Magnetic Domain. Group of magnetic atoms that, when aligned, gives a material magnetic properties; when these domains are randomly oriented, the material has no overall magnetic properties

Magnetic Field (B). A region of space in which a magnet or ferromagnetic substance is subject to a magnetic force of attraction or repulsion

Magnetic Polarity. Designation as to the location of north and south poles of a magnet

Mutual Induction. The generation of a voltage (or current) in a coil as a result of a changing magnetic field produced in an adjacent coil

Out-of-Phase. Term used to describe the phase relationship between two waves when crests and troughs of one wave do not coincide with those of a second wave

Permanent Magnet. Magnet formed from magnetized metal or ceramics

Phase. The spatial relationship of the crests and troughs of one wave to another

Primary. The input coil of a transformer

Rectification. Elimination of the negative portion of the AC cycle; this can be accomplished by half- or full-wave rectification

Ripple Factor. Numerical factor (expressed as a percentage) used to describe the maximum drop from the peak voltage value that will occur in any AC cycle

Root Mean Square (RMS) Voltage (or Current). The "effective" AC voltage (or AC current) that produces the same heating effect as a specific, nonfluctuating DC current; RMS voltage $\approx 0.707 \times$ peak voltage

Rotor. The component of an induction motor which rotates

Secondary. The output coil of a transformer

Self-Induction. The generation of an opposing voltage (or current) in a single coil as a result of the changing magnetic field produced when an AC current is run through the coil

Self-Rectification. In an x-ray circuit, rectification of an AC voltage (or current) waveform occurring when no rectifiers are placed in the x-ray circuit;

this results from the fact that the x-ray tube (a diode itself) acts as a rectifier

Solenoid. A coil of wire that behaves as a bar magnet when a current passes through the coil

Stator. Coil windings that surround the rotor in an induction motor

Step-Down Transformer. A transformer having fewer coil windings on its secondary than on its primary; a transformer having a turns ratio of less than one

Step-Up Transformer. A transformer having more coil windings on its secondary than on its primary; a transformer having a turns ratio of greater than one

Superposition. The addition of two or more waves, taking into account their amplitudes and phase relationships, to produce a single composite wave

Synchronous Motor. A special type of AC motor in which the armature rotates the same number of times per second as the frequency of the AC voltage supplied (e.g., the armature rotates 60 rps when 60-cycle AC voltage is supplied)

Tesla (T). SI unit of magnetic field strength

Transformer. An electromagnetic device used to transfer AC power from one circuit to another

Transformer Power Rating. Rating, expressed in kilowatts (kW), used to express the maximum safe output of secondary coils to avoid damage to the coil windings

Tube Current. The current expressed in milliamperes (mA) that flows between cathode and anode of an x-ray tube

Turns Ratio. The ratio of the number of coil windings on the secondary (N_s) to the number of coil windings on the primary (N_p)

Variable Transformer. A transformer whose turns ratio can be altered (e.g., the autotransformer)

60-cycle AC. AC current that changes its direction of motion 120 times each second

180° out of phase. Phase relationship existing between two waves in which the crests of one wave coincide with the troughs of the second wave.

Bibliography

Beiser, A. Modern Technical Physics, 6th ed. Reading, MA: Addison-Wesley, 1992.

Curry, T.S. III; Dowdey, J.E.; Murry, R.C., Jr. Christensen's Physics of Diagnostic Radiology, 4th ed. Philadelphia: Lea & Febiger, 1990.

Hazen, M.E. Experiencing Electricity and Electronics. Philadelphia: W.B. Saunders, 1989.

Selman, J. The Fundamentals of X-ray and Radium Physics, 7th ed. Springfield, IL: Charles C Thomas, 1985.

Weigl, W. A new high-frequency controlled x-ray generator system with multi-pulse wave shape. J Radiol Eng 1:7–19, 1989.

Review Questions

1. Indicate similarities between electric and magnetic forces.
2. Explain what is meant by the term *ferromagnetic.*
3. Explain why magnetic north and south poles cannot be separated.
4. Indicate how the direction of a magnetic field is determined.
5. Specify the direction of the magnetic field (B) lines both inside and outside a bar magnet.
6. Indicate whether each of the following has a magnetic field, an electric field, neither, or both:
   a. a stationary proton
   b. a moving electron
   c. a bar magnet
   d. a compass needle
   e. a steel bar
   f. a current-carrying solenoid
7. Indicate the magnetic polarity and the direction of the induced current when the south pole of a bar magnet is withdrawn from a solenoid.
8. Sketch the magnetic field (B) lines (refer to drawings in Table 5–2), indicating direction, for each of the following:

   a.

   b.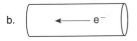

   c.   i indicates *current*

   d. 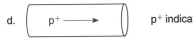   p⁺ indicates a *proton*

9. Explain or indicate the following:
   a. How can an electric charge be used to produce a magnetic field?
   b. How can a magnetic field be used to produce an electric current?
   c. How are each of the above principles put to practical application in the design of x-ray circuitry components?
10. Sketch the voltage waveforms for each of the following.
    a. standard 60-Hz AC
    b. 1ϕ, full-wave rectified voltage
    c. 1ϕ, half-wave rectified voltage

11. Sketch the voltage waveforms for each of the following. Indicate on each the duration (i.e., the length of time) of each individual pulse.
    a. 60-Hz, 1ϕ, half-wave rectified voltage
    b. 60-Hz, 1ϕ, full-wave rectified voltage
    c. 60-Hz, 3ϕ, 6-pulse, full-wave rectified voltage
12. Explain the advantage of 3ϕ over 1ϕ generators.
13. Specify the ripple factors for each of the following types of generators:
    a. 1ϕ, full-wave rectified
    b. 3ϕ, 6-pulse, full-wave rectified
    c. 3ϕ, 12-pulse, full-wave rectified
    d. 1ϕ, half-wave rectified
14. The maximum voltage of an AC waveform is 120 kV. What is the minimum voltage if this generator has a 10% ripple factor?
15. If one desires a generator that provides a near-constant voltage, should a generator with a high or low ripple factor be obtained? Explain.
16. Indicate in each case whether the transformer described is step-up or step-down:
    a. $\dfrac{N_s}{N_p} = 1000$
    b. $N_p = 100$; $N_s = 10,000$
    c. $N_p = 1000$; $N_s = 50$
    d. $\dfrac{N_s}{N_p} = 0.25$
17. The turns ratio of a transformer is 5000.
    a. If the incoming voltage is 10 V, what is the output voltage?
    b. If the current flow in the primary is 25 A, what current flows in the secondary?
18. Determine the power rating of a 3ϕ generator if it can safely supply 60 mA at 100 kV. What would its power rating be if it had been a 1ϕ unit?
19. Determine the effective, or root mean square, voltage if the peak AC voltage is 100 kVp. What is the RMS voltage when the peak voltage is 70 kVp?

Exercises

1. A simple directional compass is placed in the vicinity of each of the following:
   a. a fast-moving beam of protons
   b. a fast-moving beam of electrons
   c. a stationary proton
   d. a stationary electron

   In which of the above cases will the compass needle be deflected? Why?
2. Describe the basic design of an electromagnet and indicate how it differs from a permanent magnet.

3. Why are the coils of electromagnets usually wrapped around a ferromagnetic core?
4. A particular generator provides 50-Hz AC voltage. How many voltage pulses are produced in 0.1 sec if the voltage is
   a. 1ϕ, half-wave rectified?
   b. 1ϕ, full-wave rectified?
5. What is the time duration of each pulse produced by a 50-Hz AC generator that is
   a. 3ϕ, 6-pulse?
   b. 3ϕ, 12-pulse?
6. A particular AC generator can supply voltage at 150 kVp. What is the minimum voltage supplied if the generator is
   a. 3ϕ, 6-pulse?
   b. 3ϕ, 12-pulse?

(Hint: Use ripple factors stated within this chapter for each of these types of generators.)
7. Why do all 1ϕ generators have a ripple factor of 100%?
8. What is the advantage of using a high-frequency generator?
9. Explain why DC currents cannot be used with transformers.
10. Use the information provided to determine the unknown quantity:
    a. $N_p = 50$, $N_s = 500$, $I_p = 2$ A, $I_s = $?
    b. turns ratio = 0.002, $V_p = $?, $V_s = 10$ V
    c. $V_p = 220$ V, $V_s = 100$ kV, $I_s = 10$ A, $I_p = $?
    d. $I_p = 15$ A, $I_s = 100$ mA, turns ratio = ?
11. A high-voltage transformer (3ϕ) is rated at 30 kW. What is the maximum current it can safely supply at 70 kV?

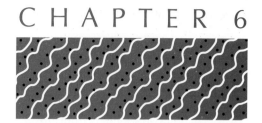

X-ray Tube Components and Design

Michael A. Thompson, M.S.

Chapter Objectives

Upon completion of this chapter, you should be able to

- Describe the general method by which x-rays are produced in an x-ray machine.
- Describe in general the functions of the console, the filament circuit, the high voltage section, and the x-ray tube.
- Identify the various components of an x-ray tube (e.g., glass envelope, cathode, anode, filament), and describe the function of each in the production of x-rays.
- Explain how the energy of the resulting x-rays is related to the voltage applied across the x-ray tube electrodes.
- Distinguish between the terms *filament current* and *tube current.*
- Explain the relationship existing between filament current and tube current.
- Describe qualitatively the type of energy conversion that occurs when fast-moving electrons strike the target anode.
- Explain why rotating anode disks are in most cases more advantageous than a stationary anode.
- Describe the general designs of stationary and rotating anodes, indicating the advantages and disadvantages of each.
- Describe the design and method of operation of an induction motor as it applies to rotating anode x-ray tubes.
- Indicate the primary methods of heat dissipation in the stationary and rotating anode x-ray tube.
- Explain why anode target faces are slanted.
- Explain the difference between the actual focal spot and apparent focal spot sizes and their relationship to angle of tilt of the target face.
- Explain the advantages and disadvantages of the line-focus principle.
- Describe the processes by which heat is transferred from the anode target to the air outside the tube housing.
- Given the mA, kVp, and exposure time, calculate the number of heat units (HU) generated during a radiographic procedure.
- Interpret and use an x-ray tube-rating chart to determine whether a particular radiographic procedure would or would not result in unacceptable thermal damage to the tube.
- Interpret and use an anode-cooling chart.
- Explain what is meant by a grid-controlled x-ray tube.
- Explain how a mammography x-ray tube differs from a standard or conventional x-ray tube.

IMPROVING X-RAY TUBE EFFICIENCY

Recall from Chapter 1 that Röntgen's discovery of x-rays resulted from his experimentation with a simple device known as a Crookes tube. The Crookes tube consisted of an evacuated tube containing two electrodes. This tube design was however neither the most efficient nor the most dependable for x-ray production. Recall that x-rays were produced when fast-moving electrons struck the glass walls of the tube, but with the Crookes tube there was no way to control the number of electrons moving between the tube electrodes. In radiographical tube terminology, the number of electrons moving between the electrodes per second is referred to as the *tube current*. Without control over the tube current, the number of x-rays produced could not be regulated. This was a serious limitation in the production of diagnostic-quality images.

In 1913 W. D. Coolidge reported on his "hot cathode" tube, which at the time represented a major redirection in basic x-ray tube design. This design change consisted of replacing the standard *cathode* (negative terminal) of the Crookes tube with a small, spiral-wound tungsten wire heated by an electric current. The heat produced in the wire provided sufficient energy to release loosely bound outer shell electrons from the tungsten atoms. This process by which the electrons are released is called *thermionic emission*. Thus the hot cathode became the new source of electrons that would travel from cathode to *anode* (positive terminal) and provided a method for operator control of tube current and subsequent x-ray emission. Tubes having this new design became known as Coolidge tubes. Hot cathode tubes subsequently replaced Crookes tubes for x-ray production and remain the primary cathode design in modern x-ray tubes. Because the x-ray tube is the heart of the x-ray machine, the major portion of this chapter concentrates on the modern x-ray tube, its components and design, and each of the major electrical components necessary for the tube's proper operation.

THE X-RAY MACHINE: AN OVERVIEW

Before concentrating on individual components, let us first take an overview of the x-ray machine and its operation. The standard x-ray machine consists of a control module, or console, a filament circuit, a high-voltage section, and the tube itself.

The modern x-ray tube normally consists of a glass envelope that serves to contain the negative electrode (the cathode) and the positive electrode (the anode). The *filament* is part of the cathode assembly and serves as the source of electrons when heated. The electrons released from the filament are then accelerated to extremely high speeds toward the positive anode by the application of a high voltage between the two electrodes. Recall that as the voltage between the electrodes is increased, the electrons move faster—that is, their kinetic energy is increased. When these fast-moving electrons strike the positive anode, their kinetic energy of motion is converted (by conservation of energy) into heat and x-rays. Each of the components of the x-ray tube mentioned previously are shown in Figure 6-1.

The energy (or penetrating ability) of the x-rays produced is determined by the voltage applied across the tube electrodes. Therefore to regulate the energy of the x-rays one must have the means to regulate the *voltage*, or potential, across the tube. The controlled variation of tube voltage is provided at the control console. It is within this section that incoming line voltage (as supplied by the local power company) can be slightly raised or lowered to obtain the required voltage across the tube. The voltage at this point, however, is usually of the order of only several hundred volts. For diagnostic energy x-rays, this voltage must be raised to the order of *kilovolts (kV)*.

Incoming voltage is raised to the kV level in the high-voltage section (also called the high-voltage generator). This is accomplished through the use of high-voltage step-up transformers. Additionally, alternating current (AC) voltage waveforms are rectified prior to application to the electrodes of the x-ray tube in an effort to make efficient use of the entire voltage waveform (recall discussions of step-up transformers and rectifiers from Chapter 5).

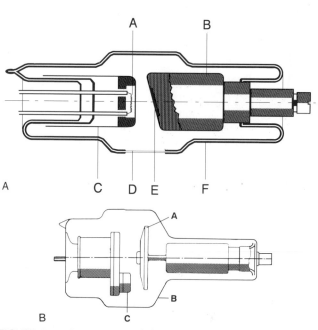

FIGURE 6-1. Components of the stationary and rotating anode x-ray tubes. *A,* For the stationary anode tube, components include the filament (A), the anode (B), the cathode (C), exit window (D), target (E), and glass envelope (F). *B,* The rotating anode tube has a rotating anode (A), a glass envelope (B), and filaments housed within a focusing cup (C). (Courtesy of Philips Medical Systems.)

A second circuit required for proper operation of today's x-ray tubes is the *filament circuit.* Coolidge's modification of the original Crookes tube was the introduction of a filament into the cathode assembly. The filament was heated by an electric current that generated sufficient heat to release loosely bound electrons from the tungsten wire. The heated filament then served as a source of electrons to be accelerated into the anode to produce x-rays. The voltage required to produce the current that heats the filament is generally lower than the incoming line voltage. Voltage for this circuit is therefore obtained with the use of a step-down transformer. (Note: Take care to distinguish between the current that passes through the filament to release electrons, or the *filament current,* and the current composed of the fast-moving electrons passing between the cathode and anode of the x-ray tube, known as the *tube current.* Although the tube current is related to the filament current, they are not the same.) For almost all x-ray units, the step-up and step-down transformers are physically located together in the transformer box of the high-voltage generator.

These components constitute the basic circuitry of the conventional x-ray machine shown schematically in Figure 6–2. Each component is discussed in greater detail in the following sections of this chapter. It is important, however, not to lose sight of this overall view of the equipment operation.

X-RAY TUBES: COMMON DESIGN FEATURES

X-ray tubes take several forms, depending on their specific applications. Obtaining specific types of radiographs, such as a single image of a stationary portion of the body, known as a *static image,* as opposed to multiple images obtained in rapid succession, or *serial exposures,* which are used in the production of motion or dynamic images, impose very different physical requirements on the x-ray tube used. As a result, two general types of x-ray tubes are commonly found in clinical use—stationary anode tubes and rotating anode tubes. Each of these general tube designs is considered separately and in more detail later. Each type of tube, regardless of which design—stationary or rotating anode—shares several common structural components. These common components include the glass envelope, the cathode, and the anode (see Fig. 6–1).

Glass Envelope

Since electrons are extremely light particles, early investigators in x-ray tube construction found that x-ray tube efficiency could be improved if the air within

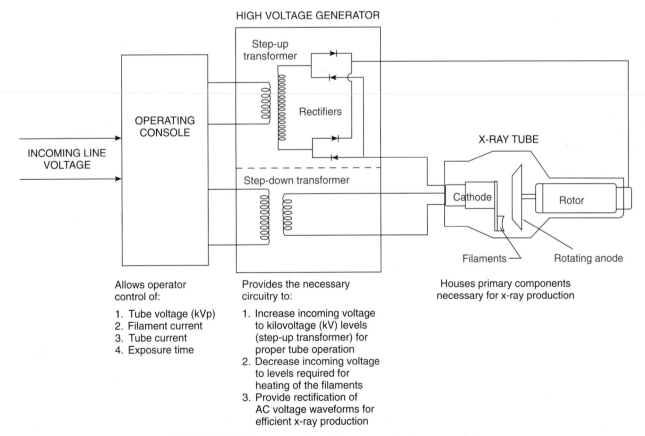

FIGURE 6–2. Basic components of the conventional x-ray machine.

an x-ray tube was removed (i.e., a vacuum was created within the tube) prior to sealing the tube. This increase in tube efficiency resulted from reducing the number of collisions between electrons and gas molecules within the tube, allowing more electrons to travel un-impeded toward the anode and resulting in production of more x-rays.

The glass portion of the tube serves several purposes, including (1) containing the vacuum necessary for efficient x-ray production, (2) providing structural support for the cathode and anode, (3) supplying a degree of electrical insulation from the high voltage applied to the tube electrodes, and (4) assisting in the removal of heat from the anode, preventing tube damage.

The material used to form the envelope in today's tubes is hard, heat-resistant glass. It must also be sufficiently thick to withstand the pressure difference created by the introduction of the vacuum inside the tube. However, the thickness is not uniform; the tube is much thinner at the site where the x-rays exit. This point is called the *exit window*. If the window is too thick, not only will it decrease the x-ray intensity (i.e., the number of x-rays) of the beam but it will also affect the average energy of the beam by removing x-rays with lower energy.

Cathode

The cathode is the negative electrode of the x-ray tube (Fig. 6–3) and consists of the filament (and its associated circuitry) and a metallic focusing cup. Recall that the purpose of the filament is to serve as the source of electrons. The electrons are liberated when heat is generated in the filament wire. The filament is a long, thin tungsten wire shaped into a spiral coil approximately 1 cm or less in length. This particular design is chosen because long, thin wires have high electrical resistance (see Chapter 4) to the flow of electric current. When the filament circuitry provides approximately 10 volts to the filament, an electric current of approximately 3 to 5 amperes flows through the high-resistance wire, generating sufficient heat to free loosely bound shell electrons. This process of electron emission is called *thermionic emission*. The electrons emitted from the filament wire form an "electron cloud" in the vicinity of the filament (often referred to as the *Edison effect*) until sufficient voltage is applied to draw the electrons into the anode.

Tungsten is the metal of choice for the filament because of its high melting point (3370°C or 6098°F) and its ability to be drawn into wire of narrow diameter. Tungsten's high melting point is especially important to the useful life of the tube. If the filament vaporizes to some degree each time it is heated, tungsten vapor within the tube compromises the vacuum conditions necessary for proper tube operation. In addition, any tungsten vapor created during the operation can create deposits on the inside of the glass envelope and produce electrical arcing (i.e., sparking, or electrical discharge). When this occurs, the useful life of the tube is greatly reduced and the tube usually requires re-

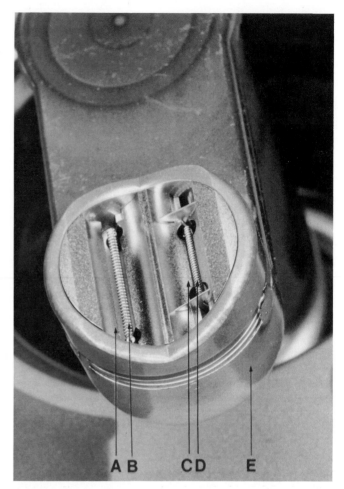

FIGURE 6–3. The filament assembly of a dual filament x-ray tube. Two filaments (B and D) are shown in focusing cups (A and C) of a typical cathode assembly (E).

placement. Vaporization of the tungsten filament is perhaps one of the most common causes of tube failure. In an effort to minimize this particular problem, *thorium* is added to the tungsten as an impurity. When thorium is added to the tungsten in a 1% to 2% concentration (the mixture is called thoriated tungsten), the effect is to lower the amount of heat energy required for thermionic emission. This allows the filament to produce the necessary number of electrons at lower operating temperatures, also minimizing filament vaporization and lengthening tube life.

Most modern x-ray tubes are *dual-filament tubes,* having two individual filaments as shown in Figure 6–3. The longer filament ($\sim$1.3 to 1.5 cm in length) is used when large numbers of electrons (i.e., high tube currents) are needed and a high degree of image detail *(resolution)* is not necessarily required. The shorter filament ($\sim$1 cm in length) is used to produce radiographs requiring lower tube currents and higher resolution. The actual filament used to produce a particular radiograph is usually chosen automatically when the tube current (i.e., the milliampere [mA] setting) is chosen.

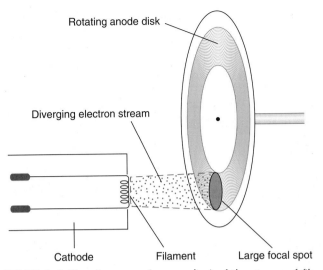

FIGURE 6-4. The divergence (or spreading) of the stream of filament electrons that occurs when a focusing cup is not used. This divergence tends to produce a large focal spot, resulting in unsharp radiographic images.

As the electrons emitted from the filament are pulled across the tube to the positively charged anode, there is a natural tendency for the electron stream to diverge, or spread apart (see Fig. 6-5). This results from the mutual repulsive force that exists between charges of like sign. This divergence produces several undesired effects. If the electrons in moving toward the anode diverge too widely, many could miss the anode entirely, resulting in fewer x-rays being produced. Also the larger the area of the anode that these accelerated electrons strike, the less sharp the radiographic image produced. To minimize these problems, the filaments are mounted in a negatively charged *focusing cup.* This focusing cup (usually made of nickel, stainless steel, or molybdenum because of their high melting points and poor thermionic emission characteristics) is specially shaped to have sharp edges around the edge of the cup. When a negative charge is placed on the cathode and is subsequently distributed over the focusing cup, the negative charge will tend to concentrate on these sharp edges. This concentration of negative charge in the region surrounding the filaments provides an electrical force that tends to counteract the natural tendency of the electrons emitted from the filament to diverge. This is illustrated in Figure 6-4. The electrical force exerted on the electrons by the negatively charged cup causes them to converge, or focus, on a smaller area of the anode. The area on which the electrons are focused is known as the *focal spot* and is indicated in Figure 6-5.

If the electrons strike only a small area of the target, the focal spot is small, and the resulting x-rays originate from only a small region of the anode. This results in radiographic images that are sharper and show greater detail. Conversely, if the stream of electrons cover a larger area of the target, the focal spot is larger, and image sharpness decreases. Focal spot size is primarily determined by the size of the filament used

(i.e., a longer versus a shorter filament) and the degree of focusing accomplished by the focusing cup.

Anode

Perhaps the greatest design variation among x-ray tubes occurs at the *anode,* or positive electrode. Electrons emitted from the filament are accelerated into the anode to produce x-rays. The electrons strike a small region of the anode known as the *target.* The target material most commonly used is tungsten (chemical symbol, W; Z number, 74) primarily because of two of its physical properties. One problem that arises at any x-ray tube anode is the problem of heat production and heat dissipation (i.e., the removal of heat once it is produced). When the fast-moving electrons originating at the filament strike the target plate of the anode, an energy conversion occurs. On striking the tungsten target, the kinetic energy of motion of the electrons is converted into heat ($\sim$99%) and x-rays ($\sim$1%). Several factors determine the quantity of heat produced at an anode:

- The voltage (kVp) between the tube electrodes: the higher the kVp, the faster the electrons move; the faster the electrons move, the greater their kinetic energy, which is primarily converted into heat
- The tube current (mA) that flows between the tube electrodes: tube current refers to the number of electrons moving per second between the tube electrodes; the greater the number of electrons striking the anode per second, the more electron kinetic energy converted into heat
- The length of time that electrons actually bombard the target anode: the longer the period of time that the electrons strike the target, the more heat produced; large quantities of heat may be produced by

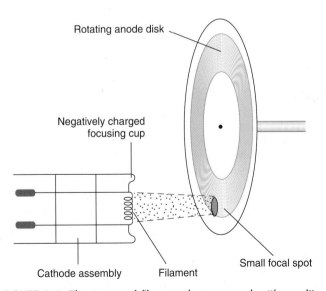

FIGURE 6-5. The stream of filament electrons can be "focused" on a smaller area of the anode target with the use of a negatively charged focusing cup surrounding the filament.

making a single, long radiographic exposure or a series of short, multiple exposures.

In addition to these factors, the type of high-voltage generator used also influences the amount of heat produced in the generation of radiographic images. More is said about heat production and its implications later in this chapter.

In sealing the components within the tube, great care is taken to assure that a high-quality vacuum is maintained. Gases trapped within the glass of the tube or its metal components could be released when the temperatures within the tube are raised to high levels during operation. To minimize this potential problem, tubes are heated in several stages while still connected to a vacuum pump (a device used to remove air or other gases from a container). As any trapped gases are released during the heating process, they are removed. If trapped gases were released during tube operation, the ionization of these gas molecules by fast-moving electrons emitted from the filament would result in varied numbers of electrons actually striking the target. This would result in fluctuating tube currents and unpredictable numbers of x-rays (related to what is known as x-ray intensity) with each exposure. Images produced under these conditions would be unpredictably light or dark. Once the tube has been "degassed" and appropriate vacuum conditions have been established, the x-ray tube is sealed.

Tube Exit Window

The useful beam of x-rays are emitted from the tube through the *exit window.* This section of the glass envelope is usually much thinner than other sections of the tube in order to minimize any reduction in x-ray beam intensity. The exit window is positioned above the tube port, through which the useful beam exits the tube shield. The tube port is usually made of glass so as to be transparent, or *radiolucent,* to the emerging x-rays.

Tube Housing (Tube Shield)

The x-ray tube is securely positioned within a protective metal *tube housing* that serves to provide mechanical support and protection for the tube. Most housings are constructed of steel, aluminum, or aluminum alloy that provides the needed mechanical support while providing a degree of protection for the patient and operator against x-rays traveling in directions other than that of the useful beam. The metal tube housing is not sufficiently thick to stop or *attenuate* a significant amount of this stray radiation, and because of this, the tube shield is lined with 3 to 4 mm thicknesses of lead at specific points. This is often referred to as "ray-proofing," but one must always remember that some x-radiation is transmitted through the tube housing during x-ray tube use. This warning emphasizes the importance of the radiographer's use of

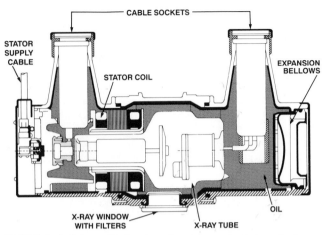

FIGURE 6–6. Schematic drawing of an x-ray tube in its tube housing. (Courtesy of Philips Medical Systems.)

adequate shielding to reduce unnecessary radiation exposure during radiographic procedures.

The tube shield must also provide sufficient electrical insulation to minimize the chance of potentially lethal shock and electrical arcing as a result of the tens of thousands of volts existing between the tube electrodes. The voltage is supplied to the tube electrodes through specially insulated high-voltage cables that are connected to the tube through designated receptacles in the tube shield. Within the tube shield, oil surrounds the tube (Fig. 6–6). In addition to providing electrical insulation, the oil also serves to assist in the removal of heat generated within the tube. More is said about this method of heat removal later in this chapter. Expandable bellows, also found with the tube shield, allow for thermal expansion of the oil as it becomes heated during tube operation. This assures a relatively constant pressure between the tube and its shield. With many x-ray units, the bellows within the tube shield are equipped with a microswitch that when activated by the compression of the bellows, automatically prevents further use of the tube if unsafe levels of heat are generated.

The following section consists of a more detailed look at the two basic anode designs.

STATIONARY AND ROTATING ANODES

Stationary Anodes

Since it is at the anode that the heat is produced, anodes have been designed to dissipate differing amounts of heat generated by various radiographic procedures. Stationary anodes (i.e., anodes that do not move) are employed when the commonly used *technical factors* of tube voltage (kVp), tube current (milliamperes, *mA*) and exposure time (seconds, sec) produce relatively low quantities of heat. When these technical factors are such that much greater quantities of heat are produced, a different type of anode design, known as a rotating anode, is the design of choice. Unlike the stationary anode tube, in which the heat energy is concentrated in the relatively small area of the tungsten target plate, a rotating anode can safely handle larger quantities of heat by distributing it over a larger surface area. This is analogous to comfortably handling the warmth of the sun's rays when they fall on a large surface area of the body but becoming most uncomfortable if these same rays are focused on a much smaller area of the skin surface with the aid of a simple magnifying glass. When this heat energy is focused, or concentrated, damage can occur to an anode just as to the skin. As a result, many of the design characteristics of x-ray tubes concentrate on methods to dissipate the large quantities of heat produced within the tube during the making of a radiographic image.

Stationary anode tubes can be found in use in the production of relatively simple radiographs not requiring the high tube currents or series of multiple exposures. The basic components of the stationary anode tube are shown in Figure 6–4. As previously described, all basic tube components (i.e., cathode, including focusing cup, filaments, and the anode with target plate) are contained in a vacuum enclosed by the glass envelope.

Electrons emitted from the filament are drawn from the cathode to the positively charged anode as a result of the high voltage applied across the tube electrodes. It should be recalled that approximately 99% of the kinetic energy of the fast-moving electrons from the filament is converted into heat on striking the anode target. Less than 1% of the incident electron kinetic energy is converted into x-rays. The stationary anode tube, the earliest and most basic design of x-ray tubes, is limited by its design to those radiographic procedures that do not generate excessive quantities of heat. For this reason, such a tube can be found in dental and some portable x-ray equipment.

The anode of any x-ray tube serves several purposes: It (1) serves as the positive electrode through which electrons from the cathode flow to complete the electrical circuit, (2) acts to provide structural support for the tungsten target plate, and (3) provides a means of dissipating heat generated at the target. A stationary anode is relatively simple in design, consisting of a tungsten target plate and a copper block and stem (Fig. 6–7).

The *target plate,* that portion of the anode actually struck by the fast-moving electrons from the filament, is usually (but not always) made of tungsten. Tungsten is generally chosen for several important reasons:

- Its ability to be shaped into many forms
- Its high melting point (3370°C compared with 1500°C or less for all other metals)
- Its high Z number (74)

Note: The efficiency of x-ray production varies directly with the Z number of the target material

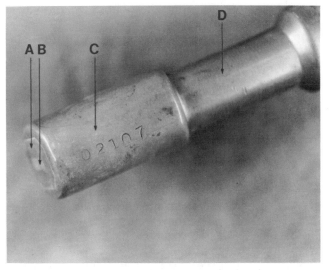

FIGURE 6–7. A stationary anode, indicating various components such as the target plate (A), focal spot (B), copper anode block (C), and anode stem (D).

struck by the incident electrons as indicated:

$$\begin{aligned} \text{X-ray production efficiency} &= \frac{\text{x-ray output} \times 100\%}{\text{power input}} \\ &= \frac{0.9 \times 10^{-9}\, ZIV^2 \times 100\%}{VI} \\ &= 0.9 \times 10^{-9}\, ZV \times 100\% \end{aligned}$$

where

Z = atomic number of target plate
I = tube current (amperes)
V = tube voltage (volts)

From the preceding relationship, it is seen that as the Z number increases, the efficiency of x-ray production also increases.

)))》)) EXAMPLE

The x-ray production efficiency obtained with a tungsten target ($Z = 74$) using electrons accelerated through 100 kV would be

$$\begin{aligned} \text{Production efficiency} &= (0.9 \times 10^{-9})\, ZV \times 100\% \\ &= (0.9 \times 10^{-9})(74)(10^5) \times 100\% \\ &\sim 0.0067 \times 100\% \\ &= 0.67\% \end{aligned}$$

Recall that less than 1% of the incident electrons' kinetic energy is converted into x-rays, as this simple calculation verifies.

- Its tendency to resist vaporization at high temperatures (recall that vaporization of the target can compromise vacuum conditions, produce electrical arcing, and shorten tube life)

- Its ability to conduct heat away from the area where it is produced
- Its density (density ~ 19.3 gm/cc at 20°C), sufficiently high for adequate absorption and interaction with incident electrons within the relatively small dimensions of the target plate
- Its ability to absorb heat without excessive rise in plate temperature
- Its availability in nature assures that its use is not cost-prohibitive

Tungsten meets most of these specific needs. However, it does have one specific shortcoming. Compared with other metals, tungsten does not conduct heat (in physics referred to as its thermal conductivity) away from its point of origin rapidly. As a result, the area of the target plate actually struck by the incident electrons (focal spot or focal area) is subjected to repeated expansions and contractions as the focal area is heated and cooled during radiographic exposures. This alternating heating and cooling of the target plate (also called thermal stress) makes the surface subject to "pitting" and cracking as shown in Figures 6–8 and 6–9. When this occurs, the anode (actually the target) is damaged irreparably, and the tube must be replaced.

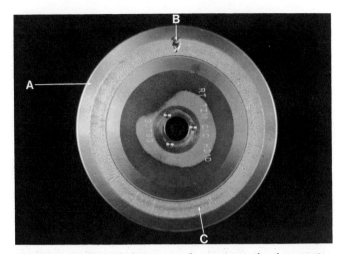

FIGURE 6–9. Thermal damage to the target track of a rotating anode (A) has led to pitting (B) and cracking (C) of the target surface.

A heat-damaged target plate results in x-ray beams of reduced intensity, resulting from scattering and absorption in the damaged, uneven surface of the target.

The target plate typically measures 1.0 to 1.5 cm in length and width with a thickness of only a few millimeters. The plate is actually larger than the focal spot, which is usually positioned toward its center. The larger target plate assists with the distribution of heat produced at the focal spot to prevent excessive temperature rise. This is based on the principle that for the same quantity of heat added, a large plate will show less rise in temperature than a smaller plate of the same material. Reducing the temperature rise of the target plate is also important in reducing its thermal expansion. Recall that metals expand on heating and that the amount of expansion observed depends on the type of metal and its change in temperature. If the temperature of the tungsten plate is allowed to change by too great a degree, it could expand to the point that it breaks away from the copper anode to which it is bonded.

To prevent thermal damage as a result of excessive heat build-up, the target plate is embedded in a large copper block. Copper, having a higher thermal conductivity than tungsten, rapidly conducts the heat away from the target plate to the exterior of the tube through the copper stem. The relatively large mass of the copper block in which the target plate is embedded serves to reduce the temperature rise of the copper, since copper has a much lower melting point (1083°C) than tungsten (3370°C). (Recall that for a given quantity of heat supplied to an object, its rise in temperature is inversely proportional to its mass.) Additional cooling may be accomplished by channeling the heat through the copper stem to metal disks with a large surface area known as cooling fins (Fig. 6–10), where heat is further removed by circulating air or oil. Methods of heat removal are discussed later in this chapter, as are the heat limitations of x-ray tubes and additional methods used to dissipate the heat.

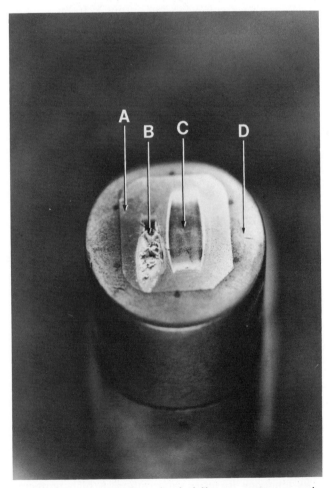

FIGURE 6–8. The target face of a dual filament, stationary anode. Damage done to the tungsten target plate (A) as a result of heat build-up is shown on both the small (B) and large (C) focal spots. The target plate is shown mounted on the copper anode block (D).

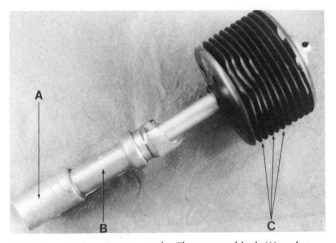

FIGURE 6–10. A stationary anode. The copper block (A) and stem (B) aid in heat dissipation by conducting heat from the target plate to cooling fins (C). Cooling fins assist in heat removal by means of convection.

Rotating Anodes

As medical science has progressed, greater demands have been placed on x-ray equipment. Equipment is not only required to make faster exposures to minimize the effects of patients' motion but also to make rapid serial exposures to trace the movement of contrast agents through body structures. To make faster exposures, tube current must be increased, thus generating the same number of x-rays in a shorter time period. However, this process generates more heat at the target plate. Rapid serial exposures also generate much greater quantities of heat, since the target plate and anode do not have sufficient time to cool between individual exposures. Therefore to reduce the chance of thermal damage to the target, changes in anode design have been required.

Perhaps one of the most important developments in x-ray tube design came in 1929 with the manufacture of the first rotating anode tube by Philips Medical Systems in Holland. Unlike the original stationary anode design, early rotating anodes consisted of a solid tungsten disk mounted on a short molybdenum stem attached at its center. The opposite end of the stem was attached to the copper rotor of an induction motor that provided rotational motion. The basic components of the rotating anode tube (i.e., glass envelope, cathode assembly, tungsten target, and anode) are essentially the same as in stationary anode tubes except for the obvious design differences of the anode.

The advantage of the rotating anode is the increased area of the target over which heat generated by electron bombardment is distributed. Unlike stationary anodes in which the total heat energy may be distributed over a rectangular area having (for discussion purposes) dimensions of 6 mm by 2 mm, or 12 mm², the same quantity of heat would typically be distributed over an approximate area of 1507 mm² on a rotating anode (see Comparison of Focal Areas of Stationary and Rotating Anodes, in box, for this calcula-

tion). This is some 125 times the area of the stationary anode, greatly increasing the heat storage capabilities of the tube.

Although most earlier anode disks were totally made of tungsten, today's x-ray tubes utilize a number of advances in rotating anode designs, the most common of which is the compound anode disk. It is so called because compound disks are made of two or more materials—a base material on which a coating layer is bonded (Fig. 6–11). The coating layer, most commonly tungsten or tungsten alloy, is the layer bombarded by filament electrons and is the one responsible for x-ray production. This coating layer on many rotating anodes is an alloy composed of 90% tungsten and 10% rhenium, a metal with good heat storage properties. The addition of rhenium reduces roughening and cracking of the target track surface that results from thermal stress. As a result of the use of this tungsten alloy, roughening of the target surface is not a major problem in these tubes. For several reasons, the backing, or base, material used with this type of anode disk normally is molybdenum. Molybdenum has good

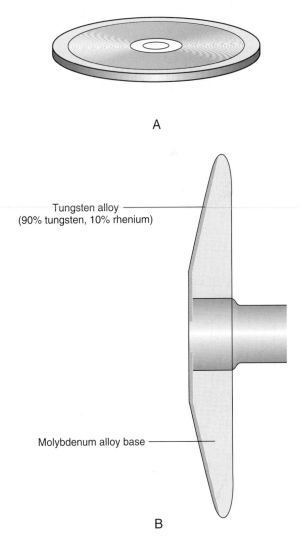

A

Tungsten alloy
(90% tungsten, 10% rhenium)

Molybdenum alloy base

B

FIGURE 6–11. A, Rotating anode disk, and B, cross-sectional view, indicating materials used in its construction.

■ COMPARISON OF FOCAL AREAS OF STATIONARY AND ROTATING ANODES

To obtain a comparison of the areas over which heat energy is distributed in a stationary and a rotating anode, first assume for calculation purposes an actual focal spot size of 2 mm by 6 mm as shown below on the stationary anode (Fig. 1). As indicated on the stationary anode, this corresponds to an area (A_s) of 12 mm^2.

Using typical dimensions of a rotating anode, shown in Figure 2 (on the right), the area covered by the tungsten focal track can be calculated by using this technique: Since the tungsten track forms a ring on the anode disk, the area of the track can be determined by first calculating the area of the

circle having radius r_1 and subtracting from it the area of the circle having radius r_2. That is,

$$\text{Area of tungsten target track, } A_R = \pi r_1^2 - \pi r_2^2$$
$$= (3.14)(43 \text{ mm})^2$$
$$\quad - (3.14)(37 \text{ mm})^2$$
$$= 5806 \text{ mm}^2 - 4299 \text{ mm}^2$$
$$= 1507 \text{ mm}^2$$

A comparison of the two areas expressed in the form of a ratio

$$\frac{A_R}{A_S} = \frac{1507 \text{ mm}^2}{12 \text{ mm}^2} = 126$$

indicates that the rotating anode has an actual focal track area approximately 126 times greater than the actual focal area on this particular stationary anode.

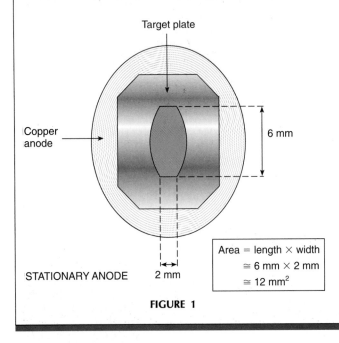

Target plate

Copper anode

6 mm

2 mm

STATIONARY ANODE

Area = length × width
$\cong$ 6 mm × 2 mm
$\cong$ 12 mm^2

FIGURE 1

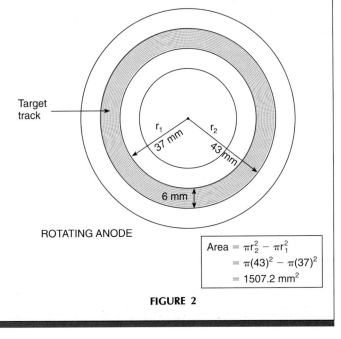

Target track

r_1 37 mm r_2 43 mm

6 mm

ROTATING ANODE

Area = $\pi r_2^2 - \pi r_1^2$
= $\pi(43)^2 - \pi(37)^2$
= 1507.2 mm^2

FIGURE 2

heat storage ability, so that it can absorb the heat generated at the coating layer but generally is a poor heat conductor, minimizing heat transferred to the rotor. The importance of this factor is discussed shortly. In addition, molybdenum is used because of its relatively low density (10.2 gm/cc compared with 19.3 gm/cc for tungsten measured at 20°C). Its lower density produces an anode disk of lighter mass, making it easier to put the disk into rotational motion.

Typical rotating anode disks range in diameter from approximately 5 cm (~2 in.) to about 12.5 cm (~5 in.). Disk size is an important factor (along with disk mass and speed of rotation), determining the

thermal loads that can safely be applied without damage to the anode disk. The disk itself is not flat but has a beveled outer rim to take advantage of the line-focus principle just as with stationary anodes. Typical angles of tilt range between 7° and 20°. A typical rotating anode design is illustrated in Figure 6–12. Because of the use of the angled target face, rotating anodes have the potential for heel effect x-ray intensity variation. Both the line-focus principle and associated heel effect are discussed later in this chapter under the topic of target plate angulation.

In this type of tube filament as shown previously in Figure 6–3, electrons are focused on the anode target

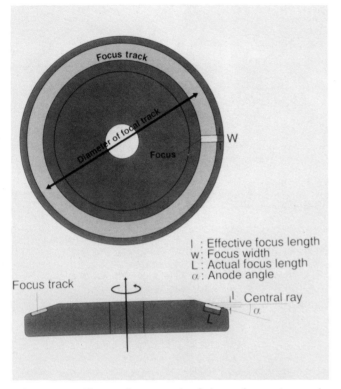

FIGURE 6–12. Plane and cross-sectional views of a rotating anode disk. (Courtesy of Philips Medical Systems.)

surface to form a small rectangular area which, as the anode disk rotates, traces out the target track (focal track) (Fig. 6–12). The rotation of the disk assures that the same area of the target track exposed to electron bombardment changes continuously. This allows heat energy generated to be distributed more evenly over the larger area. Therefore more rapid exposures can be made while minimizing possible thermal damage to the target. The proper rotation of the anode is thus an important requirement for proper tube operation.

Advances in Rotating Anode Design

The quest to produce anodes that can safely handle the quantity of heat generated by rapid, short-exposure time radiographs has led manufacturers to introduce several variations in anode disk design. In addition to solid tungsten disks and compound disks of rhenium, tungsten, and molybdenum (RTM disks), other materials such as titanium and zirconium (materials having high melting points, low densities, and relatively poor conductivity of heat) have begun to find their way into the materials used in compound disks.

It has been found that conventional RTM disks have demonstrated mechanical problems when used in making multiple serial exposures. The resulting thermal stress results in expansion and contraction (from heating, then cooling) that has led to surface distortions and even cracking of the disk. Surface distortion

of the disk can have definite, adverse effects on the anode target angle, the resulting x-ray intensity, and its distribution, along with other factors detrimental to quality image production. At least one manufacturer has attempted to remedy this problem by the production of disks with slits angulated (cut at angles) radially into the disk about its axis of rotation (Fig. 6–13) to prevent bombarding electrons from passing through the disk. Tests have shown this disk to be much more resistant to thermal distortion than disks without slits.

Another type of anode disk has been designed with grooves cut into the disk on each side of the target track. These grooves extend from the surface into the molybdenum base. The manufacturer claims that this disk can be used in conventional radiography and that when used in fluoroscopy (radiographic examination used to visualize motion), images can be produced with the disk stationary. (Note: In fluoroscopy procedures, tube currents are generally less than 5 mA, compared with tube currents ranging from 100 mA to as high as 1000 mA in conventional radiography.)

Additional modifications to disk design include compound disks composed of three layers rather than two; disks with two separate focal tracks, each at a different angle of tilt (called a double-angle, or biangular, tube); and the use of new alloys. Some of these modifications are illustrated in Figure 6–14. Another material that had seriously been considered as a base material was carbon in the form of graphite. The lighter mass of such a disk makes it easier to start and stop its rotation. However, graphite does not transfer heat as well as molybdenum, and as a result, graphite disks tend to get hotter than a comparable molybdenum disk. Additional technical problems arose in acquiring a solid bond between the tungsten coating layer and the graphite base. As a result, graphite disks have not gained widespread acceptance. These design variations are summarized in Table 6–1.

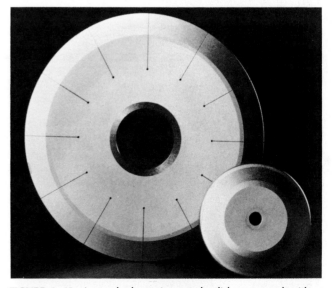

FIGURE 6–13. A standard rotating anode disk compared with a much larger rotating anode with slits. (Courtesy of Philips Medical Systems.)

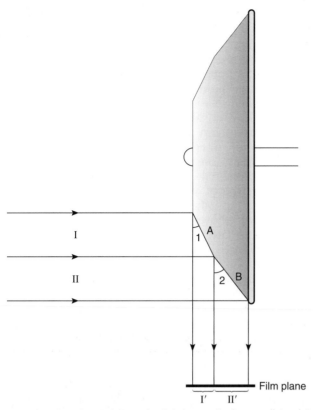

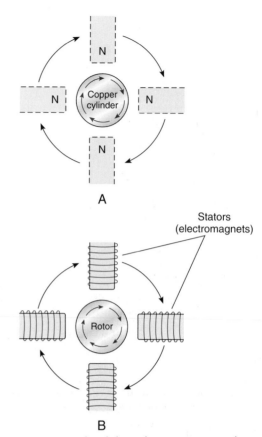

FIGURE 6–14. A biangular anode disk having both a small (angle) and large (angle 2) angle to tilt. Target area A would be used during low heat producing procedures when sharper radiographic images were required. Target area B would be used in higher heat producing procedures and image sharpness is not the major concern. (Chesney, D. N.; Chesney, M. O. X-ray Equipment for Student Radiographers. 3rd ed. ©1984, Oxford: Blackwell Scientific Publications, Ltd., 1984.)

FIGURE 6–15. Principle of the induction motor used to produce rotor rotation. *A*, A current can be induced in a copper cylinder as a result of a changing magnetic field in its vicinity. The magnetic field resulting from the induced current interacts with the changing magnetic field to cause the cylinder to rotate. *B*, The same principle can be applied using alternately activated electromagnets (solenoids), known as stators, to produce rotor rotation.

Table 6–1: SUMMARY OF X-RAY TUBE ANODE CHARACTERISTICS AND DESIGNS

Type	Design Characteristics	Primary Mode of Heat Dissipation	Advantages	Disadvantages
Stationary anode: standard type	Tungsten target plate embedded in copper block	Conduction	Heat rapidly conducted away from target plate	Unable to handle excessive heat loads resulting from long and multiple exposures
Rotating anode: older design	Solid tungsten disk	Radiation	Capable of handling higher heat loads	Rotating disk very massive —difficult to bring up to high rotational speeds quickly
More modern design (RTM compound disk)	Tungsten target track bonded to a molybdenum base	Radiation	Capable of handling high heat loads; lighter mass of disk makes rotation easier	Thermal stress can produce surface distortion of target material
Newer designs: RTM compound disk with angulated slits	RTM disk with angulated slits cut radially into disk about its axis of rotation	Radiation	Minimizes surface distortions which can result from thermal stress	None noted
Disk with grooves	Grooves cut into molybdenum base around target track	Radiation	Can be used for conventional radiography and then with disk stationary for fluoroscopy	None noted
Double-Angle or Biangular tubes	Disk has 2 focal tracks in the form of 2 concentric rings; each focal track is at a different anode angle—small angle for fine focus, larger angle for less detail focus	Radiation	Two different anode angles which can be used to advantage in radiographic production	None noted
Graphite disks	Tungsten target track bonded onto a graphite (carbon) base	Radiation	Lighter mass makes rotation easier	Does not transfer heat as well as molybdenum; disk tends to become hotter than other disks during use

Anode Rotation: The Induction Motor

Rotation of the anode disk at the required speeds is an important factor in the proper operation of any rotating anode tube. The fact that the anode disk rotates at a high speed, typically 3000 revolutions per minute (rpm) and as high as 10,000 rpm, allows the target disk to distribute evenly larger quantities of heat over its surface and thereby to minimize potential thermal damage to the anode. A somewhat different approach must however be taken in the type of motor used to produce anode rotation. Because of the vacuum that must exist within the tube, conventional motors, requiring wires exiting the tube through the glass envelope, cannot be used. Motors of this type at times require service that would be impossible if they were sealed within the glass envelope.

To avoid these problems, a different type of motor is used. It is called an induction motor, since its operation is based on electromagnetic induction and Lenz's law (see Chapter 5). To understand how rotation is produced, recall that a changing magnetic field can be used to induce a current in a conductor such as copper. According to Lenz's law, the current induced in the conductor will flow in such a direction that its magnetic field will oppose the changing magnetic field that first induced the current in the conductor. To better illustrate this concept, consider a conducting copper cylinder about which a magnet is moved (Fig. 6–15A). As the magnet is moved quickly around the

conducting cylinder, the cylinder reacts to this as a changing magnetic field, and as a result, a current is induced in the conducting cylinder. According to Lenz's law, the current induced flows in a direction to oppose the change in the magnetic field that induced it. The induced current will flow in such a direction that its magnetic field will interact with the changing magnetic field of the magnet. This will result in a force between the two interacting magnetic fields that will cause the cylinder to rotate in the same direction as the rotating magnet.

Rotation is accomplished more efficiently by surrounding the copper rotor with a series of electromagnets (i.e., current-carrying solenoids) that can be switched on and off rapidly in rotational sequence. The copper rotor reacts to this action of the electromagnets, or stators, as if they were a changing magnetic field. Currents are induced in the copper rotor, and as a result, the opposing magnetic fields cause the rotor to rotate (Fig. 6–15B). Utilizing 60-Hz alternating current (AC), anode rotational speeds theoretically approach 3600 rpm. In actuality, typical rotational speeds are assumed to fall more closely between 3000 and 3600 rpm as a result of mechanical slipping. Newer tubes supplied with higher-frequency AC have produced rotational speeds of 9000 rpm (150 Hz) and even 10,000 rpm (180 Hz).

The copper rotor rotates about the anode shank on steel ball-bearings (Fig. 6–16). Conventional methods of lubrication to minimize friction and assure ease of

A Assembled

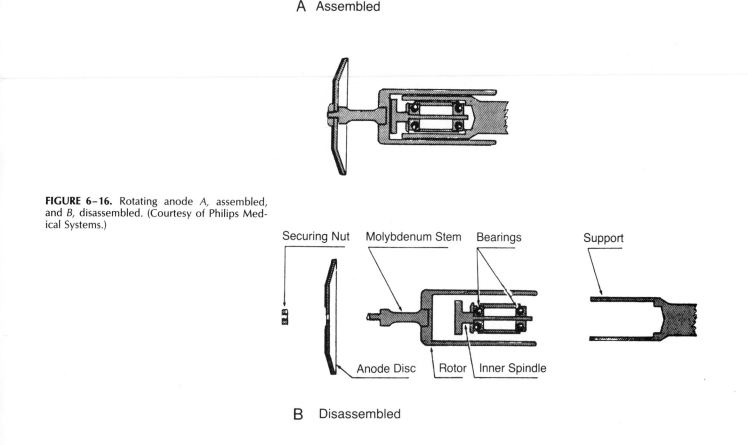

FIGURE 6–16. Rotating anode A, assembled, and B, disassembled. (Courtesy of Philips Medical Systems.)

B Disassembled

rotation cannot be used within the vacuum conditions of the x-ray tube. Liquid lubricants, upon heating, could spread into the tube and destroy the required vacuum conditions. To avoid this potential problem, bearings are lubricated with metallic silver, lead, or barium. Higher-speed rotation allows the tube to safely handle higher heat loads, but these higher rotation speeds are considerably more wearing on the rotational structures than lower rotational speeds.

The anode shank on which the rotor is supported emerges from the anode end of the glass tube and is connected to the positive side of the high-voltage power supply. An airtight and heat-resistant seal bonds the glass envelope to the anode shank.

Another important consideration in proper performance of the rotating anode is heat distribution through the anode assembly. The greater quantities of heat generated at the anode disk must not be conducted to the steel bearings, which would tend to expand and bind on heating. This would subsequently reduce optimal rotation speeds and result in thermal damage to the disk. To minimize this problem, the anode disk is linked to the copper rotor by a molybdenum stem of small diameter. Molybdenum is a relatively poor conductor of heat, and its small cross-sectional area reduces the rate of heat flow from the disk to the copper rotor. Additionally, the outer walls of the copper rotor are usually blackened to make it a more effective heat radiator, so that heat is radiated to the glass wall and away from the steel bearings.

TARGET PLATE ANGULATION

Line-Focus Principle

In the previous section, that portion of the target plate actually struck by the incident electron beam was referred to as the focal spot. In reality it is more like a focal area with dimensions of length and width as shown in Figures 6–8 and 6–9. The size of the area, imprinted on the target face, is dependent on several physical factors:

- Filament size and shape
- Physical dimensions of the focusing cup
- Position of the filament within the focusing cup
- Electrical field configuration produced by the focusing cup
- Distance between cathode and anode inside the x-ray tube

It should be recalled from previous discussions that image sharpness is improved when the focal spot is small. That is, with a dual-filament tube, the smaller filament is used when a higher degree of image sharpness is required, since it produces a smaller focal spot.

It must also be recalled, however, that more than 99% of the incident electron energy is converted to heat on striking the target plate. If this heat energy is distributed over a small area of the target plate such as

a small focal spot, there is a possibility of damage to the target plate as a result of heat build-up. This possibility increases when large quantities of heat are produced in a single exposure or a rapid succession of exposures. There is less chance of target plate damage if this heat energy is distributed over a large rather than a small area on the target plate.

This apparent conflict of needs—a large area for heat distribution but a small area to assure image sharpness—is remedied by slanting the target face. This is known as the line-focus principle. As shown in Figure 6–17A, when the anode face is parallel to the vertical (dashed) reference line, the incident electron beam is distributed over an area of the target plate determined by the width of the beam. As the anode

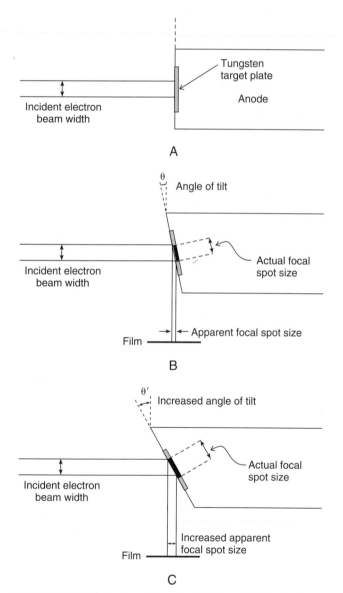

FIGURE 6–17. Effect of anode angle to tilt on effective focal spot size. *A,* Actual focal spot size is determined by the width of incident electron beam if there is no angle of tilt on the anode. *B,* When a small angle of tilt (θ) is used, a small apparent focal spot size is obtained. *C,* As the angle of tilt is increased (θ'), the apparent focal spot size also increases.

face is tilted at some angle θ (Greek letter *theta*) to the vertical reference line, the electron beam is distributed over a larger area (Fig. 6–17*B*) of the target plate. This actual area over which the electron beam is distributed is known as the *actual focal spot* and, being larger, aids in heat dissipation. However, from the plane of the film, it would appear to an observer that the electrons strike (and subsequent x-rays emerge) from a smaller area of the target plate referred to as the *apparent or effective focal spot,* indicated in the illustration. Since the apparent focal spot is smaller, image sharpness is improved. There is a limit, however, to the application of this concept.

It can be seen from Figure 6–17*C* that as the angle of tilt, θ', of the anode face is further increased, the size of the apparent focal spot also increases, thereby adversely affecting image sharpness. As a result, in almost all modern x-ray tubes, both stationary and ro-

tating anode types, anodes are slanted at angles ranging between 7° and 20°.

Heel Effect

With the face of the target plate slanted to take full advantage of the line-focus principle, another minor problem arises. As incident electrons from the filament strike the target, the electrons travel into the target plate, where they interact with target atoms in the production of x-rays. As the x-rays produced exit the target, they travel through different thicknesses of target material as a result of the slant of the target face. Those exiting through the upper surface of the target are transmitted with minimal absorption. More of those traveling through the thicker heel portion of the anode shown in Figure 6–18*A* are absorbed. This re-

■ APPARENT FOCAL SPOT SIZE AS A FUNCTION OF THE TILT ANGLE OF THE ANODE

As shown in the preceding figure, the incoming electron beam strikes the target plate at points A and C. Line AC on the diagram forms the long dimension of the actual focal spot (or focal area). The length indicated on the diagram as the dimension b is the corresponding length of the apparent focal spot. Length b is equivalent to the length of line BC.

Using the triangle ABC and the trigonometric sine function (here sin θ = BC/AC), we have

$$\sin \theta = \frac{BC}{AC}$$

$$BC = AC \sin \theta$$

Since the length of AC is fixed by the dimensions of the beam, the length BC is determined by sin θ. From the values shown here

θ	sin θ
5°	0.087
10°	0.174
15°	0.259
20°	0.342

and assuming AC is constant (i.e., beam width remains contant), the apparent focal spot size increases with increasing angle of tilt.

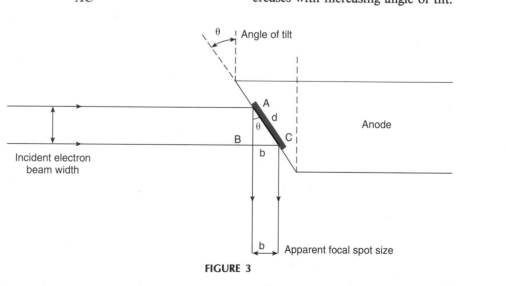

FIGURE 3

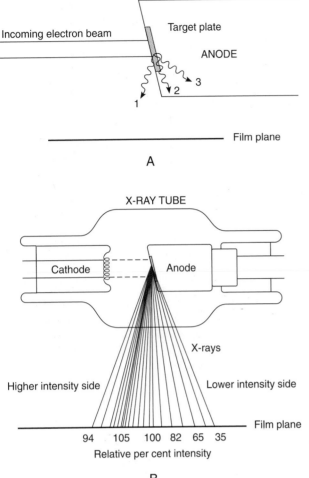

A

B

FIGURE 6–18. The heel effect. *A*, The heel effect is a variation in x-ray intensity as a result of the use of a target that is slightly tilted to the direction of the incoming electron beam. *B*, The variation in x-ray intensity as a result of the heel effect is seen as an increased intensity toward the cathode side and a decreased intensity toward the anode side of the tube.

sults in a variation in x-ray intensity along the line between the cathode and anode, the greatest intensity occurring on the cathode side of the tube. This variation in intensity (Fig. 6–18*B*) is known as the *heel effect,* since the decrease in x-ray intensity on the anode side of the tube results from a smaller number of x-rays being able to penetrate the heel of the anode. The heel effect as it would appear in a radiograph is shown in Figure 6–19.

Since radiographic images are created as a result of variations in x-ray beam intensity as the beam encounters the various structures within the body, variations in the beam intensity on exiting the tube are not desirable. The most desirable situation would be to produce an x-ray beam that is uniform in intensity. In this case, intensity variations visualized in the radiographic images as different shades of gray would result solely from anatomical structures, not from the heel effect.

The heel effect is an unavoidable phenomenon of all x-ray tubes that have beveled anodes. The degree of intensity varies significantly with changes in the angle of tilt of the anode, being more pronounced with steeper (i.e., smaller) angles of tilt compared with those anodes having larger angles of tilt. Some investigators have reported 30% to 50% variations in intensity between cathodes and anodes of several radiographic units. The degree to which intensity variance can be observed depends on a number of factors, including the angle of tilt of the anode, the size of film used, and the target-to-film distance.

Perhaps the most common way to compensate for the heel effect in the clinic is by patient positioning. Since the heel effect produces increased x-ray intensity toward the cathode side of the tube, the thicker portion of a patient's body should be positioned toward the cathode when radiographing body structures that vary significantly in thickness and tissue density along their length (e.g., the thoracic spine, chest, abdomen, and long-bone extremities). By so positioning the patient, the thicker portions of the body structure will remove or attenuate more x-ray photons than the thinner portion of the structure. In this way, more photons are removed from the high-intensity side of the beam. Now the degree of darkening, or *radiographic density,* more accurately represents variations in anatomical structure and their composition.

The influence of the heel effect on a radiograph may

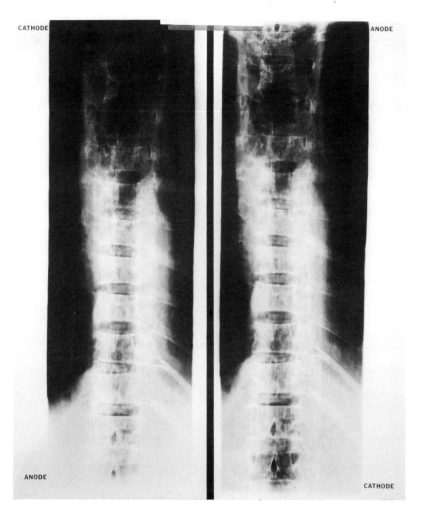

FIGURE 6–19. Visualization of the anode heel effect on a radiograph of the thoracic spine. The image on the right is of better quality, in that x-ray intensity does not vary as greatly from the upper to lower portion of the image. Detail within the image on the left is lost when the thicker portion of the patient's body is positioned toward the anode (lower intensity) side of the tube. A greater degree of darkening is also noted in the same image on the cathode (higher intensity) side of the tube. (Courtesy of the American College of Radiology Institute.)

also be minimized by proper selection of film size. Since the x-ray intensity variation resulting from the heel effect manifests itself over the area beneath the tube anode and cathode, larger films (e.g., 11 × 14 and 14 × 17) are more likely to show the effect than smaller films (e.g., 8 × 10, 9 × 9, or 10 × 12) at a specified target-to-film distance. Since the larger film records the x-ray intensity over a larger area, any variation in intensity between cathode and anode is more pronounced. This effect on larger film can actually limit the size of film used with special procedure tubes, which have steeper anode angles. Such tubes have anode angles of 7° to 10° compared with standard diagnostic tubes, which have anode angles typically ranging from 10° to 17°, the most common angle being about 12°.

An additional factor that can also affect the degree to which an anode heel effect is observed on a radiographic image is the distance between the tube's focal spot and the plane of the radiographic film (the focus-film distance, FFD; or target-film distance, TFD). Most common radiographic procedures are performed at an FFD of 40 inches (101.6 cm) or 72 inches (182.9 cm). For a specific size of film, less intensity variation can be observed when larger FFDs are used. This results from the fact that as the film is moved farther away from the tube, its area receives only the more uniform x-radiation surrounding the central ray. Each of these situations and its effect on differences in intensity resulting from the anode heel effect is illustrated in Figure 6–20.

Although the heel effect is an inherent phenomenon that occurs with all x-ray tubes having beveled anodes, the degree to which it affects a radiograph is influenced by many factors. As previously discussed, some of these factors can be controlled by the radiographer, whereas others cannot. With many of the newer radiographic units currently in clinical use, the anode heel effect does not appear to present a major problem in producing quality radiographic images. This could be a result of the angle of tilt of the anode, use of standardized technical factors, better screen-film combinations, or improvements in x-ray generators. The medical radiographer should however always be mindful of the ever-present potential problem and the techniques that can be employed to minimize its effects.

■ CONCEPT OF X-RAY INTENSITY

The term *flux* is used to describe the number of photons traveling through a unit area (e.g., 1 square meter, m²) per second as shown in the following figure.

For the example shown, the flux would be described as "three photons per square meter per second." This indicates that three x-ray photons travel through any 1 m² of area each second. By definition, flux is defined accordingly as

$$\text{Flux} = \frac{\text{number of photons}}{\text{area–time}}$$

Closely related to the concept of flux is that of intensity. Since each photon carries a specific quantity of energy, intensity is defined as

$$\text{Intensity} = \frac{\text{energy}}{\text{area–time}}$$

that is, intensity represents the amount of energy traveling through a unit of area per unit of time. In an initial example, if each x-ray photon carried 10 keV of energy, the intensity of the x-ray beam shown would be

$$\text{Intensity} = \frac{30 \text{ keV}}{1 \text{ m}^2 - 1 \text{ sec}} \quad \text{or} \quad 30 \frac{\text{keV}}{\text{m}^2 - \text{sec}}$$

This concept finds important applications in later discussions on radiation exposure, radiation protection, photon interaction with matter, and image production.

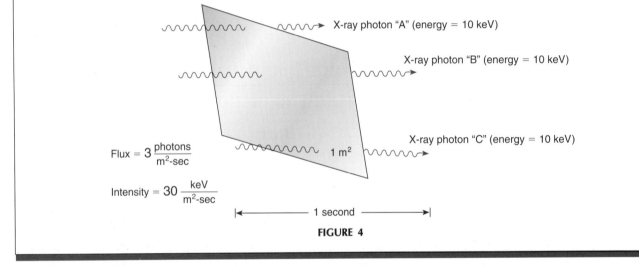

X-ray photon "A" (energy = 10 keV)

X-ray photon "B" (energy = 10 keV)

X-ray photon "C" (energy = 10 keV)

$$\text{Flux} = 3 \frac{\text{photons}}{\text{m}^2\text{-sec}}$$

$$\text{Intensity} = 30 \frac{\text{keV}}{\text{m}^2\text{-sec}}$$

1 m²

|← —————— 1 second —————— →|

FIGURE 4

HEAT DISSIPATION TECHNIQUES

Stationary Anode Tubes

The problems associated with the removal of heat generated at the anode as a result of electron bombardment are of major importance in the design and proper operation of any x-ray tube. If large quantities of heat are produced by a radiographic procedure and this heat is not adequately removed from the target, melting of the target plate, which will adversely affect x-ray beam intensity and radiographic image quality, may occur.

In stationary anode tubes, the primary mode of heat transfer is *conduction* (recall that this is the primary method by which heat is transferred in metals). Heat generated at the focal spot is conducted through the tungsten plate to the copper block on which it is mounted. Since copper is an excellent thermal conductor, the heat produced is rapidly transferred away from the target plate. Depending on the specific anode design, from this point heat may be dissipated in one of several ways. If the copper block is sufficiently massive, it may be capable of safely absorbing the heat generated without approaching the melting point of copper. In this case, the copper block and stem may not extend beyond the end of the tube's glass envelope.

For those cases in which the copper block and stem cannot adequately dissipate the heat produced, the copper stem may extend beyond the glass envelope, where it may be attached to cooling fins (large surface area metal plates over which heat may be distributed as shown in Fig. 6–10) or another copper structure that can act as an additional heat reservoir. These structures in turn are surrounded by the oil within the tube shield. Heat conducted to these structures is then transferred to the oil, which removes it from the structure by the process of *convection* (i.e., the transfer of heat by a moving fluid).

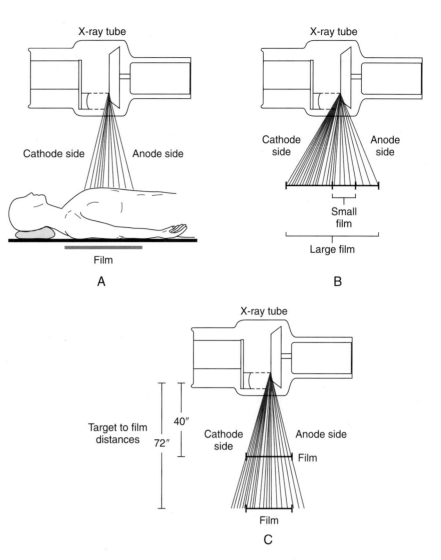

FIGURE 6–20. Factors that influence the anode heel effect. *A,* The thicker portion of the patient's body is positioned toward the cathode side to attenuate more of the higher intensity portion of the beam. *B,* Use of a small film that subtends the central portion of the x-ray beam is less likely to indicate a heel effect than a large film. *C,* Variation in x-ray beam intensity is also less noticeable for a specific size film at longer focus-to-film distances.

■ PHOTON ATTENUATION AND ITS VARIATION WITH ABSORBER THICKNESS

When photons (e.g., x-rays) strike matter such as the human body, lead shielding, or concrete, some are removed from the incident beam either as a result of scattering (redirection of a photon) or absorption (total removal of the photon from the initial beam) as shown in the following figure. These methods of reduction in incident photon intensity as a photon beam travels through an absorber medium is called photon *attenuation.*

As the photon beam travels through an absorbing medium, the number of photons removed from the beam depends on factors such as the energy of the photons, the type of absorber, and thickness of the absorber. Each of these factors is discussed in greater detail in Chapter 8. The last factor, absorber thickness, is of some importance in minimization of the heel effect.

As the thickness of absorber increases, the number of photons transmitted decreases. This can be used to the radiographer's advantage in minimizing the heel effect by positioning the thicker portion of the patient's body toward the cathode, where radiation intensity is higher. This has the overall effect of reducing intensity variations that result from use of the slant-faced anode.

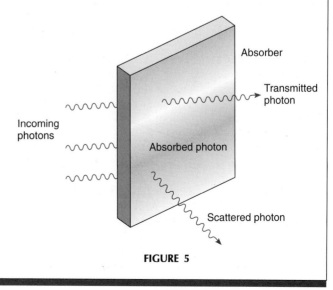

FIGURE 5

In many cases, heat is more rapidly transferred away from the tube by oil within the tube housing that is circulated by an electric motor (a process called forced convection). Heat energy removed by the circulating oil is transferred to the tube housing, where it is conducted to the outside of the housing and is finally transferred to the surrounding air by convection air currents.

Rotating Anode Tubes

With greater quantities of heat generated as a result of techniques for producing higher tube currents (mA) and rapid multiple exposures, methods must be devised to remove heat quickly from the target track where it is generated. This energy must also be dissipated in a manner that is not harmful to the x-ray tube. In the rotating anode tube, the primary method used for heat transfer is *radiation*. One should recall that when a metal is heated to high temperatures it begins to glow. At relatively low temperatures, the radiation emitted is invisible infrared (i.e., heat radiation). As the temperature increases, the radiation falls into the visible portion of the electromagnetic energy spectrum. When this occurs, the anode target track begins to give off visible light (e.g., red, yellow, blue, or even "white hot") (Fig. 6–21). Radiation does not require a medium through which to travel and therefore is free to move through the vacuum within the tube. Unlike the situation with stationary anode tubes, in which heat is transferred from the target plate by conduction through the copper block and stem, this is not desirable in rotating anode tubes. With this type of tube, any heat conducted along the anode stem and into the region of the rotor could cause thermal ex-

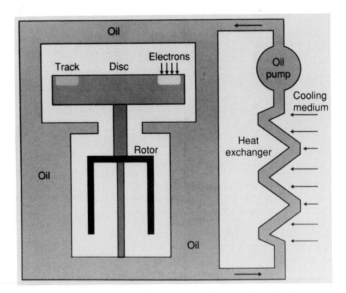

FIGURE 6–22. Heat removal, using circulating oil and a heat exchanger. (Courtesy of Philips Medical Systems.)

pansion of the rotor bearings. Any such expansion of these bearings could cause the rotor to bind and could subsequently result in thermal damage to the anode surface. For this reason, the rotating anode stem is commonly made of molybdenum, which is a relatively poor heat conductor.

Heat energy radiated from the target surface is then transferred to the glass walls of the tube. The tube is supported within a metal housing just as are stationary anode tubes. Similarly, oil surrounds the tube (as illustrated in Fig. 6–6), both for electrical insulation and to assist with heat removal. Heat within the tube's glass walls is carried away by the motion of the surrounding oil (i.e., convection). Some manufacturers utilize an oil pump that forces the oil to circulate (forced convection) around the tube in order to remove the heat. The heated oil then moves through flexible tubes to a heat exchanger outside the metal housing (Fig. 6–22), where the oil is cooled then returned to remove additional heat. Heat transferred to the metal housing is removed by the room air, which may circulate on its own or with the use of fans.

Many modern x-ray tubes are equipped with temperature-sensing devices, which are used to monitor anode disk temperatures in order to avoid potential thermal damage. One method utilizes color indicators (e.g., red, yellow, and green), whereas others use electronic displays to indicate the state of readiness of the target disk to safely handle additional heat loads.

HEAT-LOADING CAPACITIES INDICATED BY TUBE-RATING CHARTS

In previous sections, discussion focused on the fact that kinetic energy attained by the filament electrons

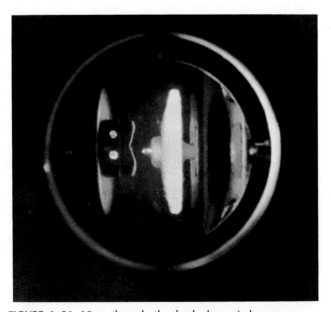

FIGURE 6–21. View through the lead glass window as an extremely hot anode disk radiates its energy to the surroundings within the tube housing. (Courtesy of Philips Medical Systems.)

as they are accelerated to the anode target plate is converted into x-rays (<1%) and heat (>99%). Unless these large quantities of heat generated by electron bombardment of the target are effectively dissipated, tube damage can result. Thus safe tube operation depends on two basic considerations: (1) the rate at which energy is incident on the anode and (2) the rate at which the resulting heat energy is dissipated by conduction, radiation, or both to other tube components or to its surroundings.

The amount of heat that can safely be delivered to the anode of an x-ray tube is dependent in general on several factors involved in tube design and associated instrumentation. These include

- Whether the tube has a stationary or rotating anode
- For rotating anode tubes, the anode rotation speed
- Focal spot size
- The type of x-ray generator (i.e., 1ϕ or 3ϕ) used

Heat Units

The amount of heat generated by any radiographic procedure also depends on several specific factors:

- kVp used in the procedure
- Tube current (i.e., mA) employed
- Length of the exposure
- Type of voltage waveform (i.e., 1ϕ, 3ϕ, type rectification) used
- Number of exposures made in rapid succession

Target anodes can only sustain finite quantities of heat before irreparable damage may occur to the tube. In order to better quantitate the amount of heat energy delivered to a target anode, the concept of the *heat unit (HU)** was devised. The heat units generated by the various types of x-ray circuits are given as follows:

HU = kVp × mA × sec	(1ϕ units)
HU = 1.35 × kVp × mA × sec	(3ϕ, 6-pulse units)
HU = 1.41 × kVp × mA × sec	(3ϕ, 12-pulse units)

))⟩⟩⟩) EXAMPLE

An x-ray machine operates at 80 kVp, 100 mA for 0.1 sec. Determine the heat units generated by

---

*Physically the heat unit, defined as the product of

kilovoltage × tube current × time,

represents in terms of more fundamental physical quantities

joules/coulombs × coulombs/sec × sec

equivalent to joules, the SI unit of energy.

a) a 1ϕ unit:
$$HU = kVp \times mA \times sec$$
$$= (80\ kVp)(100\ mA)(0.1\ sec)$$
$$= 800\ HUs$$

b) a 3ϕ, 6-pulse unit:
$$HU = 1.35 \times kVp \times mA \times sec$$
$$= (1.35)(80\ kVp)(100\ mA)(0.1\ sec)$$
$$= 1080\ HUs$$

c) a 3ϕ, 12-pulse unit:
$$HU = 1.41 \times kVp \times mA \times sec$$
$$= (1.41)(80\ kVp)(100\ mA)(0.1\ sec)$$
$$= 1128\ HUs$$

The heat storage capacity of an x-ray tube's anode and housing refers to the number of heat units that can be absorbed without thermal damage resulting. X-ray tube manufacturers combine all heat-loading characteristics and information concerning the limitations of their individual tubes in graphical representations referred to as *tube-rating charts.* These charts take into consideration anode and cathode design, their size, mass, thermal conductivity, rate of heat radiation from their surfaces, focal spot size, speed of rotation, and type of voltage waveform and tube current used. Each of these parameters plays an important role in determining whether a particular combination of technical factors (i.e., the combination of kVp, mA, and exposure time) does or does not produce unacceptable thermal damage. Other factors that must also be considered include

- Determination of the maximum heat load that can be handled safely as a result of a single exposure
- Determination of the maximum heat load that results from a series of exposures made in rapid succession
- Effect of near-continuous tube use as a result of heavy clinical use

Single-Exposure Use and Tube-Rating Chart Interpretation

Tube-rating charts are used to determine if a particular combination of exposure factors (i.e., kVp, mA, and exposure time) will produce unacceptable thermal damage to an x-ray tube. These charts are provided by tube manufacturers with their x-ray tubes. Tube-rating charts are specific to the tube manufacturer, type of anode, speed of anode rotation (if the tube is of that design), focal spot size, and type of voltage waveform used. This information, generally found on each chart, allows the radiographer to determine prior to its use if the chart is the proper one for the tube that is to be used. Tube-rating charts used for single radiographic exposure information assume that at initiation of the exposure, the anode is at room temperature and that it is rotating at normal speed.

Tube-rating charts such as those shown in Figure 6–23 usually take the form of a series of curves drawn

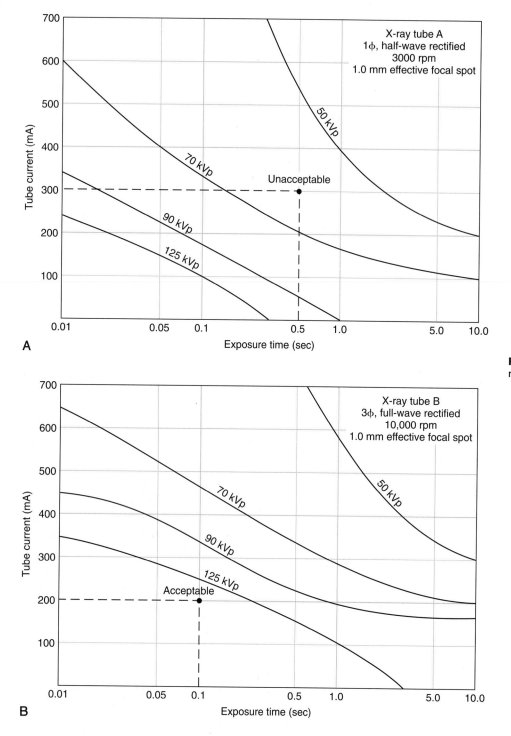

FIGURE 6–23. *A* and *B,* X-ray tube rating charts.

on a semilog graph (i.e., the vertical scale may be linear, whereas the horizontal scale is a logarithmic scale or vice versa). Commonly, tube current (mA) is represented on the vertical (linear) axis and exposure time in seconds, on the horizontal (logarithmic) axis. It is important to remember that when reading a logarithmic scale, each cycle on this scale represents a different power of ten, as discussed in Chapter 2 and as seen on both charts in Figure 6–23. The series of curves shown on both these charts represent the various peak kilovoltages (i.e., kVp settings) at which

the tube may be operated. To determine whether a particular set of technical factors will result in unacceptable damage to the target at the focal spot, first find the desired tube current on the vertical axis and the exposure time on the horizontal axis. Next, trace horizontally and vertically upward to find the point of intersection of these two values. If this point of intersection lies above the chosen kVp curve, the procedure is unacceptable and the technical factors are unsafe for the tube. If the point of intersection lies below the kVp curve, the procedure is considered acceptable.

Two examples of such a determination are illustrated here.

)))))) EXAMPLE

Use Figure 6–23 to determine if a procedure which calls for technical factors of 300 mA, 90 kVp, and 0.5 sec would be acceptable or unacceptable. This radiograph is to be made using x-ray tube A, utilizing 1ϕ, half-wave rectification and having a 1.0 mm effective focal point.

Solution. From the rating chart in Figure 6–23A, the point at which 300 mA and 0.5 sec intersect is above the 90 kVp curve.

Therefore, according to the tube rating chart, this procedure would be unacceptable and would likely result in thermal damage to the target surface.

)))))) EXAMPLE

Use Figure 6–23 to decide if a procedure calling for technical factors of 125 kVp, 200 mA, and 0.1 sec would be acceptable or unacceptable. This radiograph is to be made using an x-ray tube, a 1.0 mm effective focal spot with 3ϕ, full-wave rectification.

Solution. Using rating chart in Figure 6–23B the point at which 200 mA and 0.1 sec intersect is under the 125 kVp curve. According to the tube-rating chart, this procedure would be acceptable and would not result in unacceptable thermal damage to the tube.

It is important to realize that tube-rating charts such as those illustrated in Figure 6–23 can provide the safe limits for single-exposure radiographic procedures. This assumes sufficient time exists between exposures to allow the necessary cooling of the target, anode, and tube housing.

When rapid serial exposures are made within a short time period, as in angiography, even larger quantities of heat are generated. In these procedures, tube damage can result from several factors:

● Insufficient cooling of the target surface
● Insufficient cooling of the entire anode assembly
● Insufficient cooling of the tube housing

Charts for finding single-exposure limits can be used to determine whether a tube can safely handle the heat generated by a multiple-exposure procedure. In order to do this, remember the following principle:

> The total number of heat units generated in a rapid serial exposure cannot be greater than the number of heat units allowed for a single exposure with a total elapsed time equivalent to that required to complete the series of exposures.

This principle is demonstrated in the following example:

)))))) EXAMPLE

X-ray tube B is to be used to make 10 exposures in rapid succession using technical factors of 300 mA, 70 kVp, and 0.2 sec. If the 10 exposures are to be made within 5 sec, can the procedure be performed without damage to the tube?

Solution. Using the tube rating chart for tube B and the technical factors chosen (300 mA, 70 kVp, and 0.2 sec), it is determined that a single exposure using these technical factors will not result in tube damage.

Next, calculate the number of heat units generated by a single exposure having these technical factors:

$$HU = 1.41 \times kVp \times mA \times sec$$
$$= (1.41)(70)(300)(0.2)$$
$$= 5922 \ HU$$

The number of heat units generated by 10 such exposures would then be

$$Total \ HU = 10(5922)$$
$$= 59220 \ HU \ in \ a \ time \ interval \ of \ 5 \ sec$$

From tube B's rating chart, the maximum permissible heat load this tube could safely withstand for a 5-sec exposure is 70 kVp when the tube current is approximately 210 mA. This corresponds to a maximum heat load of

$$HU_{max} = (1.41)(70)(210)(5)$$
$$= 103,635 \ HU$$

Thus the 59,220 HU delivered in 5 sec is much less than the 103,635 HU the tube is capable of withstanding.

This particular determination assumes that a sufficient time is allowed between multiple exposures to allow for some cooling to take place. Specially formulated charts provided by manufacturers of tubes used in procedures such as angiography and cineradiography should always be checked for more accurate information when using these tubes to make rapid serial exposures. Many tubes in clinical use today have both a normal rotor speed (~3000 rpm), which is used for procedures that produce relatively low quantities of heat and a high rotor speed (~10,000 rpm) for those procedures in which higher quantities of heat are produced. Many of the more modern x-ray units do not allow exposures to be made if an unsafe combination of technical factors are used.

Anode-Cooling Charts

Heat energy generated at the target as a result of electron bombardment is transferred to structures of the tube anode. When this occurs, the heat storage capability of these structures becomes an important consideration. Anode thermal characteristics can be

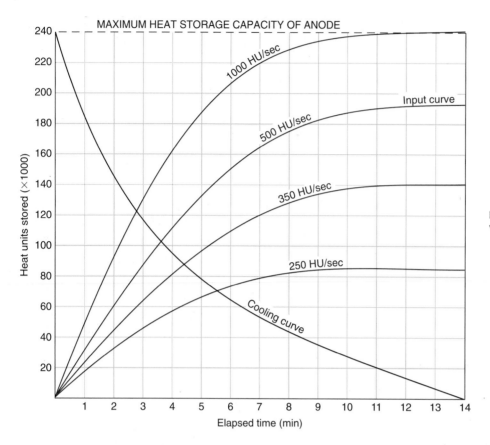

FIGURE 6-24. An anode cooling chart with input curves.

represented graphically (Fig. 6–24). Such a chart consists of two distinct types of curves.

1. Input curves, designated in heat units per second, indicate the amount of heat units stored in the anode as a result of a single exposure or a series of rapid multiple exposures. In the graph (Fig. 6–24), four input curves are shown. The anode represented by this chart has a maximum heat storage capacity of 240,000 HU, indicated by the uppermost number on the vertical axis. For the four input curves shown, the procedure that delivers 1000 HU/sec will result in this maximum heat storage capacity being attained after 14 min of use (i.e., since this uppermost input curve reaches the 240,000 HU maximum limit in 14 min). Procedures delivering 500 HU/sec, 350 HU/sec, and 250 HU/sec could be used for longer periods of time since their input curves do not approach the 240,000 HU maximum limit.

2. The anode-cooling curve, also shown in Figure 6–24, is used to describe the amount of heat remaining in the anode after periods of cooling have occurred. The anode described by the curve shown has a maximum heat storage capacity of 240,000 HU. The curve indicates that if the maximum heat storage capacity is attained it will take 14 min (i.e., that time when the cooling curve drops to zero) to completely cool, or come into thermal equilibrium with its surroundings. If procedures are conducted that deposit, for example, 132,000 HU, several important facts are obtained from the curve:

a. Only an additional 108,000 HU can be deposited (i.e., 240,000 HU − 132,000 HU) in the anode, assuming no cooling is allowed.
b. It will take approximately 11.6 min (i.e., 14 min − 2.4 min) for the anode to completely cool when 132,000 HU have been deposited.

Not that the rate of cooling is initially much greater than at later times after some cooling has occurred. This is evidenced by the fact that the cooling rate during the first minute is ~52,000 HU/min (i.e., [240,000 HU − 188,000 HU]/1 min), but drops to ~14,000 HU/min (i.e., [80,000 HU − 66,000 HU]/1 min) after 5 min of cooling. This more rapid rate of initial cooling occurs when the anode temperature is highest, since it is at this time that significant heat loss occurs by radiation (recall that heat loss by radiation is proportional to T^4).

Similar cooling curves exist for x-ray tube housings and the technique for using such curves generally is the same. Becoming proficient in the use of such curves is not as important today as it was at one time. Most modern radiographic equipment contains sufficient safeguards to prevent the chance of thermal damage to the unit.

VARIATIONS IN X-RAY TUBE DESIGN

The previous sections have discussed the basic design of the conventional stationary anode and rotating anode x-ray tubes. Several variations in conventional tube design have now been introduced either as an improvement of tube performance or for x-ray tube use for other than conventional applications. Some of the more important design variations are discussed here.

Grid-Controlled Tubes

Whereas most x-ray tubes contain only two electrodes (i.e., cathode and anode), this type of tube contains a third electrode known as a control grid. In grid-controlled tubes, the focusing cup, which is usually negative to assist with electron focusing, is maintained at ~1.5 kV to 3.0 kV negative with respect to the filament. The more negative the control grid, the more difficult it is for electrons to move from the filament to the anode. In this way by rapidly raising and lowering this negative bias voltage, the control grid can be used as an electronic switch to control the passage of filament electrons to the anode and thereby to regulate the production of x-rays. This is in comparison with conventional tubes in which x-ray production is controlled by regulating the high voltage across the electrodes. (Recall that if the voltage across the electrodes drops to zero, no electrons are pulled across the tube, and no x-rays are produced.) Thus with grid-controlled tubes, the grid allows the tube itself to control x-ray production. The advantage of the grid-controlled tube is that it allows extremely short exposures (as short as 1 msec) to be made. This makes it most useful in angiography and special fluoroscopic procedures.

Tubes With Metal Envelopes

Conventional x-ray tubes with glass envelopes have certain limitations imposed on their efficient operation when tungsten deposits become attached to their glass walls. These deposits adversely affect the tube's ability to dissipate heat efficiently. In an effort to minimize this particular problem, certain manufacturers have developed rotating anode tubes with metal envelopes. The advantage of such tubes is the fact that they are unaffected by these metal deposits throughout the life of the tube. Metal tubes (Fig. 6–25) also have several additional features:

- Higher tube current capabilities for shorter radiographic exposures
- More substantial support structures, allowing the use of more massive anode disks (e.g., a 2000 gm disk compared with a conventional disk of less than 700 gm); this increased mass allows greater heat storage capability and more efficient heat dissipation
- The use of two exit windows—one beryllium and the other aluminum; the beryllium (Z = 4) window is almost transparent to the x-rays produced, whereas the aluminum (Z = 13) window, located just below it, filters out lower-energy less penetrating

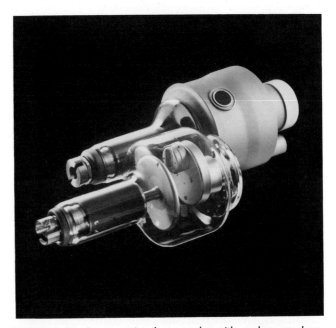

FIGURE 6–25. A conventional x-ray tube with a glass envelope. Shown together with a high-output tube having a combined glass and metal envelope. (Courtesy of Philips Medical Systems.)

x-rays that contribute only an additional radiation dose to the patient; these windows also act to reduce off-focus radiation (scattered electrons and x-rays from scattered electrons that strike nonfocal track areas of the anode disk) and scattered x-rays from within the tube

These tubes are most useful in both conventional and special procedure radiography when short exposure times and sustained tube use are required.

Metal and Ceramic Tubes With Double Bearings

Philips Medical Systems has developed a specially designed metal-cased tube with several advantages over conventional tubes. This tube, the Super Rotalix Ceramic tube (Fig. 6–26), has an anode disk that rotates on an axle supported at each end of the tube (Fig. 6–27). The axle itself rotates on bearings located at each end. This method of mechanical support allows the use of more massive anode disks with greater heat capacities than the lighter disks used in conventional tubes.

Additionally, this tube is characterized by the use of three ceramic insulators (aluminum oxide is the most commonly used material) to provide electrical insulation between the tube's high-voltage components and its metal envelope. These insulators, also shown in Figure 6–27, surround the points of attachment of high-voltage leads to the tube's anode and cathode. An additional ceramic collar supports the anode stem. This added support provides the extra stability needed for the more massive anode disks used in these tubes.

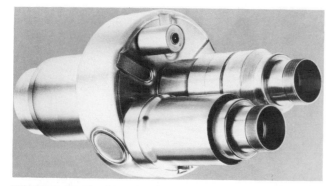

FIGURE 6-26. The Super Rotalix metal/ceramic x-ray tube. (Courtesy of MedicaMundi.)

More recent developments in the metal-ceramic tube have included the introduction of bearings having spiral grooves. These bearings are lubricated with liquid metal (a special gallium alloy) and have several advantages over conventional rotor bearings, including

- Longer bearing life
- Less noise
- Improved heat dissipation

Additionally, when the lifetime of conventional tubes is determined to a great part by wear on the anode bearings, the anodes of such tubes are rotated only during the actual exposure in an effort to minimize wear. Within a typical 1 to 3 sec time period, these anodes are brought to rotational speeds ranging from 3000 to 9000 rpm then decelerated rapidly on termination of the exposure. However, tubes utilizing the new design of spiral-groove bearings with liquid metal lubricant can rotate continuously, needing to be brought up to operational speed only once each day. This feature, along with the tube's increased heat storage capability and its ability to dissipate heat rapidly (by conduction through the bearings as well as by radiation), makes this tube most suitable for imaging procedures in which numerous exposures in rapid succession are required to trace the swift movement of blood through vessels, as is the case in coronary angiography. Rapid serial exposures such as this are called ciné exposures, derived from the term cinema, or motion picture.

Mammography Tubes

The diagnostic quality of radiographs of soft tissue structures such as the breast are dependent on the energy of the x-rays used. The primary reason for this is that both normal and pathological structures tend to interact with x-rays in a similar manner. As a result, there are extremely small differences in the number of x-rays passing through each type of structure. If the energy of the x-rays used is too high (i.e., too penetrating), the radiographic appearance of the two types of structures would almost be indistinguishable. Thus in order to maximize the differences, low-energy x-rays are used.

Low-energy x-rays can be produced by operating the tube at lower kVp settings and by properly choosing the anode target material. X-ray tubes used exclusively for mammography (Fig. 6-28) have targets made of molybdenum rather than tungsten, since these targets produce an increased number of x-rays having energies of 17.5 keV and 19.5 keV (known as characteristic x-rays discussed in greater detail in Chapter 9. It is x-rays in this general low-energy range (~20 keV to 30 keV) that are most useful in producing diagnostic-quality mammograms. These x-ray tubes may have either stationary or rotating anodes.

Since these tubes are used to produce relatively low-energy x-rays, the tube exit port must be designed so that it does not filter out or attenuate the x-rays as they pass through. This is accomplished in one of two ways. Some tubes utilize beryllium (Z = 4) windows that because of their low atomic number do not substantially remove x-rays from the beam as it passes through. Other tubes simply use thinner than normal borosilicate glass windows. Using thinner windows restricts the maximum kilovoltage levels that can be

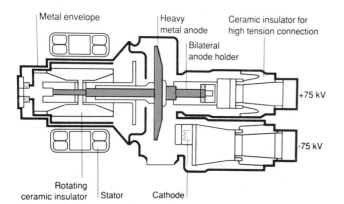

FIGURE 6-27. Diagrammatic cross-section through a Super Rotalix Ceramic tube showing the double-bearing rotor with anode disk and the ceramic insulator that rotates with it. (Courtesy of Philips Medical Systems.)

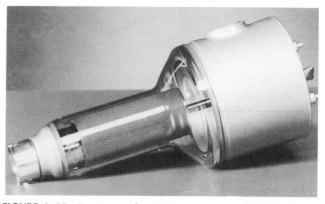

FIGURE 6-28. An x-ray tube used for mammography. In most mammographic examinations, very low energy radiation is used to obtain soft tissue contrast. This is best achieved with molybdenum filtration, a molybdenum anode, and operating voltages between 25 kV and 30 kV. (Courtesy of Philips Medical Systems.)

used with tubes of this design. However, this does not pose any major problem, since mammography tubes are usually not operated above 50 kVp.

Chapter Summary/ Important Concepts and Relationships

X-rays are produced when fast-moving electrons strike high atomic (Z) number targets

The greatest percentage (>99%) of the energy carried by the incident electrons moving within the x-ray tube is converted into heat with only a small percentage (<1%) being converted into x-rays

X-ray tubes generally contain two electrodes—the cathode (negative electrode) that acts as the source of electrons and the anode (positive electrode) that acts as the target—mounted within a glass envelope from which air has been evacuated

The filament of an x-ray tube produces electrons by thermionic emission

Electrons emitted from the filament are accelerated to high speeds by the kilovoltage applied between the tube electrodes

Thermal limitations set on an x-ray tube are represented graphically on tube-rating charts, which are used to determine if a specific set of technical factors will result in unacceptable thermal damage to a specific tube

The most commonly used target material is tungsten (W) because of its high atomic number (Z = 74) and its high melting point (~3370°C)

The use of rotating anodes increases the capability of an x-ray tube to handle larger quantities of heat without incurring unacceptable thermal damage to the target anode

Target anodes are commonly slanted at angles ranging between ~7° to 20° to minimize the chance of thermal damage to the target while decreasing the size of the tube's effective focal spot; this is known as the line-focus principle

The use of slant-face targets can produce a variation in x-ray intensity, known as the heel effect, across the x-ray beam produced; the beam may tend to have a higher intensity toward the cathode side of the tube and a lower intensity toward the anode side

The actual focal spot refers to the actual area on the target plate struck by the beam of incident electrons from the cathode, whereas the effective focal spot refers to the smaller area on the target plate from which x-rays appear to originate from the view point of the x-ray image receptor (e.g., film)

Heat energy generated at the target during x-ray production must be effectively removed to minimize the chance of permanent damage to the x-ray tube

Stationary anode tubes primarily utilize conduction to remove heat from the anode target

Rotating anode tubes distribute heat over a larger target surface and then primarily utilize radiation as a means of heat transfer

The number of heat units (HU) generated by a specific radiographic procedure is determined by the number of exposures made in rapid succession; the kVp, the mA, the length of the exposure; and the type of generator used. For single exposures, the number of heat units produced is given by the following formulas:

$$HU = (kVp) \times (mA) \times seconds) \qquad 1\phi$$

$$HU = 1.35 \times (kVp) \times (mA) \times seconds \qquad 3\phi, \text{6-pulse}$$

$$HU = 1.41 \times (kVp) \times (mA) \times seconds \qquad 3\phi, \text{12-pulse}$$

Important Terminology

Actual Focal Spot. The actual area of the target plate struck by incident electrons from the filament in the production of x-rays; this area tends to be somewhat larger when the target face is slanted.

Anode. The positive electrode of the x-ray tube

Anode-Cooling Chart. A graphic description of the cooling characteristics of the anode of a specific x-ray tube

Attenuation. The partial removal of x-rays from an x-ray beam as a result of absorption or scattering in a material through which the beam passes

Cathode. The negative electrode of the x-ray tube

Conduction. Method in which heat energy is transferred from atom to atom by atomic collisions; this method is characteristic of heat transfer in metals

Convection. Heat transfer by a moving fluid, either gas or liquid

Dual-Filament Tube. X-ray tube having two filaments —one large (for high-mA procedures in which fine image detail is not required) and one small (for low-mA procedures in which greater image detail is required)

Dynamic Image. Image used to visualize motion, produced by making serial exposures and playing them back in rapid succession

Edison Effect. The formation during thermionic emission of a "cloud" of electrons in the vicinity of the filament in the absence of a sufficiently high voltage

Effective (Apparent) Focal Spot. The small area on the anode target from which x-rays appear to originate during x-ray production as a result of the angle of tilt of the anode target

Exit Window. Structure on an x-ray tube through which x-rays emerge; it is usually made of materials relatively transparent to x-rays

Filament. The thin, coiled tungsten wire that when heated by the current, produces the electrons that are accelerated into the anode target during x-ray production

Filament Circuit. Portion of the x-ray circuitry that controls the current flowing through the x-ray tube filament

Filament Current. The electrical current that flows through the x-ray tube filament, releasing the electrons necessary for x-ray production

Focal Spot (Focal Area). Area on the anode target that is struck by stream of electrons emitted from the filament

Focusing Cup. The negatively charged metal cup that surrounds the x-ray tube filament; its purpose is to minimize the divergence, or spreading, of the electrons as they are emitted from the filament and move toward the anode target

Heat Unit (HU). An artificial unit of heat energy used to describe the thermal characteristics and limitations of x-ray tube targets, anodes, and housings

Heel Effect. Variation in x-ray beam intensity from the cathode to the anode side of the x-ray tube as a result of x-ray attenuation by the heel of the tilted anode

Kilovoltage, Kilovolts (kV). The voltage placed across the x-ray tube electrodes in order to accelerate electrons into the anode target; used to regulate the energy of the resulting x-rays

Line-Focus Principle. Use of an anode target that is tilted at an angle to assist in minimizing thermal damage to the anode target

mA (see also Tube Current). Abbreviation for *milliamperes;* refers to the current (electrons) flowing between cathode and anode of an x-ray tube during x-ray production

Radiation. General term used to describe any of the various types of electromagnetic radiation (i.e., photon radiation such as infrared, x-ray, visible, ultraviolet, etc.) or particulate radiation (i.e., alpha and beta particles, positrons, neutrons, etc.) that are emitted from unstable nuclei or nuclear processes

Radiographic Density. Degree of darkening of a radiographic film

Radiolucent. Transparent, or capable of being penetrated by x-rays

Radiopaque. Cannot be penetrated by x-rays

Resolution. Depiction of closely spaced structures as separate rather than as a single structure.

Serial Exposures. Images made in rapid succession

Static Image. Image of a body structure that does not depict motion

Target. Portion of the anode that is struck by fast-moving electrons during x-ray production

Technical Factors. The combination of kilovoltage (kVp), tube current (mA), and exposure time chosen for a specific radiographic procedure

Thermionic Emission. Process by which electrons are emitted from the tube filament as a result of heat generated within the filament by the filament current

Thorium. Metal added to tungsten in the production of filament wires as a 1% to 2% impurity to improve efficiency of thermionic emission, reduce filament vaporization, and thereby lengthen tube life

Tube Current. Current consisting of electrons moving between the x-ray tube cathode and anode during x-ray production

Tube Housing. Metal support structure in which an x-ray tube is encased

Tube-Rating Charts. Graphic representations describing the thermal characteristics of the target of an x-ray tube

Tungsten. Metal used for x-ray tube filaments and target plates because of its high melting point ($\sim 3370°C$) and relatively low degree of vaporization and ductility; tungsten has an atomic number of 74, and its chemical symbol is W (for wolfram, its original name)

Voltage. Difference in electrical potential that is necessary in conventional electrical circuits in order to move an electric charge from one point (high potential) to another (low potential)

Bibliography

Abbott, D., ed. Physicists. New York: Peter Bedrick Books, 1984.

Balter, S., ed. The Technical History of Radiology (monograph). Radiographics 9:1095–1283, 1989.

Carroll, Q.B.; Thomas, C.C. Fuchs's Principles of Radiographic Exposure, Processing, and Quality Control, 3rd ed. Springfield, IL: Charles C Thomas, 1985.

Clifford, A.H., ed. The Encyclopedia of the Chemical Elements. New York: Reinhold Book Corporation, 1968.

Coulam, C.M.; Erickson, J.J.; Rollo, F.D.; James, A.E., Jr. The Physical Basis of Medical Imaging. New York: Appleton-Century-Crofts, 1981.

Cullinan, A.M. Producing Quality Radiographs. Philadelphia: J.B. Lippincott, 1987.

Curry, T.S. III; Dowdey, J.E.; Murry, R.C., Jr. Christensen's Physics of Diagnostic Radiology. Philadelphia: Lea & Febiger, 1990.

Gratale, P.; Wright, D.L.; Daughtry, L. Using the anode heel effect for extremity radiography. Radiol Tech 61:195–198, 1990.

Hendee, W.R. Medical Radiation Physics, 2nd ed. Chicago: Year Book Medical Publishers, 1979.

Hendee, W.R.; Chaney, E.L.; Rossi, R.P. Radiologic Physics, Equipment, and Quality Control. Chicago: Year Book Medical Publishers, 1977.

Hill, D.R., ed. Principles of Diagnostic X-ray Apparatus. Philips Technical Library. London: The MacMillan Press, 1975.

Ridgway, A.; Thumm, W. Physics of Medical Radiography. Reading, MA: Addison-Wesley, 1968.

Seeram, E.; Thomas, C.C. X-ray Imaging Equipment. Springfield, IL: Charles C Thomas, 1985.

The Illustrated Science and Invention Encyclopedia, Vols 15 and 20. Westport, CT: H.S. Stuttman, 1983.

⚡ Review Questions

1. Briefly explain the importance of maintaining x-ray tube components under vacuum conditions within the x-ray tube.
2. Explain the purpose of each of the following x-ray tube components:
   a. glass envelope
   b. cathode
   c. filament
   d. target
   e. anode
   f. focusing cup
3. Indicate the advantage of rotating over stationary anode tubes.
4. Explain the relationships among the magnitude of the kilovoltage applied, the speed of the electrons as they move from cathode to anode, and the penetrating ability of the resulting x-rays.
5. How does the use of fans or circulating oil assist in the dissipation of heat?
6. Indicate two ways the line-focus principle assists the radiographer in terms of improving heat-handling capabilities of the anode and improving radiographic image sharpness.
7. Determine the number of heat units (HU) generated by each of the following radiographic procedures, using the equipment indicated:
   a. 200 mA, 70 kVp, 0.5 sec, using 3ϕ, 6-pulse equipment
   b. 100 mA, 80 kVp, 100 msec, using 3ϕ, 12-pulse equipment
   c. 800 mA, 100 kVp, 0.5 sec, using 3ϕ, 12-pulse equipment
   d. 300 mA, 100 kVp, 1 sec, using 1ϕ equipment
   e. 1000 mA, 60 kVp, 0.8 sec, using 3ϕ, 6-pulse equipment
8. Using the tube rating charts shown in Figure 6–23, determine whether each of the following radiographic procedures would result in acceptable or unacceptable thermal damage to the anode:
   a. Tube A: 200 mA, 70 kVp, 1 sec
   b. Tube A: 300 mA, 50 kVp, 0.5 sec
   c. Tube A: 200 mA, 90 kVp, 1/5 sec
   d. Tube B: 300 mA, 125 kVp, 0.03 sec
   e. Tube B: 500 mA, 70 kVp, 0.1 sec
   f. Tube B: 250 mA, 125 kVp, 0.2 sec
   g. Tube B: 100 mA, 125 kVp, 0.6 sec
9. Use the anode-cooling chart shown in Figure 6–24 to determine how long it will take the anode to completely cool after absorbing
   a. 180,000 HU
   b. 76,000 HU
   c. 20,000 HU

Exercises

1. Indicate how each of the following factors affects the ability of the anode to satisfactorily handle large quantities of heat without incurring unacceptable damage:
   a. the mass of the copper block of a stationary anode
   b. the diameter of the rotating anode disk
   c. the rotational speed of a rotating anode
2. Keeping in mind the function of the filament, why does the filament take the form of a long, thin wire rather than a short, thick wire?
3. Use the anode thermal characteristic curves shown in Figure 6–24 to answer each of the following questions:
   a. Could a procedure that delivers 350 HU/sec to the anode be conducted without exceeding the anode thermal storage capacity for 14 min? How many heat units would be stored in the anode at the end of 14 min? How long would it take the anode to completely cool?
   b. A procedure delivers 500 HU/sec to the anode. How many heat units are stored in the anode after 9 min? How long will it take the anode to completely cool?
   c. How long will it take a procedure that delivers 250 HU/sec to deliver 80,000 HU to the anode?
   d. Compare the rate of heat loss (in HU/min) when the anode contains 180,000 HU and when it contains 20,000 HU. How do you explain this difference in the rate of heat loss?

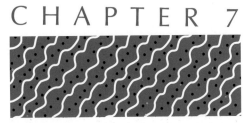

CHAPTER 7

X-ray Machine Operation: The X-ray Circuit

Michael A. Thompson, M.S.

Chapter Outline

Chapter Objectives

Upon completion of this chapter, you should be able to

- Identify the two major subcircuits of the x-ray machine and explain their purpose in x-ray production.
- Explain what is meant by line voltage.
- Describe the purpose of line-voltage compensation.
- Describe the components of the high-voltage circuit and the role each plays in efficient x-ray production.
- Describe how voltage across the x-ray tube electrodes is varied by the technologist.
- Explain the importance of rectification to efficient x-ray production.
- Describe the various types of timers used in x-ray units and their methods of operation.
- Demonstrate how a spinning-top is used to check the accuracy of an x-ray timer.
- Describe the components of the filament circuit and the role each plays in x-ray production.
- Indicate factors that affect x-ray tube current.
- Describe three types of x-ray generators used in portable x-ray units and their respective advantages and disadvantages.
- Explain what is meant by the "ripple factor" and its effect on the x-rays produced by an x-ray unit.
- Describe the principle of operation of a falling-load generator.

X-RAY MACHINE CIRCUITRY: AN OVERVIEW

In the previous chapter it was shown that x-rays are produced when electrons emitted by the filament are accelerated to extremely high speeds and slam into the anode target plate. For this process to occur, a sufficiently large electrical current must be directed through the appropriate filament in order to generate sufficient heat so that electrons are released from the filament surface by the process known as *thermionic emission*. Since the number of electrons emitted from the filament directly relates to the number of x-rays produced, the radiographer must have a way to control electron production by the filament. This control is provided by the *filament circuit*. This circuit allows the radiographer to adjust the current that flows through the filament (i.e., the *filament current*), thereby regulating electron emission. By controlling electron emission, *tube current* (i.e., the electron flow between cathode and anode) and the subsequent number of x-rays produced can also be regulated.

On release of electrons from the filament, no x-rays are generated within the x-ray tube, unless a sufficiently high voltage exists between the tube electrodes. For diagnostically useful x-rays to be produced, voltages must be raised from several hundred volts (typical incoming *line voltage*) to tens of thousands of volts, which is accomplished by the *high-voltage circuit.* This circuit also allows the voltages across the tube to be adjusted by the radiographer. Adjustment is most important when one recalls that the energy or penetrating ability of the x-rays produced by the x-ray tube is determined by the voltage across the tube electrodes. It is the appropriate combination of number of x-rays (defined by the tube current and tube voltage) and the energy of the x-rays produced (defined by the tube voltage) that determines whether or not a diagnostically useful radiograph is obtained.

In addition to the filament and high-voltage circuits, additional circuitry and circuit components are needed to perform specific tasks. These include

- A *timing circuit,* which allows x-rays to be produced for only a specific period of time
- A means to electronically monitor and to compensate for variations or fluctuations that can occur in the incoming line voltage
- An appropriate number of high-voltage *rectifiers* for more efficient x-ray production
- Appropriate meters, such as *ammeters* (to monitor tube current) and *voltmeters* (to measure tube voltage)

Each of these circuits and circuit components is shown in the overall x-ray circuit illustrated in Figure 7–1. This overall circuit is broken down into its components for closer inspection.

THE X-RAY GENERATOR

Overview of Generator Components

In Chapter 5, the term *generator* is used to describe a device that converts mechanical energy of motion into electrical energy by using changing magnetic fields to generate an electric current. When applied to x-ray equipment the term *x-ray generator* refers to those electrical components and circuits involved in supplying electrical power to the x-ray tube. Generally, x-ray generators consist of the following components:

- A source of electrical power supplied to the x-ray imaging room by the local power company. In the United States, it typically is 120 to 480 volts (V), 60-Hz alternating current (AC). The AC power supply is represented by the symbol
- *Line-voltage compensation,* or correction for voltage fluctuations —⊙—
- A high-voltage circuit that provides appropriate voltage across the x-ray tube electrodes. This circuit takes incoming line voltage and allows the radiographer to make slight modifications in its initial

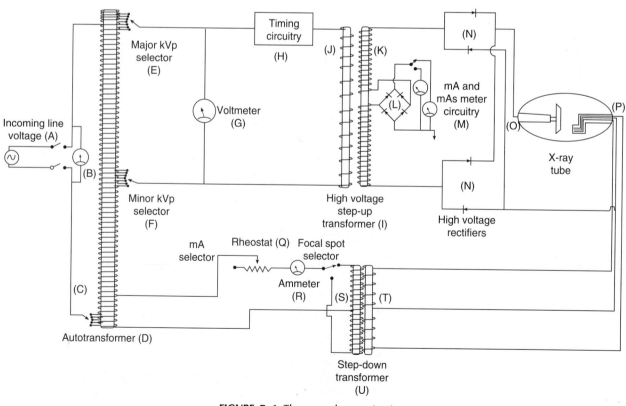

FIGURE 7–1. The general x-ray circuit.

value by using the autotransformer. This relatively low voltage is then greatly increased in value to the appropriate kilovoltage by using a fixed turn *step-up transformer*. In order to make the most efficient use of the electrical energy supplied, appropriate voltage rectification must also occur within this circuit. The primary purpose of this circuit is to provide sufficiently high voltage to accelerate filament electrons from cathode to anode

● A timer circuit that allows the radiographer to accurately control the length of time x-rays are produced by the x-ray unit. This is accomplished by controlling the length of time the high voltage is applied across the x-ray tube electrodes

● A circuit that supplies sufficient voltage to the tube filament to liberate electrons by thermionic emission allows the radiographer to regulate tube current. This is accomplished by controlling the current that flows through the filament (i.e., by controlling the filament current). This circuit, the filament circuit, contains a number of individual resistors or a variable resistance (i.e., a rheostat). This allows the radiographer to control incoming voltage that can be lowered to an appropriate level by using a step-down transformer

All of these listed circuits and electrical components make up the conventional x-ray generator. Newer high-frequency generators differ somewhat in design; these differences are discussed later in the chapter. Typically, the generator components previously listed are found in two separate sections of the x-ray unit — *the control console* (Fig. 7–2) and the *transformer box*, or transformer assembly (Fig. 7–3).

Control console appearance varies considerably

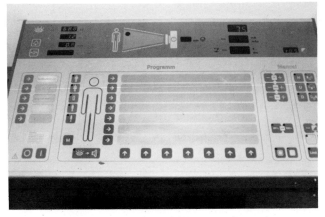

FIGURE 7–2. An x-ray machine control console.

among equipment manufacturers. Here, the controls allowing the radiographer to select specific values for kVp, mA, and exposure time are located. Appropriate voltmeters (to measure kVp) and ammeters (to measure mA) are also found in this part of the equipment, providing readings during the radiographic exposure. Two buttons are also found on the control console. The first button (designated standby, or prep) has two important functions. First, it brings the rotating anode up to required speed, and, second, it sends the appropriate current through the filament to release electrons by thermionic emission. The second button provides the necessary high voltage across the tube electrodes to draw electrons into the target and produce the radiographic exposure.

The transformer box, a grounded metal case containing the step-up and step-down transformers sub-

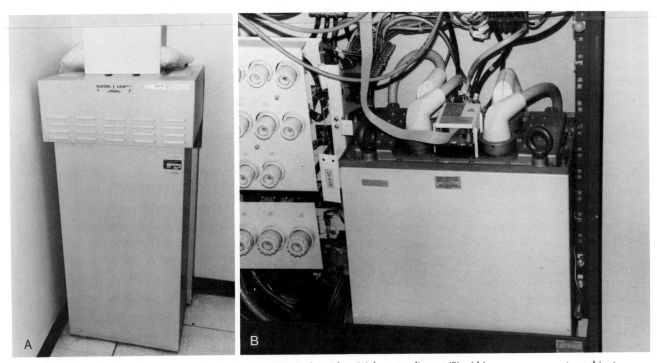

FIGURE 7–3. An x-ray unit transformer box. These may be either (A) free-standing or (B) within an x-ray generator cabinet.

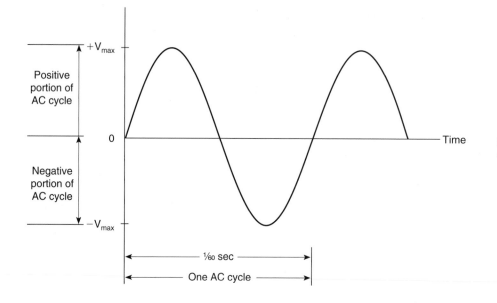

FIGURE 7–4. Sinusoidal 60-Hz AC waveform (1 cycle).

merged in oil, may stand alone in the imaging room or may be located in an equipment cabinet in a room adjacent to the x-ray unit.

Each component of the x-ray generator is now considered in more detail and for a better understanding of the operation of the x-ray unit.

Source of Electrical Power

Electrical power is supplied commercially by local power companies to residences, businesses, and medical facilities in the form of *alternating current* (AC). On the North American continent, the current reverses its direction of flow 60 times per second and is therefore described as 60-cycle, or 60-Hertz (Hz), AC. (Re-

call that the Hertz is a unit of frequency and is equivalent to cycles per second, or simply second⁻¹). This frequency refers to the variation in voltage (and current) that occurs in time (Fig. 7–4). As shown in the diagram of the single-phase (1ϕ) AC voltage waveform, the voltage varies in time from zero to some maximum or peak voltage (V_{max}). If 60-Hz AC voltage is used, there will be 60 voltage cycles each second, and therefore the duration, or length of time, of each individual cycle is 1/60 sec. If 50-Hz AC voltage had been supplied (as commonly used in Europe), the duration of each AC cycle would have been 1/50 sec.

In Figure 7–4, with single-phase AC power sources, several important factors must be noted:

● Voltage starts at zero, rises to some V_{max}, then falls to zero again

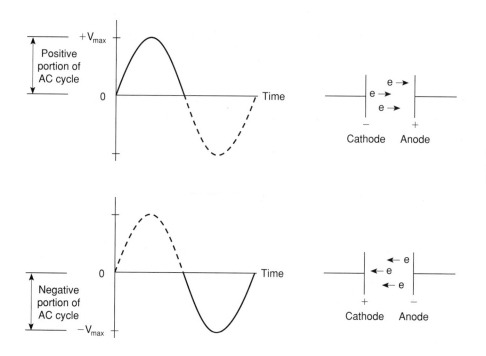

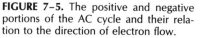

FIGURE 7–5. The positive and negative portions of the AC cycle and their relation to the direction of electron flow.

- The single-phase AC voltage waveform has a positive and negative portion in each AC cycle; the positive portion occurs when the anode is positive, the cathode is negative, and electrons move from the cathode to the anode of the x-ray tube; the negative portion occurs when the anode is negative and the cathode is positive, and electrons would move from anode to cathode (Fig. 7–5) if it were possible

Recall from Chapter 6 how x-rays are produced in the x-ray tube, and realize that these factors can produce nonbeneficial effects during x-ray production. These negative aspects arise from the fact that

- As the voltage varies across the x-ray tube electrodes, so does the energy of the x-rays produced; variations in tube voltage affect not only x-ray energy but also the number of x-rays produced within a specified time period
- X-rays can be produced only when electrons emitted from the filament are accelerated into the target anode; this can occur during the positive portion of the AC cycle but not during the negative portion

when electrode polarity reverses; thus with 1ϕ AC voltage, x-rays are produced only during the positive half of each cycle, which is inefficient use of the electrical energy provided

This does not imply that single-phase AC voltage cannot be used to power an x-ray unit, but if it is used, voltage rectification (see Chap. 5) can make more efficient use of the electrical energy supplied to the unit.

Commercial electrical power is commonly supplied as three-phase (3ϕ), 60-Hz AC. It should be recalled from Chapter 5 that 3ϕ AC indicates that rather than a single AC voltage waveform, three AC voltage waveforms are produced simultaneously, but each typically is 120° out of phase with the other. When appropriately rectified and depending upon how the 3ϕ AC voltage is generated, 6- or 12-pulse voltage waveforms that have significant advantages in x-ray production over 1ϕ units are produced. A comparison of the various voltage waveforms is summarized in Figure 7–6. One obvious advantage of 3ϕ power is that, un-

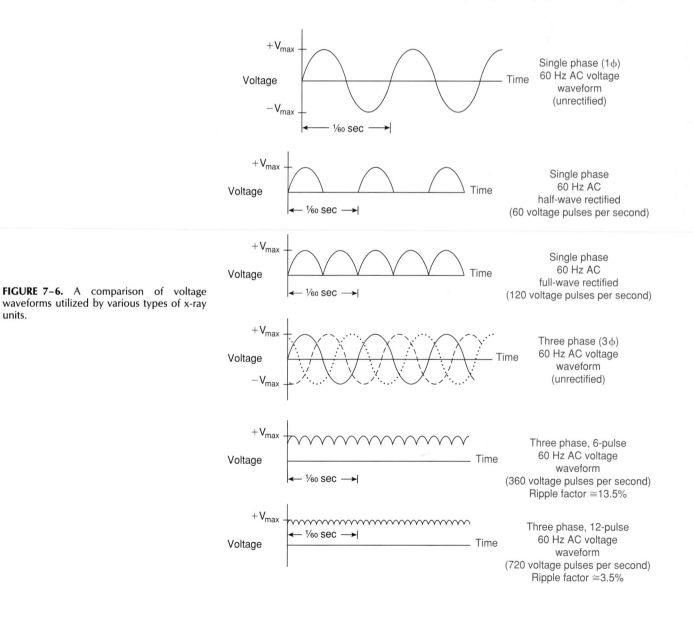

FIGURE 7–6. A comparison of voltage waveforms utilized by various types of x-ray units.

■ THE AC CYCLE

It is important to recall from previous discussions (Chapter 5) that the power supplied to medical facilities by local power companies is AC. AC voltage fluctuates, or varies, from zero to some maximum voltage (V_{max}) then back to zero. The voltage then becomes negative (corresponding to electrical polarity reversal) and returns to zero after reaching a minimum (V_{min}). The voltage variation *(AC cycle)* repeats itself in time (in the United States it repeats itself 60 times each second) and can be represented by the type of curve shown below.

When the voltage variation is plotted as a function of time, as indicated in the illustration, it is referred to as the AC voltage waveform. If only one AC waveform is sent out (as shown), it is a single-phase (1ϕ) waveform.

Several important features about the waveform should be specifically noted:

- The voltage waveform consists of a positive and negative portion to each cycle. The positive portion corresponds to the tube anode being positive and the cathode negative. The negative portion corresponds to polarity reversal in which the tube anode is negative and the cathode is positive.
- When 60-cycle (or 60-Hz) AC is used, each cycle lasts 1/60 sec.

- During each AC cycle, voltage fluctuates from zero to some *peak voltage* (V_{peak} in the illustration) during both positive and negative portions of the cycle, then returns to zero.
- In making comparisons between AC and DC currents, AC effective voltages are useful. The effective voltage is defined as

$$V_{eff} = \frac{V_{peak}}{\sqrt{2}} = 0.707\ V_{peak}$$

(By definition V_{eff} is the voltage that would produce an effective current, I_{eff}, so that a DC current of this magnitude would generate heat in a resistor at the same rate as the AC current.) When the magnitude of AC voltage is quoted as 220-V, 60-cycle AC, this means that the actual voltage fluctuates from zero to

$$+V_{peak} = +\frac{V_{eff}}{0.707} = +1.414 V_{eff}$$
$$= +(1.414)(220\ V)$$
$$\approx +311\ V$$

then back to zero. During the negative portion of the cycle, the AC voltage would fluctuate from zero to -311 V then back to zero.

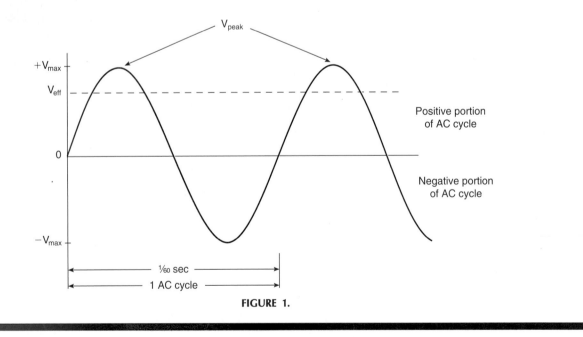

FIGURE 1.

like 1ϕ power, the supplied voltage never drops to zero. More is said about 1ϕ and 3ϕ power and its effect on x-ray production later in the chapter.

Line-Voltage Compensation

Line voltage refers to the voltage supplied to the x-ray imaging room by the local power company. Typically, these voltages range from approximately 120 V to 480 V, 60-Hz AC. To obtain diagnostically useful x-rays, these voltages must be raised to the kilovoltage (kV) range by the use of appropriate transformers. Since it is the incoming line voltage that will eventually be raised to kV levels by multiplying its incoming value by specific transformer constants, it is most important that this incoming voltage be provided at a constant known value. If this voltage is allowed to randomly vary during a radiographic exposure, voltages applied to all parts of the x-ray unit will also vary, and the radiographer can no longer depend on the accuracy of chosen technical factors such as the kVp and the mA. Obviously, this could adversely affect the image quality of the radiograph produced.

Line voltage is subject to fluctuations occurring when other pieces of equipment operating in the same electrical circuit are switched on or off. Since the number of times this might occur is subject to a variety of factors (e.g., specific working hours and patient load), the variations in incoming line voltage occur randomly. Such variations in voltage are monitored by a *voltmeter* (B in Fig. 7–1), which is used to indicate when the correct number of volts per turn on the primary side of the autotransformer is within the required limits. To better understand this concept, consider the following example.

)))))) EXAMPLE

a) An x-ray unit is supplied with an incoming line voltage of 220 V. If there are 110 turns on the primary side of the autotransformer as shown below, determine the number of volts per turn as would be measured by the voltmeter.

$$Volts\ per\ turn = \frac{line\ voltage}{turns\ on\ primary\ (n_p)}$$
$$= \frac{220\ V}{110\ turns}$$
$$= 2\ V/turn$$

b) If the incoming voltage drops to 200 V, how many turns should there be on the primary in order to maintain 2 V/turn?

$$Volts\ per\ turn = \frac{line\ voltage}{turns\ on\ primary\ (n_p)}$$
$$Turns\ on\ primary\ (n_p) = \frac{line\ voltage}{volts/turn}$$
$$= \frac{200\ V}{2\ V/turn}$$
$$= 100\ turns$$

Therefore the switch (C in Fig. 7–1) can be adjusted appropriately so that $n_p = 100$ turns. Accordingly, if incoming line voltage had risen to 240 V, the switch could have been adjusted such that $n_p = 120$ turns in order to maintain the same number of volts per turn. This process of correcting, or compensating, for these voltage fluctuations is referred to as *line-voltage compensation*. On older x-ray units, line-voltage compensation can be accomplished manually as described in the previous example. On such units, the meter used to monitor voltage fluctuations may display only a region on a scale in which the needle of the meter should be maintained. On modern x-ray units, line voltage is monitored and compensation is accomplished automatically.

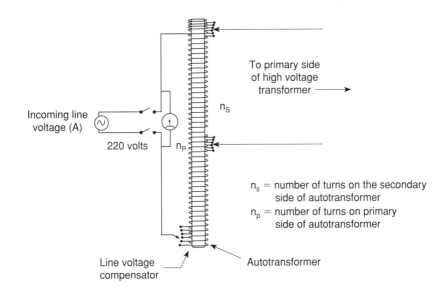

Incoming line voltage (A)

220 volts

n_p

n_s

To primary side of high voltage transformer →

n_s = number of turns on the secondary side of autotransformer
n_p = number of turns on primary side of autotransformer

Line voltage compensator

Autotransformer

The High-Voltage Circuit: Converting Volts to Kilovolts

The primary purpose of the *high-voltage circuit* is to convert incoming line voltage from volt to kilovolt levels in order to obtain diagnostic energy x-rays. The circuit must also allow the radiographer to change accurately the kilovoltage applied across the x-ray tube electrodes. This process is accomplished through the use of an *autotransformer* with a variable turns ratio and a high-voltage, step-up transformer with a fixed turns ratio. After voltage amplification, the voltage waveform is rectified to optimize x-ray production.

The high-voltage circuit (Fig. 7–7) consists of the incoming line-voltage connections, the autotransformer, appropriate voltmeters and ammeters, the high-voltage step-up transformer, and an appropriate number of rectifiers.

A timing circuit, which consists of one of several types of timers and a switching mechanism, determines the moment at which the exposure is terminated. It is most important to note the location of the timing circuit in relation to the overall x-ray circuit. The production of x-rays is controlled by regulating the voltage across the x-ray tube electrodes. Within the x-ray tube, x-ray production could theoretically be controlled by either of two techniques:

1. Controlling electron emission from the filament by making rapid changes in the filament current; only if electrons are emitted from the filament can x-rays be produced

2. Controlling the high voltage across the tube electrodes; if there is no voltage, electrons will not be drawn into the anode target and no x-rays will be produced

Of the two methods described, the second is the method of choice, since it occurs instantaneously. This is not the case with the first method. After the filament is heated by the filament current to the point at which thermionic emission occurs, emission does not suddenly stop if the filament current drops to zero, since the tungsten filament does not cool instantaneously. Electrons continue to be released, and if high voltage remains across the tube electrodes, x-rays continue to be produced, resulting in a higher patient radiation dose and potentially overexposed radiographs. For this reason, timers are located in the high-voltage circuit rather than in the filament circuit. Specific types of timers and methods of operation are discussed in more detail later in the chapter.

The Autotransformer

The first major circuit component encountered by the incoming line voltage is the autotransformer. This component is designated *D* in Figure 7–7. Recall that the autotransformer is a transformer with several specific properties:

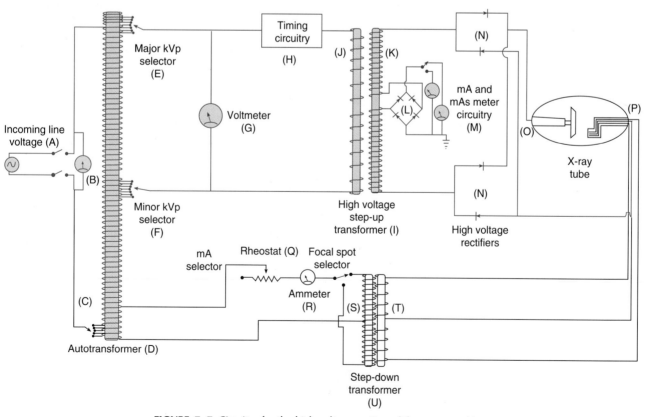

FIGURE 7–7. Circuitry for the high-voltage section of the x-ray machine.

Table 7–1. DIAGNOSTIC-ENERGY X-RAY PRODUCTION

Incoming Line Voltage	×	Autotransformer Turns Ratio	=	Autotransformer Output Voltage	×	Step-Up Transformer Turns Ratio	=	Final Output Voltage Across Tube Electrodes
220 V	×	1.364	=	300 V	×	500	=	150 kV
220 V	×	1.091	=	240 V	×	500	=	120 kV
220 V	×	0.91	=	200 V	×	500	=	100 kV
220 V	×	0.727	=	160 V	×	500	=	80 kV
220 V	×	0.636	=	140 V	×	500	=	70 kV

kV = kilovolts, V = volts.

- It is a special type of transformer with only a single winding on a laminated iron core (operates on the principle of self-induction)
- It has a variable turns ratio dependent on the specific electrical contacts (or taps) made on the primary and secondary sides of the coil
- Because of its variable turns ratio, the autotransformer can be used as either a step-up or step-down transformer, allowing for minor variations in incoming line voltage

Within the high-voltage circuit, there are two transformers—an autotransformer that allows the radiographer to select the kVp and a high-voltage step-up transformer (indicated by I in Fig. 7–7) having a fixed *turns ratio* that is responsible for elevating the incoming line voltage to the kilovolt level. It is important to recall that there is a direct relationship between voltage and number of turns on the transformer coil. That is,

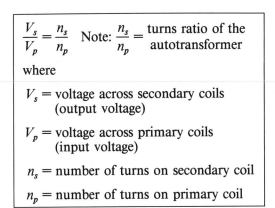

$$\frac{V_s}{V_p} = \frac{n_s}{n_p} \quad \text{Note:} \frac{n_s}{n_p} = \text{turns ratio of the autotransformer}$$

where

V_s = voltage across secondary coils (output voltage)

V_p = voltage across primary coils (input voltage)

n_s = number of turns on secondary coil

n_p = number of turns on primary coil

Therefore if the voltage is raised by the high voltage step-up transformer by a factor of 500, the turns ratio of the autotransformer need vary over only a relatively narrow range of values. In this way, voltages across the tube electrodes can be raised to the levels required for diagnostic-energy x-ray production (i.e., ~70 kV to 150 kV). This can be seen from the values of the turns ratio shown in Table 7–1. In the table, incoming line voltage has an assumed value of 220 V. Also assuming a typical value of 500 for the turns ratio of the high-voltage step-up transformer, it can be seen that the required turns ratio of the autotransformer need only range from approximately 0.5 to 1.5. This relatively low turns ratio requirement indicates that relatively few coils of wire are actually needed on the autotransformer compared with the high-voltage step-up transformer. Notice that even with variations, incoming line voltage at the level of the autotransformer is still relatively low (from Table 7–1, autotransformer output voltages range only from 140 V to 300 V). Autotransformers being somewhat less bulky are found in the control console. The radiographer directly adjusts the autotransformer's turns ratio, using the major and minor kVp selectors.

)))))) EXAMPLE

Incoming line voltage to an x-ray unit is 220 V. If there are 100 turns on the primary side of the autotransformer and kVp selectors on the control console are adjusted such that there are 60 turns on the secondary side (shown below), what will be the output (secondary) voltage?

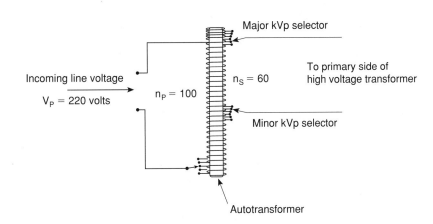

Major kVp selector

Incoming line voltage

V_P = 220 volts

n_P = 100

n_S = 60

To primary side of high voltage transformer

Minor kVp selector

Autotransformer

Using the transformer law given by

$$\frac{V_s}{V_p} = \frac{n_s}{n_p}$$

where

$$V_p = 220 \text{ V}$$

$$n_s = 60 \text{ turns}$$

$$n_p = 100 \text{ turns}$$

$$V_s = ?$$

$$\frac{V_s}{220 \text{ V}} = \frac{60 \text{ turns}}{100 \text{ turns}}$$

$$V_s = \left(\frac{60}{100}\right)(220 \text{ V})$$

$$V_s = 132 \text{ V}$$

(Note: This is the voltage that is then provided to the high-voltage step-up transformer to produce a final output voltage across the x-ray tube electrodes.)

High-Voltage Step-Up Transformer

After incoming line voltage has been slightly raised or lowered by using the kVp selectors on the autotransformer, its output voltage becomes the input voltage across the primary of the high-voltage step-up transformer. This second transformer (designated *I* in Fig. 7–7) is required to bring line voltage to the kilovoltage level. Typically, this transformer has a turns ratio of between 500 and 600. As a result, it is more massive, since significantly more coils of wire are needed on the secondary side and requires more electrical insulation since its output voltage is of the order of kilovolts. For these specific reasons, this transformer is typically located in an electrically grounded metal container close to the x-ray unit. The transformer box may stand alone within the imaging room or may be located within a larger equipment cabinet (see Fig. 7–3). The contents of such a transformer box are shown in Figure 7–8. These structures are usually easily identified by the high-voltage cables running from the transformer box to the x-ray unit. The box usually contains not only the high-voltage transformer but also associated rectifiers and the filament transformer. (More is said about these other circuit components later in this chapter.) All circuit components within the box are totally immersed in a thin, purified, transformer oil that serves as both electrical insulation and coolant, because heat is generated during heavy tube use. The box is sealed with an air-tight lid. The metal transformer box, its associated high-voltage cables, and the metal housing that provides structural support for the x-ray tube are all electrically grounded to minimize the chance of electrical shock. It should be noted that in smaller x-ray units (e.g., portable and dental units) in which procedures do not generate significant quantities of heat, the high-voltage transformer is found in

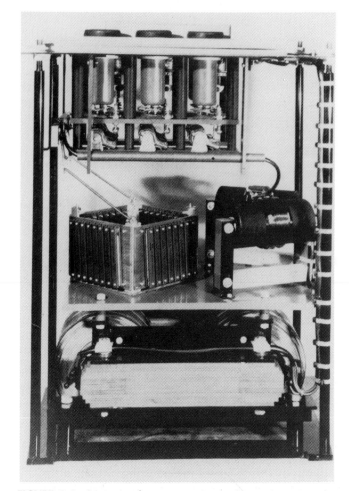

FIGURE 7–8. Contents of an x-ray unit transformer box, showing rectifiers and filament transformer (*on second shelf*) and the high-voltage step-up transformer (*on lower shelf*). (Courtesy of Picker International, Inc.)

a somewhat different arrangement. With most smaller units, the high-voltage transformer is found in the same housing as the x-ray tube. Lighter electrical insulating materials used with these units surround both the transformer and the x-ray tube. Materials that have been used with success include certain semisolid plastics and a combination of resin-impregnated paper and oil.

It is also important to remember that the high-voltage step-up transformer has a fixed turns ratio—that is, N_s/N_p. Once the incoming line voltage has been appropriately adjusted by using the autotransformer, it is then stepped-up to the required kilovoltage by this second transformer. A brief review of transformer laws as applied to this type of transformer is now provided.

))))))) EXAMPLE

The high-voltage step-up transformer for a particular x-ray unit has 25 turns on its primary and 13,000 turns on its secondary coil. If the voltage provided from the autotransformer is 154 V, what voltage could be placed across the x-ray tube electrodes?

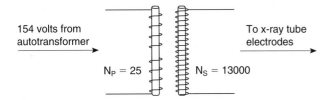

154 volts from autotransformer →

$N_P = 25$ $N_S = 13000$

→ To x-ray tube electrodes

Given:

$$V_p = 154 \text{ V}$$
$$N_p = 25 \text{ turns}$$
$$N_s = 13{,}000 \text{ turns}$$
$$V_s = ?$$

Recall the direct relationship that exists for transformers between voltage and the number of turns on the respective coils:

$$\frac{V_s}{V_p} = \frac{N_s}{N_p}$$

$$V_s = \left(\frac{N_s}{N_p}\right) V_p$$
$$= \left(\frac{13{,}000}{25}\right) (154 \text{ V})$$
$$= (520)(154 \text{ V})$$
$$= 80080 \text{ V}$$

or $\approx 80 \text{ kV}$

)))))) EXAMPLE

The high-voltage transformer of a second x-ray unit has a turns ratio of 600. If 200 V are supplied by the autotransformer, what will be the output voltage?

Given:

$$\text{Turns ratio} = \frac{N_s}{N_p} = 600$$
$$V_p = 200 \text{ V}$$
$$V_s = ?$$
$$\frac{V_s}{V_p} = \frac{N_s}{N_p}$$
$$V_s = \left(\frac{N_s}{N_p}\right)(V_p)$$
$$= (600)(200 \text{ V})$$
$$= 120{,}000 \text{ V or } 120 \text{ kV}$$

As the high-voltage transformer is used to produce the necessary voltage across the x-ray tube electrodes, heat is generated. This heat arises from several sources:

- Heat is produced as current flows through the primary and secondary coils of the transformer; this is referred to as resistive heating, since the wire coils have electrical resistance
- Heat is generated within the iron core as its direction of magnetization is continuously changed by the AC current flowing through its coils (called hysteresis)
- Heat is produced by currents generated in the iron core (known as eddy currents) by the changing magnetic fields associated with the coil windings

To minimize this last source of heat production, transformer coils are typically wound on laminated cores (i.e., cores composed of stacks of individual metal plates). These sources of heat loss indicate that transformers are not 100% efficient, since some of the input electrical energy is "lost" in the form of heat energy during operation. The insulating oil surrounding the transformers also assists in the removal of heat from the transformer assembly.

The energy losses that occur in the transformer serve as reminders that previously used "transformer laws" relating voltages and currents to the transformer turns ratio are valid only for ideal transformers, where these energy losses do not occur. Thus for accurate voltages to be supplied to the tube electrodes, voltages are regulated within the circuit to compensate for these energy losses.

On the primary (low-input voltage) side of the high-voltage transformer is a voltmeter that is used to indicate the kVp across the x-ray tube electrodes. This voltmeter is actually located on the operator's control panel, but its location in the high-voltage circuit is indicated as G in Figure 7–7. Recognize that since the output voltage of the high-voltage transformer is merely the product of the output voltage of the autotransformer and the turns ratio of the high-voltage transformer, then the voltmeter can be so calibrated that its final output reading can be determined based on the output voltage of the autotransformer. When this meter is calibrated in such a manner, it can indicate the kVp before it is actually placed across the tube electrodes to make the radiographic exposure. For this reason, the meter is often referred to as a prereading kVp meter.

An ammeter that is used to measure tube current in milliamperes (mA) is found in the secondary circuit of the high-voltage transformer. Located on the high-voltage side of the transformer, it is positioned in the circuit at the point where the transformer is grounded (at the coil center). This assures that the meter is at zero potential difference with respect to ground and can therefore be safely placed on the operator console without risk of electrical shock. The mA meter provides an average value of the tube current and does not reflect the variation of tube current that occurs when using a varying AC voltage. It is important to note that with the mA meter connected as shown in Figure 7–7, it will measure the current across the tube electrodes, since it is in the same circuit as the x-ray tube.

Since a great number of radiographic exposures are made with exposure times of less than a second, the mA meter may not always have adequate response time to even register a reading. For those cases of extremely short exposure times, a milliampere-second (mAs) meter may be employed. mAs is the product of current (expressed in mA) and time (expressed in seconds). Recall the definition of current:

$$\text{Current} = \frac{\text{charge}}{\text{time}}$$

then

$$\text{Current} \times \text{time} = \frac{\text{charge}}{\text{time}} \times \text{time}$$
$$= \text{charge}$$

Thus mAs physically indicates the amount of charge (or number of electrons) passing between the tube electrodes. Meters can be designed to register the magnitude of this current in terms of mAs regardless of the length of the exposure time. These are known as milliampere-seconds (mAs) meters. X-ray units such as the circuitry shown in Figure 7–7 may contain both mA and mAs meters. When exposure times are greater than one second, the mA meter is used, since it has adequate response time. For exposures of less than a second, the switch position is changed, and the mAs meter is brought into the circuit. Once the mAs reading has been determined, the value of the tube current can be obtained by dividing the mAs by the exposure time in seconds as indicated in the following example.

)))))) EXAMPLE

A radiographic exposure registers 200 mAs. Determine the tube current (mA) if the exposure time is 250 msec.

The exposure time must first be converted to seconds:

$$250 \; \text{msec} \times \frac{1 \; \text{sec}}{1000 \; \text{msec}} = \frac{250}{1000} \; \text{sec} = 0.25 \; \text{sec}$$

Then use the relationship

$$\text{mAs} = \text{tube current (mA)} \times \text{exposure time (sec)}$$

or

$$\text{Tube current (mA)} = \text{mAs/exposure time (sec)}$$
$$= 200 \; \text{mAs}/0.25 \; \text{sec}$$
$$= 800 \; \text{mA}$$

Rectifiers

Transformers require changing magnetic fields generated by AC currents in order to operate properly. Although x-ray tubes can operate on high-voltage AC, they operate most efficiently on high-voltage DC. Recall from Figure 7–5 that AC stands for alternating current, which travels first in one direction (during the first half of the AC cycle) and then turns and travels in the opposite direction (during the second half of the AC cycle). If an AC voltage is supplied across the x-ray tube electrodes, for the tube current (i.e., electrons emitted from the filament) to change its direction of flow, the tube electrodes must reverse their electrical polarity each half-cycle. For example, during the first half of the cycle, the cathode is negative and the anode positive. Electrons move from the cathode into the anode, and x-rays are produced. However, during the second half of the cycle, the cathode becomes positive and the anode negative. Electrons emitted from the filament now do not move into the negatively charged anode, and as a result, x-rays are not produced. In this case, the x-ray tube allows current to flow in only one direction. Devices that allow current to flow in only one direction are known as *rectifiers*. When the x-ray tube acts alone as a rectifying device, the circuit is said to be *self-rectified*. It should be noted that vacuum tubes, consisting of two electrodes (like the x-ray tube itself) and called diodes, act as rectifiers since they allow current to flow in only one direction. For many years, vacuum tubes, known as *valve tubes*, were used as rectifiers in the x-ray circuit. Valve tubes have been replaced in modern x-ray equipment by *solid-state rectifiers*.

Unlike the antiquated vacuum diode, which contained a heated filament to supply electrons and a positively charged anode within an evacuated glass envelope, solid-state rectifiers are much simpler in their overall design. Valve tubes, because of their construction, allowed current to flow only when the cathode was negative and the anode positive. In comparison solid-state rectifiers generally consist of two types of semiconductors:

1. n-Type semiconductors: semiconductors to which an impurity has been added in order to produce a surplus of negative charge within the material; typically, germanium or silicon with phosphorus added as the impurity; these are referred to as the donor materials
2. p-Type semiconductors: semiconductors to which an impurity has been added to produce a deficiency of negative charge, referred to as a hole; this type of material is called an acceptor material; typically, silicon and germanium with boron or indium added as impurities

The general design of a solid-state rectifier (known also as a semiconductor diode) is to join a layer of n-type material with a layer of p-type material. When voltage is applied, electrons flow easily from the n-type (which has a surplus of negative charges) to the p-type material. If the voltage polarity is reversed, electrons cannot flow easily in the opposite direction, thus making it an effective rectifier. The symbol used to designate the solid-state rectifier is →|; the arrowhead indicates the direction of allowed current flow.

The region in which the n- and p-types of materials are joined is called the junction, or barrier layer. Single-barrier layers of silicon can typically withstand only several hundred volts, and as a result, several hundred of these junction layers may be needed to rectify the kilovolt levels applied to the x-ray tube. Usually, these

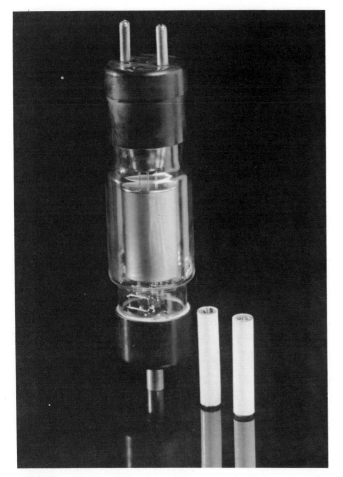

FIGURE 7–9. Comparison of an older valve tube *(left)* and smaller solid-state rectifiers *(right)*.

- *Half-wave rectification:* obtained when zero, one, or two rectifiers are used; the use of a single rectifier prevents the redirection of any electrons emitted from a heated anode back into the cathode filament, causing its destruction; use of two rectifiers not only prevents this "reverse current" flow but also provides an additional safeguard against electrical insulation breakdown in the high-voltage cables leading from the transformer to the tube electrodes
- *Full-wave rectification:* obtained when at least four rectifiers are used in the circuit; this type of rectification makes the most efficient use of both halves of the AC cycle by assuring that the cathode is always negative and by using the negative portion of the AC cycle; this is the most common type of rectification used in modern x-ray units

A summary of circuit characteristics for conventional circuits containing different numbers of rectifiers is contained in Table 7–2. The type of rectification used in this portion of the circuitry is most important, since it is the characteristics of the voltage placed across the x-ray tube electrodes that primarily determines the energies of the x-rays produced. Several specific effects of voltage rectification on the x-rays generated should carefully be reviewed:

- Half-wave rectified equipment that utilizes 1ϕ, 60-Hz AC line voltage produces 60-DC voltage pulses each second across tube electrodes. This voltage varies from zero to some peak value then back to zero during each pulse. Since the energy (or penetrating ability) of the x-rays generated depends on the voltage across the tube electrodes, the energy

(Continued on page 182)

junction layers are linked and encased in cylindrical ceramic tubes. A solid-state rectifier is shown in comparison with a valve tube in Figure 7–9. A radiograph of two solid-state rectifiers (Fig. 7–10) shows the linked junction layers within the ceramic casing. The smaller size of solid-state rectifiers compared with older valve tubes makes them most useful in the design of more compact radiographic equipment. Additional advantages of solid-state rectifiers include the following:

- Longer useful life span because there are no elements that must be heated for electron production
- Since electrons are not accelerated into an anode (as with valve tubes), x-rays are not produced, and therefore no special shielding is required
- They tend to be more efficient than valve tubes

The type of rectification occurring in an x-ray circuit is dependent on the number of rectifiers within the circuit. Rectifier requirements for each type of rectification are summarized as follows:

- *Self-rectification:* no rectifiers within the circuit other than the x-ray tube itself; tube current limited to approximately 100 mA, thus restricting its use to dental and other low-power x-ray units

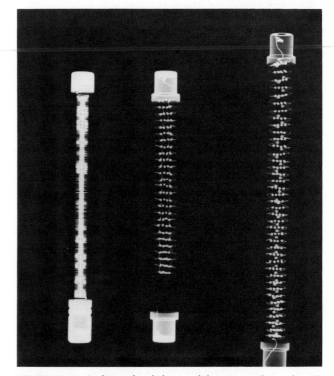

FIGURE 7–10. Radiograph of three solid-state rectifiers, showing numerous junction layers within the rectifier cases.

■ CURRENT FLOW IN X-RAY RECTIFIER CIRCUITRY

Since the voltage supplied to the x-ray tube by the high-voltage transformer is AC voltage, voltage rectification is required to make the most efficient use of the AC voltage waveform. Rectifiers allow current to flow in only one direction. It should be remembered however that the movement of electrons forms an electric current but current flow is defined as being in the opposite direction. These concepts are elaborated below in relation to the rectifier symbol.

Rectifier

Direction of allowed *current* flow

Direction of allowed *electron* flow

One-Rectifier Circuit

When a single rectifier is used in the circuit as shown below, current is allowed to flow in the direction indicated only during the first half of the AC cycle. This assures that electrons move from cathode to anode and that x-rays are produced.

When the polarity is reversed during the second half of the cycle, no current is allowed to flow, and no x-rays are produced. Half-wave rectification is achieved.

Two-Rectifier Circuit

If two rectifiers are placed in the circuit as shown below, again, current is allowed to flow only in the direction indicated.

With the rectifiers connected as shown, during the first half of the AC cycle electrons can flow only from cathode to anode when the cathode is negative and the anode is positive. It is only during this portion of the cycle that x-rays are generated. When electrical polarity of the electrodes changes during the negative portion of the AC cycle, no current flows and no x-rays are produced. The circuit is again half-wave rectified.

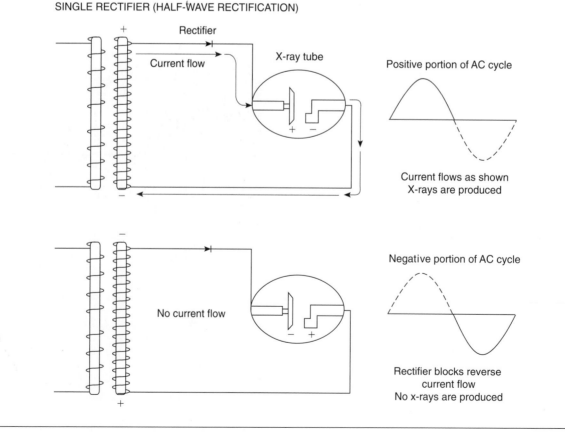

SINGLE RECTIFIER (HALF-WAVE RECTIFICATION)

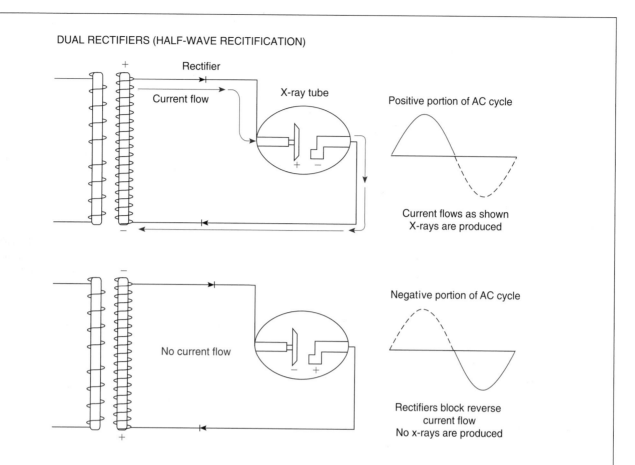

DUAL RECTIFIERS (HALF-WAVE RECITIFICATION)

Four-Rectifier Circuit

When single-phase AC voltage is supplied to circuits containing one or two rectifiers connected as previously shown, half-wave rectified voltage is obtained. With this type of rectification, x-rays are produced only during the positive half of each AC cycle. To more effectively use the entire AC cycle, four rectifiers can be connected in any one of the ways shown below.

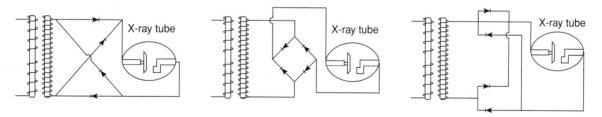

FOUR RECTIFIER CONFIGURATIONS (SINGLE PHASE, FULL-WAVE RECTIFICATION)

Each of these types of connections allows current to flow in only one direction (shown below for a representative configuration) during both halves of the AC cycle. This indicates that throughout the cycle, the cathode remains negative and the anode remains positive, assuring that electrons emitted from the filament always travel toward the anode, resulting in x-ray production. This type of rectifier circuitry produces full-wave rectification.

(continued)

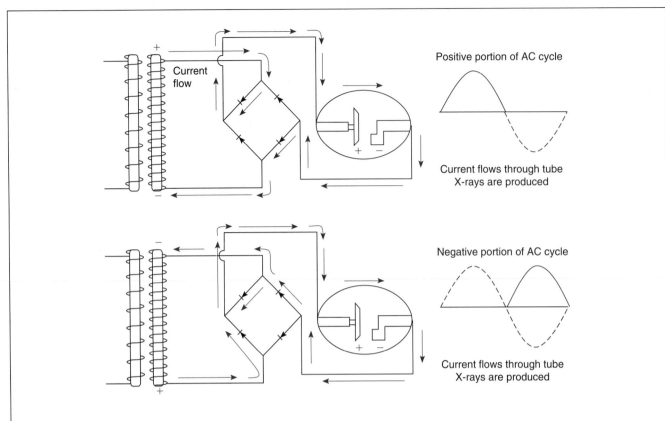

Positive portion of AC cycle

Current flows through tube
X-rays are produced

Negative portion of AC cycle

Current flows through tube
X-rays are produced

Three-Phase Rectifier Circuits (Full-Wave Rectification)

As described in Chapter 5, in an effort to obtain a more constant voltage across the x-ray tube electrodes, three-phase (3φ) electrical power is used. Three-phase power transformers contain three sets of primary and secondary coils arranged in one of several configurations. With appropriate rectification provided by either 6 or 12 rectifiers, 6- or 12-pulse, full-wave rectified voltage waveforms can be achieved. The resulting voltage waveform in each of these cases is shown below with a description of the associated x-ray beam.

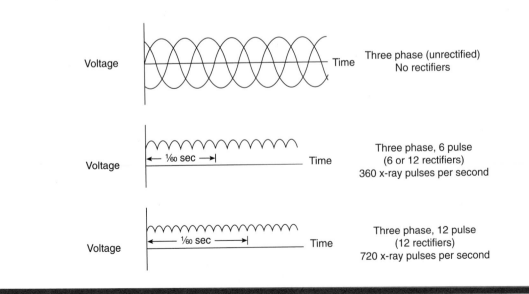

Three phase (unrectified)
No rectifiers

Three phase, 6 pulse
(6 or 12 rectifiers)
360 x-ray pulses per second

Three phase, 12 pulse
(12 rectifiers)
720 x-ray pulses per second

Table 7-2. CIRCUIT CHARACTERISTICS FOR DIFFERENT NUMBERS OF RECTIFIERS

Type of Power Supplied	Number of Rectifiers in Circuit	Type of Rectification Achieved	Voltage Waveform Appearance	Advantages	Disadvantages	Comments
1φ	0	Half-wave	60 pulses/sec	• Most simple of rectification circuits • May allow smaller, more compact units to be designed	• Only half of the AC voltage supplied is used; exposure times are thus twice as long as for full-wave rectification • Any reverse current flow during negative portion of cycle can destroy the tube filament • Generally limited to low-power mobile or dental x-ray units	Circuit said to be self-rectified since x-ray tube itself acts as a rectifier; 100% ripple
1φ	1	Half-wave	60 pulses/sec	• Prevents potential damage to filament by any reverse current during negative portion of AC cycle	• Uses only half of the AC voltage waveform supplied • May result in breakdown of electrical insulation in high-voltage cable from transformer to tube	Does not make effective use of the electrical energy supplied to produce x-rays; 100% ripple
1φ	2	Half-wave	60 pulses/sec	• Prevents potential breakdown of high-voltage cable insulation • Has back-up rectifier in circuit in event of a rectifier failure	• Uses only half of the AC voltage waveform supplied	Does not make effective use of the electrical energy supplied to produce x-rays; 100% ripple
1φ	4	Full-wave	120 pulses/sec	• Produces x-rays during both portions of the AC cycle, resulting in shorter exposure times • Current across tube electrodes is a pulsating DC current (120 pulses/sec for 60-Hz AC) • Allows the use of higher mA and kVp	• Voltage across tube electrodes drops to zero during each cycle • More expensive • More massive equipment • More complex electrical circuitry	Although makes more effective use of entire AC voltage waveform, 100% ripple still results in significant quantity of low-energy x-rays and in heat generated at anode
3φ	6 or 12	Full-wave	360 pulses/sec 720 pulses/sec	• Makes most effective use of both portions of the AC voltage waveform • Voltage across tube electrodes remains near peak throughout exposure, resulting in higher-energy x-rays • Can supply higher mA than 1φ units • Higher x-ray output	• More complex electrical circuitry • More expensive • More massive equipment	Theoretical ripple factors for these units range from ∼ 13.5% (6-pulse) to ∼ 3.5% (12-pulse)

varies from zero (when the voltage is zero) to some peak value (determined by the peak voltage). The significant number of low-energy x-rays produced under these conditions of 100% ripple factor would be absorbed within the patient's body and would contribute significantly to the patient's radiation dose

● Full-wave rectified equipment utilizing 1ϕ, 60-Hz AC line voltage produces 120–DC voltage pulses across the tube electrodes. As in half-wave rectified equipment, tube voltage fluctuates from zero to some peak value then returns again to zero. The energy characteristics of the x-rays produced are identical to those from half-wave rectified units. In this case, however, twice as many x-rays are produced per time unit, since both positive and negative portions of the AC cycle are used in x-ray production

● Three-phase (3ϕ) equipment produces a DC voltage across the tube electrodes that fluctuates within narrow limits, determined by whether the unit is a 6- or 12-pulse unit. Theoretically, the voltage drops by approximately 13.5% (6-pulse) or 3.5% (12-pulse) from the peak voltage during tube operation. Three-phase equipment, again theoretically, produces many fewer, lower-energy x-rays and should result in lower radiation dose to the patient. It is explained later that not only does this type of equipment tend to produce more x-rays but it also produces x-ray beams of higher average energy than 1ϕ units

These factors are considered again when factors that affect x-ray quality (i.e., the energy of the x-rays produced) and x-ray quantity (i.e., the number of x-rays produced) are investigated.

In Figure 7–7 appears an additional set of rectifiers (denoted by L) needed to rectify the current passing through the milliammeter (or mAs meter), which is used to read the tube current. Recall that currents (and voltages) coming from the secondary side of the high-voltage transformer are alternating. The type of meter used to measure tube current (mAs) requires that these quantities be rectified before passing through the device for measurement. The illustrated rectifiers serve that purpose. And although the current flowing through the tube and the mA meter is now DC, the current still fluctuates, since the voltages across the tube electrodes also fluctuate to varying degrees in both single- and three-phase units. These meters are therefore designed to provide a reading of the average current.

Timing Circuitry

In addition to producing enough x-rays with sufficient energy to penetrate the patient's body, an important component in the making of quality radiographs is an accurate timing mechanism to terminate the exposure at a predetermined time. A variety of timing mechanisms exists—from relatively simple designs to quite complex ones. The complexity of the timing circuitry is determined by the degree of accuracy required. With many low-power x-ray units, exposure times may last for a second or more. Most likely a timer with an accuracy to 0.01 sec is not needed, and in this case, a less complex, less expensive timer can be used. On the other hand, in a trauma situation or in certain special radiographic procedures, exposure times may approach 0.01 sec or less. In these situations, if a timer is inaccurate by 0.01 sec, the radiograph can be adversely affected, since the error is of the order of the actual exposure time. Here, a more accurate and more complex timer is required. As technology has advanced, a variety of timing mechanisms have been developed. Each is considered separately.

Mechanical Timers. *Mechanical timers* are perhaps the least complex but least commonly used of all timing devices. This type of timer is usually based on a clockwork mechanism employing a coiled spring. As the timer dial is rotated to a specific time on its scale, the coiled spring becomes more tightly wound, and a set of electrical contacts within the circuit is closed. When the exposure switch on the operator's control is pressed, a second set of electrical contacts are closed, and the coiled spring is allowed to unwind. During this time, with both sets of contacts closed, voltage is supplied to the primary of the high-voltage transformer and subsequently to the x-ray tube electrodes, and assuming electrons are available from the filament, x-rays are generated. As the coil unwinds and the dial returns to its zero position, the electrical contacts open, and voltage is no longer supplied to the transformer and the x-ray tube. As a result, the exposure is terminated. This type of timer is reasonably accurate to approximately 1/4 sec (i.e., 0.25 sec, or 250 msec). Mechanical timers are essentially obsolete and for the most part have been replaced by more accurate devices.

Synchronous Timers. *Synchronous timers* are also an older type of timing mechanism; they are based on the use of a special motor known as a synchronous motor. This motor turns in synchronization with the incoming AC current on which it operates. As an example, a synchronous motor that utilizes 60-Hz AC could be designed to rotate a shaft at a speed of 60 revolutions per second (i.e., 60 rps). With such a motor, the shortest time that can be designated is 1 revolution of the shaft, corresponding to 1/60 sec. Other designated time periods found on this type of timer are whole number multiples of 1/60 sec such as 2(1/60 sec), or 1/30 sec; 3(1/60 sec), or 1/20 sec; and so forth. The action of closing and opening the circuit in order to supply voltage to the transformer and tube in order to generate x-rays is similar to techniques used with mechanical timers. These timers, too, are becoming obsolete but may still be found on older pieces of equipment. They do not lend themselves to making rapid serial exposures, since they must be reset prior to each exposure.

Impulse Timers. An *impulse timer* is an accurate timing device whose operation is based on counting periodic events (i.e., events that repeat at regular intervals) such as voltage pulses. For example, if a 1ϕ, half-wave

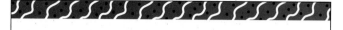

■ CHARGING A CAPACITOR

A capacitor does not instantaneously become fully charged. The length of time required to charge a capacitor depends on its capacitance (C) measured in farads and the resistance (R) in the circuit measured in ohms. The product of R × C is known as the RC time constant (Note: R × C = seconds). The length of time required to reach a certain percentage of full charge, shown by the graph below, depends upon the value of the RC time constant which can be varied by varying the value of the resistance, R.

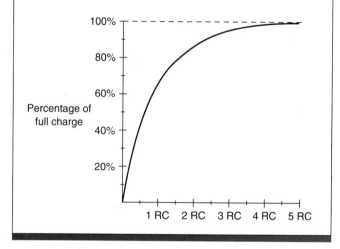

rectified unit is used, 60 voltage pulses per second can be observed. One pulse therefore represents 1/60 sec. If a 1ϕ, full-wave rectified unit is used, 120 voltage pulses are produced each second, and one pulse therefore represents a shorter time period, namely, 1/120 sec. The higher the frequency voltage used, the shorter and more accurate are the measurable time periods. This type of timer can accurately make time measurements in milliseconds (msec).

Electronic Timers. *Electronic timers* were designed to provide accurate determinations of extremely short exposure times. The basic components of this type of timer consist of (1) a capacitor, (2) a variable resistance, and (3) a switching device to terminate the exposure.

It should be recalled from Chapter 4 that a capacitor is a device used to store electrical charge. The length of time it takes a capacitor to reach a certain percentage of full charge is determined by the capacitance (C) of the capacitor and the resistance (R) in the circuit (see Charging a Capacitor, in box). The product of resistance and capacitance is known as the RC time constant. This time constant can be varied (by changing the resistance, using a rheostat) to obtain a range of exposure times. Depending on the RC time constant

used, when the capacitor reaches a certain "critical voltage," an electronic switch is activated, so that the exposure is terminated. In older equipment, an electronic switch known as a thyratron (actually a gas-filled triode tube) was used, but this is now being replaced with solid-state switches known as silicon-controlled rectifiers (SCRs).

More recent designs of electronic timers utilize microprocessor clocks to accurately measure exposure times. Electronic timers are capable of making exposures as short as 1 msec.

Milliampere-Second (mAs) Timers. mAs Timers are a specially designed type of electronic timer that also uses a capacitor and an electronic switching device. The difference between this type of timer and other electronic timers is that this timer uses the tube current (mA) flowing between the x-ray tube electrodes to charge a capacitor. Since the mAs simply represents the product of mA and exposure time, the time to charge the capacitor becomes the exposure time. Since it is the mAs that is actually being monitored, the shortest exposure times are those corresponding to the highest mA that is safe for the tube. Since this type timer uses the mA passing through the x-ray tube circuit, it is found on the secondary side of the high-voltage transformer.

Automatic Timers. None of the timers previously discussed monitor the amount of radiation that actually strikes the film. As a result, factors such as variations in patient thickness must adequately be taken into consideration by the radiographer in order to assure a quality radiograph. The radiographer must therefore carefully adjust the technical factors (i.e., mA, kVp, exposure time) to each individual patient. *Automatic timers* (or autotimers) link the exposure times more directly to the amount of x-radiation actually striking the radiographic film, which is known as automatic exposure control (AEC), or phototimer. This device was designed in an attempt to minimize operator error in radiograph production.

In general, autotimers consist of some type of device that can convert the radiation penetrating the patient's body into a measurable current. The amount of current produced is directly related to the quantity of radiation reaching the film. The current produced can then be used to charge a capacitor. When the capacitor reaches a specified level of charge, an electronic switch is opened, and the exposure is terminated.

Two basic variations in autotimer design are commonly found in today's x-ray units. One design uses a *photomultiplier tube* (PMT) (see the discussion of this topic in the box that follows), whereas another uses an ionization chamber as a means of detecting x-rays transmitted through the patient's body. Each design is considered separately.

Autotimers Using Photomultiplier Tubes. The basic arrangement of components of this type of timer is shown in Figure 7–11. As x-rays pass through the patient's body and the film cassette (note: cassettes here must be made of radiolucent materials so as not

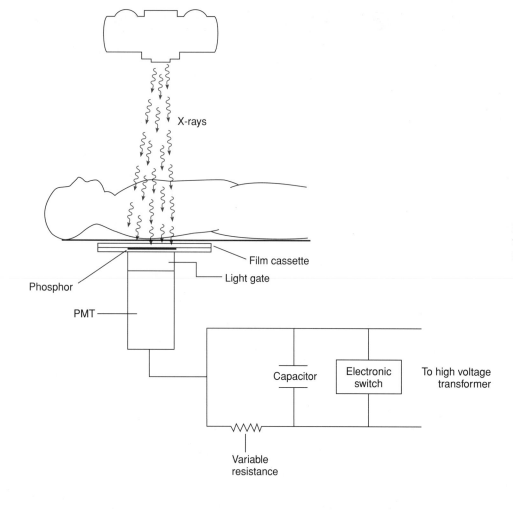

X-rays

Film cassette

Light gate

Phosphor

PMT

Capacitor

Electronic switch

To high voltage transformer

Variable resistance

FIGURE 7–11. Schematic of an autotimer that utilizes a photomultiplier tube (PMT).

to attenuate the x-rays), they strike detectors, commonly made of lucite, a material that readily transmits light. Usually, three areas, or paddles ($\sim$ 100 cm² each), are made radiation-sensitive by coating the lucite with a phosphor that emits light when x-rays strike its surface. The intensity of the light emitted is proportional to the intensity of the x-rays striking the phosphor. The light emitted from the phosphor is transmitted through the lucite and channeled to the photomultiplier tube through structures known as light gates, or light pipes. On entering the PMT, the light is converted into an electric current, which is then used to charge a capacitor through a variable resistor (rheostat). When the charge on the capacitor reaches a predetermined value, corresponding to a desired degree of film darkening (commonly specified by the radiologist at the time of installation), an electronic switch is activated to terminate the exposure. Adjustments to the degree of film darkening can be made by varying the resistance in the circuit, thus altering the RC time constant and the length of time required to charge the capacitor.

The lucite detector used with this type of timer may be located either before the cassette (called an entrance-type phototimer) or behind the cassette (referred to as an exit-type phototimer), possible since the lucite is radiolucent to diagnostic-energy x-rays. One potential problem that could arise with such a timer is the effect of kVp variations on the response of the detector. Low-kVp (e.g., 60 kVp) x-rays are more likely to be absorbed by the phosphor and to produce the emission of light than are higher-energy x-rays, which may pass through the detector without producing any emission of light. This circumstance could result in underexposure in low-kVp procedures as a result of insufficient irradiation of the radiographic film. This possibility is usually corrected by special sensors that monitor the kVp used and makes appropriate adjustments in detector sensitivity (i.e., the detector's response to the radiation it detects).

Autotimers Using Ionization Chambers. Rather than utilizing a photomultiplier tube as a means of converting the incident x-rays into an electric current, this type of autotimer uses a radiation detector known as an ionization chamber. A diagram of the general arrangement of components of this type autotimer is shown in Figure 7–12. As depicted, x-rays passing through the patient's body enter the ionization chamber, which is a radiation detector consisting of two conducting plates. Between the plates is a gas, usually air, that acts as the detection medium. Charge is placed on the plates of the ionization chamber as shown in Figure 7–13.

■ THE PHOTOMULTIPLIER TUBE (PMT)

The photomultiplier tube (PMT) is a device used in the detection of photon radiation (e.g., x-rays) by the conversion of light into electricity. In the detection process, x-rays are first allowed to interact with a phosphor that converts the x-ray photon into a light photon (i.e., visible or UV light). The PMT shown below consists of a negative electrode known as the photocathode because electrons are emitted from its surface when it is struck by light. Along the length of the tube are a series of positively charged metal plates called dynodes, each more positive than the preceding. Near the base of the tube is the positive electrode or anode.

On emission from the phosphor, the light photon travels into the PMT, where it strikes the photocathode and ejects an electron (known as a photoelectron). The photoelectron is then attracted to the first dynode. On striking the dynode, two electrons are ejected from its surface. These electrons are then attracted to the second dynode, where each ejects two additional electrons. This "multiplication" process continues until the electrons are collected at the anode of the tube. This collection of electrons is now large enough to be used to charge a capacitor, which can be used to trigger an electronic switch to terminate a radiographic exposure.

One important characteristic of the PMT is that the amount of charge produced at the anode is proportional to the amount of incident x-rays striking the phosphor. Thus the more x-rays striking the phosphor, the more charge collected at the anode. The greater the charge collected, the less time it takes to charge the capacitor and to terminate the exposure.

The purpose of using the photomultiplier is for amplification of the initial number of electrons ejected from the photocathode. Recall that in this method of radiation detection, the x-ray photons are first converted into light photons in the phosphor, and then the emitted light photons eject photo electrons from the photocathode surface. Only one or two electrons initially emitted from the surface per light photon striking the photocathode represents such a small amount of charge (charge on electron $= -1.6 \times 10^{-19}$ coulomb) that it would essentially be immeasurable as a current in a wire. Thus the PMT provides the necessary amplification of the initial electrical charge, allowing it to be effectively used in the circuit to charge a capacitor.

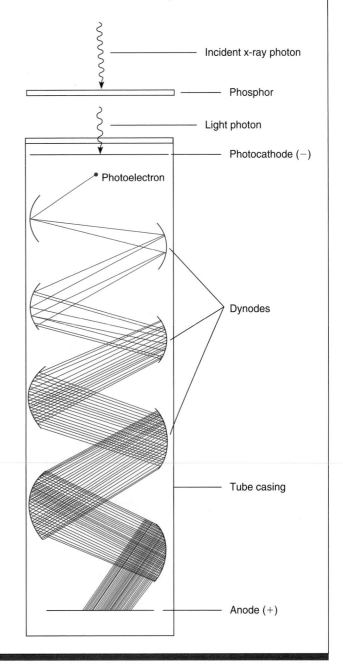

Incident x-ray photon

Phosphor

Light photon

Photocathode (−)

Photoelectron

Dynodes

Tube casing

Anode (+)

Recall that by doing so, a voltage is produced across the plates. As x-rays enter the chamber, ion pairs (i.e., electric charge) are produced in the air between the plates as gas atoms are ionized. The voltage on the plates of the chamber pull positive ions to the negatively charged plate, and negative ions are pulled to the positively charged plate. As the ions created by the x-rays reach the oppositely charged plates, charges on the plates are neutralized, and the voltage is reduced. When the voltage is reduced to a predetermined value, an electronic switch is activated, and the exposure is terminated.

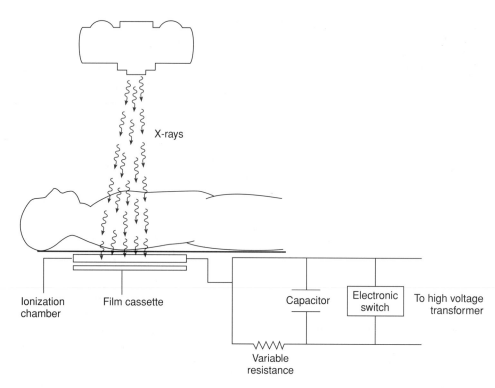

FIGURE 7–12. Schematic of an autotimer that uses an ionization chamber.

The ionization chamber is most commonly located in front of the film cassette (an entrance-type autotimer). As a result, the chamber itself may cast a faint image on the radiographic film, but this does not interfere with the diagnostic information in the image.

Autotimers Using Solid-State Detectors. Although the photomultiplier tube and the ionization chamber are the two most common types of detectors used with autotimers, newer units have begun to use solid-state detectors, which have the advantages of being more compact with rapid response and minimal x-ray beam attenuation. Autotimers were designed with the intention of producing consistent, quality radiographs having the correct radiographic density regardless of the patient's size or body thickness. However, since technical factors such as mA and kVp chosen by the technologist have an effect on the exposure time, a back-up timer is normally incorporated in autotimers. The back-up timer is included in the circuitry to terminate the exposure and to prevent a higher than acceptable radiation dose to the patient or thermal damage to the x-ray tube.

CHECKING TIMER ACCURACY

The accuracy of the radiographic timer is obviously important in the production of diagnostic-quality ra-

diographs. If the timer is slow in terminating the exposure, the result is an overexposed (i.e., too dark) radiograph. Conversely, if the timer is too fast in terminating the exposure, this can result in an underexposed radiograph (i.e., one that is too light). This is not to say that only a faulty timer can result in overexposed or underexposed radiographs, but this potential problem can be easily checked by the radiographer if 1ϕ equipment is being used. The way this is done is to use a simple device known as a spinning top, illustrated in Figure 7–14.

The spinning top disk is usually made of steel or brass several millimeters thick. The disk is constructed to revolve freely on a central peg mounted on its base. Toward the edge of the disk is a small hole that allows x-rays to pass through. The disk is set spinning and placed on top of a loaded film cassette. An exposure is then made for a specific time period (e.g., 0.5 sec). When the film is processed, an image like that shown in Figure 7–15A is obtained. By counting the number of "dashes" on the film, one can determine whether the timer is functioning properly. The key to this technique is realizing that 1ϕ equipment produces discrete pulses of x-rays. The number of x-ray pulses produced per second depends on the type of rectification used. Recall from Figure 7–6 that a 1ϕ, half-wave rectified unit produces 60 x-ray pulses per second, whereas a full-wave rectified unit produces 120 pulses per second.

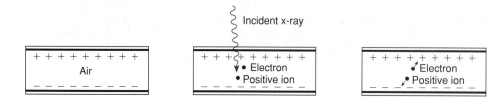

FIGURE 7–13. The process by which voltage is reduced across the plates of an ionization chamber as a result of ionization of gas atoms by incoming x-rays.

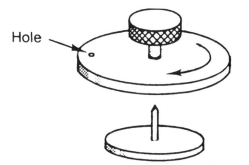

FIGURE 7–14. Schematic drawing of a spinning top used to manually check an x-ray timer. (Courtesy of Philips Medical Systems.)

Hole

With this information, an appropriate determination can be made as the following examples show.

)))))) EXAMPLE

A 1ϕ, full-wave rectified x-ray unit has its timer checked using a spinning top. When a 0.1 sec exposure is made, 12 dashes are observed on the film. What can be said about the accuracy of this timer?

Single-phase, full-wave rectified equipment produces 120 x-ray pulses per second (assuming 60-Hz AC). Therefore the number of x-ray pulses produced in 0.1 sec would be

$$120 \text{ pulses/see} \times 0.1 \text{ see} = 12 \text{ pulses}$$

Since 12 dashes were observed, this agrees with the number of pulses produced. Therefore the timer is accurate.

)))))) EXAMPLE

A 1ϕ, half-wave rectified x-ray unit is used to make a 0.25 sec exposure of a spinning top. Ten dashes are observed on the film when it is processed. What can be said about this timer?

Single-phase, half-wave rectified equipment produces 60 x-ray pulses per second (assuming 60-Hz AC). The number of x-ray pulses produced in 0.25

seconds would be:

$$60 \text{ pulses/see} \times 0.25 \text{ see} = 15 \text{ pulses}$$

The timer on this unit allowed only 10 pulses when 15 pulses should have been observed. Therefore the timer terminated the exposure prematurely; the timer is fast (i.e., it terminated the exposure too early).

Use of the spinning top is a relatively simple way for the technologist to check timer accuracy, provided the unit is 1ϕ. The 100% ripple factor of a 1ϕ unit produces "bursts" of x-rays rather than a continuous beam, thus allowing individual dots or dashes to be formed on the film. X-ray units using 3ϕ power, high-frequency generators, or capacitor discharge generators produce a more uniform, continuous beam of x-rays that do not produce discernible dots on the film when the spinning top is used. In this case, because the x-ray beam is more continuous, arcs are formed (Fig. 7–15B) as the spinning top turns through fractions of a revolution during the designated exposure time.

If the spinning top could be made to turn at a designated rate, such as 1 rps, then it would turn through 1/2 revolution in 1/2 sec, 1/4 revolution in 1/4 sec, and so forth. A motorized spinning top such as that described is known as a synchronous spinning top. Such a device would allow the technologist a method by which to check timer accuracy. More accurate techniques for checking timer accuracy (such as the use of oscilloscopes) is usually beyond the training of most technologists and is left to be performed by the department's service engineer. The more complex the timing mechanism, the more likely its proper operation is monitored by qualified service personnel or a physicist.

The Filament Circuit: Generating Heat for Electron Production

The x-ray tube contains filaments that must be heated to incandescence (i.e., to a temperature at which a filament begins to glow) in order to emit electrons from its surface. The production of x-rays

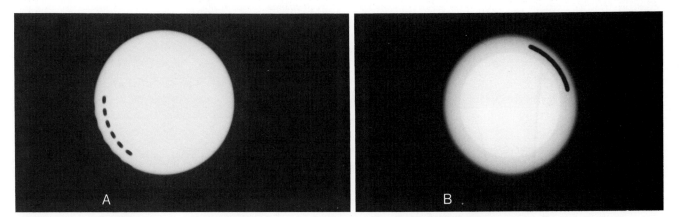

FIGURE 7–15. A, Radiograph of a spinning top made using a single-phase, full-wave rectified unit with exposure time set at 1/20 sec. B, Radiograph of a spinning top made using a three-phase x-ray unit. Here, an arc rather than individual dots is obtained.

depends on the emission of these electrons. As the temperature of the filament rises, more electrons are emitted. As the temperature is lowered, fewer electrons are released. These electrons are drawn into the tube anode in the production of x-rays. Therefore by controlling the number of electrons emitted from the filament, the number of x-rays produced during an exposure is controlled. The filament circuit (Fig. 7–16) contains the electrical components necessary to generate the heat required for electron emission in a manner that can be controlled by the radiographer.

Typically, voltages of only 5 to 10 V across the filament are needed to produce a filament current sufficiently high ($\sim$3 to 5 amps) for thermionic emission. Incoming line voltage ($\sim$110 V to 220 V) must therefore be reduced to obtain the required voltages. As shown in Figure 7–16, line voltage is supplied to the filament circuit through connections from the autotransformer. In order to reduce the voltage to the desired levels, a step-down transformer (U in Fig. 7–16) is utilized. Recall that the turns ratio is defined as N_s/N_p relating the number of turns on the secondary coil to that on the primary coil; these transformers typically have turns ratios ranging between 1:20 and 1:10. (Recall that step-down transformers have turns ratios of less than 1, since $N_s < N_p$.) Since this type of transformer provides such low power (recall that P = VI), it is common to find the secondary coil wound on top of the primary coil, which itself is wound around a laminated soft-iron core. Even if the secondary coil is at a relatively low voltage (i.e., 5 to 10 V), it is con-

nected to the cathode assembly, which is at a high (kV) negative potential with respect to ground. This can result in a large potential difference between the primary and secondary coils of the filament transformer. To prevent any electrical arcing that could then result between these two coils, an insulating cylinder of a material such as porcelain is placed over the primary coil, and the secondary coil is then wound around the insulating cylinder. For additional insulation, the filament transformer is commonly found in the oil-filled transformer box along with the high-voltage transformer. Characteristically, the filament transformer is of a smaller size than the high-voltage transformer.

Tube current (i.e., the movement of electrons between the cathode and anode) directly depends on the release of adequate numbers of electrons from the filament. In turn, the number of electrons released from the filament depends on the magnitude of the current flowing through the filament and the subsequent heat that is generated in the high-resistance wire. The magnitude of the filament current is regulated by the voltage supplied from the secondary coil of the filament (step-down) transformer. The voltage provided by the secondary coil is controlled by varying the voltage across the primary coil. The radiographer controls the primary voltage, using the mA selector, which is a rheostat (variable resistance). By varying the resistance, the voltage across the primary coil can effectively be varied. Recall that when resistances are connected in series, the voltages across each resistance must be

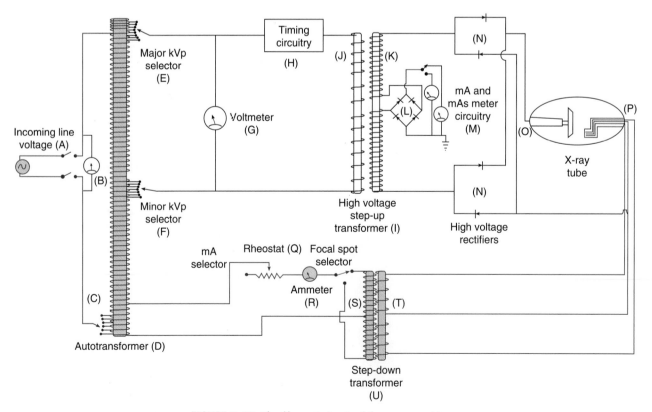

FIGURE 7–16. The filament circuit of the x-ray machine.

added to give the total incoming voltage. Thus the choice of either a high or low resistance by use of the mA selector alters the voltage across the primary coil. In modern x-ray units, the mA selector allows the radiographer to enter into the circuit specific values of resistance that correspond to specific values of the tube current, such as 100 mA, 200 mA, 500 mA, 1000 mA, and so forth.

Another factor concerning x-ray tube design that was originally discussed in Chapter 6 must also be mentioned here. The magnitude of the tube current depends not only on the amount of filament current but also on the kVp. As electrons are released from the filament, small changes in the kVp can result in large changes in the tube current. This is called the space-charge effect, and it can result in higher mA values as the kVp increases, even though the mA selector remains unchanged. An example is a situation in which the radiographer sets the mA selector for 200 mA at 70 kVp but obtains 150 mA at 60 kVp and 250 mA at 100 keV as shown in Figure 7–17. To correct for this condition a space-charge compensator is included in the filament circuit. This component functions automatically to lower the voltage on the primary coil (thereby lowering the heat produced in the filament and the number of electrons released) as the kVp is raised. As kVp is lowered, the voltage is raised to increase electron emission. This type of correction pro-cess is needed to assure that the same mA is obtained for various kVp settings.

An additional component known as a voltage stabilizer is included in the circuit in order to minimize the effects of any fluctuations in the incoming line voltage supplying the filament circuit. Any significant random variation in the voltage supplying the primary coil of the filament transformer could produce significant variations in the number of electrons emitted from the filament, which could in turn affect tube current.

GENERATOR DESIGNS USED WITH PORTABLE X-RAY UNITS

There are numerous instances in which a patient in need of a medical radiograph is unable to have the study conducted within the radiology department. The radiographer is commonly called on to make radiographs in the emergency room, intensive care unit, or operating room, and even in the patient's own hospital room. Such situations require x-ray units that are mobile and small enough to be easily maneuvered by a single individual. This means that certain modifications to previously described circuitry are required to meet the specific needs of the mobile, or *portable,*

FIGURE 7–17. Graphical representation of a typical tube current variation with filament current and kVp.

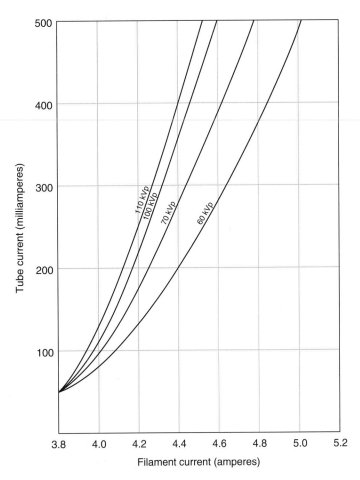

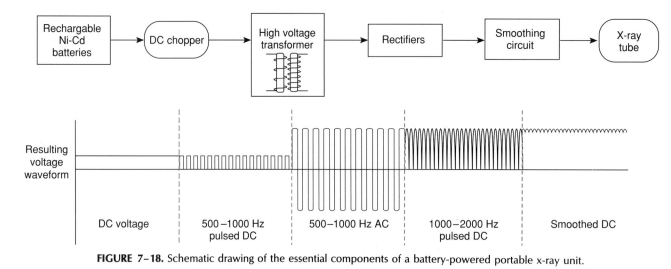

FIGURE 7–18. Schematic drawing of the essential components of a battery-powered portable x-ray unit.

x-ray unit. Several specific types of portable units are considered in the following paragraphs.

Battery-Powered Mobile Units

This type of mobile unit utilizes large-capacity nickel-cadmium (Ni-Cd) batteries as their power source. Batteries are generally charged whenever the unit is not in use. Charging is accomplished by connecting the unit to an appropriate power outlet. Once it is fully charged, the batteries provide the total power for the unit (i.e., power to energize the tube, spin the rotor, propel the unit, and so on), which does not require connections to an outside electrical energy source during use. For this reason, these units are often referred to as cordless x-ray units. Recall that batteries provide only DC current (i.e., current that flows in only one direction). Batteries alone cannot however supply the necessary kilovoltage required for diagnostic energy x-ray production. Therefore in order

to attain kilovoltage levels, a high-voltage transformer is needed, but transformers require a changing current, such as AC, for proper operation. To obtain this current, the DC battery current is fed into a DC chopper, which produces 500- to 1000-Hz pulsed DC current. This pulsed DC current is then supplied to the primary coil of the high-voltage transformer. The output from the transformer's secondary coil is 500- to 1000-Hz pulsed AC (Fig. 7–18). This resulting AC voltage is then rectified to produce 1000- to 2000-Hz pulsed DC (100% ripple). This output voltage is then smoothed to minimize ripple before its application across the x-ray tube electrodes. Advantages and disadvantages of this type of unit are summarized in Table 7–3.

Capacitor-Discharge Units

Another type of portable unit is the capacitor-discharge design. As shown in Figure 7–19, the capaci-

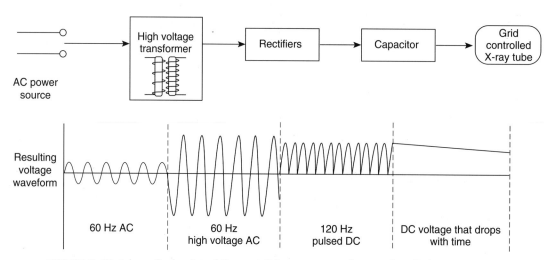

FIGURE 7–19. Schematic drawing of the essential components of a capacitor discharge x-ray unit.

Table 7–3. ADVANTAGES AND DISADVANTAGES OF VARIOUS UNITS

Type of Unit	Special Features	Advantages	Disadvantages
Battery-powered units	Uses rechargeable Ni-Cd batteries as a power source and a DC chopper to convert DC voltage from battery into high-frequency, pulsed DC	• "Cordless" unit does not require power outlet for operation once batteries have been charged • Provides constant kV and mA throughout the radiographic exposure • Batteries supply electrical energy for all aspects of instrument operation	• Batteries must be adequately charged before each use • Units tend to be somewhat heavy from weight of batteries
Capacitor-discharge unit	Incoming AC line voltage is stepped up using a high-voltage transformer; the voltage is rectified and used to charge a bank of capacitors; the capacitor bank is then discharged across the tube electrodes at the time of the exposure	• Usually smaller and easier to move about than battery-powered units • Does not require long periods of charging before use as do battery-powered units	• Each exposure starts at a preselected kV, but kV drops during the exposure; therefore may not provide sufficient x-rays of adequate energy for thick body structures • Must be connected to an external power outlet for instrument operation • Capacitors require time for charging (order of seconds) before each exposure • Older units could possibly pose electrical shock hazard
High- (or medium-) frequency units	Converts 60-Hz AC into high-frequency (kHz), pulsed DC, using a DC chopper; the resulting high-frequency voltage is stepped-up to kV levels, rectified, and supplied to the x-ray tube electrodes	• Provides a near-constant, ripple-free voltage to x-ray tube electrodes • Does not require special power supplies • Use of high-frequency electricity allows units to be smaller and more maneuverable • Electrical components such as transformers tend to be somewhat more efficient at higher-frequency levels	• Units tend to be somewhat more expensive

Ni-Cd = nickel-cadmium.

tor-discharge unit feeds standard incoming line voltage into the primary coil of the high-voltage transformer. The output of the secondary coil is then rectified and used to charge a bank of capacitors. Charging is accomplished with the individual capacitors connected in parallel so that the voltage is equal across each set of capacitor plates. When the capacitors are discharged across the x-ray tube electrodes, they are connected in series in such a way that their voltages add to provide the necessary kV for the radiographic exposure. Typically, a grid-controlled tube is used. Recall that grid-controlled x-ray tubes contain a third electrode, or grid, which surrounds the filament. As the grid is made more electrically negative, electron flow from the filament to the anode can be effectively stopped, thus allowing the grid to act as a switch to start and stop exposures.

In this design, the capacitor bank is located on the secondary side of the high-voltage transformer. When the tube is in use, voltage is drained from the capacitors to provide the necessary kV for radiographic exposure. Recall that charge does not drain from a capacitor instantaneously but does so exponentially, which indicates that the voltage across the electrodes tends to drop throughout the exposure.

With the capacitors discharging directly across the x-ray tube electrodes, it is also possible that residual charge could remain on the electrodes at the conclusion of an exposure, and electric shock is a possibility. To minimize the chances of electric shock and the further production of x-rays, residual charge on the electrodes can be removed by using the discharge switch on the console control panel.

Capacitor-discharge units have their own distinctive characteristics. Although less massive than battery-powered units, these units must be charged prior to each exposure. Therefore an appropriate external AC power outlet must be available when using these units. Also, recall that kV and mA are constant throughout an exposure made with a battery-powered unit but that it is not the case with a capacitor-discharge unit. As a capacitor is discharged, the voltage across its plates drops as charge leaves the capacitor plates. As a result,

units of this type are typically limited to radiographic procedures of 50 mAs or less. The explanation of such a limitation is that approximately 1 kV drop per unit mAs can be observed. That is, a radiographic exposure requiring 20 mAs and starting at 70 kV would have dropped to approximately 50 kV by the end of the exposure.

For this reason, capacitor-discharge units may not always be appropriate when making radiographs of thick body parts for which higher penetrating power is required. Advantages and disadvantages of this type of unit are also summarized in Table 7–3.

Medium- or High-Frequency Units

The term *high-frequency* generator indicates to many persons any x-ray generator that uses voltages having frequencies greater than standard 60-cycle AC. The term *medium-frequency* may also be used to describe such generators, depending on the manufacturer. An increasing number of x-ray units employ DC choppers to convert 60-Hz AC into voltages with frequencies in the kilohertz range. A schematic drawing of a typical high-frquency unit is illustrated in Figure 7–20. Here, standard AC line voltage is rectified and smoothed, then converted into higher-frequency (e.g., 6500-Hz), pulsed DC (necessary for proper transformer operation), which is fed to the primary side of the high-voltage transformer. The output of the secondary side is again rectified, now producing 1300-Hz, pulsed DC that is smoothed to provide an almost constant voltage across the x-ray tube electrodes.

A more recent design, designated as a modified high-frequency unit is schematically shown in Figure 7–21. In this design, standard AC line voltage is first rectified then used to charge a capacitor bank. The capacitor is then discharged, and the resulting voltage is fed into the DC chopper and converted into high-frequency pulsed DC, to supply the primary side of the high-voltage transformer, which produces the necessary kilovoltage levels on its secondary side. The resulting kilovoltage is then rectified and supplied to the x-ray

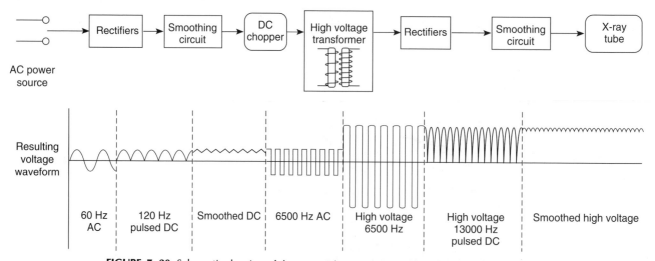

FIGURE 7–20. Schematic drawing of the essential components of a high-frequency x-ray unit.

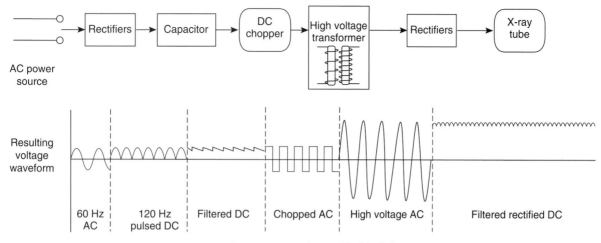

FIGURE 7–21. Essential components of a modified high-frequency x-ray unit.

tube as pulsed DC. With this design, the capacitor is charged after each exposure, charging times typically taking approximately 30 sec.

The one major advantage of using higher-frequency voltage is that it allows production of smaller, more compact x-ray units. When higher-frequency voltage is used, less bulky transformers can be used to step up

voltages to desired levels. In certain models of high-frequency portable units, the high-voltage transformer is small enough to fit within the x-ray tube housing. Another advantage of high-frequency units is the minimization of voltage ripple (Fig. 7–22). Advantages and disadvantages of this type of unit are also summarized in Table 7–3.

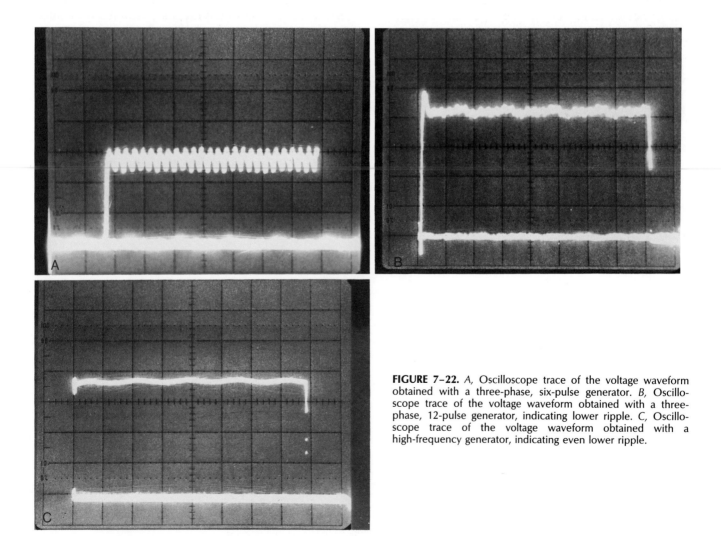

FIGURE 7–22. A, Oscilloscope trace of the voltage waveform obtained with a three-phase, six-pulse generator. B, Oscilloscope trace of the voltage waveform obtained with a three-phase, 12-pulse generator, indicating lower ripple. C, Oscilloscope trace of the voltage waveform obtained with a high-frequency generator, indicating even lower ripple.

FALLING-LOAD GENERATORS

The falling-load generator is designed to produce radiographic exposure in the shortest possible time by operating the x-ray tube at the highest mA settings without exceeding the heat-loading capabilities of the tube. Recall from previous discussions that it is the combination of mA, kVp, and exposure time that determines the heat load generated at an x-ray tube anode. When making a radiographic exposure with a designated mAs, the appropriate tube-rating chart can be used to illustrate two methods by which exposure factors can be determined. A theoretical tube rating chart is shown in Figure 7–23.

Fixed-Tube mA Method

Suppose that a radiograph of 300 mAs, such as for a lateral lumbosacral projection, using an x-ray tube operating at 90 kVp, is desired. In Figure 7–23, it can be seen that 300 mAs can safely be obtained, using a tube current of 100 mA with an exposure time of 3 sec. If a shorter exposure time is desired, notice from the graph that if 300 mA is used, the longest exposure time that can be used is 0.6 sec, which would result in only 180 mAs. Also, higher tube currents do not allow the production of 300 mAs. Therefore for this tube, operated in this manner, the shortest exposure time that can be used to obtain a radiograph of 300 mAs is 3 sec with a tube current of 100 mA.

Falling-Load Method

A falling-load generator obtains the 300 mAs radiograph in a much different way. With this type of generator, a specific exposure time is not designated. However, mAs is set, and the unit acquires the desired mAs through a series of steps, always using the highest mA for the longest period of time allowed without exceeding the tube-loading limit. This is illustrated in the following calculation example.

Again, if a radiograph of 300 mAs using the same x-ray tube operated at 90 kVp is desired, a falling-load generator would first start with a tube current of 500 mA as shown in Figure 7–23. The tube would operate at 500 mA for 0.04 sec, since this is the maximum length of time it could operate at this mA and kVp without damaging the tube. From Figure 7–23 it can be seen that this would result in only 20 mAs. The unit would then drop to 400 mA, at which it could operate safely for an additional 0.35 sec, resulting in an additional 140 mAs. Once again tube current would drop, now to 300 mA for 0.2 sec (an additional 60 mAs), then finally to 200 mA for 0.4 sec (for an additional 80 mAs). The total mAs acquired by each of these individual stages would be 20 mAs + 140 mAs + 60 mAs + 80 mAs = 300 mAs in a total time of 0.04 sec + 0.35 sec + 0.2 sec + 0.4 sec = 0.99 sec. This is less than the 3 sec required if the tube is to be operated at a fixed 100 mA to attain the same radiographic density. This type of generator is not without its own specific problems, including the following:

- Falling-load generators were designed to use the shortest exposure time by operating the tube at the

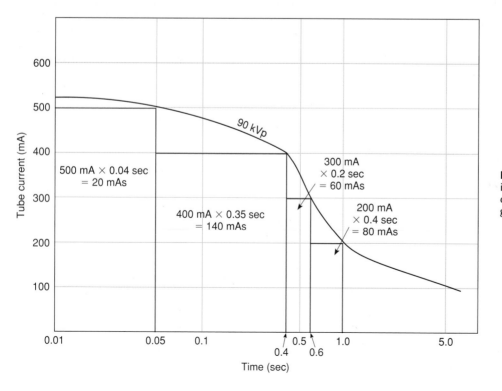

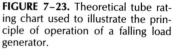

FIGURE 7–23. Theoretical tube rating chart used to illustrate the principle of operation of a falling load generator.

highest mA without producing unacceptable damage to the tube. Repeatedly operating the tube at high mA values can tend to shorten x-ray tube life.

- Since this type of generator uses the highest mA values for time periods determined by the tube's anode cooling curve, the tube focal spot can have a tendency to change in size and shape. This is referred to as focal spot blooming. Although the degree to which this occurs varies with the x-ray tube used, the effect becomes more pronounced at higher mA values. This is an important consideration; recall that image sharpness is affected by focal spot size.
- Rapid serial exposures may result in longer exposure times at lower mA values as a result of residual heat in the anode from previous exposures. This can lead to problems with repeatability when images with the same technical factors are desired.
- This type of generator also tends to be relatively expensive.

Falling-load generators were primarily developed to work in conjunction with automatic exposure timers when there were no predetermined exposure times.

rectifiers are used to convert AC to DC voltages. Also found within the high-voltage circuit is a timing circuit. The timing circuitry is located on the primary side of the high-voltage transformer in order to allow immediate termination of an exposure. A variety of timers exists, allowing varying degrees of accuracy. Timers must be checked periodically to ensure that they function properly. Timers may be checked by the technologist using a spinning top or by service personnel using more sophisticated instrumentation.

The control console is the portion of the x-ray circuitry that allows the technologist to control exposure factors such as kVp, mA, and exposure time.

A variety of portable x-ray units exists. These include battery-powered units, capacitor-discharge units, and high-frequency units. Each has its own advantages and disadvantages. Another type of generator is the falling-load generator, designed for use with automatic exposure control. It uses the shortest exposure time while operating the tube at maximum mA without exceeding the heat-loading limits of the tube.

⚋⚋ Chapter Summary/ Important Concepts

The general x-ray circuit consists of a control console, a filament circuit, and a high-voltage circuit

The purpose of the filament circuit is to provide the electrons that will be accelerated between the x-ray tube electrodes to produce x-rays. Voltage is supplied to the filament circuit from the autotransformer. The voltage supplied from the autotransformer is altered by using variable resistances. Selected voltages are then supplied to the primary side of a step-down transformer, in which the supplied voltage is reduced from approximately several hundred volts to about 10 V. The lowered voltage, when supplied to the x-ray tube filament, produces the filament current. The filament current generates heat as it flows through the tungsten filament. Electrons are emitted from the tungsten filament by the process known as thermionic emission. Tube current and the number of x-rays subsequently produced are a function of the filament current

The high-voltage circuit converts incoming line voltage, which is of the order of 100 V, to the kilovoltage levels required for diagnostic x-ray production. Voltage supplied by the autotransformer is stepped-up to the kilovoltage range by using a high-voltage step-up transformer. To make the most efficient use of the resulting AC voltage waveforms,

Important Terminology

AC Cycle. Sinusoidal variation of AC voltage (and current) consisting of one consecutive positive and negative pulse; in the United States, 60 AC cycles are generated each second with 60-Hz AC line voltage

Alternating Current (AC). Current that continuously alternates, or changes, its direction of flow a specified number of times per second (referred to as its frequency)

Ammeter. Meter used to determine the amount of current that is flowing

Automatic Timer. A specific type of x-ray timing device designed to end a radiographic exposure when a predetermined quantity of radiation has been detected; ideally, it allows for the production of radiographs of uniform density regardless of the patient's size

Autotransformer. A single-coil transformer that acts as both primary and secondary coils and is used to produce small variations in incoming (primary side) voltage; used primarily in the x-ray circuit as a kVp selector

Control Console. Portion of the x-ray unit containing the controls that allow the technologist to vary radiographic technical factors such as kVp, mA, and exposure time together with various meters for monitoring purposes

Electronic Timer. An x-ray timing device whose operation is based on the time to charge a capacitor through a variable resistance; one of the most accurate of timers used in x-ray circuitry

Filament Circuit. Portion of the x-ray circuit that supplies the necessary current to the x-ray tube filaments necessary for the ejection of electrons from the filament surface

Filament Current. Current that flows through the x-ray tube filament and results in electron production by thermionic emission; measured in amperes

Full-Wave Rectification. Rectification of an AC voltage waveform that results in the conversion of all negative portions of the AC cycle into positive portions; this type of rectification, using 1ϕ 60-Hz AC, results in 120 positive voltage pulses each second

Half-Wave Rectification. Rectification of an AC voltage waveform that results in the elimination of all negative portions of the AC cycle; this type of rectification, using 1ϕ 60-Hz AC, results in 60 positive voltage pulses each second

High-Frequency Generator. A type of x-ray generator that takes standard 60-Hz AC voltage from an incoming line source and converts it into high-frequency (usually kHz) electricity; the advantage of this conversion is that it allows the use of smaller transformers and more efficient use of electrical energy in the production of x-rays

High-Voltage Circuit. Portion of the x-ray circuit responsible for providing the high voltage necessary for the production of x-rays to the electrodes of the x-ray tube

Impulse Timer. X-ray timing device designed to end a radiographic exposure by counting the number of periodic electronic pulses (i.e., pulses which occur at identically spaced time intervals)

Line Voltage. Voltage supplied to a facility by the electric power company

Line-Voltage Compensation. Adjustments that are made to assure a constant incoming line voltage when fluctuations occur

mAs. Product of tube current (mA) and exposure time in seconds (s); physically, this relates to the number of electrons traveling between the x-ray tube electrodes during a radiographic exposure

Mechanical Timer. A timing device designed to end a radiographic exposure by using a simple coiled spring or clockwork mechanism; usually not accurate for time less than 0.25 second

Peak Voltage. The maximum value of a fluctuating or varying voltage

Photomultiplier Tube (PMT). Electronic device used to convert light into electricity

Portable X-ray Unit. X-ray unit capable of being moved from one location to another; a mobile unit

Rectifier. Tube or solid-state device used to convert AC to DC

Self-Rectification. Rectification that occurs when the only rectifier in the x-ray circuit is the x-ray tube itself

Solid-State Rectifier. Device found in modern x-ray circuitry that allows current flow in only one direction through the use of special combinations of semiconducting materials; the term *solid state* refers to the fact that movement of electrons takes place through solid, semiconducting materials rather than through the vacuum of older valve tube designs

Spinning Top. A simple, notched metal disk that can be used to check the accuracy of an x-ray timing device

Step-Up Transformer. Transformer having more coils on its secondary than its primary side, allowing it to take low-voltage input and convert it to high-voltage output

Synchronous Timer. X-ray timing device whose operation is based on an electric (synchronous) motor that turns a drive shaft at a constant rate of 60 revolutions each second; timing of this design provides exposure times in multiples of 1/60 sec, since the voltage supplied is 60-Hz AC

Thermionic Emission. Process by which electrons are released from the filament of an x-ray tube as the filament is heated by an electric current

Timing Circuit. Portion of the x-ray circuit that terminates the radiographic exposure after the passage of a specified period of time

Transformer Box. Metal box containing x-ray unit transformers and other circuit components submerged in oil for electrical insulation and thermal convection

Tube Current. Current, referred to as and measured in mA, that flows between the x-ray tube electrodes during x-ray production

Turns Ratio. Ratio of the number of turns on the secondary (N_s) to the number of turns on the primary (N_p) side of a transformer, that is, N_s/N_p

Valve Tube. Older type of rectifier, consisting of a positive and a negative electrode within an evacuated tube; also known as a vacuum diode

Voltmeter. Meter designed to measure the potential difference (voltage) across two points in an electric circuit

X-ray Generator. Combination of electrical components in an x-ray circuit that is required to supply electrical power to an x-ray tube for x-ray production

Bibliography

Buchmann, F. Mobile radiography systems. Med Mundi 3:26–32, 1992.

Bushong, S.C. Radiologic Science for Technologists, 4th ed. St. Louis: C.V. Mosby, 1988.

Chesney, D.N.; Chesney, M.O. X-ray Equipment for Student Radiographers, 3rd ed. Boston: Blackwell Scientific Publications, 1984.

Curry, T.S. III; Dowdey, J.E.; Murry, R.C., Jr. Christensen's Physics of Diagnostic Radiology, 4th ed. Philadelphia: Lea & Febiger, 1990.

Hendee, W.R. Medical Radiation Physics, 2nd ed. Chicago: Year Book Medical Publishers, 1979.

Kelsey, C.A. Essentials of Radiology Physics. St. Louis: Warren H. Green, 1985.

Seeram, E. X-ray Imaging Equipment—An Introduction. Springfield, IL: Charles C Thomas, 1985.

Wilks, R. Principles of Radiological Physics. New York: Churchill Livingstone, 1981.

Review Questions

1. Briefly indicate the function of each of the following within the x-ray circuit:
   a. autotransformer
   b. step-up transformer
   c. step-down transformer
   d. rectifier
   e. variable resistance
   f. voltmeter
   g. ammeter
2. What is meant by the term *line voltage?*
3. Briefly explain how current flow through the filament is used to control the numbers of electrons emitted from the surface of the tungsten filament.
4. Describe the process by which voltage across the x-ray tube electrodes is varied.
5. Recalling your answer to the preceding question, indicate the importance of line-voltage compensation.
6. Indicate a major difference between the turns ratio of an autotransformer and that of other transformers found in the x-ray circuit.
7. Why are step-up and step-down transformers submerged in oil and usually housed in grounded transformer boxes?
8. Briefly explain why the voltage supplied by a battery cannot be used directly with a conventional step-up transformer.
9. Why are x-ray timing devices always located in the high-voltage circuit rather than the filament circuit?
10. Describe the physical differences between the following quantities:
    a. filament current
    b. tube current
    c. mAs (i.e., tube current × time)
11. If 60-Hz AC voltage is initially supplied by the incoming line voltage, describe the voltage waveform supplied to the x-ray tube when the x-ray circuit is
    a. self-rectified
    b. half-wave rectified
    c. full-wave rectified
12. Describe the voltage waveform supplied by each of the following and explain how the ripple factors compare in each case:
    a. a single-phase generator
    b. a three-phase generator
    c. a high-frequency generator
13. Indicate the advantage of three-phase (3ϕ) and high-frequency generators over single-phase (1ϕ) generators in regard to the energy of the x-rays produced by each.
14. In each of the following cases, indicate whether the radiographic image produced would be overexposed, underexposed, or correctly exposed:

a. the timer is set for 1/20 sec, and the exposure is terminated after 0.05 sec.
b. the timer is set for 1/5 sec, and the exposure is terminated after 1/10 sec.
c. the timer is set for 1/4 sec, and the exposure is terminated after 250 msec.
d. the timer is set for 1/2 sec, and the exposure is terminated after 0.8 sec.
15. Indicate the number of x-ray pulses that would be observed each second using
    a. 60-Hz AC line voltage; 1ϕ, full-wave rectified equipment
    b. 60-Hz AC line voltage; 1ϕ, half-wave rectified equipment
    c. 60-Hz AC line voltage; 3ϕ, 6-pulse equipment
    d. 60-Hz AC line voltage; 3ϕ, 12-pulse equipment
16. Compare the units used to measure tube current and filament current.
17. Indicate the practical advantages of high-frequency generators over the more conventional type of generators.
18. List three types of generator systems used with mobile x-ray units.
19. Describe the principle of operation of a falling-load generator.

Exercises

1. Determine the final output voltage across the x-ray tube electrodes when the incoming line voltage is 120 V, the turns ratio of the high voltage transformer is 600, and the turns ratio of the autotransformer is
   a. 0.97 c. 1.389
   b. 1.25
2. Calculate the ripple factor for each of the voltage wave forms shown below:

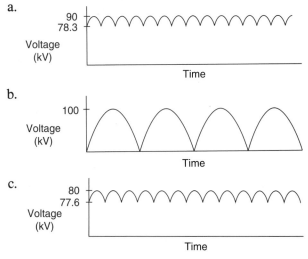

3. If V_p = input (primary) voltage, V_s = output (secondary) voltage, N_p = number of turns on the primary coil, and N_s = number of turns on the secondary coil, determine the unknown quantities in

each of the following:

a. $V_p = 80$ kV, $N_p = 100$, $N_s = 5000$, $V_p = ?$
b. $V_p = 220$ V, turns ratio $= 500$, $V_s = ?$
c. $V_p = 120$ V, $V_s = 66$ kV, turns ratio $= ?$
d. $V_p = 150$ V, $N_p = 200$, $N_s = 80,000$, $V_s = ?$
e. $V_p = 190$ V, $N_p = 125$, $V_s = 95$ kV, $N_s = ?$

4. Determine the number of electrons moving between the x-ray tube electrodes each second when there are tube currents of 100 mA, 300 mA, and 1000 mA. (Recall that the charge on an electron is 1.6×10^{-19} coulomb and that 1 ampere = 1 coulomb/sec).

5. A spinning-top is used to check the timer on the equipment indicated, and the stated number of "dots" is observed on the resulting radiograph. Determine from the information provided whether the timer is too slow, too fast, or accurate. Assume 60-Hz AC line voltage is used in each case.

a. timer is set for 1/10 sec; equipment used is 1ϕ, half-wave rectified; 8 dots are observed
b. timer is set for 1/5 sec; equipment used is 1ϕ, full-wave rectified; 10 dots are observed
c. timer is set for 1/20 sec; equipment used is 1ϕ, full-wave rectified; 6 dots are observed
d. timer is set for 0.5 sec; equipment is 1ϕ, half-wave rectified; 35 dots are observed

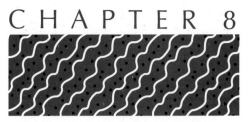

Photon Interaction in Matter

Michael A. Thompson, M.S.

Chapter Outline

Chapter Objectives

On completion of this chapter, you should be able to

- Explain how photons differ from other forms of radiation in the manner in which they interact with matter
- Describe qualitatively what occurs in each of the following photon interactions:
  - *classical scattering events*
  - *photoelectric interactions*
  - *Compton scattering interactions*
  - *pair-production events*
  - *triplet-production events*
  - *photodisintegration events*
- Perform simple calculations, given adequate date, regarding
  - *photoelectric interactions*
  - *Compton scattering events*
  - *pair-production events*
- Indicate factors affecting the ways in which photons interact with matter.
- Indicate the primary ways in which diagnostic-energy photons interact with soft tissue.
- Describe the effect of scatter radiation on
  - *image quality*
  - *radiation safety concerns for technologists*
- Describe factors that determine whether or not scatter radiation will interact with the image receptor.
- Describe methods that can be used to reduce the amount of scatter radiation reaching the film.
- List the ways in which photons are removed from an x-ray beam as it passes through matter.
- Perform simple calculations regarding x-ray beam attenuation.
- Determine the half-value layer (HVL) thickness for an x-ray beam, given sufficient data or a graphic representation of intensity versus absorber thickness.

PHOTON VS. PARTICLE RADIATION

In Chapter 3, because of their applications in medical imaging and therapy, forms of radiation other than x-rays are discussed. These other forms of radiation include alpha particles (positively charged helium nuclei), negative beta particles (negatively charged nuclear electrons), and positrons (positively charged nuclear electrons). Each of these are described as forms of ionizing radiation, that is, radiation with the ability to create *ion pairs* in matter through which it passes. These particles create ion pairs as they pass neutral atoms, because the particles are electrically charged. Negatively charged beta particles can eject loosely bound outer-shell electrons as a result of electrical repulsive forces. Positively charged particles can eject loosely bound outer-shell electrons as a result of electrical attractive forces.

Unlike these charged particle radiations, photons such as x-rays carry no electrical charge. Since x-rays do produce ion pairs, the process by which the latter are created is very different. When a photon strikes matter such as tissue or shielding material any of several possibilities may occur:

● The photon may pass through the material completely without interaction (recall that on the atomic level atoms contain much empty space)
● It may momentarily be absorbed by an atom then be re-emitted with little or no change in its energy and only a slight change in its original direction of motion
● It may be totally absorbed within the material
● It may be partially absorbed, resulting in the production of a lower energy scattered photon
● It may result in the production of an electron-positron pair
● It may be absorbed by the nucleus, resulting in the ejection of a nuclear particle

With all of these possibilities, how can the manner of interaction of any photon be determined? There is no simple answer to this question. The way in which a photon interacts with matter is a complex function of factors such as photon energy and properties of the material into which it passes. For this reason, it is not possible to say with 100% accuracy exactly how any one photon will interact as it passes through matter. It is more correct to describe the probability, or "chance," that a photon will behave in a specific way.

One important factor that influences how a photon interacts with matter is its incident energy, that is, its initial energy prior to interaction. For convenience photons can be classified according to their energy (Table 8–1). It should be pointed out that these energy ranges are somewhat arbitrary for there are no clear dividing lines between low-, medium-, and high-energy photons. The ranges in Table 8–1 were chosen for their usefulness in describing x-ray interactions in matter. Each of the various modes of photon interaction in matter are now considered in greater detail.

CLASSICAL (COHERENT) SCATTERING

Classical (coherent) scattering is typically a low-energy ($E \leq 10$ keV) photon interaction when it occurs in tissue, which has a relatively low effective atomic number ($Z_{eff} \approx 7.4$). This interaction occurs when an incoming or incident photon is momentarily absorbed either by a shell electron (Thomson scattering) or the atom as a whole (Rayleigh scattering). The absorbed energy is re-radiated in the form of a photon with no change in its energy but a change only in its direction of motion. This type of interaction is illustrated in Figure 8–1. The interaction does not result in ionization of the atom with which the incident photon interacts.

Although this type of interaction can occur with photons having energies as high as 200 keV in materials with higher Z numbers, it occurs less frequently (less than 5 interactions in 100) with diagnostic x-ray photons in tissue. Coherent scattering events contribute no diagnostically useful information to the radiograph, rather only overall darkening of the film called film fog.

PHOTOELECTRIC INTERACTIONS

Photoelectric interaction results when an incident photon, having an incident energy (E_i) just somewhat greater than the binding energy (E_b) of an inner-shell electron, is completely absorbed, resulting in the ejection of an inner shell electron from the atom with which it interacts. Any energy above this electronic binding energy is transferred as kinetic energy of motion (E_e) of the ejected *photoelectron*. This type of interaction is illustrated in Figure 8–2.

Energies of the ejected photoelectrons, important in calculations of patient dose, can easily be determined by using the law of conservation of energy, which states that the total energy before the interaction must

Table 8–1. PHOTON CLASSIFICATIONS ACCORDING TO ENERGY

Photon Classifications	Approximate Energy Range
Non-ionizing	≤ 33 eV to 35 eV
Low energy	~35 eV to ~10 keV
Intermediate energy	~10 keV to ~1 MeV
Low	~10 keV to ~100 keV
High	~100 keV to ~1 MeV
High energy	>1 MeV
Diagnostic-energy x-rays	~25 keV to 110 keV
Therapeutic x- and γ-rays	~50 keV to 10 MeV

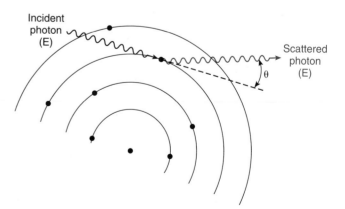

FIGURE 8–1. A classic, or coherent, scattering event. The incident photon is momentarily absorbed then re-emitted with a change in its direction but no change in energy.

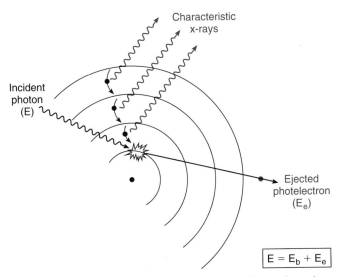

Characteristic
x-rays

Incident
photon
(E)

Ejected
photelectron
(E_e)

$$E = E_b + E_e$$

FIGURE 8-2. A photoelectric absorption event. The incident photon is totally absorbed with the ejection of an inner shell electron. This is followed by the emission of characteristic x-rays.

equal the total energy after the interaction or in equation form

Total energy before = total energy after

that is,

$$E_i = E_b + E_e$$

where

E_i = incident photon energy

E_b = electronic binding energy

E_e = kinetic energy of ejected photoelectron

))))))) EXAMPLE

A 90-keV x-ray photon interacts photoelectrically with the K-shell electron (E_b = 88 keV) of a lead (Pb) atom. What is the kinetic energy of the ejected photoelectron?

From the law of conservation of energy we have

$$E_i = E_b + E_e$$

$$90 \text{ keV} = 88 \text{ keV} + E_e$$

$$E_e = 90 \text{ keV} - 88 \text{ keV} = 2 \text{ keV}$$

Several K-shell–binding energies for materials of interest in radiography are provided in Table 8-2. As indicated in the table, electronic binding energies increase with increasing atomic number. Thus higher-energy photons can also interact photoelectrically as they encounter materials with high Z numbers. This fact is one reason lead (Z = 82) is commonly used in radiography as a means of radiation protection. It has the ability to completely absorb diagnostic-energy x-rays

by photoelectric interactions. Also, photoelectric interactions with biological materials (e.g., bone) and contrast agents (e.g., barium and iodine) provide increased contrast in the radiographic image.

Each time a photoelectric interaction occurs, an incident photon disappears, and an ion pair is created. In addition to the creation of the ion pair, the event is followed by the emission of characteristic x-rays as electrons from higher-energy states fall to fill in lower–energy state vacancies produced by the ejection of the photoelectron.

In considering the probability, or chances, that a photon will interact photoelectrically, the following factors are important to note:

- The probability of a photoelectric interaction decreases as the energy of the incident photon increases. Photoelectric events are more likely to occur when the incident photon energy is just a little greater than the shell electron–binding energy; however, as the incident photon energy increases, the chance of a photoelectric event drops quickly, or to be more specific,

$$\text{Probability of photoelectric event} \propto \frac{1}{(\text{energy})^3}$$

Note: This proportionality simply indicates that as the energy of the incident photon increases, the chance of a photoelectric event drops sharply.

- The probability of a photoelectric event increases as the Z number of the absorber increases.
- As the Z number of the material with which the photon interacts increases, there are more electrons per atom, and the inner-shell electrons are held more tightly; photoelectric events occur more often with electrons that have relatively high binding energies; in equation form

$$\text{Probability of photoelectric event} \propto Z^3$$

Note: The preceding proportionality indicates that as the Z number of the absorber increases, the chance of a photoelectrical event greatly increases.

Table 8-2. K-SHELL–BINDING ENERGIES FOR MATERIALS OF INTEREST IN RADIOGRAPHY

Element/Material	Z Number	K-Shell–Binding Energy
Biological Elements		
Carbon (C)	6	284 eV
Nitrogen (N)	7	400 eV
Oxygen (O)	8	532 eV
Calcium (Ca)	20	4.04 keV
Contrast Agents and Shielding		
Iodine (I)	53	33.2 keV
Barium (Ba)	56	37.4 keV
Tungsten (W)	74	69.5 keV
Lead (Pb)	82	88 keV

■ CHARACTERISTIC X-RAYS FROM PHOTOELECTRIC EVENTS (SECONDARY RADIATION)

Recall from Chapter 3 that characteristic x-rays are produced when an inner-shell electron is dislodged from an atom. When this occurs, electrons in higher-energy shells fall to fill in the vacancy. When the higher-energy electron makes this electronic transition, energy is given off in the form of a photon called a characteristic x-ray. The energy of the characteristic x-ray is just the difference in the binding energies of the two shells between which the transition occurred, as shown in the figure below.

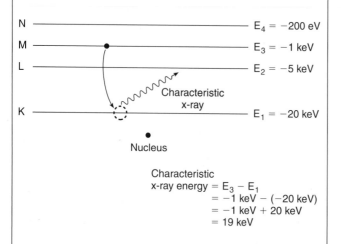

Characteristic
x-ray energy = $E_3 - E_1$
= -1 keV $-$ (-20 keV)
= -1 keV $+ 20$ keV
= 19 keV

This process was also discussed in relation to production of the characteristic x-ray portion of the x-ray spectrum produced when high-speed electrons strike the tungsten target. Here, the shell electrons are ejected by fast-moving electrons, and the characteristic x-rays produced are considered part of the primary radiation produced by the x-ray unit.

In a photoelectric event, the inner-shell electron of an atom is ejected by an incident photon (in this case, an x-ray photon). The characteristic x-rays emitted following this event are referred to as *secondary radiation.*

It should be pointed out that of the primary elements found in the body (i.e., hydrogen, oxygen, nitrogen, carbon, and calcium), the maximum-energy characteristic x-ray is approximately 4 keV. This is extremely low energy compared with diagnostic-energy x-rays. Therefore it is safe to say that any secondary radiation resulting from a photoelectric interaction in the body is absorbed within the tissue of the body. Only a photoelectric interaction with a K-shell electron of contrast agents such as iodine or barium could produce secondary radiation having sufficient energy (33.2 keV and 37.4 keV, respectively) to contribute to film fog.

This latter factor is important in understanding why high Z number materials such as lead (Z = 82) and tungsten (Z = 74) are highly efficient shielding materials. Similarly, this also aids in understanding the choice of relatively materials with high Z numbers such as barium (Z = 56) and iodine (Z = 53) as commonly used radiographic contrast agents.

The production of high-quality radiographs depends on the presence of significant natural tissue contrast in the image. Contrast relies on the fact that certain tissues absorb more of the incident x-rays than do others. This occurrence produces the various shades of gray in the radiographic image. As an x-ray beam passes into a body structure in which there are tissues of significantly different Z number, such as bone and soft tissue, contrast is enhanced. This enhancement results from increased occurrence of photoelectric events within bone, which has a higher effective Z number (~ 13.8) than soft tissue (~ 7.4).

A photoelectric event does not produce scatter radiation, which contributes only to film fog. However, although it enhances image contrast, a photoelectric event represents complete absorption of the incident photon energy and contributes to radiation dose received by the patient. This is an undesirable effect. Thus in making quality diagnostic images, the radiographer must carefully adjust the kVp to produce the desired image contrast but to minimize radiation dose to the patient.

COMPTON SCATTERING INTERACTION

The Interaction

The *Compton scattering interaction,* also referred to as incoherent scattering, is the predominant mode of interaction in soft tissue for photons within the approximate energy range of 30 keV to 10 MeV. This interaction occurs when a higher-energy photon within the previously described energy range ejects an outer shell electron from an atom of the medium through which it is moving. Unlike the photoelectric interaction, in which the total energy of the photon is consumed in the ejection of the shell electron, in Compton scattering events only a portion of the incident photon energy is used to eject the shell electron. Recall that Compton scattering events occur with outer-shell electrons whose binding energies are much lower than those of inner shells; in addition to an ejected shell electron, this type of interaction also results in lower-energy scattered photons. This is commonly referred to as *scatter,* or scattered radiation, since it is not only of lower energy but also travels in a direction different from that of the original incident photon. The interaction is illustrated in Figure 8–3.

For Compton scattering events, the law of conservation of energy requires the following relationship:

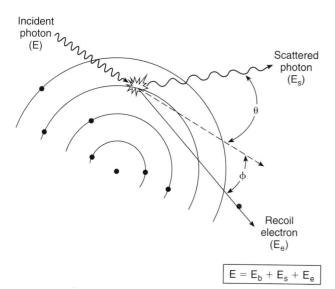

Incident
photon
(E)

Scattered
photon
(E$_s$)

θ

φ

Recoil
electron
(E$_e$)

$$E = E_b + E_s + E_e$$

FIGURE 8–3. A Compton scattering interaction. The incident photon is partially absorbed with the ejection of an outer shell electron. The interaction also results in the release of a lower-energy, scattered photon.

Total energy before interaction =
total energy after interaction, that is

$$E_i = E_b + E_e + E_s$$

where

E_i = incident photon energy

E_b = binding energy of shell electron

E_e = kinetic energy of the ejected shell electron

E_s = energy of the scattered photon

)))))) **EXAMPLE**

An incident x-ray photon having an energy of 70 keV undergoes a Compton scattering event with a shell electron having a binding energy of 100 eV. If the Compton scattered electron has a measured energy of 25 keV, what is the energy of the scattered photon?
Given

$$E_i = 70 \text{ keV}$$
$$E_b = 100 \text{ eV} = 0.1 \text{ keV}$$
$$E_e = 25 \text{ keV}$$
$$E_s = ?$$

From the law of conservation of energy, we must have

$$E_i = E_b + E_e + E_s$$
$$70 \text{ keV} = 0.1 \text{ keV} + 25 \text{ keV} + E_s$$
$$E_s = 70 \text{ keV} - 25.1 \text{ keV} = 44.9 \text{ keV}$$

Note: This 44.9-keV–scattered photon possibly could Compton scatter again with another shell electron, could be totally absorbed in a photoelectric interaction, or could pass through the patient and interact with the image receptor (e.g., film). If this scattered radiation reaches the image receptor, it does not contribute useful diagnostic information to the image.

The relationship that determines the amount of energy carried off by the Compton-scattered photon depends on the angle at which the radiation is scattered, or the scattering angle. (This process is described in the boxed material.)

It is important to note several generalizations regarding scatter radiation:

● In the diagnostic-energy range (~60 keV to 150 keV), the greatest percentage of x-ray photons that interact with tissue in a Compton event tend to scatter in the forward direction, as illustrated in Figure 8–4. In the illustration, this scatter is directed toward the image receptor (film). Methods employed to reduce the amount of scatter radiation reaching the film are discussed in greater detail in Chapter 13. As the incident photon energy increases, a greater percentage of the scatter occurs in the forward direction.

● In general, the greater the scattering angle, the lower the energy of the scatter radiation. That is, for the same incident energy, a photon scattered through 90° angle has lower energy than a photon scattered through a 20° angle. From a radiation protection perspective, this is important. Radiation scattered toward a radiographer standing by an imaging table is of lower energy and has a greater probability of being absorbed in a photoelectric event. This can occur within the radiographer's body unless precautions, such as wearing a lead apron or using other appropriate shielding, are taken.

● The scattered photons of lowest energy, occurring at a scattering angle of 180°, are referred to as *backscatter*. This scattering angle also is the one at which maximum energy is transferred to the Compton-scattered electron (also known as the *recoil electron*).

● As the energy of the incident photon is increased, the greater the energy of the scatter radiation.

● At low-incident energies (e.g., 10 keV), the probabilities of photons being scattered forward and being backscattered are almost equal.

● At high-incident energies (>1 MeV), the probability of scattering through large angles is greatly decreased. At these high energies, photons tend to be extremely penetrating, and if they do scatter, they tend to scatter in the forward direction.

At this point, it is important to mention that the term *secondary radiation* has historically meant radiation emitted from an atom after it has absorbed a photon (either x-ray or γ ray), and it typically has included

● Characteristic x-rays (following a photoelectric interaction), also known as fluorescence

- Ejected photoelectrons (also as a result of a photo-electric interaction)
- Compton-scattered or recoil electrons (from a Compton scattering event)
- Electron-positron pairs and annihilation radiation (following a pair-production event, discussed later in the chapter)

On the other hand, scattered radiation has typically referred to photons that undergo a change in original direction of motion after interacting with atoms. However, several recognized authors tend to use the terms *secondary* and *scattered radiation* interchangeably. It is important for the student to recognize that this interchange of terminology occurs in the literature. It

■ DETERMINATION OF ENERGY OF SCATTER RADIATION BASED ON SCATTERING ANGLE (θ) AND INCIDENT PHOTON ENERGY

Problem. An 80-keV x-ray photon undergoes a Compton scattering event. If the photon is scattered at an angle of 90°, determine the energy of the scattered photon.

Solution. First determine the wavelength (λ) of the incident photon by using the following relationship:

$$\lambda(\text{Å}) = \frac{12.4}{E(keV)}$$
$$= \frac{12.4}{80 \text{ keV}}$$
$$= 0.155\text{Å} \quad \leftarrow \text{wavelength of incident photon}$$

The wavelength of the scattered photon is longer than that of the incident photon (since it is of lower energy) by an amount $\Delta\lambda$ given by

$$\Delta\lambda = 0.024 \, (1 - \cos\theta)$$
$$= 0.024 \, (1 - \cos 90°)$$
$$= 0.024 \, (1 - 0)$$
$$= 0.024 \text{ Å} \quad \leftarrow \text{amount by which wavelength increases}$$

The wavelength of the scattered photon is

$$\lambda' = \lambda + \Delta\lambda$$
$$= 0.155\text{Å} + 0.024\text{Å}$$
$$= 0.179\text{Å} \quad \leftarrow \text{wavelength of scattered photon}$$

To determine the energy of the scattered photon, then use

$$E'(keV) = \frac{12.4}{\lambda'(\text{Å})}$$
$$= \frac{12.4}{0.179\text{Å}}$$
$$\approx 69.3 \text{ kev} \quad \leftarrow \text{energy of scattered photon}$$

If the binding energy of the ejected shell electron is considered negligible, the energy given to the ejected electron would be

$$E_e = E_i - E_s$$
$$= 80 \text{ keV} - 69.3 \text{ keV}$$
$$= 10.7 \text{ keV} \quad \leftarrow \text{energy of Compton electron}$$

This technique can be used to determine the energy of the scattered photon (E'), given the incident photon energy (E) and the scattering angle (θ). Assuming negligible electronic binding energies, the energy imparted to the Compton or recoil electron (E_e) can be calculated based on conservation of energy. Several of the values for different incident energies and different scattering angles are shown in the following table.

ENERGIES OF COMPTON-SCATTERED PHOTONS (E_s) AND RECOIL ELECTRONS (E_e) AS A FUNCTION OF INCIDENT PHOTON ENERGY (E) AND SCATTERING ANGLE (θ)

Incident Energy (E)	$\theta = 10°$	$\theta = 30°$	$\theta = 60°$	$\theta = 90°$	$\theta = 180°$
40 keV	$E_s = 39.95$ keV $E_e = 0.05$ keV	$E_s = 39.59$ keV $E_e = 0.41$ keV	$E_s = 38.5$ keV $E_e = 1.5$ keV	$E_s = 37.1$ keV $E_e = 2.9$ keV	$E_s = 34.6$ keV $E_e = 5.4$ keV
60 keV	$E_s = 59.79$ keV $E_e = 0.21$ keV	$E_s \approx 59$ keV $E_e \approx 1$ keV	$E_s = 56.6$ keV $E_e = 3.4$ keV	$E_s = 53.7$ keV $E_e = 6.3$ keV	$E_s = 48.6$ keV $E_e = 11.4$ keV
80 keV	$E_s = 79.79$ keV $E_e = 0.21$ keV	$E_s = 78.4$ keV $E_e = 1.6$ keV	$E_s = 74.3$ keV $E_e = 5.7$ keV	$E_s = 69.3$ keV $E_e = 10.7$ keV	$E_s = 61.1$ keV $E_e = 18.9$ keV
100 keV	$E_s = 99.68$ keV $E_e = 0.32$ keV	$E_s = 97.5$ keV $E_e = 2.5$ keV	$E_s = 91.2$ keV $E_e = 8.8$ keV	$E_s = 83.8$ keV $E_e = 16.2$ keV	$E_s = 72.1$ keV $E_e = 27.9$ keV

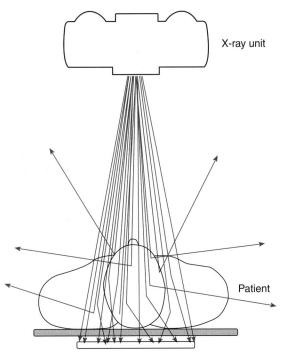

X-ray unit

Patient

Image receptor

FIGURE 8-4. Scattered radiation from a diagnostic x-ray unit. The greatest probability of scattered radiation occurs in the forward direction (i.e., toward the image receptor).

should also be noted that although scattered radiation may be considered under the general heading of secondary radiation, not all secondary radiation is scattered radiation.

Factors Affecting the Probability of Compton Interaction

When a photon interacts with a shell electron in matter through which it passes, the chance that it will interact with an electron appears to depend on several factors:

- The binding energies holding shell electrons to the atom; these values strongly depend on the Z number of the atoms that make up the material
- The total number of electrons in the absorbing medium (in turn related to the density of the medium and the number of electrons per gram)
- How closely the atoms of the medium are packed together (i.e., the density of the medium)
- The energy of the incident photon (since photons of high energy tend to be more penetrating)

When these factors are more closely analyzed, several conclusions as to their influence on Compton scattering events are drawn:

1. Unlike photoelectric interactions occurring with tightly bound, inner-shell electrons (binding ener-

gies are strongly dependent on the Z number of the atom), Compton events occur with loosely bound outer-shell electrons. These are often referred to as free electrons, the term *free* indicating that the binding energy is low compared with the energy of the incident photon. Since it is these electrons with which Compton scattering occurs, the probability of a Compton scattering event is found to be independent of the atomic number of the medium.

> Compton probability is independent of the Z number of the absorber

2. The number of electrons available to interact with the incident photon influence the chances of this interaction's occurring. However, calculations indicate that all elements contain about the same number of electrons per gram regardless of their Z number (Table 8–3). With the exception of hydrogen, which contains about twice the number of electrons per gram as do other elements, most materials contain about the same number. Substances that contain considerable amounts of hydrogen, such as water and soft tissue, have increased probability for Compton interactions.

> Probability for Compton interaction is increased for materials containing considerable amounts of hydrogen (e.g., water and soft tissues)

3. Compton interaction probability is also increased when the number of electrons per unit volume (i.e., electrons/cc) of the medium increases. The number of electrons/cc is related to the number of electrons/gm (known as the electron density) as indicated below:

Number of electrons/cc = electrons/gm × density

Since it has been shown that most materials (except hydrogen) contain about the same number of elec-

Table 8-3. PHYSICAL DATA FOR MATERIALS OF INTEREST IN RADIOGRAPHY

Element or Tissue	Atomic Number (Z or Effective Z)	Density (gm/cc)	Electrons/gm
Hydrogen (H)	1	$\sim 9 \times 10^{-5}$	$\sim 6.0 \times 10^{23}$
Carbon (C)	6	2.62	$\sim 3.0 \times 10^{23}$
Oxygen (O)	8	$\sim 1.4 \times 10^{-3}$	$\sim 3.0 \times 10^{23}$
Aluminum (Al)	13	2.7	$\sim 2.9 \times 10^{23}$
Lead (Pb)	82	11.3	$\sim 2.4 \times 10^{23}$
Water*	~ 7.4	1.0	$\sim 3.4 \times 10^{23}$
Muscle*	~ 7.4	~ 1.0	$\sim 3.4 \times 10^{23}$
Air*	~ 7.6	$\sim 1.3 \times 10^{-3}$	$\sim 3.0 \times 10^{23}$
Bone*	~ 13.8	~ 1.85	$\sim 3.0 \times 10^{23}$
Barium	56	3.5	$\sim 2.5 \times 10^{23}$
Iodine	53	4.92	$\sim 2.5 \times 10^{23}$

* Data for tissues taken from values given in Johns, H.E.; Cunningham, J.R. The Physics of Radiology, 3rd ed. Springfield, IL: Charles C Thomas, 1974.

trons/gm, density tends to affect the Compton interaction probability.

> The probability of a Compton interaction tends to increase with increases in density of the medium

4. The probability that any x-ray photon will interact with matter in a Compton scattering event is a complex function of incident photon energy. As incident photon energy increases, the chance of a Compton interaction decreases and there is a greater probability of transmission.

> The probability of a Compton interaction tends to decrease with increases in incident photon energy

From this analysis, it can be seen that the chance an incident x-ray photon will undergo a Compton scattering event depends on its energy and the density of the material into which it passes. In addition, if the material contains significant amounts of hydrogen, the probability of a Compton interaction is enhanced.

Clinical Significance of Scattered Radiation

When an incident x-ray undergoes a Compton scattering event, a portion of its energy is transferred to a Compton-scattered electron while another portion is carried off by a lower-energy scattered photon. The amount of energy carried off by each depends on the scattering angle, represented by θ, and the incident photon energy. Calculations and physical measurements indicate the following facts:

- The scattered photon with the lowest energy occurs when the scattering angle is 180° (known as *backscatter* radiation); in such an instance, maximum energy is transferred to the Compton-scattered electron
- For a specific incident photon energy, as the scattering angle increases, the energy of the scattered photons decrease (Fig. 8–5)
- As the energy of the incident photon increases, the energy of the scattered radiation at all scattering angles also increases

As an x-ray beam exits the x-ray tube, its photons may produce scatter radiation when they encounter tube housing, filters, collimators, beam-restriction devices, patient, imaging table, and even floor surfaces. Of all these potential scattering objects, the greatest source of scatter is the patient's body. This scatter not only poses a problem for image quality but also causes a radiation protection problem for radiography personnel.

Recall that scattered radiation is of lower energy and that this in turn increases its chances of being totally absorbed in a photoelectric interaction. If this scattered

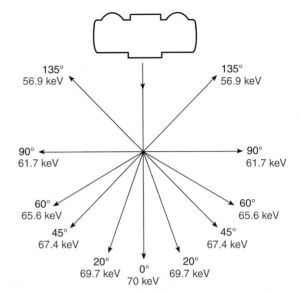

FIGURE 8–5. Energy of scattered radiation as a function of scattering angle. The energy of the scattered radiation tends to decrease as the scattering angle increases.

radiation is absorbed by the radiographer's body, his or her radiation dose is increased. It is for this reason that the radiographer typically stands behind a lead shield and not beside the imaging table during a radiographic procedure. In those cases in which a technologist must be close to the patient during a procedure (e.g., emergency situations and special fluoroscopic examinations), appropriate shielding (e.g., lead aprons, lead gloves, lead drapes, tableside shields) must be used to reduce his or her radiation dose.

In addition to radiography personnel, adequate protection from scattered radiation should also be provided for the patient in the form of gonadal shielding. This can simply take the form of a lead apron draped over that part of the body during common radiographic procedures.

Regarding the effect of scatter radiation on the radiographic image, as indicated earlier, most of the scatter that takes place with diagnostic-energy x-rays occurs in the forward direction, toward the image receptor. Since this scatter does not contribute diagnostically useful information, it must be minimized, especially when it has the potential to interact with the film and to affect the resulting image.

In the study of radiography, you will learn of several techniques employed by radiographers to minimize the effect of scattered radiation. These include such methods as

- Restriction of beam size. Reducing the x-ray beam size to the area of specific interest diminishes the amount of scattering material in the beam
- Use of physical barriers. Lead strips, known as grids, are located in front of the image receptor to reduce the amount of scatter reaching the film
- Increasing the distance between the patient and the image receptor. As the image receptor is moved a

distance away from the scatter source (i.e., the patient), some of the scattered radiation misses the film

● Effective use of kVp. The chosen kVp must be sufficiently high to penetrate the anatomical part and reduce radiation dose to the patient; however, if kVp is too high, it tends to increase the amount of scatter reaching the film and will degrade the radiographic image

Each of these, along with other techniques used to reduce scatter, is discussed in greater detail in later chapters.

OTHER PHOTON INTERACTIONS IN MATTER

Within the diagnostic-energy range, photoelectric and Compton scattering interactions are most common and most important to radiography. However, these interactions are not the only ways in which photons interact with matter. Discussion of additional types of interaction, restricted to high-energy photons (>1 MeV), is included for those radiographers who may later work in the field of radiation therapy, which uses higher-energy photon beams, as well as for general information. All professionals who use radiation should have a basic knowledge of all types of radiation and their mode of interaction.

Pair Production

In this type of photon interaction, a high-energy photon interacts with the electromagnetic field of an atomic nucleus. When the interaction, known as a *pair-production event,* occurs, the photon disappears in the vicinity of the nucleus, and in its place appears an *electron-positron pair.* Recall the law of conservation of energy—energy (in this case, the incident photon) can be neither created nor destroyed but can be changed in form. In this case, the photon is converted into an electron-positron pair (Fig. 8–6). This represents a conversion of energy into mass, since both particles have mass. The amount of energy required to produce the two particles is 1.022 MeV. This is the energy equivalent of two electron masses (i.e., $2\ m_e c^2$, where m_e is the mass of a single electron), which is obtained using Einstein's rest mass–energy equation. Therefore in order for this type of interaction to have any probability of occurrence, the incident photon must have at least 1.022 MeV of energy. This is an energy requirement for pair-production events. Any energy of the incident photon in excess of 1.022 MeV appears as kinetic energy of the electron-positron pair. This excess energy may or may not be equally divided between the electron and positron. Based on the law of conserva-

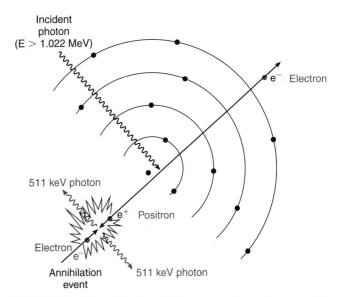

FIGURE 8–6. Pair production. A high-energy photon interacts with the electromagnetic field of an atomic nucleus to produce an electron-positron pair. The positron soon encounters an electron, resulting in annihilation radiation.

tion of energy, this interaction can be expressed as

Total energy before interaction
$$= \text{total energy after interaction}$$

$$E_i = 1.022\text{ MeV} + E_e + E_{e^+}$$

E_i = incident photon energy

E_e = electron kinetic energy

E_{e^+} = positron kinetic energy

))❭❭❭) EXAMPLE

A 6.5-MeV photon interacts in a pair-production event. Determine the kinetic energy of the electron-positron pair of the electron takes 60% of the available energy and the positron takes the remainder.

$$E_i = 1.022\text{ MeV} + E_e + E_{e^+}$$
$$6.5\text{ MeV} = 1.022\text{ MeV} + E_e + E_{e^+}$$
$$E_e + E_{e^+} = 6.5\text{ MeV} - 1.022\text{ MeV} = 5.478\text{ MeV}$$
$$E_e = 0.60(5.478\text{ MeV}) \approx 3.287\text{ MeV}$$
$$E_{e^+} = 5.478 - 3.287\text{ MeV} \approx 2.191\text{ MeV}$$

The result of this type of interaction is the release of an electron and a positron that travel into the absorbing medium. Both produce ionization events until they lose their kinetic energy. As the positron comes to the end of its path, it interacts with an electron in an annihilation event to produce two 511-keV photons that travel in roughly opposite directions. These two photons may either penetrate or interact with the absorber through Compton and photoelectric events.

This type of photon interaction becomes important in tissue at energies greater than about 10 MeV.

Triplet Production

If a pair-production event occurs in the electromagnetic field of a shell electron (rather than an atomic nucleus) such that the shell electron is also ejected, the interaction event is called *triplet production* (Fig. 8–7). Like pair production, triplet production requires a minimum incident photon energy. However, triplet production requires the incident photon to have an energy of at least 2.04 MeV. With this type of interaction, two electrons, are released into the absorber along with a positron. The positron again produces *annihilation radiation* (i.e., two 511-keV photons traveling in opposite directions) as it comes toward the end of its path.

Photodisintegration

When incident photons have energies that exceed approximately 7 MeV, the photon may be absorbed by a nucleus that can momentarily make the atom radioactive. In an attempt to achieve stability, particles (e.g., protons, neutrons, alpha particles, or clusters of nuclear particles) can be ejected from the unstable nucleus. This type of photon interaction with matter is known as *photodisintegration*.

Although this type of interaction does not occur in the diagnostic-energy range, it can occur with high-energy photons used in radiation therapy. The use of photons in the MeV energy range can make certain machinery components used in therapy radioactive for a short period of time after use. Even walls of rooms in which high-energy photon radiation is used for therapy may become slightly radioactive as a result of photodisintegration interactions. The effect is usually short-lived and not a radiation hazard for personnel.

RELATIVE IMPORTANCE OF PHOTON INTERACTIONS TO RADIOGRAPHY

A radiograph is produced when an x-ray beam is incident on a specific part of a patient's body. As the x-ray beam enters the tissue, many photons are transmitted and interact with the film, causing the film to darken. These are areas of increased radiographic density.

As the lower-energy photons (e.g., 20- to 30-keV) pass into tissue, there is a greater probability of total absorption through photoelectric interactions, especially with higher Z number absorbers such as bone. Total absorption results in high contrast between soft tissue and bone but also in increased absorbed radiation dose to the patient. Using the Z^3 dependence of photoelectric probabilities, image contrast can be further enhanced between different types of tissue by the introduction of a *contrast agent*. Two of the most common contrast agents used in radiography are barium (Z = 56) and iodine (Z = 53). Their high Z numbers make them extremely effective in absorbing higher-energy photons in the x-ray beam through photoelectric interactions, yielding higher contrast in the radiographic image.

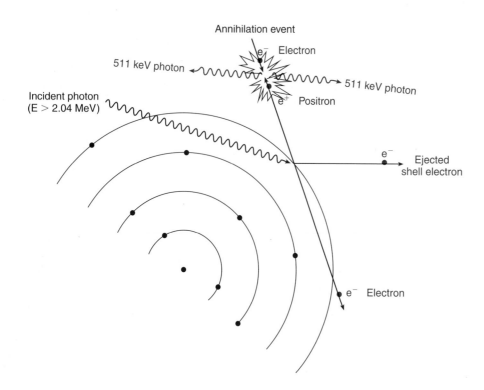

FIGURE 8–7. Triplet production. A high-energy photon interacts with the electromagnetic field of an atomic electron to produce an electron-positron pair along with the ejection of the shell electron. Annihilation radiation results when the positron encounters an electron in matter.

Compton scattering events, however, represent the most common type interaction of diagnostic-energy x-rays in body tissues. Not only do these interactions produce scatter radiation that acts to degrade the radiographic image, the scattering process also removes photons from the primary beam as it passes through body structures. This absorption reduces the number of photons that strike the radiographic film in those areas in which the scattering events occur. The combination of transmission, photoelectric absorption, and Compton scattering events results in the varying shades of gray making up the composite radiograph. The combined process by which the radiographic image is formed is called *differential absorption.*

The radiographer can significantly change the degree of differential absorption shown in a radiograph by varying the energy (i.e., the kVp) of the x-ray beam. If the kVp is set too low, low-energy photons will be produced and too many will be photoelectrically absorbed, increasing radiation dose to the patient and resulting in a radiograph that is too light. If the kVp is set too high, high-energy photons will be produced, and too many will be transmitted. This transmission will reduce the radiation absorbed dose to the patient but will result in little if any tissue contrast and a radiograph that is too dark. Thus the production of a quality diagnostic radiograph is the result of the "best" combination of transmission, absorption, and scattering events occurring within the structures being radio-

graphed. This concept is illustrated in Figure 8–8. One must keep in mind that x-ray beams are *polyenergetic,* meaning that they consist of photons having many energies. As a result, other factors influence the choice of kVp needed to provide the best degree of differential absorption. These other factors, such as effects of filtration, type of equipment used (1ϕ or 3ϕ), and grids are discussed in later chapters.

Another important factor that affects differential absorption is density (i.e., the gm/cc) differences among the tissues involved. Density, defined as mass per unit volume, provides a measure of the "compactness," or amount of matter, compressed into a unit volume. The greater the numerical value of the density, the more atoms (and electrons) compacted into a unit volume. Since x-ray photons interact with shell electrons in both photoelectric and Compton events, the more electrons per unit volume, the greater the probability of a photon interaction. As a result of density differences, there is sufficient differential absorption to allow visualization of certain body structures such as air-containing soft tissues. Structures such as the lungs can be visualized as a result of differential absorption resulting from density differences between soft tissue and air. The introduction of air or other gases into body structures is used in a variety of examinations such as contrast arthrography and double-contrast gastrointestinal radiography to outline structures and enhance visualization.

PHOTON ATTENUATION

In the preceding section, the various methods by which photons interact with matter are discussed. It is shown that the probability of a photon interacting in a specific way depends on the energy of the incident photon and is influenced in many cases by the material constituting the absorber. The relative percentages of different photon interactions with water (soft tissue equivalent) as a function of photon energy is shown in Figure 8–9.

As an x-ray beam passes through an absorber, whether it is a patient's body or a piece of lead shielding, whichever interactions occur, most will tend to remove photons from the incident beam (Fig. 8–10). The process by which photons are removed from an x-ray beam as it passes through an absorber is known as *attenuation.* It is important to distinguish between this term and the term *transmission,* which refers to those photons that pass through the absorber unhindered.

In describing a photon beam as it passes through an absorbing medium, the percentages transmission and attenuation must add together to yield the total beam, or 100%. The general relationship that must exist is

$$\boxed{\% \text{ attenuation} + \% \text{ transmission} = 100\%}$$

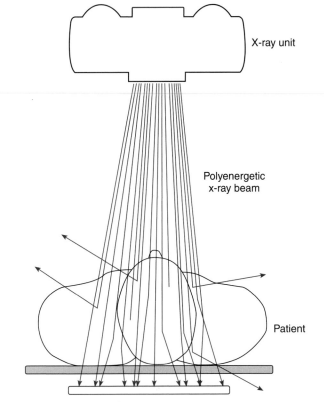

FIGURE 8–8. Effect of incident photon energy on differential absorption.

X-ray unit

Polyenergetic x-ray beam

Patient

Image receptor

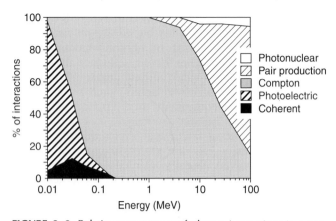

FIGURE 8-9. Relative percentages of photon interactions in water as a function of photon energy. (From Stanton, R.; Stinson, D. An Introduction to Radiation Oncology Physics. Madison, WI: Medical Physics Publishing, 1992.)

This simple relationship is based on the concept that whatever fraction or percentage of an incident beam is not attenuated is transmitted.

)))⟩⟩⟩) EXAMPLE

45% of an x-ray beam is attenuated as it passes through an aluminum absorber. What percent of the beam is transmitted?

$$45\% + \% \text{ transmitted} = 100\%$$

$$\% \text{ transmitted} = 100\% - 45\% = 55\%$$

It is also extremely important to predict what percentage of an x-ray beam will be transmitted when it passes through a given thickness of absorber. This is necessary not only for image production but also for radiation protection in which shielding material thickness must be determined in order to reduce radiation exposure.

A simple experiment, illustrated in Figure 8–11, can determine how such predictions can be made. Begin with a *monoenergetic* beam (i.e., a single-energied photon beam) having an initial intensity, I_0. The beam is allowed to strike several known thicknesses, t, of an absorber, and the transmitted intensity in each case is then measured. The transmitted intensity is designated as I. It should be noted that when written as a ratio, I/I_0 represents the fraction of the beam transmitted (which can also be represented as a percentage), since I_0 is the intensity of the beam when there is no absorber in the beam.

Sample data is collected using the monoenergetic (or *monochromatic*) beam, and the data is presented and plotted on linear graph paper (Fig. 8–12*A*). When it is plotted in this manner, a typical negative exponential decay curve is obtained. Recall from Chapter 2 that if this same data is plotted on semilog graph paper, a straight-line graph is obtained (Fig. 8–12*B*). From a practical standpoint, the semilog plot is usually preferred, since greater accuracy can be achieved by drawing a straight line rather than a curve. However, if care is taken, both graphs can provide the desired information. The following examples show how the graphs can be used to provide useful information.

)))⟩⟩⟩) EXAMPLE

What thickness of absorber used in Figure 8–12*B* is required to measure a transmission of 150 mR?

Using the semilog graph, sketch a straight line (using a ruler for greater accuracy) across from the 150 mR point on the vertical axis until it intersects the straight line. Then draw a straight line down from this point to the horizontal axis. The value on this axis indicates that approximately 3.55 mm of absorber is needed.

)))⟩⟩⟩) EXAMPLE

What intensity would be measured when the beam passes through 6.5 mm of absorber?

Again using the semilog graph, find 6.5 mm on the horizontal axis. Draw a vertical line from this point until it intersects the straight line. From this point, draw a horizontal line and find its point of intersection with the vertical axis. From the graph, 6.5 mm of absorber will transmit an intensity of approximately 66 mR.

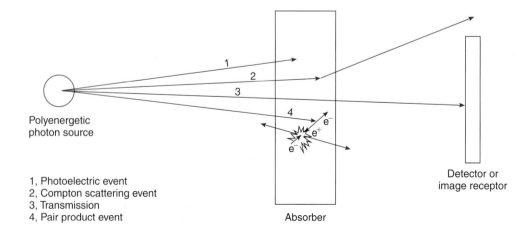

1, Photoelectric event
2, Compton scattering event
3, Transmission
4, Pair product event

Polyenergetic photon source

Absorber

Detector or image receptor

FIGURE 8-10. Processes by which photons are removed from a photon beam as it passes into matter.

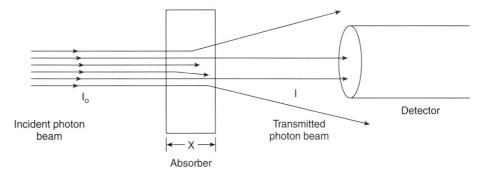

FIGURE 8–11. Experimental set-up for photon attenuation determinations.

I_o

Incident photon beam

Absorber

X

Transmitted photon beam

I

Detector

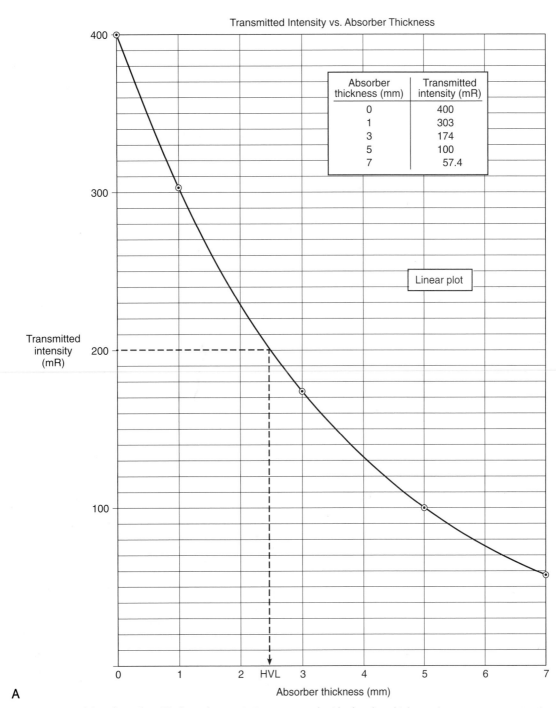

Transmitted Intensity vs. Absorber Thickness

Absorber thickness (mm)	Transmitted intensity (mR)
0	400
1	303
3	174
5	100
7	57.4

Linear plot

Transmitted intensity (mR)

Absorber thickness (mm)

HVL

A

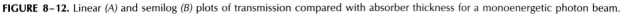

FIGURE 8–12. Linear (A) and semilog (B) plots of transmission compared with absorber thickness for a monoenergetic photon beam.

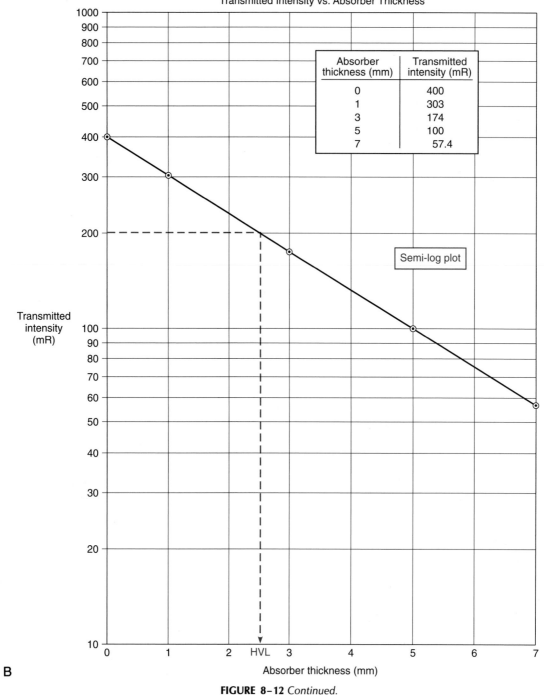

FIGURE 8–12 Continued.

The form the data takes when plotted on semilog graph paper (i.e., a straight line) indicates that the relationship between transmitted intensity (I) and absorber thickness (x) can be written in the following form:

$$\frac{I}{I_0} = e^{-\mu_L x}$$

or

$$I = I_0 e^{-\mu_L x}$$

where

I = transmitted intensity

I_0 = initial intensity

μ_L = linear attenuation coefficient

x = absorber thickness

The preceding equation is known as an attenuation equation. The one new term which has been introduced here is μ_L, which is the linear attenuation coef-cient. This is a numerical value found in tables such as those in *The Radiological Health Handbook.* These attenuation coefficients vary with the energy of the incident photon and the material composing the absorber.

Perhaps a somewhat easier form of the attenuation equation to use is one based on the *half-value layer* (HVL) concept. The HVL is the thickness of a material that is required to reduce the beam intensity to 50% of its original value. The HVL varies with photon energy and the material constituting the absorber. This concept is illustrated in Figure 8–13 with a beam of 140-keV photons having an HVL of 0.2 mm of lead. As illustrated, each time the beam passes through a 0.2 mm thickness of lead, the beam is attenuated by 50%. This concept can be extended to produce an attenuation equation of the following form:

$$\boxed{I = I_0(0.5)^N}$$

where

I = transmitted intensity

I_0 = initial intensity

$N = \dfrac{x}{\text{HVL}}$ (i.e., the thickness of the material in terms of half-value layers)

)) **)))**) EXAMPLE

A monoenergetic beam consisting of 140-keV photons produces an initial intensity reading of 250 mR when no absorber is placed in the beam. If its HVL in lead is 0.2 mm, what will be the beam intensity when it passes through a thickness of 0.55 mm?

First find N, the thickness of the absorber in HVLs:

$$N = \frac{x}{HVL}$$

$$= \frac{0.55 \text{ mm}}{0.2 \text{ mm/HVL}} = 2.75 \text{ HVLs}$$

Now simply substitute numerical values in the equation and solve:

$$\begin{aligned}
I &= I_0(0.5)^N \\
&= (250 \text{ mR})(0.5)^{2.75} \\
&\approx (250 \text{ mR})(0.15) \\
&\approx 37.5 \text{ mR}
\end{aligned}$$

Thus the transmitted intensity is approximately 37.5 mR.

Given sufficient information, the same equation can be used to determine the HVL, as shown in the following example. This involves solving the equation for the HVL. (You may wish to review Solving Logarithmic and Exponential Equations in Chap. 2).

)) **)))**) EXAMPLE

A photon beam produces an initial intensity reading of 350 mR when no absorber is placed within the beam. If 1.5 mm Pb is placed in the beam, the intensity reading drops to 225 mR. What is the HVL of this photon beam in lead?

Given

$$I_0 = 350 \text{ mR}$$

$$I = 225 \text{ mR}$$

$$x = 1.5 \text{ mm}$$

Substituting these values in the equation yields

$$I = I_0(0.5)^N$$

$$225 \text{ mR} = (350 \text{ mR})(0.5)^N$$

$$\frac{225 \text{ mR}}{350 \text{ mR}} = (0.5)^N$$

$$0.643 \approx (0.5)^N$$

Taking the ln of both sides now gives

$$\ln(0.643) = \ln(0.5)^N$$

$$-0.442 = N \ln(0.5) = N(-0.693)$$

$$N = \frac{-0.442}{-0.693} \approx 0.638$$

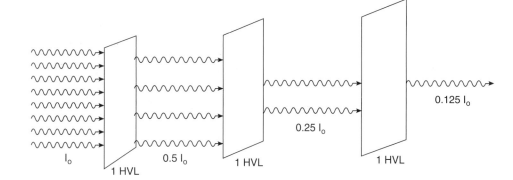

FIGURE 8–13. Concept of the half-value layer (HVL) using 140 keV photons having a 0.2 mm HVL in Pb.

I_0

1 HVL

$0.5\ I_0$

1 HVL

$0.25\ I_0$

1 HVL

$0.125\ I_0$

But

$$N = \frac{x}{HVL}$$

therefore

$$\frac{x}{HVL} \approx 0.638$$

$$HVL = \frac{x}{0.638} = \frac{1.5 \text{ mm}}{0.638} \approx 2.35 \text{ mm Pb}$$

The HVL thickness can also be determined graphically. As shown in Figure 8–12, the HVL can be determined by taking the initial intensity, 400 mR, and reducing it by 50%. Draw a horizontal line from this point to the curve (or straight line). Then draw a vertical line from this point to the horizontal axis. The point of intersection is the HVL thickness as shown in Figure 8–12*A* and *B*. For the data presented, the HVL corresponds to 2.5 mm. It is important to note that the HVL thickness varies with the energy of the incident photons and the material composing the absorber.

If the HVL thickness of a particular absorber is known, much useful information can be obtained from another type of graph. In this case, using semilog graph paper (at least two-cycle), on the vertical axis represent Percentage Transmission and on the horizontal axis, Absorber Thickness. The difference here is the choice to express the thickness in terms of HVLs. No data is needed to draw a graph such as this. Only two data points, shown in Figure 8–14, are needed. These two data points represent 100% transmission when there is zero thickness and 50% transmission at 1 HVL thickness. A straight line is drawn through these points, and the graph is complete. The use of such a graph is shown in the following examples.

))))) EXAMPLE

A beam containing only 100 keV photons has an HVL of 0.15 mm of copper (Cu). What thickness of copper would be needed to reduce this beams intensity from 500 mR to 150 mR?

First determine the percent transmission desired:

$$\% \text{ Transmission} = \frac{150 \text{ mR}}{500 \text{ mR}} \times 100\%$$
$$= 30\%$$

From Figure 8–14, 30% transmission corresponds to approximately 1.74 HVLs. Therefore

Thickness of Cu needed = 1.74 HVLs
$$= (1.74 \text{ HVLs}) \left(\frac{0.15 \text{ mm Cu}}{HVL} \right)$$
$$\approx 0.26 \text{ mm Cu}$$

))))) EXAMPLE

How many HVLs are needed to attenuate 90% of a photon beam?

To attenuate 90% or transmit 10% (recall that attenuation + transmission must equal 100%). Transmission of 10% corresponds on the graph (Fig. 8–14) to approximately 3.32 HVLs.

Therefore approximately 3.32 HVLs are needed to attenuate 90% (or transmit 10%) of the incident beam.

Up to this time only monoenergetic radiation has been considered. Recall, however, that an x-ray beam consists of photons ranging in energy from zero to some maximum energy determined by the kVp setting. The x-ray beam produced by a standard x-ray tube is therefore *polyenergetic*. As a result, a deviation from graphs previously plotted can be expected. Figure 8–15 shows a semilog plot of transmitted intensity versus absorber thickness (mm of aluminum) for a 90-kVp x-ray beam. Note that rather than obtaining a straight line, there is a slight turn upward at the upper left side of this graph. This is because lower-energy photons within the beam have been filtered out in the first several thicknesses of absorber, thus increasing the average energy of the beam. As a result, the first and second HVLs determined from the graphic data are not the same. In Figure 8–15, halving the initial intensity of 259 mR to 129.5 mR, indicates a first HVL of approximately 3.5 mm of aluminum. Halving the second intensity value to obtain $1/2(129.5 \text{ mr}) \approx 64.75 \text{ mR}$, the second HVL is (8 mm − 3.5 mm) = 4.5 mm of aluminum. The fact that a somewhat larger second HVL is obtained is not unusual, since the beam has now been "hardened" (i.e., its average energy has been raised) after its passage through the first HVL. The HVL is commonly used to describe an x-ray beam's penetrating ability—the thicker the HVL, the more penetrating the beam. This application is discussed again in Chapter 17 when a homogeneity coefficient, defined as

$$\text{Homogeneity coefficient } (HC) = \frac{\text{first } HVL}{\text{second } HVL}$$

is used to describe the energy characteristics of an x-ray beam. The closer the HC is to 1.0, the closer is the beam to being monoenergetic.

Not only is use of the HVL important in describing beam penetrating power and x-ray beam characteristics, but as seen earlier, it is also important in radiation protection in reducing radiation intensities to acceptable levels. HVLs can be measured in units of thickness of aluminum, copper, lead, tissue or any other material. In the range of diagnostic energies used in radiography references state

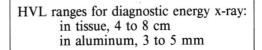

HVL ranges for diagnostic energy x-ray:
  in tissue, 4 to 8 cm
  in aluminum, 3 to 5 mm

Chapter Summary/ Important Concepts

Unlike charged particle radiation, which loses its energy through electrical interactions, photons are uncharged and tend to lose their energy by direct interaction with shell electrons, atomic nuclei, or atoms as a whole

When photons pass into matter they may be transmitted or totally or partially absorbed. Although exactly how any one specific photon will interact with matter cannot be predicted, the probability that it will interact in a specific manner can be described. The manner in which a photon interacts with matter strongly depends on the energy of the incident photon.

Photon radiation may interact with matter by the following methods:

a. Classical scattering. A low-energy photon is momentarily absorbed by a shell electron or an atom and is then re-emitted with a change in its direction but no change in energy
b. Photoelectric absorption. A photon is completely absorbed by an inner-shell electron, resulting in the ejection of the shell electron
c. Compton (incoherent) scattering. The incident photon interacts with an outer-shell electron; this results in the ejection of the shell electron and a lower-energy, scattered photon
d. Pair production. High–energy (>1.022 MeV) photon interaction in which the incident photon interacts with the electromagnetic field of an atomic nucleus and is converted into an electron-positron pair
e. Triplet production. A high-energy (>2.04 MeV) photon interacts with a shell electron to eject the shell electron and produces an electron-positron pair
f. Photodisintegration. Absorption of a high-energy (>7 MeV) incident photon by an atomic nucleus, resulting in the ejection of a nuclear particle

In the diagnostic-energy range, the two most important methods of interaction in tissue are photoelectric absorption and Compton scattering. Compton scattering is the primary mode of interaction of diagnostic x-rays in tissue

Since the probability of a photoelectric absorption event is strongly dependent on the Z number of the absorber, materials with relatively high Z numbers such as barium ($Z = 56$) and iodine ($Z = 53$) are used in radiography as contrast agents to enhance image contrast

Scatter radiation does not add any diagnostically useful information to the radiographic image, rather, it contributes only to film fog. In the diagnostic-energy range, the greatest portion of scatter radiation tends to be in the forward direction (i.e., toward the film). As the energy of the incident photons increases, the scatter is more energetic and has a greater chance of reaching the film. For a given energy photon, backscatter (i.e., photons scattered through a 180° angle) represents the lowest energy scattered radiation

The different shades of gray seen on a radiographic image are a result of the varying degrees of interaction and types of radiation interaction that occur as the x-ray beam passes through body tissues, a process referred to as differential absorption

Attenuation refers to the removal of photons from an x-ray beam as it passes through matter. All of the individual methods of photon interaction (i.e., photoelectric, scattering, and so forth) are the processes by which photons are removed from a beam as it passes through matter. Attenuation varies as a negative exponential

A concept useful for describing the attenuation process is the half-value layer (HVL), which is the thickness of material that transmits only 50% of an incident radiation beam; this value varies with the material and energy of the incident radiation

Important Terminology

Annihilation Radiation. The two 511-keV photons (emitted in opposite directions) produced when a positron encounters an electron
Attenuation. The process of removal of photons from an x-ray beam as it passes through an absorber; attenuation result from photoelectric absorption, Compton scattering, pair or triplet production, or photodisintegration processes; the last three of these are high-energy photon interactions and do not occur in diagnostic radiology
Backscatter. Photon radiation that has been scattered through a 180° angle; for a given incident photon energy, this is the lowest-energy scatter radiation
Classical (Coherent) Scattering. Low–energy photon interaction in matter in which the incident photon is momentarily absorbed by a shell electron or the atom as a whole then re-emitted with no change in its energy but a change in direction of motion
Compton Scattering Interaction. Medium–energy photon interaction in matter in which the incident photon ejects an outer-shell electron, resulting in only partial absorption of the incident photon; in addition to the Compton-scattered electron, a lower-energy, scattered photon is also produced; also called incoherent scattering

Contrast Agent. Substance such as barium, iodine, or air introduced into the body to improve radiographic image contrast

Differential Absorption. Process by which a quality radiographic image is produced as a result of photons in an x-ray beam interacting in various ways (i.e., transmission, absorption, or scatter) to varying degrees as they pass into different tissues

Electron-Positron Pair. Electron and positron created when 1.022 MeV of energy is converted into matter in a pair-production event

Half-Value Layer (HVL). Thickness of material required to transmit only 50% of an incident radiation beam; it varies with the material and the energy of the incident photons

Ion Pairs. What remains after an atom undergoes an ionizing event, usually an ejected electron and a positive ion

Monochromatic. Literally, one color; it refers to having a single wavelength or single energy

Monoenergetic. Having a single energy

Pair-Production Event. A high–energy ($E_i > 1.022$ MeV) photon interaction with matter in which the incident photon interacts with the electromagnetic field of an atomic nucleus; the incident photon disappears, and in its place appears an electron-positron pair

Photodisintegration. High–energy photon (>7 MeV) interaction in matter in which the incident photon is absorbed by an atomic nucleus, causing the ejection of a nuclear particle

Photoelectric Interaction. Photon interaction in matter in which the incident photon is completely absorbed by an inner-shell electron, resulting in the ejection of the shell electron, followed by characteristic x-ray emission

Photoelectron. Ejected shell electron resulting from a photoelectric interaction in matter

Polyenergetic. Having many energies

Recoil (Compton-scattered) Electron. Outer-shell electron ejected during a Compton scattering event

Scattered Radiation (Scatter). Lower–energy photon radiation that has been redirected as a result of a Compton scattering event

Secondary Radiation. Radiation emitted from an atom after it has absorbed a photon; generally thought to include characteristic x-rays, photoelectrons, recoil electrons, positron-electron pairs, and annihilation radiation; this term may also include scatter radiation

Transmission. Portion of an x-ray beam that passes through an absorber; when the absorber is the patient's body, it is called exit radiation

Triplet Production. High–energy (>2.04 MeV) photon interaction in matter in which the incident photon interacts with the electromagnetic field of a shell electron; the photon is converted into an electron-positron pair, and a shell electron is ejected

Bibliography

Anderson, D.W. Absorption of Ionizing Radiation. Baltimore: University Park Press, 1984.

Bushong, S.C. Radiologic Science for Technologists—Physics, Biology and Protection, 4th ed. St. Louis: C.V. Mosby, 1988.

Curry, T.S. III; Dowdey, J.E.; Murry, R.C. Jr. Christensen's Physics of Diagnostic Radiology, 4th ed. Philadelphia, Lea & Febiger, 1990.

Dendy, P.P.; Heaton, B. Physics for Radiologists. Chicago: Blackwell/Year Book Medical Publishers, 1987.

Hendee, W.R. Medical Radiation Physics, 2nd ed. Chicago: Year Book Medical Publishers, 1979.

Hendee, W.R. Radioactive Isotopes in Biological Research. New York: John Wiley & Sons, 1973.

Khan, F.M. The Physics of Radiation Therapy. Baltimore: Williams & Wilkins, 1984.

Lapp, R.E.; Andrews, H.L. Nuclear Radiation Physics, 4th ed. Englewood Cliffs, NJ: Prentice-Hall, 1972.

Meredith, W.J.; Massey, J.B. Fundamental Physics of Radiology, 3rd ed. Chicago: Year Book Medical Publishers, 1977.

Selman, J. The Fundamentals of X-ray and Radium Physics, 7th ed. Springfield, IL: Charles C Thomas, 1985.

Sprawls, P. Principles of Radiography for Technologists. Rockville, MD: Aspen Publishers, 1990.

Sprawls, P. The Physical Principles of Diagnostic Radiology. Baltimore: University Park Press, 1977.

Ridgway, A.; Thumm, W. The Physics of Medical Radiography. Reading, MA: Addison-Wesley, 1968.

Stanton, R.; Stinson, D. An Introduction to Radiation Oncology Physics. Madison: Medical Physics Publishing, 1992.

Webb, S. The Physics of Medical Imaging. New York: Adam Hilger, 1988.

Review Questions

1. Why do photons interact differently with matter from alpha or beta particles?
2. List five ways that photons can interact with matter.
3. List the modes of photon interaction with matter resulting in an ionization event.
4. Indicate the manner in which diagnostic x-rays can interact with body tissues.
5. Of the five ways photons interact in matter, which ones result in complete absorption of the incident photon?
6. Which of the five photon interactions in matter would be considered high–energy (> 1 MeV) photon interactions?
7. How does the wavelength and frequency of the scattered photon compare with that of the incident photon in a Compton scattering event?
8. Indicate two factors that determine the energy of scatter radiation resulting from a Compton scattering event.
9. At what angle in a Compton scattering event
   a. is maximum energy transferred from the incident photon to the recoil electron?
   b. does the scattered photon have the least energy?
10. Why is scatter radiation of concern from a radiation safety perspective?
11. Of the high–energy photon interactions in matter, which
    a. results in an ionization event?
    b. requires that the incident photon have a minimum energy of 1.022 MeV?
    c. causes the target nucleus to emit a nuclear particle?
    d. requires the incident photon to have a minimum energy of 2.04 MeV?
12. For diagnostic-energy x-rays, specify the range of values for the HVL in tissue and aluminum.
13. Indicate two factors that influence the numerical value of the HVL for a photon beam.
14. What percentage of an incident photon beam is
    a. attenuated by HVL thicknesses?
    b. transmitted by 2 HVL thicknesses?
15. What is the most common method of diagnostic x-ray interaction
    a. in soft tissue?   c. in bone?
    b. with contrast agents?

Exercises

1. A 50-keV photon travels into a piece of lead (Pb) shielding. Can it interact with a K-shell electron of a Pb atom whose binding energy is 88 keV? Why or why not?
2. A 90-keV x-ray photon interacts with the K-shell electron of a Pb atom (binding energy = 88 keV).

What is the kinetic energy of the ejected photo-electron?

3. An x-ray photon having an incident energy of 70 keV interacts with an outer-shell electron in a Compton scattering event. If the binding energy of the shell electron is considered negligible and the recoil electron acquires 25 keV of kinetic energy, what is the energy of the Compton-scattered photon?
4. An incident x-ray photon has an energy of 85 keV and interacts with an outer-shell electron whose binding energy is 800 eV. If the photon is scattered through a 90° angle, determine the energy of the Compton-scattered photon and the kinetic energy of the recoil electron.
5. Calculate the energy of the scattered photon in each of the following cases:
   a. incident photon energy = 60 keV, scattering angle = 25°
   b. incident photon energy = 90 keV, scattering angle = 25°
   c. incident photon energy = 120 keV, scattering angle = 25°
   d. incident photon energy = 160 keV, scattering angle = 25°

   What can be said about the energy of the scattered radiation as incident photon energy increases? Since in each of the above cases, scatter is in the "forward" direction, how does the scatter affect the radiographic image?
6. A 2.5-MeV photon interacts in a lead sheet by a pair-production event. If the electron carries off 60% of the available energy, determine the kinetic energy of the electron and the positron.
7. Explain the difference between pair and triplet production in terms of where each event is initiated.
8. A monoenergetic photon beam has an HVL in lead of 1.3 mm. If the incident beam with no absorber has an intensity of 120 mR, determine the intensity after it passes through 3.5 mm of lead.
9. A monoenergetic photon beam has an intensity of 800 mR when there is no absorber in the beam. Beam intensity drops to 620 mR when it passes through 0.8 mm of aluminum (Al). What is the HVL of this photon beam in Al?
10. The HVL in lead (Pb) is 2.2 mm for a monoenergetic photon beam. What thickness of Pb is required to reduce the incident beam intensity from 950 mR to 2 mR?
11. Use a 2-cycle semilog graph as shown in Figure 8–14 (Transmission vs Absorber Thickness in HVLs) to answer the following:
    a. What percentage of an incident beam is transmitted by 2.5 HVLs?
    b. What percentage of an incident photon beam is attenuated by 3.8 HVLs?
    c. If the HVL of an incident photon beam is 2.4 cm of aluminum (Al), what thickness of Al would be needed to attenuate 30% of the incident beam?
    d. If the HVL of an incident beam is 0.6 mm of

lead (Pb), how much Pb is needed to transmit 65% of the incident beam?

e. If the HVL of an incident photon beam is 0.15 mm Pb, what thickness of Pb is needed to reduce the incident beam from 1200 mR to 20 mR?

12. Given the following attenuation data using a 100-kVp x-ray beam: 100 kVp, 200 mA, 0.2 sec

Thickness (mm Al)	Intensity (mR)
0	253
1	204
2	164
3	128
4	112
5	95
6	83
7	72

a. Plot this data on semilog graph paper to obtain a transmission vs absorber thickness graph.

b. Use your graph to obtain first and second HVLs for this beam.

c. From your results, calculate the homogeneity coefficient (HC). What can be said about the beam based on your results?

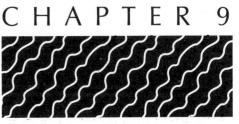

CHAPTER 9

Factors Affecting the X-ray Spectrum

Michael A. Thompson, M.S.

Chapter Objectives

On completion of this chapter, you should be able to

- Explain what is meant by the x-ray emission spectrum.
- Describe the two components of the x-ray spectrum.
- Explain the origin of the two components of the x-ray spectrum.
- Indicate how the graphic representation of the x-ray spectrum (continuous and discrete) changes when
  - *the energies of the emitted x-rays change*
  - *the number of x-rays emitted changes*
- Describe how the graphic representation of the x-ray emission spectrum, both continuous and discrete, changes with changes in
  - *kVp*
  - *mA*
  - *mAs*
  - *filtration*
  - *Z number of the target*
  - *voltage waveform used (i.e., 1φ or 3φ)*
  - *distance from the x-ray source*

THE X-RAY SPECTRUM

X-rays are produced by two distinct processes when electrons are accelerated into the target of the x-ray tube:

1. X-rays are produced when fast-moving electrons are rapidly decelerated in and around target atoms; the x-rays thus created are referred to as *bremsstrahlung* (i.e., braking radiation).
2. X-rays are also generated when fast-moving electrons eject inner-shell electrons from target atoms; this results in the production of *characteristic x-rays* having energies that are characteristic of the target material.

These processes of x-ray production result when electrons emitted from the filament are accelerated to high velocities by the voltage applied across the tube electrodes. For a given kVp, typical electron velocities can be determined as indicated:

))))) EXAMPLE

Determine the maximum velocity of an electron accelerated through a potential difference of 90 kVp.
Given

$$\text{Electron mass} = m_e \cong 9.1 \times 10^{-31} \text{ kg}$$

$$1 \text{ eV} = 1.6 \times 10^{-19} \text{ J}$$

An electron accelerated through a potential difference of 90 kVp has a maximum kinetic energy of 90 keV by definition of the electron volt. The 90 keV must be first converted to joules (J), the SI unit of energy. Then, electron velocity can be determined from the kinetic energy formula

$$KE = \frac{1}{2} mv^2$$

$$90 \; keV \times \frac{1.6 \times 10^{-16} \; J}{keV} = \frac{1}{2} \, m_e v^2$$

$$1.44 \times 10^{-14} \; J = \frac{1}{2} (9.1 \times 10^{-31} \; kg) \, v^2$$

$$1.44 \times 10^{-14} \; J = (4.55 \times 10^{-31} \; kg) \, v^2$$

$$v = \sqrt{1.44 \times 10^{-14} \; J/(4.55 \times 10^{-31} \; kg)}$$

$$v \cong \sqrt{3.16 \times 10^{16} \; m^2/sec^2}$$

$$v = 1.78 \times 10^8 \; m/sec \; (\sim 110,000 \; miles/sec)$$

Recall that light travels at a speed of 3×10^8 m/sec in vacuum; therefore this velocity corresponds to

$$\frac{1.79 \times 10^8 \; m/sec}{3 \times 10^8 \; m/sec} \times 100\%$$

or 59% of the speed of light.

The high velocities of these electrons attest to the large amount of kinetic energy they possess as they approach the anode target. As these fast-moving electrons enter the target, the interactions that give rise to bremsstrahlung and characteristic x-rays convert their kinetic energy into heat and x-rays.

The combination of bremsstrahlung and characteristic x-rays together forms what is known as the x-ray emission spectrum. Recall that the term *spectrum* refers to a representation of the range of numerical values that can be observed. An example is the visible spectrum of light. When we refer to the visible spectrum we mean only those photons whose wavelengths are between 4000 Å and 7000 Å. These wavelengths correspond to the colors that are observed when white light is passed through a prism. In the case of the x-ray emission spectrum graphical representations are developed that indicate not only the range of x-ray energies emitted from the tube as technical factors are changed but also relative number of these x-rays that have specific energies.

Bremsstrahlung: The Continuous Spectrum

As fast-moving electrons enter the target, they may interact with either orbital electrons or nuclei of the target atoms. Several possible types of interaction that result in the loss of their original kinetic energy can occur:

- Incident electrons may undergo numerous collisions with the orbital electrons of target atoms, resulting

in the release of excitation radiation; this excitation radiation may be in the form of visible light or, more commonly, in the form of heat (recall that approximately slightly more than 99% of the energy of incident electrons is converted into heat on interaction with the target)
- An incident electron may directly interact with only one target atom nucleus, resulting in the emission of an x-ray photon having the same energy as the incident electron
- An incident electron may lose various amounts of its kinetic energy as it is deflected in multiple interactions with nuclei of target atoms; these energy losses are emitted in the form of x-ray photons of various energies
- An incident electron may cause the ejection of an inner-shell target atom electron resulting in the emission of characteristic x-rays

Each of these forms of interaction is illustrated in Figure 9–1. The first three of the above-described interactions are most common. The x-rays produced when the incident electrons interact directly with a target atom nucleus or when they are deflected are referred to as bremsstrahlung (German for *braking radiation*).

Typically, an incoming electron interacts with many target atoms before finally giving up all of its kinetic energy. This results in a spectrum of energies for the x-rays produced in this manner. On those occasions when an incoming electron imparts all of its energy to a target atom nucleus on its first and only interaction with the target, an x-ray with the same energy as the incoming electron is emitted. This maximum energy photon has an energy dependent on the kVp across the tube electrodes. That is,

$$E_{max} \, (keV) = V_{max} \, (kVp) \tag{1}$$

This indicates that the energy of the maximum energy photon expressed in keV is equivalent to the numerical value of the peak voltage across the tube electrodes. (Note: This relationship in no way equates units of energy with units of voltage.) Recall that for photons

$$\lambda(\text{Å}) = \frac{12.4}{E \, (keV)} \tag{2}$$

then utilize equation (1) in equation (2), to obtain the relationship for the minimum wavelength (λ_{min}):

$$\lambda_{min} \, (\text{Å}) = \frac{12.4}{E_{max} \, (keV)} = \frac{12.4}{V_{max} \, (kVp)} \tag{3}$$

)))))) EXAMPLE

Determine the maximum energy and the minimum wavelength of the x-ray photons produced by bremsstrahlung when the maximum applied voltage is 80 kVp.

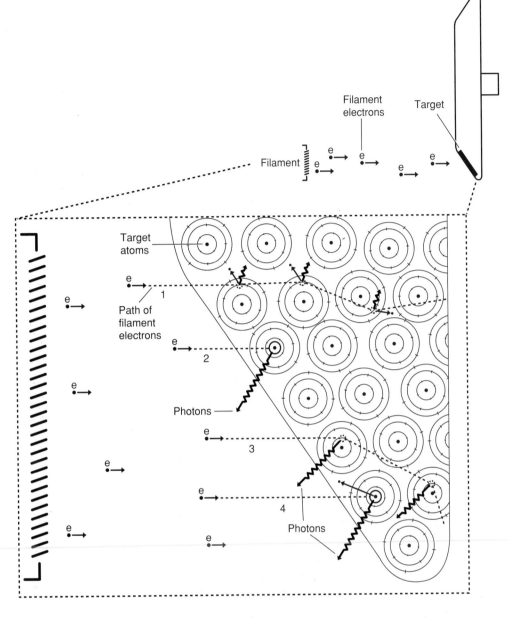

FIGURE 9–1. Types of target interactions that generate x-rays. These include (1) multiple target interactions, (2) direct interactions with target atom nuclei, (3) multiple deflections by target atom nuclei, and (4) ejection of inner-shell target atom electrons.

The maximum energy photons have a maximum energy given by

$$E_{max} = 80 \text{ keV}$$

The minimum wavelength of these photons is

$$\lambda_{min} = \frac{12.4}{80 \text{ keV}} = 0.155 \text{ Å}$$

Note. All other photons produced by bremsstrahlung at this kVp will have lower energies and longer wavelengths.

Bremsstrahlung x-rays therefore range in energy from some E_{max} dependent on the kVp to approximately zero. It should be pointed out that the minimum photon energy of the spectrum is not zero if the

emergent or useful beam that actually strikes the patient is considered. In this case, the very low end of the bremsstrahlung spectrum is absorbed by the glass envelope and added filtration (the effect of filtration on the x-ray spectrum is discussed in greater detail later in this chapter). Thus x-rays produced in this manner form the *continuous* portion of the x-ray *spectrum*. Here, the term *continuous* implies that x-rays produced as bremsstrahlung are emitted with energies ranging uninterruptedly from approximately zero to some E_{max}. This portion of the spectrum is illustrated graphically in Figure 9–2. Since a typical x-ray beam consists primarily of bremsstrahlung radiation, the beam can be described as being *polyenergetic* (i.e., consisting of many energies) or *polychromatic* (i.e., consisting of many wavelengths).

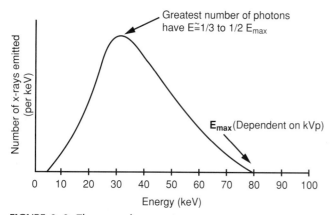

FIGURE 9–2. The general or continuous x-ray emission spectrum produced by bremsstrahlung. The spectrum shown assumes some inherent filtration.

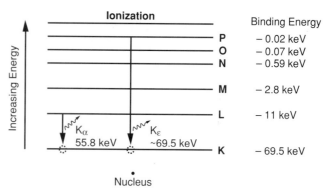

FIGURE 9–3. Binding energies for shell electrons of tungsten (W). Two K-characteristic x-rays are indicated which result from electronic transitions.

Characteristic X-rays: The Discrete Spectrum

If the fast-moving incident electron has sufficient energy, it can cause the ejection of an inner-shell electron of the target atom. Recall that when an inner-shell electron is ejected from an atom, electrons in higher-energy orbitals fall to fill in the vacancy followed by the emission of characteristic x-rays. These x-rays are emitted with specific energies characteristic of the element of which the target is made. Characteristic x-rays are emitted having specific (or discrete) energies, not with a continuous band of energies as

with bremsstrahlung production. Characteristic x-rays form the *discrete spectrum.*

The energy of the characteristic x-ray is the difference in the binding energies of the two shells between which the electron moves. Figure 9–3 indicates binding energies for tungsten. In order to eject a K-shell electron from tungsten, an incoming electron must have an energy of at least approximately 70 keV. Incoming electrons need to have at least 11 keV to eject an L-shell electron. If an incoming electron has sufficient energy to eject a K-shell electron and the vacancy is filled by an electron in the L shell, a characteristic x-ray with 58.5 keV of energy [i.e., $E_L - E_K = -11$ keV $- (-69.5$ keV$) = -11$ keV $+ 69.5$ keV] will be emitted. This characteristic x-ray is designated as a K_α

Table 9–1: POSSIBLE CHARACTERISTIC X-RAYS EMITTED FROM A TUNGSTEN TARGET

Characteristic X-ray Designation	Shell Transition From Which It Originates	Binding Energy Difference	X-Ray Energy
K–x-rays:			
K_α	L $\longrightarrow$ K	69.5 keV − 11 keV	~ 58.5 keV
K_β	M $\longrightarrow$ K	69.5 keV − 2.8 keV	~ 66.7 keV
K_γ	N $\longrightarrow$ K	69.5 keV − 0.59 keV	~ 68.9 keV
			E_{eff}: **~69 keV**
L–x-rays:			
L_α	M $\longrightarrow$ L	11 keV − 2.8 keV	~ 8.2 keV
L_β	N $\longrightarrow$ L	11 keV − 0.59 keV	~ 10.4 keV
L_γ	O $\longrightarrow$ L	11 keV − 0.07 keV	~ 10.9 keV
			E_{eff}: **~12 keV**
M–x-rays:			
M_α	N $\longrightarrow$ M	2.8 keV − 0.59 keV	~ 2.2 keV
M_β	O $\longrightarrow$ M	2.8 keV − 0.07 keV	~ 2.7 keV
M_γ	P $\longrightarrow$ M	2.8 keV − 0.02 keV	~ 2.8 keV
			E_{eff}: **~2 keV**
N–x-rays:			
N_α	O $\longrightarrow$ N	0.59 keV − 0.07 keV	~ 0.52 keV
N_β	P $\longrightarrow$ N	0.59 keV − 0.02 keV	~ 0.57 keV
			E_{eff}: **~0.6 keV**

x-ray (Table 9–1). This table summarizes characteristic x-rays that could possibly be produced when a tungsten target is used. It is important to remember that the energies of the x-rays produced by this method are characteristic of the material of which the target is made.

Also shown in Table 9–1 are the effective energies (E_{eff}) of the K, L, M, and N characteristic x-rays of tungsten. It should be noted that x-rays produced by electronic transitions to the L, M, and N shells result in low-energy x-rays that are not useful in diagnostic radiography because of their low penetrating ability. Most of these low-energy x-rays are absorbed by the glass envelope or added filtration. However, the K–characteristic x-rays, with an effective energy of approximately 70 keV, have sufficient energy to be useful to radiography.

The relative number of characteristic x-rays appearing in the spectrum of x-rays produced by the tube depends on the kVp used (Table 9–2). Typically, within the voltage range of approximately 80 to 150 kVp, characteristic x-rays may represent from 10% to as much as 28% of the useful beam.

When characteristic x-rays are included as part of the spectrum in the useful beam, there is an increase in the number of x-rays at approximately 70 keV. At this energy, a "spike," or line, is superimposed on the bremsstrahlung spectrum as shown in Figure 9–4. This spike indicates that an increased number of x-rays is produced at this specific energy. Characteristic x-rays form the discrete portion of the x-ray spectrum, because characteristic x-rays are produced at specific energies as opposed to the continuous spectrum produced by bremsstrahlung. Although characteristic x-rays do not constitute a major portion of the x-ray spectrum in conventional x-ray units, mammography units, which use molybdenum targets and typically operate between 25 kVp and 50 kVp, produce an x-ray spectrum that predominately consists of characteristic x-rays. Molybdenum produces K–characteristic x-rays having an effective energy of about 18 keV.

Bremsstrahlung production is extremely inefficient at such low operating voltages, and the low-energy characteristic x-rays become a dominant portion of this special x-ray spectrum.

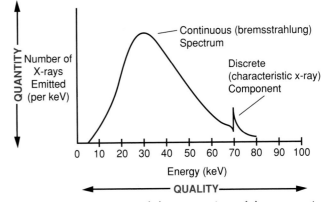

FIGURE 9–4. Continuous and discrete portions of the x-ray emission spectrum.

QUALITY AND QUANTITY

The terms *quality* and *quantity* are terms used to describe x-ray beam characteristics. *Quality* is the term used to describe the overall energy of the beam. Recall that an x-ray beam is polyenergetic; therefore any factors that increase or decrease the average energy of the photons in the beam affect x-ray beam quality. Quality is directly affected by

● Changes in kVp
● Changes in the material (i.e., Z number) of the target
● Changes in filtration
● The type of voltage waveform used (i.e., 1ϕ, 3ϕ, or high-frequency)

Quantity is a term used to describe the number of x-ray photons in the beam. It should be noted that although the number of photons in an x-ray beam is related to beam intensity, quantity and intensity are not the same thing. Recall from previous chapters that

$$\text{Intensity} = \frac{\text{energy}}{\text{area} - \text{time}}$$

$$= \text{number of photons} \times \left(\frac{\text{energy/photon}}{\text{area} - \text{time}}\right)$$

The equation indicates that as the number of photons increases, so does the beam intensity. However, another important factor here is the energy of each photon (i.e., energy/photon). Thus a beam consisting of 100-keV photons has a greater intensity than a beam consisting of the same number of 60-keV photons.

By definition any factors that affect the number of x-ray photons in the beam influence x-ray beam quantity. Quantity is affected by

● Changes in mA (i.e., tube current)
● Changes in filtration
● Changes in the material (i.e., Z number) of which the target is made
● Changes in kVp

Table 9–2: RELATIVE PERCENTAGE COMPOSITION OF X-RAY BEAM PRODUCED WITH TUNGSTEN TARGET AT VARIOUS kVp

kVp	Useful Beam Composition
≤ 70 kVp	~ 100% bremsstrahlung
80 kVp	~ 10% K–characteristic x-rays ~ 90% bremsstrahlung
150 kVp	~ 28% K–characteristic x-rays ~ 72% bremsstrahlung
> 300 kVp	~ 100% bremsstrahlung

- The type of voltage waveform used (i.e., 1ϕ, 3ϕ, or high-frequency)
- Changes in distance from the tube (FFD or SID)

Knowledge of these factors is important to the radiographer, because beams of adequate energy and a sufficient number of photons are needed for the production of quality radiographs. Each of these factors is considered in somewhat greater detail in terms of its influence on each component (i.e., bremsstrahlung and characteristic x-rays) of the x-ray spectrum.

INTERPRETING CHANGES IN THE X-RAY SPECTRUM

Discussion of the previously listed factors in terms of their effects on x-ray quality and quantity also includes how these changes affect the height (amplitude) and the position along the energy axis of each component of the spectrum. In Figure 9–4, only two important concepts need to be noted:

1. Change in the height or amplitude of either component indicates a change in the number of x-rays (i.e., quantity) having a specific energy
2. Change in the position of the peaks of either component along the horizontal (energy) axis represents a change in the energy (i.e., quality) of the x-ray photons within the beam

It is also important to remember that x-rays emitted from the x-ray tube are polyenergetic, consisting of many energies, ranging from approximately zero (for an unfiltered beam) to some maximum value dependent on the kVp. Any factor that changes the number of photons of a specific energy within the beam affects the overall average energy of the beam.

EFFECT OF CHANGES IN kVp

Recall that changes in kVp allow the radiographer to vary the energy of the incoming electrons prior to striking the target. The chosen kVp determines the maximum energy of the x-ray photons in the bremsstrahlung spectrum. Therefore as kVp increases, more higher-energy photons are included in the beam, raising the average energy of the beam.

In addition to increasing the average energy of the beam, increases in kVp increase the speed with which incoming electrons strike the target. This increases the chances of more incoming electrons interacting with multiple target atoms before losing their kinetic energy within the target plate. Each time an incoming electron undergoes a deceleration about a target atom nucleus, bremsstrahlung photons are produced. This results in an increase in the overall number of brems-

strahlung x-ray photons in the beam. Note that this enhancement of the number of photons produced at higher kVps results in more high-energy photons than low-energy photons being produced.

An increase in kVp also means more ejections of inner-shell electrons from target atoms. This results from the fact that more incoming electrons have sufficient energy to overcome inner-shell binding energies. This increases the number of characteristic x-rays in the beam but does not affect their energy. These effects are graphically demonstrated in Figure 9–5.

Summary of Effects of kVp Changes
- In the bremsstrahlung spectrum shifts in energy (quality) and changes in amplitude (quantity) occur; typically, more high-energy photons are produced as kVp is increased
- In the characteristic x-ray portion of the x-ray spectrum changes result in amplitude (quantity) but not in energy shifts (quality)

EFFECTS OF CHANGES IN mA

For a particular radiographic exposure, as the tube current (mA) increases, the number of incoming electrons striking the target also becomes greater. Recall that mA stands for milliampere, a unit of electric current. This unit indicates the amount of charge, or number of electrons moving past a given point per second. When the mA changes, the number of electrons striking the target and thus the number of x-ray photons produced in both the bremsstrahlung and characteristic x-ray portions of the x-ray spectrum is also altered. This direct relationship between mA and the number of photons produced directly affects the amplitude of the resulting x-ray emission spectrum. For example, doubling the tube mA doubles the number of x-ray photons produced and vice versa. Changes

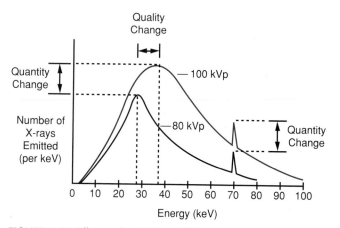

FIGURE 9–5. Effects of variation of kVp on the x-ray emission spectrum.

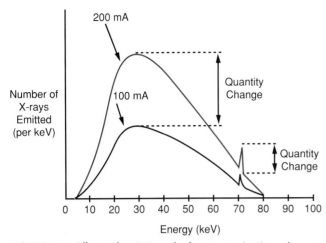

FIGURE 9–6. Effects of variation of tube current (mA) on the x-ray emission spectrum.

in mA produce no energy shifts in either portion of the spectrum as illustrated in Figure 9–6.

Summary of Effects of Changes in mA:
- In the bremsstrahlung spectrum, changes occur in amplitude (quantity) but not in energy
- In the characteristic x-ray portion of the spectrum, changes occur in amplitude (quantity) but not in energy (quality)

EFFECTS OF CHANGES IN TARGET MATERIALS

Recall that bremsstrahlung radiation is produced when fast-moving charged particles such as electrons undergo rapid decelerations on impact with an appropriate target. Typically, as the Z number of the target material is raised, the amount of bremsstrahlung radiation produced is increased. As illustrated in Figure 9–7, although the effect of using a higher Z number target is more apparent on the high-energy side of the bremsstrahlung peak, in many ways the spectra are the same. Note that the minimum and maximum energies are the same and that the greatest number of x-rays produced—that is, the peak of the bremsstrahlung spectrum—occurs at the same position on the energy axis. Therefore a change in the quantity but not the quality of the bremsstrahlung portion of the x-ray spectrum can be observed. This statement assumes that the same tube voltage (kVp) is applied and only the Z number of the target is changed.

The most obvious consequence of a change in the Z number of the target is the shift occurring in the discrete portion of the x-ray spectrum. As the Z number of the target becomes larger so do the binding energies of shell electrons. This increase in electronic binding energies results in higher-energy characteristic x-rays.

Low–Z number target materials, such as molybdenum (Z = 42), tend to produce not only characteristic x-rays with lower energy but also lower quantities of bremsstrahlung x-rays. Low-energy characteristic x-rays of molybdenum (K_α = 17.5 keV and K_β = 19.6 keV) are most useful in soft tissue imaging such as mammography.

Summary of Effects of Changes in Z Number of Target Material
- In the bremsstrahlung spectrum, changes occur in amplitude (quantity) but not in energy
- In the characteristic x-ray portion of the spectrum, only shifts in energy (quality) take place

---

Also note that the discrete energy characteristic x-rays are always added to the continuous bremsstrahlung spectrum. Since there is an overall increase in bremsstrahlung x-ray production with the use of high Z number targets, the number of these higher-energy x-rays, corresponding to the energy of the emitted characteristic x-rays, is increased. Thus when comparing the two spectra shown in Figure 9–7, do not conclude that there is also a change in quantity in the discrete portion of the spectrum. The apparent difference in amplitude results from change in amplitude of the bremsstrahlung portion of the spectrum.

EFFECTS OF CHANGES IN mAs

Recall that mAs refers to the product of tube current (measured in mA) and exposure time (measured in seconds). From the definition of the ampere, it is seen that the product of amperes and seconds (sec) is

$$\text{Amperes} \times \text{seconds} = \frac{\text{coulombs}}{\text{sec}} \times \text{sec}$$
$$= \text{coulombs}$$

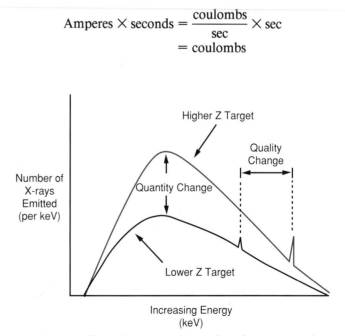
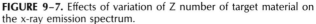

FIGURE 9–7. Effects of variation of Z number of target material on the x-ray emission spectrum.

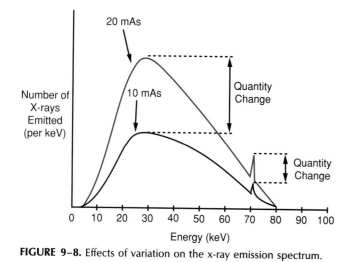

FIGURE 9-8. Effects of variation on the x-ray emission spectrum.

Here, coulombs (C) refers to the charge carried by individual electrons as they move toward the target plate. The exact number of electrons flowing between the tube electrodes can be determined by dividing the total charge in coulombs by the charge on an individual electron. Therefore as mAs is increased, the number of electrons striking the target increases. The more electrons that strike the target, the more x-rays are produced in both the continuous and discrete portions of the x-ray spectrum (Fig. 9-8). Changes in mAs do not affect the quality of either component of the x-ray spectrum.

Summary of Effects of Changes in mAs
- In the bremsstrahlung portion of the x-ray spectrum, changes can be seen in amplitude (quantity) but not in energy (quality)
- In the characteristic portion of the x-ray spectrum, shifts occur in amplitude (quantity) but not in energy (quality)

EFFECTS OF CHANGES IN ADDED FILTRATION

Filtration refers to the process by which photons in a polyenergetic beam are selectively removed by materials placed in the path of the emerging x-ray beam. These materials may be part of the equipment *(inherent filtration),* such as the glass envelope of the tube, the insulating oil surrounding the tube, or the tube housing window.

Of the equipment material listed, the glass envelope provides the greatest amount of filtration because of its higher atomic number. Inherent filtration in most tubes is approximately the same as a 1-mm *aluminum equivalent* (Al eq)—that is, it provides the same amount of filtration as a 1-mm thickness of alumi-

num. Beryllium (Z = 4) windows are used in x-ray tubes when it is not desirable to completely filter out low-energy photons. Such a case is mammography, in which lower-energy photons are needed to provide soft tissue contrast (i.e., maximum differential absorption).

Added filtration consists of additional filters placed in the path of the emerging beam to absorb low-energy photons. These low-energy photons contribute only radiation dose to the patient. The National Council of Radiation Protection and Measurements has made specific recommendations (NCRP Report #102), as indicated, for the minimum total filtration for diagnostic x-ray units:

Tube Potential	Required Minimum Filtration
< 50 kVp	0.5 mm Al (or 0.03 mm Mo for molybdenum target tubes)
50–70 kVp	1.5 mm Al
>70 kVp	2.5 mm Al

Specific requirements for diagnostic x-ray units in the United States are found in Title 21 of the Code of Federal Regulations (21 CFR, Part 1020).

There are several effects of added filtration. One is to increase the average energy of the x-ray beam. As low-energy photons are removed by the added filters, high-energy photons constitute a greater percentage of the beam. This has the effect of increasing the average energy of the beam, which is referred to as *beam hardening.* (See Beam Hardening, in box.) In addition to hardening the beam, the number of photons in the beam is reduced as a result of photon attenuation by the added filters. This reduction in photon number is more prominent in the low-energy portion of the bremsstrahlung spectrum (recall that photoelectric absorption events are more probable for lower-energy photons). In general, there is an overall reduction in photon number in all portions of the spectrum, but it is more evident for those photons of lower energy. These effects are demonstrated in Figure 9-9.

Although most filters used in radiography are made of aluminum (Z = 13), which is excellent for removing lower-energy (< 20-keV) photons, other materials such as copper can also be used. Copper, having a Z number of 29, is a more efficient filter for high-energy x-rays. Whenever copper is used, it is always in the form of a *compound filter* with aluminum. The reason for using copper is primarily to reduce the thickness of the filter. If such a compound filter is used, the highest Z number material (in this case, copper) is positioned facing the tube. The reason for this is to allow higher-energy characteristic x-rays from the first filter to be absorbed by the lower Z number filter. For example, copper can produce characteristic x-rays of approximately 8 keV. An x-ray of this energy is too low to be diagnostically useful, but it could result in an increased dose of radiation to the skin of the patient. However, the aluminum layer absorbs these x-rays and thereby reduces the patient's radiation dose. There may be concern with characteristic x-rays from aluminum.

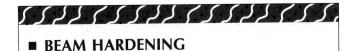

■ BEAM HARDENING

Beam hardening refers to the process in which the quality, or energy, of an x-ray beam is increased by removing lower-energy x-ray photons with appropriate filtration. To illustrate this concept, assume that an x-ray beam consists of 10 photons having these energies:

10, 20, 30, 40, 50, 60, 70, 80, 90, and 100 keV

If these energies are averaged, a beam energy of 55 keV is obtained. Now, if filtration that removes all photons having energies of 40 keV or less is added, the only photons now in the beam are those with

50, 60, 70, 80, 90, and 100 keV energies

The average of the remaining photons is now a beam energy of 75 keV. Thus the average beam energy has been raised 20 keV by removing the lower-energy photons.

It should be noted that this is a simplistic example for the number of photons in the beam with these specific energies was not considered. The concept of beam hardening, however, should be evident.

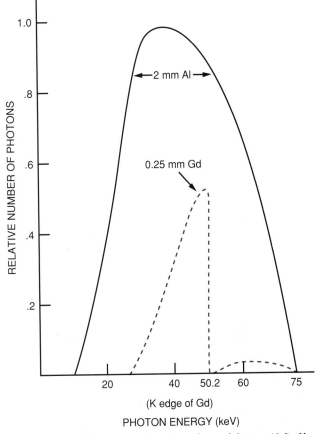

FIGURE 9–10. A heavy metal, such as the gadolinium (Gd), filter transmits a significantly narrower spectrum of x-ray energies (~ 25 keV to 50.2 keV) than does an aluminum (Al) filter. This may result in reduced radiation dose to patients and improved image contrast because of less scatter from higher-energy photons. (From Curry, T.S. III; Dowdey, J.E.; Murry, J.E., Jr. Christensen's Physics of Diagnostic Radiology ©1990. Philadelphia: Lea & Febiger. Reprinted with permission of the publisher.)

However, recall that as the Z number of the material decreases, so does the energy of the characteristic x-rays emitted. Aluminum can produce a characteristic x-ray of energy of approximately 1.5 keV, which is typically absorbed in the air before reaching the patient.

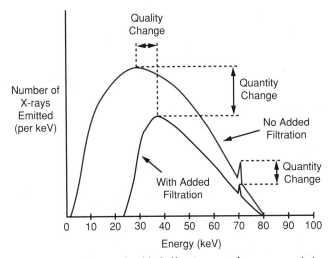

FIGURE 9–9. Effects of added filtration on the x-ray emission spectrum.

Another type of filtration, the *heavy-metal filter,* has now been introduced into clinical use as a way to improve image contrast in procedures with which barium and iodine contrast agents are used. Heavy-metal filters employ materials such as gadolinium (Gd, Z = 64) and holmium (Ho, Z = 67) among others. Use of such a filter has several advantages:

- Heavy-metal filters tend to narrow the spread of energies typically found in the bremsstrahlung spectrum, both high- and low-energy photons (shown in Fig. 9–10); the removal of low-energy photons assists in reducing the patient's radiation dose, and the removal of higher-energy photons tends to reduce the amount of scatter as a result of Compton scattering events
- By carefully matching the energies transmitted by the heavy-metal filters with energies that are highly absorbed by barium or iodine (Fig. 9–11), images containing less scatter and improved contrast can be obtained

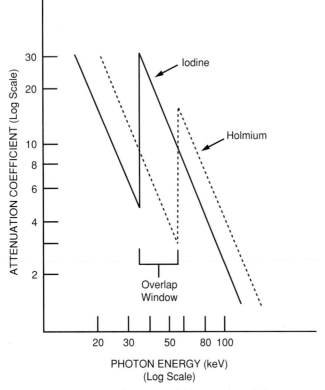

FIGURE 9–11. By using heavy-metal filters such as holmium (Z = 67) one can match the x-ray energies transmitted (~ 33 keV to 55.6 keV) to those that are highly absorbed by contrast agents such as iodine to obtain images containing less scatter. The overlap window shown represents the x-ray energy range transmitted by holmium but highly absorbed by iodine. (From Curry, T.S. III; Dowdey, J.E.; Murry, R.C., Jr. Christensen's Physics of Diagnostic Radiology ©1990. Philadelphia: Lea & Febiger. Reprinted with permission of the publisher.)

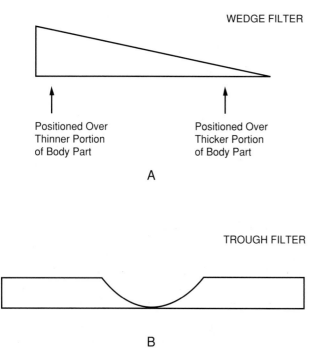

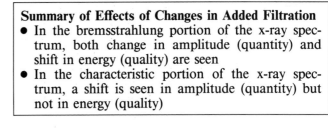

FIGURE 9–12. *A,* Schematic drawing of a wedge filter. *B,* Side view of a trough filter.

Filters are also used in radiography to obtain images having a more uniform radiographic density. Filters thus employed are particularly useful when imaging body parts that vary significantly in thickness or tissue density. Filters used for this purpose are called *compensating filters,* since they compensate for variations in x-ray transmission through the body part. Examples of compensating filters include wedge and trough filters (Fig. 9–12). These are typically made of aluminum or leaded plexiglass.

Wedge filters are designed to allow greater x-ray transmission through the thinnest section and less transmission through the thickest portion. The wedge can be used to produce a more uniform radiograph when it is positioned with its thickest portion over the thinnest section of the body part being imaged. Although not commonly employed, wedge filters have found some use in the making of posteroanterior and lateral projections of the chest. Proper use of such filters can also result in reduced radiation dose to the patient.

Trough filters allow the greatest x-ray transmission through the trough running through the center. They have been found useful in producing more uniform radiographs of the chest and spine. The shape of the trough filter allows production of radiographs having sufficient radiographic density in the area of the spine without increasing the radiation dose to surrounding soft tissue. In radiographs of the chest, filters of this type allow penetration of the mediastinum without overpenetrating the lungs.

The use of such compensating filters typically requires an increase in technical factors for a specific radiographic density. A higher kVp setting may in turn result in an undesirable loss of image contrast. It therefore is the decision of the radiologist as to whether contrast or uniform density is more useful in image interpretation and diagnosis.

Summary of Effects of Changes in Added Filtration
- In the bremsstrahlung portion of the x-ray spectrum, both change in amplitude (quantity) and shift in energy (quality) are seen
- In the characteristic portion of the x-ray spectrum, a shift is seen in amplitude (quantity) but not in energy (quality)

EFFECTS OF CHANGES IN VOLTAGE WAVEFORM: SINGLE-PHASE (1ϕ) VERSUS THREE-PHASE (3ϕ)

Recall that the phase of the x-ray generator also affects the x-ray spectrum. Single-phase generators produce a voltage waveform that begins at zero, reaches a maximum, then drops back to zero—a cycle repeated throughout the exposure. As the voltage across the tube electrodes fluctuates, the number of x-rays also

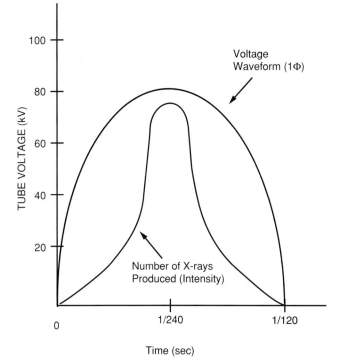

FIGURE 9–13. Variation of x-ray production with tube voltage.

With newer generators, the voltage never drops below approximately

- 87% of the kVp for 3ϕ, 6-pulse units (corresponding to ~ 13% ripple)
- 96% of the kVp for 3ϕ, 12-pulse units (corresponding to ~ 4% ripple)
- 99% of the kVp for high-frequency units (corresponding to ~ 1% ripple)

With the voltage across the tube electrodes remaining significantly higher throughout the exposure time, not only are more x-rays produced (i.e., a quantity change) but the average energy of the beams produced also is higher (Fig. 9–14). This effect on x-ray quality affects only the bremsstrahlung portion of the spectrum, since the average energy of the beam rises as a result of the removal of lower-energy photons from the continuous portion of the x-ray spectrum. Typically, an approximate 12% increase in the number of x-rays produced is observed with three-phase units compared with single-phase units. Similarly an approximately 16% increase is observed with high-frequency units, again compared with older single-phase units. The kVp values used for procedures with single-phase units can be reduced by the previously mentioned percentages when the same procedures are performed on three-phase and high-frequency units.

rises and falls but not proportionately with these voltage variations (Fig. 9–13). As seen in the illustration, when the voltage rises from zero, x-ray intensity (related to x-ray quantity) gradually increases. As the voltage becomes even higher, x-ray intensity increases significantly and reaches a peak as peak voltage (kVp) is attained. Recall that as the voltage increases, there is an increased probability of multiple interactions between incoming electrons and target atoms. Each interaction produces x-rays. During the second half of the cycle, x-ray intensity drops sharply until the voltage reaches zero.

Summary of Effects of Changes in Voltage Waveform from 1ϕ to 3ϕ or High-Frequency Units
- In the bremsstrahlung portion of the x-ray spectrum, increases in amplitude (quantity) and shifts in energy (quality) are seen
- In the characteristic x-ray portion of the x-ray spectrum, increases in amplitude (quantity) but no shifts in energy (quality) are seen

---

EFFECT OF DISTANCE FROM THE X-RAY SOURCE

Although the distance from the x-ray source does not actually affect the x-ray emission spectrum, it does have an effect on the measured value of x-ray intensity. In most radiographic procedures, the tube is located a specific distance from the patient and the image receptor, but always remember the effect of distance on the number of x-rays reaching the image receptor. On occasion, situations will arise when standard distances cannot be used, and the radiographer will need to adjust technical factors to assure a diagnostically useful radiograph.

As the distance from any point source of radiation increases, the number of photons traveling through a representative area (e.g., 1 m²) decreases as the square of the distance. This is known as an *inverse square*

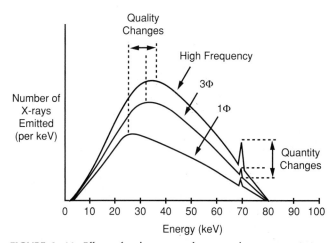

FIGURE 9–14. Effect of voltage waveform on the x-ray emission spectrum.

*law** and can be written as

$$I_1 d_1{}^2 = I_2 d_2{}^2$$

or in a form to see the inverse square nature,

$$\frac{I_1}{I_2} = \frac{d_2{}^2}{d_1{}^2}$$

where

$$I_1 = \text{initial intensity}$$
$$I_2 = \text{new intensity}$$
$$d_1 = \text{original distance}$$
$$d_2 = \text{new distance}$$

Although this relationship is expressed in terms of intensities, these terms can be replaced by either exposure (in mR) or numbers of photons per unit area per unit of time, since these quantities are directly related.

))))))) EXAMPLE

At a distance of 4 m from an x-ray unit, an x-ray beam is determined to have

$$10^3 \frac{\text{photons}}{m^2 - sec}$$

How many photons travel through the same area per second if measured at a distance of 1.5 m from the source?
Using the inverse square law,

$$I_1 d_1{}^2 = I_2 d_2{}^2$$

$$\left(10^3 \frac{\text{photons}}{m^2 - sec}\right)(4\ m)^2 = I_2\ (1.5\ m)^2$$

$$I_2 = \left(10^3 \frac{\text{photons}}{m^2 - sec}\right)\left(\frac{4\ m}{1.5}\right)^2$$

$$= \left(10^3 \frac{\text{photons}}{m^2 - sec}\right)(2.67)^2$$

$$= \left(10^3 \frac{\text{photons}}{m^2 - sec}\right)(7.1)$$

$$\cong 7100 \frac{\text{photons}}{m^2 - sec}$$

This concept is illustrated in Figure 9–15.

))))))) EXAMPLE

One clinical application of the inverse square law is a situation in which a technique chart for a portable unit calls for technical factors of 5 mAs and 80 kVp to produce a radiograph for a femur. This assumes, as do most techniques, a source-image distance of

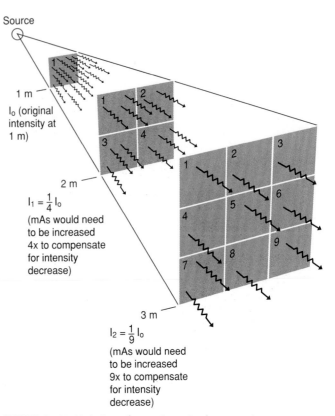

Source

1 m

I_0 (original intensity at 1 m)

2 m

$I_1 = \frac{1}{4} I_0$
(mAs would need to be increased 4x to compensate for intensity decrease)

3 m

$I_2 = \frac{1}{9} I_0$
(mAs would need to be increased 9x to compensate for intensity decrease)

FIGURE 9–15. Variation of x-ray intensity from a point source as a function of distance from the source.

40 inches. As the radiographer arrives to make the radiograph, the patient is found to be in traction. As a result of the overhead bars and associated equipment, a distance of only 32 inches can be obtained. How must the technical factors be adjusted to compensate for the decreased distance?

The inverse square law can be used in this case to determine how the technical factor mAs should be changed. Recall that mAs represents the number of photons produced during a radiographic exposure. Therefore using the inverse square law

$$\frac{I_1}{I_2} = \frac{d_2{}^2}{d_1{}^2}$$

As in the previous example, as distance decreases, the intensity or number of photons traveling through any unit area increases; then, in order to compensate for these changes in distance, the new mAs can be determined by using the inverse square law altered in the following manner:

$$\frac{mAs_1}{mAs_2} = \frac{d_1{}^2}{d_2{}^2}$$

(Note how this differs from the original form of the inverse square law.)
Therefore the mAs should be changed as follows:

$$\frac{5\ mAs}{mAs_2} = \frac{(40\ \text{inches})^2}{(32\ \text{inches})^2}$$

---

* Valid only for point radiation sources. It is also valid when the distance from the source is at least seven times the longest dimension of the source.

Emulsion Layer

The *emulsion layer* is the "active" layer that contains the image (Fig 10–1). The emulsion contains fine crystals of silver bromide evenly suspended in a gelatin medium. The silver bromide is formed by dissolving the silver metal in nitric acid, producing silver nitrate. The silver nitrate is then combined with potassium bromide, thus creating silver bromide. It was found that when silver iodide was present, the crystal had a much greater sensitivity to photon energy. Therefore in medical x-ray film, approximately 90% to 99% is silver bromide and about 1% to 10% is silver iodide. Collectively, these are referred to as silver *halides.*

The light- and x-ray–sensitive silver bromide exists in the form of crystals in the emulsion. The crystals are suspended in a medium that acts to prevent the crystals from coalescing, making for a more uniform crystal size and a more even distribution of crystals.

The characteristics of the emulsion depend on a number of factors. The composition of the silver crystals, their shape, size, and distribution all have an effect. The process of mixing, the choice of components of the emulsion, and the coating of the emulsion on the film base all help in determining the characteristics of the film. Such properties as film speed, exposure latitude, graininess, and sharpness of detail are governed by the composition and processing techniques during the formation of the emulsion.

The crystals must be suspended in a medium so that they can be evenly and uniformly spread on the film base. The viscosity of the medium must be such that the crystals will remain in suspension. *Gelatin* has been found to be the ideal medium. Gelatin is a particulate material that will not settle out when mixed with water or other solute. Other materials have been tried, but the gelatin colloid continues to be favored for film emulsion. The gelatin is obtained from collagen, which is found in the skins and hoofs of animals, mainly cattle. This clear protein gel is similar to the familiar culinary item used in desserts and salads. Cattle hides retain some of the microscopic traces of sulfur ingested from eating food containing mustard. The sulfur in the gelatin makes the silver bromide crystals more sensitive to the action of x-ray and light. Manufacturers have found that mustard oil can be used to provide the necessary sulfur to sensitize the silver bromide crystals.

Gelatin is universally used as the emulsion medium because of its unique characteristics. Gelatin prevents the silver halide crystals from adhering to one another and thus prevents clumping, which has the effect of making the crystals appear larger. When wet, gelatin can be made into a solid gel, and when dry, it serves to protect the silver bromide grains. However, the gelatin has no effect on the silver halide. In the manufacture of the gelatin emulsion, it can be made sufficiently hard and yet remain porous so that the processing solutions can seep into the deeper recesses of the emulsion and permit chemical action on the underlying silver bromide crystals. The gelatin can swell without dissolving and then shrinks and hardens, retaining the silver.

LATENT IMAGE FORMATION

When a radiographic film is exposed to radiation, the image is not immediately visible, hence the term *latent image.* When converted to metallic silver, the silver bromide crystals constitute the latent image of the radiograph. The crystals, uniformly mixed in the gelatin and spread evenly on the surface of the film base, ultimately form the radiographic image. The crystals are small—on the order of 1.0 to 1.5 μm in diameter. Most of the silver bromide crystals contain microscopic amounts of impurities or imperfections that act as photosensitive "specks." These specks, mainly on the surface of the crystals, provide the future sites for the beginning of the visible image. The following Gurney-Mott hypothesis is generally accepted as the mechanism of latent image formation.

On exposure to radiation, the crystals absorb the energy and electrons are emitted or move from their normal orbital position and travel at random throughout the crystal. The electrons may move in the crystal for a relatively long distance, but in the random motion some are trapped or captured by the "speck." The speck is now negatively charged. When this occurs, the

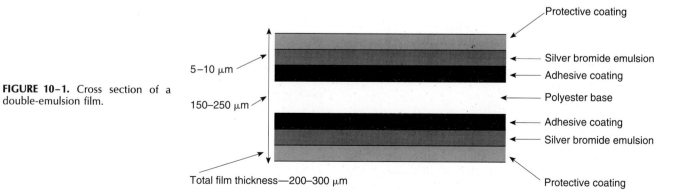

FIGURE 10–1. Cross section of a double-emulsion film.

5–10 μm

150–250 μm

Total film thickness—200–300 μm

Protective coating

Silver bromide emulsion

Adhesive coating

Polyester base

Adhesive coating

Silver bromide emulsion

Protective coating

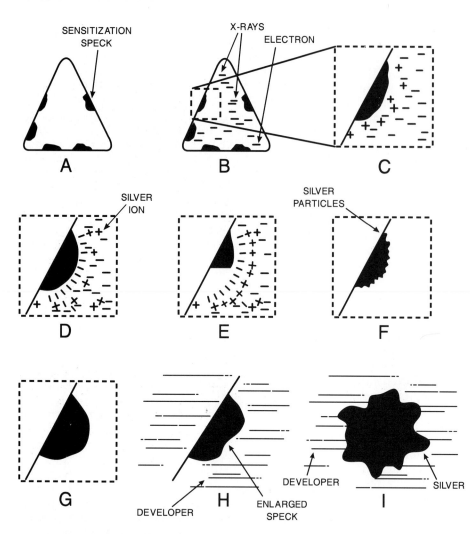

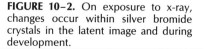

FIGURE 10–2. On exposure to x-ray, changes occur within silver bromide crystals in the latent image and during development.

positive ions of silver gravitate to the speck, since unlike charges attract. Here, the negative and positive charges unite and neutralize, forming atoms of metallic silver. The bromine portion of the crystal is absorbed in the gelatin. As more silver ions are neutralized, the speck grows in size in response to the amount of radiation energy absorbed, as indicated in Figure 10–2. This physical change in the silver bromide crystals produces the latent image. During processing the development of the visible image begins. The chemicals in the processing solution act first at the specks, resulting in a clumping of the silver to form the image. The silver bromide crystals react in this manner when exposed to x-rays or to light rays.

Radiographic Density

In the developer chemicals, the energized crystals are reduced to metallic silver. The chemicals are often referred to as the *reducing agents* for this reason. The amount of metallic silver depends on the degree of energy absorption. Silver is opaque to light and when distributed on the film gives the appearance of being black. For this reason, the blackness of a radiograph is spoken of when describing density. *Density* can be defined as the logarithm, to the base 10, of the opacity. The *opacity* of a film is the ratio of the amount of light incident on the film to the amount of light transmitted through the film. For example, a radiograph placed on the view box allows only 1/10 of the light to pass through; therefore the opacity is 10, and the density is 1. A radiograph that allows 1/100 of the view box light to be transmitted would have an opacity of 100 and a density of 2. It follows, then, that a radiograph allowing 1/1000 of the incident light to be transmitted would have an opacity of 1000 and a density of 3. Expressed in equation form, these terms can be defined as

$$\text{opacity} = \frac{I_{\text{incident}}}{I_{\text{transmitted}}}$$

and

$$\text{density} = \log_{10} (\text{opacity})$$
$$= \log_{10} (I_0/I_T)$$

where

$$I_0 = \text{incident light intensity}$$

$$I_T = \text{transmitted light intensity}$$

The following simple examples serve to illustrate the use of the above equation:

)))))) EXAMPLE

A radiograph placed on a viewbox transmits only 1/10 of the light incident on the film.

$$\text{Opacity} = \frac{I_{incident}}{I_{transmitted}} = \frac{I_0}{(1/10)I_0} = 10$$

Then, using the defining equation for density, we have

$$\begin{aligned}\text{Density} &= \log_{10} \text{opacity} \\ &= \log_{10} (10) \\ &= 1\end{aligned}$$

Thus for this case, the opacity is 10 and the density is 1.

Densitometers, instruments used to measure density, are calibrated to read the log of opacity or density directly. Densitometers indicate the relationship of the incident light intensity and the *intensity* of the light passing through the film. *Radiographs* with very little density allow a greater amount of light to be transmitted; conversely, extremely dense radiographs allow little light to pass through as shown in Figure 10–3.

The density of a radiograph is determined by the amount of radiation striking the film. In medical radiography, the amount of radiation emerging from the patient, that is, the exit radiation, is carefully controlled so that the density will be in the optimal diagnostic range.

EVALUATING FILM

Film is evaluated from the aspect of its ability to respond to radiation and latitude. By response we mean physical change in the silver bromide crystals necessary to produce the latent image and chemical changes during processing to form the visible image. The visible image is of serious concern because of its diagnostic value. Some films have the ability to respond to radiation more readily than others; this response is spoken of as its *speed*, or sensitivity.

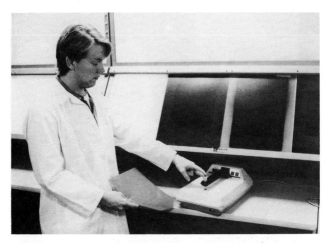

FIGURE 10–3. A typical densitometer, an instrument that measures the light transmitted through the radiograph. (Courtesy of Scott R. Gurley; photographer, A. T. Canaday.)

Film Sensitivity

The radiation exposure required to produce a specific density is a measure of film speed or sensitivity. Film coated with emulsion on both sides requires much less radiation to produce a specific density than does film coated only on one side. The thickness of the emulsion layer and size of the silver bromide crystals also affect the film's ability to respond to radiation. Generally, the thicker the emulsion layer and the larger the crystals, the greater the film response, that is, the less the radiation required to produce a specific density. Film, therefore, is described as fast or slow according to its ability to respond to radiation. Figure 10–4 is a diagram of slow, medium, and fast film based on the size of the crystals.

Today films are seldom rated independently. Most medical x-ray films are constructed to be used in combination with *intensifying screens*. Screens intensify the formation of the latent image by converting the x-ray energy to light energy. When x-radiation strikes an intensifying screen, light is emitted. The light rays are of much lower energy than x-rays but nonetheless have sufficient energy to effectively interact with the silver bromide crystals on the film to produce a latent image. Intensifying screens are mounted inside a lightproof, rigid *cassette,* and the film is placed in the cassette between the two screens. Figure 10–5 illustrates the intensifying screens placed in the front and back of a

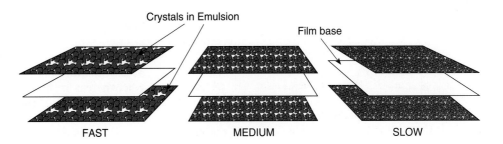

FIGURE 10–4. Diagram of slow, medium, and fast film.

Crystals in Emulsion

Film base

FAST   MEDIUM   SLOW

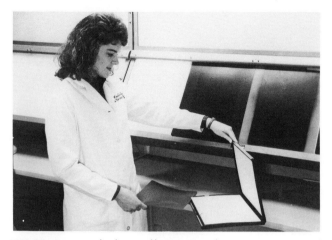

FIGURE 10–5. Medical x-ray film cassettes have screens mounted in front and back of the holder. (Courtesy of Sheree Crouch Guyer; photographer, A. T. Canaday.)

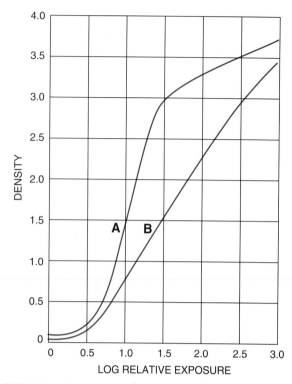

FIGURE 10–7. Comparison of exposure and density relationships for two types of film.

cassette. This is the typical method for mounting screens, although some cassettes may contain one screen only.

Because most medical radiographs are made with intensifying screens, the most useful measurement of film response is with a film–screen combination arrangement. In this arrangement, the film's response is mainly from light rays emitted from the screens, although the film also responds to the direct action of x-rays.

Long before Röntgen's discovery of x-ray, Dr. Ferdinand Hurter and V. C. Driffield attempted to quantify the light sensitivity of silver halide emulsion coated

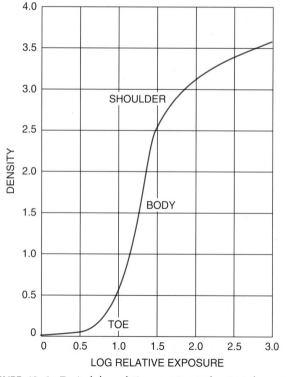

FIGURE 10–6. Typical log-relative exposure showing the major portions of the curve.

on glass plates. They reported a relationship between metallic silver deposited and exposure. This relationship is sometimes expressed by a curve that even today is called the *H&D curve* to give credit to these early investigators. The curve, also called a *sensitometric curve,* is drawn by making controlled exposures and measuring the several densities on the radiograph. Figure 10–6 is an example of such a curve. You will note that the beginning of the curve (the toe portion) represents very little density, approximately 0.25. This density can be attributed to the dye in the film base and to *fog.* Fog is almost always present, even in the most carefully controlled conditions. It is unwanted, but during the development of the film some crystals are reduced to silver even when the area is unexposed.

The straight-line portion of the curve is the useful range for diagnostic radiology. The toe portion is too light to be diagnostic, and the shoulder portion is too dense to be useful. Also note that the line levels off at the shoulder portion. This is a result of all the crystals available on the film being reduced to metallic silver; thus regardless of the amount of radiation exposure, the film will not increase in density.

With curves such as this, films can be compared for exposure-density relationships. In Figure 10–7, there are two curves for film comparison. It is clear that film A is faster than film B. For example, to reach a density of 2.5 in film A, the log relative exposure required is 1.3, whereas in film B an exposure of 2.2 is required. A closer inspection of the curve can be made by labeling various points on the curve as shown in Figure 10–8. In the A portion of the curve, the slight density is caused by fog and the dye in the film base. A small

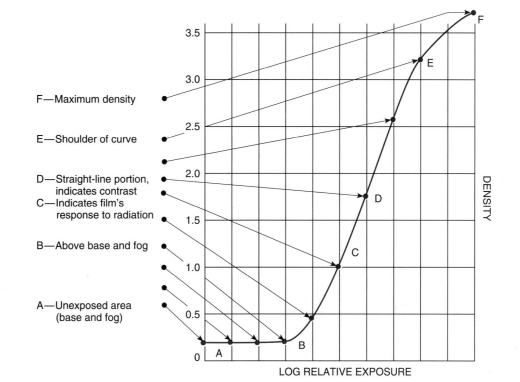

FIGURE 10–8. Key points of an H&D curve. (Redrawn from Technical Film, courtesy of 3M, St. Paul, MN.)

F—Maximum density

E—Shoulder of curve

D—Straight-line portion, indicates contrast
C—Indicates film's response to radiation

B—Above base and fog

A—Unexposed area (base and fog)

DENSITY

LOG RELATIVE EXPOSURE

number of crystals have developed spontaneously. In practice, emulsion or developer does not act ideally. Thus fog is the density produced in the unexposed areas. This is unwanted density, because it does not contribute to the information on the radiograph.

The B region, commonly called the toe of the curve, is the region of density above the base-plus-fog, generally thought to be in the density range of 0.25 to 0.50. This area is sometimes called the threshold density area and is the most susceptible to the effects of scatter radiation.

The C portion of the curve is the speed, or quantity of exposure required to achieve a designated density. This space on the curve indicates response of the film to radiation, generally measured at the density of 1.00 plus (base-plus-fog).

The D portion of the curve determines the film *contrast*. The steepness of the straight-line portion indicates the contrast quality of the film; the steeper the slope, the higher the contrast and the shorter the gray scale.

The E portion, called the shoulder of the curve, varies from the straight-line portion and tends toward the horizontal. The density at the shoulder of the curve is generally in the range of 2.75 to 3.25.

Maximum density is reached at the F portion of the curve and is achieved when all the silver bromide crystals have been converted to metallic silver; thereafter further exposure does not produce additional density.

Recorded Radiographic Detail

Detail, sometimes referred to as sharpness of the image, is the degree to which the smallest structural

lines of the anatomy can be recorded on film. In practice, detail is evaluated on two levels: (1) by the sharpness of the image recorded and (2) by the visibility of the detail. Visibility of detail is of most concern, because the detail recorded on film is significant only when it can be perceived by the human eye. The exception is the rare case when detail too small to be seen by the human eye can electronically be "seen" and analyzed on the basis of density differences. Practical application of this highly technical procedure has not yet been developed. Thus when discussing detail and visibility of detail, think in terms of what the human eye can perceive. In radiographic imaging many factors are involved with the perception of detail.

Grain size affects the detail that can be recorded, but as stated earlier, films today are made of such finely grained crystals that all medical film can record minute detail the unaided eye cannot perceive. However, it is clear that grain size must be considered, because detail smaller than grain size cannot be shown. Because intensifying screens are used in most medical radiography, the practical discussion of radiographic detail concerns the film-screen combination.

Screens make a dramatic difference in recording detail. Screen crystals are much larger than film crystals (compared in Fig. 10–9). However, it is not so much the size of the crystals (about 4 to 5 μm) that causes the image to lack sharpness. Rather, it is the light leaving the crystals in all directions and diverging over a larger area that causes the detail of structural lines to be unclear and indistinguishable as illustrated in Figure 10–10.

Making the image visible involves factors external to films and intensifying screens. These factors are dis-

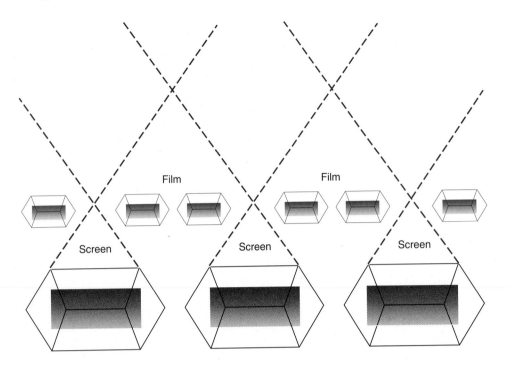

Film

Film

Screen

Screen

Screen

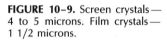

FIGURE 10–9. Screen crystals— 4 to 5 microns. Film crystals— 1 1/2 microns.

cussed in detail in a later chapter. The acuity of the eye, for example, must be considered. By acuity is meant the visual power of the eye. Although this varies among individuals, it is accepted that objects must be of a certain size to be seen, and on a radiograph, density differences between objects must possess a certain minimum value to be perceived. Another way of stating this is to say that the radiographed object must be large enough to be seen and that its contrast with respect to its surrounding density must be great enough to be discerned.

Other factors, such as patient motion, equipment characteristics, and technical exposure methods affect the sharpness of structural lines and thus the visibility of detail. These factors, too, are discussed in other chapters.

Films and film-screen combinations can be evaluated for detail by use of radiographic test objects (Fig. 10–11). Figure 10–12 demonstrates excellent detail of the 50-μm (diameter) wire with single-coated industrial film.

Figure 10–13 shows diminished detail with the use of conventional medical film coated on both sides. Figure 10–14 shows the dramatic loss of detail when an intensifying screen is used. Other test objects may be useful for evaluating the film's recording ability.

A typical test object is the parallel-line type (Fig. 10–15). The parallel lines are of various thicknesses and spacing, allowing for a numerical reading in terms of the largest number of line pairs that can be resolved. A line pair consists of the light space and the adjacent dark space. In fine detail film, some of the line pairs recorded are not discernible unless the image is magnified. The distance between the lines becomes smaller and smaller, so that the eye cannot separate or resolve them. However, with magnification it can be determined whether or not the lines were recorded. When intensifying screens are used, fine lines with close spacings may not be recorded as separate entities but appear fused, or blended together, diminishing resolution. The two test patterns discussed here are merely examples of instruments for measuring the recording ability of film or film/screen combinations; there are many others. However, no evaluation of film is adequate unless the recording ability of the film is known.

Latitude and Contrast in Film

Latitude and contrast are interrelated, so that it is difficult to separate the two. *Latitude* is the film's ability to display many shades of gray, ranging from light

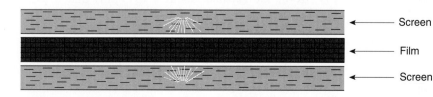

Screen

Film

Screen

FIGURE 10–10. Light given off in all directions diverges over an area larger than the crystal.

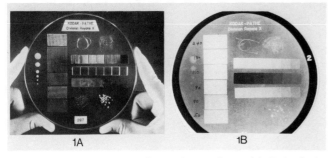

FIGURE 10-11. One type of test object: The Kodak Pathe lucite phantom (left) and a radiograph of it (right), showing embedded wire mesh sections to the left. The diameter of the wire is listed in micrometers (μm). The wire in the lower left screen measures 50 μm in diameter. The screen directly above it contains wire measuring 70 μm, and so forth. (From Gurley, L. T.; Whitfield, S. Technique for baseline mammography. Radiologic Technology 44:140–141, 1972.)

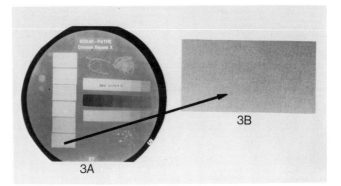

FIGURE 10-13. Radiograph of the phantom, using conventional medical film (A), and the cutout section of the radiograph, showing the 50-μm wire mesh (B). (From Gurley, L. T.; Whitfield, S. Technique for baseline mammography. Radiologic Technology 44:140–141, 1972.)

to black. Contrast may be defined as a variation in density. Latitude and contrast are sometimes discussed as if they were separate properties, but as the definition of contrast implies, the interdependence of the two is obvious. Although it is possible to have density without latitude, it is not possible to have latitude without density, because latitude, like contrast, consists of variations in density.

Radiographic contrast is usually described as *long scale* (low contrast) or *short scale* (high contrast). The concept of contrast scale is in effect an expression of latitude of the film. This can be demonstrated by radiographing an aluminum *step-wedge*. Films with wide latitude (long scale) record many shades of gray, ranging from white to black (Fig. 10–16A). Films with little latitude (short scale) show few shades of gray in the white-to-black range (Fig. 10–16B). It is evident from this comparison that latitude varies inversely with film contrast. Film is manufactured with more or less inherent contrast. The inherent contrast can be determined by the shape of the H&D curve. Recall that the position of the curve on the graph is a measure of film speed. In measuring contrast, the position of the curve is not significant; it is the shape, or slope, of the curve that reflects the inherent contrast. A gradual slope in-

dicates a gradual change in shades of gray and thus a greater exposure latitude. In Figure 10–17, film B indicates a gradual slope. Film A shows a very steep slope, indicating less exposure latitude and thus short-scale contrast.

Because radiographic film is the topic of this chapter, discussion has been limited to contrast inherent in the film because of the manufacturing process. In the following chapter, contrast is discussed from the aspect of subject contrast and the effect of kilovoltage on the scale of contrast. The subject is the object being radiographed. Because of differences in tissue density and thickness of anatomical parts, contrast in human anatomy is the crux of radiographic contrast. Without subject contrast, factors such as kilovoltage and film contrast are irrelevant. For example, if a container of water is the subject to be radiographed, there will be no contrast on the radiograph regardless of the voltage used or the inherent contrast of the film. Water is homogenous, and no differences in atomic density are seen. Water seeks its level, and thus no differences in thickness are present. The human body, on the other hand, consists of several radiographic densities and several thicknesses. When discussing radiographic contrast, it is obvious that all aspects in the production of

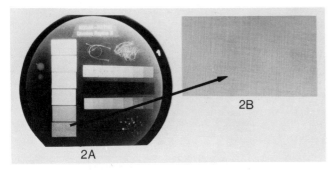

FIGURE 10-12. Radiograph of the phantom, using industrial film (A), and a cutout section showing the 50-μm wire mesh (B). (From Gurley, L. T.; Whitfield, S. Technique for baseline mammography. Radiologic Technology 44:140–141, 1972.)

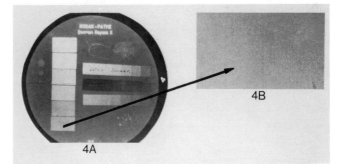

FIGURE 10-14. Radiograph of the phantom, using conventional film and one detail screen (A), and the cutout section of the 50-μm wire mesh (B). (From Gurley, L. T.; Whitfield, S. Technique for baseline mammography. Radiologic Technology 44:140–141, 1972.)

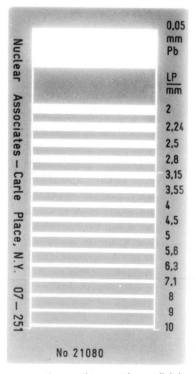

FIGURE 10-15. Typical test object with parallel lines of various spacing and thickness.

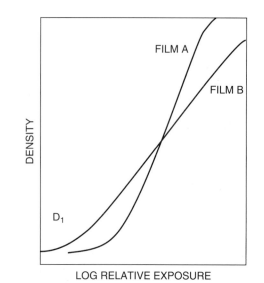

FIGURE 10-17. The characteristic curve for Film A has a steep slope, indicating short scale contrast. The curve for Film B is gradual, indicating its ability to record many shades of gray. (Redrawn from Technical Film, courtesy of 3M, St. Paul, MN.)

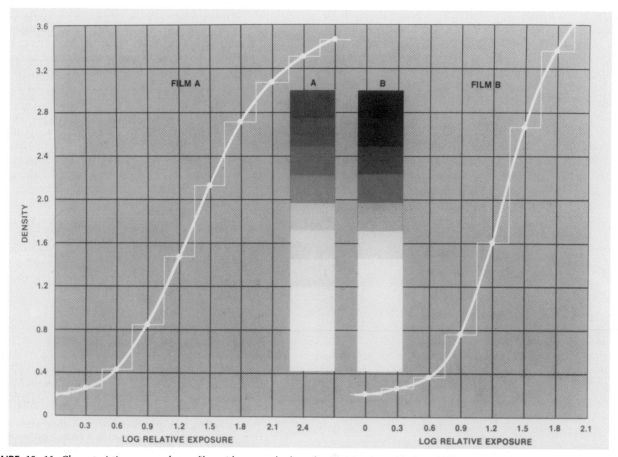

FIGURE 10-16. Characteristic curves of one film with many shades of gray (A). Film with few shades of gray (B). A has low contrast and wide latitude. B has high contrast and little latitude. (Reprinted courtesy of Eastman Kodak Company.)

a radiographic image must be considered. Contrast in film and subject and technical exposure factors all contribute to radiographic contrast.

TYPES OF FILM

Nonscreen Film

Nonscreen film requires a much larger dose of radiation for adequate density than do films used in combination with screens. Nonscreen film is rarely used in general radiographic procedures in today's practice. It is useful for imaging specimens from the morgue or surgery and in special diagnostic problems. Nonscreen film yields extremely sharp images with well-defined structural lines. Intraoral exposure in dental radiography is also performed with nonscreen film.

The emulsion is basically the same as that for other film but it is thicker so that more radiation is absorbed. The emulsion may be coated on both sides as for dental film or on only one side. Nonscreen film depends on the direct absorption of x-ray energy for its photographic effect. The thicker emulsion requires a longer developing time. This, coupled with the high dose required, has caused it to be replaced almost entirely in general radiography.

Nonscreen films are placed in lightproof envelopes or in packets with lead foil backing to prevent backscatter radiation from fogging the film and in the case of intraoral dental radiography, to reduce the patient's dose.

Screen Film

Screen films are designed to be exposed by light rays emitted from the *phosphors* making up the screens. All film will respond to light or x-radiation, but screen film is designed to respond readily to visible light. The film is placed in close contact with a radiolucent sheet of material made of phosphors that fluoresce when struck by x-radiation. The energy of the radiation photons is converted to light energy. To simplify this concept, imagine one photon of x-radiation with 30 units of energy striking a phosphor crystal in the screens. The crystal gives off 30 light rays, each with one unit of energy. In this way, the resultant photographic effect is intensified by a factor of 30 (Fig. 10–18). This illustration may be taking considerable liberty with reality, but it serves to make the point. Because light rays have sufficient energy to darken the film, it is not necessary to depend on x-ray energy to produce the photographic effect.

The disadvantage of using screens to intensify the density is that the sharpness of structural lines or detail is considerably sacrificed. However, the advantage gained by reducing the patient dose to approximately 1/30 of the dose required without screens more than offsets this loss.

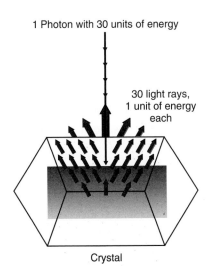

FIGURE 10–18. The intensifying effect of screens is the result of x-ray energy being converted to light energy.

Mammography Film

The mammary gland has always presented a unique radiographic problem because of its low tissue contrast. In the past, industrial double-emulsion film was used in *mammography* because of its inherent contrast and fine detail–recording properties. However, the radiation dose with industrial film was high, sometimes as much as 12 roentgens (R). The long exposure time required to obtain adequate density resulted in patient motion that quite often rendered the radiograph nondiagnostic, making repeat exposures necessary. Beating of the heart and coursing of blood through veins caused motion ranging from 300 to 750 μm. It was found that by using one screen, the exposure time could be reduced, and, consequently, motion was reduced to 100 to 300 μm (Fig. 10–19). These findings led to the development of specialty films to overcome these two problems—high patient dose and patient motion.

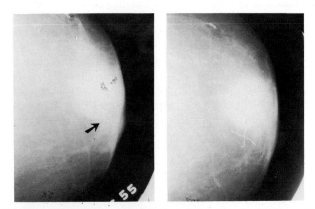

FIGURE 10–19. Radiographs of the breast: *A,* Industrial film with crosswire almost obliterated because of motion, and *B,* conventional film with one detail screen. (From Gurley, L. T.; Whitfield, S. Technique for baseline mammography. Radiologic Technology 44:144, 1972.)

Duplicating Film

Making a copy of a radiograph is a convenience for patient care and for teaching purposes. Special film made for this purpose, coated on one side with emulsion, is placed in a duplicating unit along with the original radiograph. The film is exposed to ultraviolet light; no x-radiation is needed. *Duplicating film* comes in several sizes, and the size can be matched with the original radiograph.

Ciné Film

Ciné film is used in fluorography for dynamic studies recording the fluoroscopic image. Currently, this film is used mainly in the cardiac catheterization laboratory. Ciné film is roll film of movie type and is supplied in two sizes, 16 mm and 35 mm, the 35 mm dominating the market. This film is exposed by the light from the output phosphor of the image intensifier through an optical system of lenses and mirrors and can be exposed at a rate of 8 to 60 frames per second. The 16 mm film records 40 individual frames per foot. The 35 mm film, being larger, records only 16 frames per foot. Furthermore, because the surface area of the 35 mm film is larger, a greater radiation exposure is required to produce the desired density.

Ciné films are viewed with a projector to magnify the image in the same manner as other movie film. The processing and handling of ciné film is critical, because artifacts are also magnified. Defects, dirt, dust, and even fingerprints may show on the magnified image, considerably reducing image quality.

Video Film

With the advent of computer-assisted imaging — for example, computed tomography, magnetic resonance imaging, digital radiography, ultrasound, and nuclear medicine — image receptors other than film are increasing in use. The image may be displayed by a television tube, that is, a cathode-ray tube (CRT). The image displayed in this manner is fleeting and temporary. Therefore the physician may want a permanent image of the CRT display or video image. The *video film* designed for this purpose may be marketed in several sizes, yielding either a single image or several images per film. The film is coated on only one side. There is no concern regarding patient's dose here, because the film is exposed by the light emitted from the video display and is independent of the exposure received by the patient.

Subtraction Film

Subtraction film is manufactured with high inherent contrast to accentuate the contrast existing in the subject. The film is coated on one side only. This improves detail and is independent of patient dose. Subtraction film, mainly used in angiography, is falling into disuse with the advent of digital fluorography.

PROCESSING THE LATENT IMAGE

When films are exposed to light or x-radiation energy, a latent image is formed in the emulsion. It is not visible in this state and must be developed into a silver image. The formation of a visible image by chemical means has been known for years, and the chemistry has changed very little over time. Automated film-processing equipment has required only minor changes in chemicals such as concentration of solutions and change in temperature.

The basic steps in processing the latent image are (1) development, (2) fixation, (3) washing, and (4) drying. The sequence of the process is the same for manual as for automatic processing and is illustrated in Figure 10–20. Processing takes place in the darkroom. The exposed film is protected from light during the processing cycle. The film is first placed in *developer* solution, then into the *fixer* chemicals. Thereafter the film is washed and, finally, dried.

Development

Development is the reduction of the silver halide molecules around the site of the silver *nuclei* of the latent image. Development is selective in that the areas not exposed to radiation are not significantly affected during the normally prescribed development time. However, as development continues, the amount of metallic silver increases, and if radiographs remain in the solution long enough, all the silver halide will be reduced to metallic silver. The active ingredients in the developing solution are *hydroquinone* and *metol*. A chemical similar to metol, phenidone, was discovered in 1940 and is used in automatic processors. These

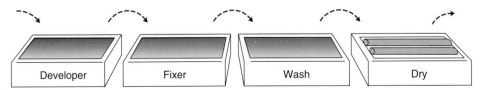

| Developer | Fixer | Wash | Dry |

FIGURE 10–20. The sequence of steps in film processing remains basically the same whether processing is manual or automatic.

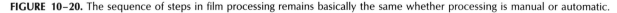

chemicals require other agents in the formula for the production of the visible image.

Hydroquinone

Hydroquinone is the most commonly used developing agent, but it is usually used in combination with another developing agent. It is slow to take effect and is quite sensitive to changes in temperature. It is practically inactive at temperatures below 59°F. Hydroquinone produces high contrast but under some conditions tends to produce fog. To prevent fog, other chemical agents are added to the formula.

Metol and Phenidone

Metol is another commonly used developing agent. It is known by a variety of names, such as elon, petcol, and photol. Unlike hydroquinone, metol starts its developing action almost immediately. It retains much detail in technical images, is quite stable in solution, and thus is not readily exhausted. Phenidone, being similar to metol is also used, mainly in combination with hydroquinone. The latter combination results in an improved working effect during processing.

Accelerators

Developing agents require a strong alkaline solution to be effective. The compounds sodium carbonate and sodium hydroxide provide an alkaline base for developer action. Sodium hydroxide, commonly known as lye, is extremely corrosive and must be handled with care. The alkaline solution in the developer serves two extremely important purposes: (1) It provides the medium required for the action of hydroquinone and (2) it swells the emulsion, allowing the developing agents to seep deep into the recesses of the emulsion for more effective development.

Preservatives

Developer solutions contain minute amounts of air because of agitation during mixing and handling. The developer reacts with the oxygen in the air and can become weak and incapable of reducing the silver bromide to metallic silver. To prevent the aerial *oxidation,* a *preservative* is added to the solution. Sodium sulfite is most often used for this purpose. Sodium sulfite prevents the formation of the colored stain that results from oxidized developer agents and also prevents or retards the oxidation process. Sodium sulfite removes air from the solutions before oxidation can take place.

Restrainer

As stated earlier, if development is carried too far, all the silver halide is reduced to metallic silver. Thus time is a critical factor. The diagnostic value of a radiograph depends on the development of only the exposed silver bromide. Without a restrainer agent in the developer formula, there will not be sufficient differentiation between the exposed and unexposed silver halide. The chemical potassium bromide selectively retards action on the unexposed silver halide grains without preventing the exposed grains from developing. This retardation has the effect of increasing the differentiation between exposed and unexposed silver bromide grains.

Other Factors in Development

The four essential ingredients previously discussed can act only in a solvent, and water is universally used for this purpose. Some formulas may add a wetting agent to "make the water wetter" in order to assure uniform covering of the film emulsion and to improve swelling of the emulsion.

In automatic processing, a hardener is added to control the swelling, preventing the emulsion from becoming too soft. The radiograph increases in thickness when the emulsion swells, and if the swelling is carried too far, the processor rollers cannot transport the film properly. In most instances, the hardener chemical is glutaraldehyde, and its presence in the developer solution for automatic processing is important.

The concentration of the developer solution components is a factor to be considered. The concentration of the chemicals influences the rate of development. In automatic processors, the concentration is higher, and this in part accounts for the shorter development time required.

Development time is a critical factor in film processing. The chemicals must have time to react, and the film emulsion requires time to swell so that the developer can penetrate and reach the deeper silver halide grains. The time required for optimum development is greatly influenced by the concentration of the solution and in the case of automatic processing, by the replenishment rate. The replenishment rate is adjusted to retain a constant concentration of chemicals and to replace the water carried out by the film. Merely wetting a dry 14- × 17-inch film requires a significant amount of water, and the replenishment rate must be adjusted to replace the water in addition to the other chemicals consumed in the developing process. For the developer processing time to remain constant, the chemical solution must remain constant or nearly so.

Temperature is another factor having a considerable influence on film development. As mentioned earlier, hydroquinone is relatively inactive at temperatures below 59°F (15°C). At higher temperatures, hydroquinone is highly responsive. Metol and phenidone are less affected by changes in temperature, but when used in combination with hydroquinine, a temperature adjustment is made so that both chemicals participate in the development process. Generally, the higher the temperature, the faster is the rate of development. The rule of thumb is that the rate of development doubles with a temperature increase of 18°F (10°C). This means that with every 10°C increase in temperature, the development time can be cut in half. Typically, automatic processors develop at 90° to 95°F, and the entire processing time, including the drying, can be reduced to 90 seconds.

The three factors—concentration of solution, development time, and temperature—work in concert and must be considered in maintaining uniform and consistent film development.

Fixer

Under ideal development conditions, the silver halide grains exposed to radiation are reduced to metallic silver, and the unexposed crystals remain unaffected. The latent image then becomes visible. However, the unexposed silver halide is *opaque* to light just as is the converted metallic silver. Eventually, it, too, will become black. This makes viewbox inspection for interpretation impossible. Additionally, the metallic silver image must be "fixed" to the film base. The fixer solutions must therefore remove the unexposed and thus undeveloped silver halide and harden the emulsion to fix the silver image to the film base.

Fixing Agent

The active ingredient in the fixing solution is *thiosulfate*—sodium thiosulfate in powdered fixer or ammonium thiosulfate in liquid. At one time, sodium thiosulfate was called hyposulfite of soda. The term was shortened to "hypo," which even today is in common usage. The temperature of the fixer solution is not as critical as that of the developer, but both solutions are usually kept approximately the same temperature.

The fixer solution requires a preservative just as the developer does and for the same reason. The chemical sodium sulfite provides the essential functions of preserving and maintaining the chemical composition of the solution.

Neutralizer

The strong alkaline base in the developer clings to the film even though the rollers remove most of it while transporting the film from the developer to the fixer. Minute amounts may be trapped in the deeper recesses of the emulsion, and unless these are neutralized, development will continue. Prolonged development gives a foggy appearance to the radiograph that seriously impairs the diagnostic usefulness of the film.

An acid is needed to neutralize an alkali. The *neutralizer* may be acetic or sulfuric acid. Acetic acid, found in vinegar, is capable of neutralizing the alkali and thus stopping the action of the developer. Additionally, the water–acetic acid mixture provides a suitable medium for the fixer chemicals.

Hardening Agent

When placed in the fixer the radiograph is easily scratched and damaged, because the emulsion is soft

from swelling. Alum is commonly used to prevent this damage. Potassium alum, chromium alum, or aluminum chloride shrink and harden the emulsion.

Washing

Residual chemicals must be removed from the film to prevent fading and discoloration of the image. The wash water temperature is generally in the same range as that of the developer and fixer. In most instances, the water circulates or is discarded and replenished at a constant rate to facilitate removal of the chemicals.

Drying

Drying can be as simple as placing the film on a hanger and air drying it. However, the process is accelerated considerably by blowing hot air over the surface of the film. In automatic processors, the air temperature may be as high as 135°F (57°C), making the drying time a matter of a few seconds. Automatic processors have alleviated the need for *wet reading,* a term seldom heard today. With manual processing, the time from developer through the entire cycle requires approximately an hour. Formerly, in this situation, physicians often looked at the radiograph before drying and made a temporary interpretation, called wet reading, which was particularly frequent in emergency situations. With modern processing, a film can be completely processed and dried in a matter of seconds. This has been a significant technical advance in improving the efficiency of processing radiographs, and, additionally, the quality of the processed films has increased.

▰▰▰ Chapter Summary/ Important Concepts

Medical radiographic film has undergone some extremely significant developments since film first took the place of glass plates. The changes have been most apparent in the film base. The film base material is now safe from spontaneous ignition, is stronger, and thus can be made thinner, and shelf life is longer. The active ingredients of the film emulsion remain basically the same. The components of the film emulsion are put together in different ways and in varying amounts, which in part accounts for differences in such properties as film speed, latitude, and recorded detail.

The film, after exposure, contains the latent image. The inherent qualities of the film and exposure technique used to produce the latent image determine the radiograph's density, detail, and contrast. These qualities, which ultimately determine the radiograph's diagnostic value, are inherent in the latent image. However, before the image becomes visible, a chemical process must take place. This process is called development. Standard, optimum development of film does not improve on the inherent qualities of the latent image. However, poor, substandard processing can and often does have a deleterious effect on the latent image. Improper temperature affects density; thus detail and contrast are affected. Chemicals with depleted strength, an improper concentration mix, or contamination can greatly affect the quality of the radiograph. It can therefore be seen that optimum processing is essential to maintenance of the inherent radiographic qualities of the latent image.

Important Terminology

(Film) Base. The layer of a film that provides the strong, flexible surface and support for the sensitive emulsion

Cassette. Lightproof device for holding x-ray film for exposure; it is composed of two intensifying screens in a rigid case

Ciné Film. Movie-type roll film for recording dynamic physiology during fluorography

Contrast. The difference in density of shades of gray present on a radiograph

Density. Degree of opaqueness or blackness of a radiograph; also defined as $\log_{10} (I_0/I_T)$

Detail. Sharpness of a radiographic image, often referred to as resolution; it can be measured in line pairs recorded per millimeter

Developer. Chemical solution used to make the latent radiographic image visible; also called a reducing agent

Development. Reduction of silver halide molecules around the site of silver nuclei containing the latent image to black metallic silver

Dose. Amount of radiation received by a patient during exposure

Duplicating Film. FIlm coated on only one side designed for copying radiographs with light exposure

Elon. The chemical in developer that starts action on the exposed film emulsion

Emulsion Layer. Portion of radiographic film that is sensitive to light and x-rays; the emulsion contains the latent image before processing and the visible image after processing

Exposure (Radiographic). The process of subjecting film to a given amount of x-radiation

Film. Medium on which the image is recorded

Fixer. The chemicals in solution that remove unexposed and undeveloped silver bromide crystals from the film after the exposed silver bromide has been reduced to silver in the developer

Fog. Unwanted additional density that covers part or all of the film, obscuring image detail

Gelatin. A jelly-like protein substance used in x-ray film emulsion; its viscosity provides a means for holding the silver bromide crystals in suspension

Halide. A compound that contains any of the following elements: fluorine, chlorine, bromine, iodine, or astatine

H&D Curve. See Sensitometric Curve

Hydroquinone. Active ingredient in the developing solution; generally used in combination with the chemical metol

Image (Radiographic). Pictorial record of the subject being radiographed; it consists of deposits of black metallic silver in the emulsion of the film

Intensifying Screen. Screen used in combination with film; it consists of fluorescent crystals coated on a rigid base to convert x-radiation into light

Intensity (Light). Rate or quantity of light striking a unit area per unit of time

Latent Image. Image of an object present in film emulsion after exposure to radiation and before the film is chemically processed; the image is not visible until the film is processed

Latitude (Exposure). Range of exposure between the minimum and maximum that yields a scale of varying densities from light to black

Long Scale. Refers to a large number of density areas (grays) within an image; usually infers a smaller difference in the density values from density area to density area, or low radiographic contrast

Mammography. Radiographic study of the mammary gland

Metol. An active ingredient in the developing solution; generally used in combination with the chemical hydroquinone

Molecule. Composed of two or more atoms; the smallest possible quantity of a substance that can exist independently and still retain the chemical properties of the substance

Neutralizer. An agent that causes another to be ineffective

Nucleus (plural, Nuclei). The positively charged central portion of an atom that constitutes nearly all of the atomic mass

Opacity. Ratio of the amount of light incident on the film to the amount of light transmitted through the film

Opaque. Impenetrable by light; the opposite of *translucent*

Oxidation. A chemical reaction that results in the removal of electrons from atoms

Parallax Effect. Outcome seen only with double emulsion films: the separation of images by the film base gives the impression of unsharpness when viewed at an angle

Phosphor. Substance that emits light when excited by radiation

Preservative. Substance added to another material to limit or prevent a change that could otherwise occur

Reducing Agent. Chemical capable of transferring electrons to silver ions of the latent image, causing them to become atoms of silver

Screen. See Intensifying Screen

Sensitivity. Ability of a film emulsion to respond to radiation; also referred to as film speed

Sensitometric Curve. A measure of film characteristics in relation to exposure; first developed by Hurter and Driffield (often called an H&D curve)

Short Scale. Refers to the presence of a small number of density areas (grays) within an image; usually infers a greater difference in the density values from density area to density area, or high radiographic contrast

Solution. A liquid containing substances dissolved in water used for developing and fixing radiographs

Speck (Sensitivity Speck). Impurity added to the silver halide crystal that is needed to facilitate the formation of a latent image

Speed. See Sensitivity

Step-Wedge. A penetrometer; a device consisting of a series of uniform absorbers that increase in thickness in definite steps

Subtraction Film. Film coated on only one side and manufactured with a high inherent contrast

Thiosulfate. The active ingredient of a fixing solution; may be sodium thiosulfate or ammonium thiosulfate

Video Film. Film specifically made to be used with light exposure emitted from the video display and thus coated on only one side

Bibliography

Bushong, S.C. Radiologic Science for Technologists: Physics, Biology and Protection, 4th ed. St. Louis: C.V. Mosby, 1988.

Cullinan, A.M. Producing Quality Radiographs. New York: J.B. Lippincott, 1987.

Curry, T.S. III; Dowdey, J.E.; Murry, R.C., Jr. Christensen's Physics of Diagnostic Radiology, 4th ed. Philadelphia: Lea & Febiger, 1990.

Fodor, J. III; Malott, J.C. The Art and Science of Medical Radiography, 6th ed. St. Louis: The Catholic Health Association, 1987.

Gurley, L.T.; Harwood, S.W. A practical technique for baseline mammography. Radiol Technol 44:140, 141, 144, 1972.

Health Sciences Markets Division. The Fundamentals of Radiography, 12th ed. Rochester, NY: Eastman Kodak Company, 1980.

Selman, J. The Fundamentals of X-ray and Radium Physics, 7th ed. Springfield, IL: Charles C Thomas, 1985.

Technical Film 2. St. Paul, MN: 3-M Company, Diagnostic Imaging Products, Imaging System Division, 1989.

van der Platts, G.J. Medical X-ray Techniques in Diagnostic Radiology: A Textbook for Radiographers and Radiological Technicians, 4th ed. The Hague: Martinus Nyhoff Publishers, 1980.

Review Questions

1. What material was first employed as a base for medical radiographic images?
2. List the characteristics of the polyester film base that make it preferable as a film base.
3. List the advantages of gelatin in the film emulsion.
4. Name the primary components of the film emulsion.
5. Describe the Gurney-Mott theory for the formation of the latent image.
6. Define radiographic density.
7. What is meant by film speed, or sensitivity?
8. List the film characteristics that a H&D curve can express.
9. What is film latitude? How does it relate to contrast?
10. Why are medical films used in combination with intensifying screens for most examinations?
11. List the sequence of basic steps in developing the latent image.
12. List the active ingredients of the developer.
13. List the active ingredients of the fixer.
14. Why are preservatives used in the developer and fixer solutions?
15. Name two main reasons why automatic processors can develop films in a shorter time than manual processing.

CHAPTER 11

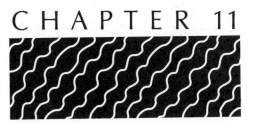

Production of the Radiographic Image

Marian P. Hattaway, B.S., R.T.(R.)

Chapter Outline

Chapter Objectives

On completion of this chapter, you should be able to

- Define all terms in the glossary list
- Describe generally the method of producing radiographs of human anatomic parts
- Describe completely the radiographic qualities of an ideal radiograph
- In relation to an exposure technique chart
  - *discuss its purpose*
  - *identify all items of information it contains about exposure factors and conditions*
  - *demonstrate an acceptable method of use (in order of procedure)*
- Name the basic qualities a radiograph should possess; define and give reason, and in general terms, state to what extent each is needed
- Differentiate between
  - *long-scale contrast and short-scale contrast*
  - *low radiographic contrast and high radiographic contrast*
  - *subject contrast and film contrast*
  - *primary, exit, and scatter radiation*
  - *a bright image and a dark, gray image*
  - *low-energy x-rays and high-energy x-rays*
- List the primary exposure factors; discuss the radiographic effect of each
  - *determine the minimum kVp required to penetrate a specific part for a stated projection*
  - *given the original exposure factors, determine the exposure factors necessary to alter the scale of radiographic contrast within an image of a specific part*
- List questions to which the radiographer should have an answer before and during the performance of any radiographic study; give the probable source of the answer for each
- State in mathematical terms the
  - *inverse square law of radiation intensity*
  - *relationship between mAs and radiographic density*
  - *relationship between the mAs and the kVp used to obtain a specific radiographic exposure (density)*
  - *relationship between the mA and the exposure time used for a specific radiographic exposure (density)*
  - *relationship between the mA and the exposure time or the mAs and the source-image distance (SID) for a specific radiographic exposure (density)*
- Use the relationships in the preceding objective to determine the value of the exposure factors necessary to satisfy the specific exposure conditions.
- State reasons the source-image distance (SID) should
  - *not be manipulated to compensate for density changes resulting from changing the exposure condition(s)*
  - *be manipulated for density changes as a result of limitations in other exposure factor(s)*
- Given the exposure factors for a radiographic image, determine the exposure factors that will produce minor but visible changes in the radiographic quality of the image; demonstrate the answer, using exposures of a phantom segment or a penetrometer

The use of *x-rays* to produce a medical image on a sensitive emulsion is called *radiography.* The purpose of the process is to produce an image of the normal or abnormal anatomy of the body part that is within the limits of the irradiated area. The image produced is a *radiograph,* similar in its basic components to Figure 11–1. The person who produces the image is a *radiographer.*

The radiographer uses the physical principles of x-ray production to correctly adjust the exposure factors that control the x-ray energy for production of an image. Those factors include voltage (kilovoltage, kV, and peak kilovoltage, kVp), amperage (milliamperage, mA), exposure time expressed in seconds (sec) or *milliseconds (ms),* and distances (source-image distance, SID, and object-image distance, OID). These four are referred to as the primary exposure factors. Their values are controlled by the radiographer for each radiographic exposure. The relationship of these factors to image production is discussed in this chapter.

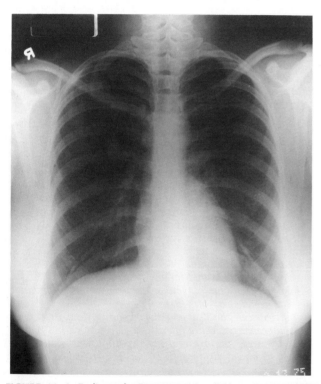

FIGURE 11–1. Radiograph: Posteroanterior (PA) projection of the chest. Image possesses all of the basic anatomical tissue densities. The air-filled lung tissues are the darker images surrounded by the relatively bright images of the ribs and vertebrae; the density (grays) of the adipose tissues about the thoracic cage and at the axilla includes a number of shades of gray; the heart muscle is of a lighter density than the lung fields but not as bright as the bony shadows. This radiograph does not meet all the criteria for a good chest radiograph. The sternoclavicular joints are not symmetrical, indicating rotation of the part and distortion of the thoracic cavity's internal structures.

RADIOGRAPHIC IMAGE PRODUCTION

Medical radiographic images of anatomical parts are produced by the passage of x-rays through the parts. X-rays, *ionizing radiation,* may produce biological damage as they pass through living tissue. For this reason a "good", diagnostic-quality radiograph must be produced for each radiographic examination using technical factors that permit the patient to absorb the least amount of radiation possible. The goal of the radiographer should always be to produce the best radiographic image each time a patient receives a radiographic exposure.

Radiographic *density* refers to the degree of darkening of a radiographic film that occurs when the film is exposed to varying intensities of x-rays. A dark area on a film is referred to as a high-density area and corresponds to a high intensity (or high number) of x-ray interactions with the film. A light area on the film is referred to as a low-density area and corresponds to a low intensity (or low number) of x-ray interactions with the film. Therefore a good, diagnostic-quality radiograph is one that demonstrates the largest number of radiographic density shades with the greatest difference between adjacent densities as in Figure 11–2. A radiograph satisfying these conditions reveals everything there is to visualize about the part imaged. A delicate balance of exposure factors for each body part and each condition is required to demonstrate the desired information. To provide this, the radiographer must understand exposure factors and their interrelationships, patient position and *patient architecture,* and pathology and the effect each has on radiographic images.

Control of X-ray Production for Radiography

Recall from previous chapters that x-rays are produced when electrons from the filament are accelerated through *kilovoltage* (kVp) potentials and strike the anode target. A much lower voltage is first applied to the filament in order to produce a sufficiently high current flow to release electrons by thermionic emission. The current that flows through the filament is known as the filament current. Controlling the filament current and the kVp allows the radiographer to control the number of electrons moving between the tube electrodes (known as the *tube current,* or mA). This in turn allows control of the *radiation* (x-ray) *intensity,* or numbers of x-rays produced.

In addition, control of the kVp allows the radiographer to vary the energy or penetrating ability of the x-rays produced. Increasing the kVp increases the average energy of the x-rays produced and gives the x-ray beam more penetrating power. Reducing the kVp does just the opposite. This becomes an impor-

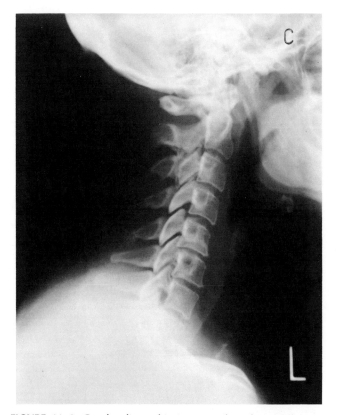

FIGURE 11–2. Good radiographic image: A lateral cervical spine. All seven cervical vertebral bodies, the lower five articular facets, and the intervertebral articulations and spinous processes of all seven vertebrae are visible. The first thoracic vertebral body is partially visible. Visible anteriorly are the air passage, the hyoid bone, the thyroid cartilage, vague outlines of the cartilages of the trachea and other soft tissues. (From the University of Alabama at Birmingham Radiographer Program Teaching Files.)

tant factor in producing the optimum contrast in the radiographic image.

The length of time that the x-ray machine actually produces x-rays is controlled by the timer. The longer the exposure time, the more x-rays produced. Thus the combination of tube current (mA) and exposure time, measured in seconds known as mAs, determines the number of x-rays produced during a radiographic exposure. It is the radiographer's responsibility to choose the best combination of technical factors (i.e., kVp, mA, and exposure time) to produce the best diagnostic quality radiograph.

Effects of Photon Energy on the Radiographic Image

Lower–energy (low kVp–produced) x-ray photons are not as penetrating as higher–energy x-ray photons. Because lower–energy x-ray photons are less penetrating, more of them are absorbed in the tissue. In this case, more photons must be used to obtain sufficient radiographic density in the image. The radiographic contrast as well as the absorbed radiation dose in-

creases. The more dense areas in the image on the film are darker. The less dense areas of the film are not penetrated as well, and their images appear brighter by comparison. The density difference between the major areas of the object in the image is more obvious, but small tissue densities in these major areas may not be visible. When an image looks like the two to the left in Figure 11–3 (or see the left image in Fig. 11–16), the radiograph contains incomplete information. This is particularly true in images *kB* and *mB*, of Figure 11–3.

Higher–energy x-ray photons penetrate the object well and allow for sufficient overall density in the radiographic image with the use of a smaller quantity of x-rays (less mAs, or mA and exposure time). The x-ray photons thus produced have a shorter wavelength and are more penetrating. Fewer of these photons are absorbed by the patient.

It is understandable that kVp is considered by some to be more important to radiographic image production than the other primary factors. This status depends upon the presence of an appropriate radiographic density, or overall blackening, of the film. *Milliamperage* (mA) and *exposure time* (seconds, sec) are the primary exposure factors that determine the radiographic density (usually considered as one unit, *milliampere-seconds, mAs*). The mAs and kVp exposure factors must be closely integrated to provide sufficient radiographic density and optimal penetration of the object. mAs alone will not result in penetration of the part nor will there be sufficient radiographic density throughout the image if the part is not properly penetrated. Rules to compensate for maintaining sufficient image density are given later in this chapter.

The use of low–energy x-ray photons is not recommended because of the increased radiation dosage to the patient. The use of excessively high–energy x-ray photons is equally undesirable. At energy levels near or above 100 kVp, all tissues of the human body become well penetrated and appear to merge in the image. As a result, the ability of the viewer to distinguish one structure from the other is lessened. There may be sufficient density but insufficient difference between adjacent densities for small or thin structures to be clearly distinguished from surrounding tissues. These small, thin structures may seem to fuse into the density of the surrounding image, differences becoming vague and ill-defined. This appearance may be caused by scattered radiation reaching the film or by over-penetration of the anatomical part. The result is a loss of information and a "gray, hazy" appearance of the image. This situation is illustrated in the two images on the right in Figure 11–3.

Low–energy x-ray photons may not properly penetrate the anatomical part. The result is an image with extremely dark areas, contrasting with other areas that are exceedingly bright. The dark areas represent areas that are easy to penetrate; those that are bright represent parts that are harder to penetrate. If two or three of the easily penetrated areas are adjacent to each other, they may appear to be one black or excessively

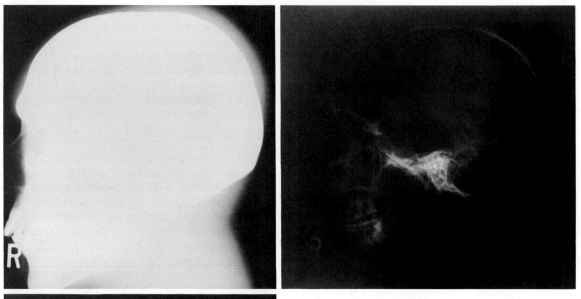

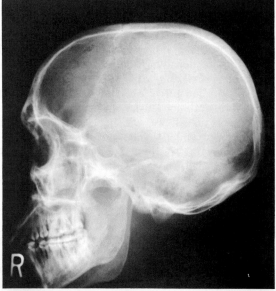

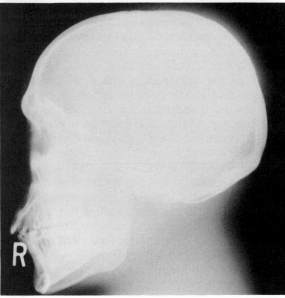

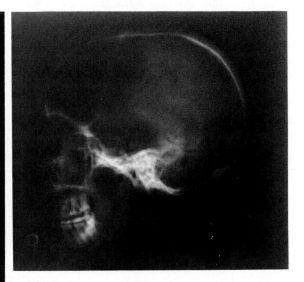

FIGURE 11–3. Underexposure and overexposure of a radiographic image. *A*, A generally acceptable image. The other images represent *A* as it undergoes changes in the single factor specified. The upper row of images represent changes made only in the kilovoltage (k*B*, k*C*), and the lower row has changes only in the milliamperseconds (m*B*, m*C*).

dark image. The same problem can result with adjacent structures that are hard to penetrate. These appear as a single bright structure in the image.

TECHNIQUE CHARTS: PURPOSE AND USE

Technique, or exposure, charts similar to that in Figure 11–4 can be found throughout most radiography departments. Each radiographic room is different. Therefore, each has a *technique chart* that if it is properly designed, will yield a diagnostic-quality radiograph in that specific room. The technique charts in radiographic rooms are devised for the normal, average-sized patients usually examined in the radiology department and the physical characteristics of the x-ray generator and x-ray tube located in that room. A radiographer should refer to the technique chart in the room used for the radiographic procedure. A chart from one room may or may not be capable of producing quality images in another radiographic room.

There are several types and designs of exposure technique charts. Fixed kVp and the variable kVp charts are common. The fixed kVp chart has a specific kilovoltage for each body part and the projection performed, using a specific set of conditions. On this chart, the mAs values vary, depending on the thickness in centimeters (cm) of the anatomical part. The mAs values are usually listed for sets of measurements in centimeters. A set consists of a range between one measurement in centimeters and another.

The variable kVp chart has specific mAs values established for sufficient radiographic density of each anatomical part and projection, using a specific set of conditions. The kVp variants are listed for specific measurements in centimeters. The measurements for which kVp values are listed are usually 2 cm apart (e.g., 10 cm, 12 cm, 14 cm), although in the sample depicted in Figure 11–5, factors are listed for each centimeter.

Conditions of exposure other than the primary exposure factors that are given by each chart usually include the following:

- Anatomical part to be radiographed
- Projection to be performed
- Screen-film (S/F) combination to be used (this may not appear if the exposure condition is standardized for the department)
- Use of grid (Bucky) or nongrid exposure is specified; if a grid-exposure technique, the type of grid is specified by its line count, grid ratio, whether moving (Bucky) or stationary, the focal range (if a focused grid), and so forth
- Correction factors for the mA or exposure time, selected to produce the necessary density if applicable

The following is a procedure using a variable kVp technique chart:

1. Determine the thickness in centimeters by measuring the anatomical part to be radiographed. The measurement must be along the path of the central portion of the x-ray beam (central ray) through the part.
2. Locate on the chart the name of the anatomical part and the projection to be performed. This part of the technique chart is shown in Figure 11–6.
3. Listed with the part and projection are various measurement values (in centimeters) with corresponding primary technical factors (mA value, kVp value, etc.). The measurement value of the part for a particular projection is usually listed, increasing from left to right in *increments* of 2 cm. For each measurement value, a kVp value that will penetrate the part and a corresponding mAs value to provide the correct radiographic density is listed. The value for an AP projection of an abdomen 20 cm thick is given in Figure 11–7. The mAs value is usually given as a single number that represents the product of the mA and exposure time (in seconds) to be used, but some technique charts list the mA value and the exposure time separately.
4. If the machine is equipped for checking and adjusting the accuracy of the line voltage to the x-ray generator, do this before proceeding with the radiographic examination. The line voltage adjustment is automatic in most modern equipment.
5. At the control panel, select the correct kVp and mAs values required for the exposure.
6. Go into the radiographic room. Make sure the source-image distance (SID) is as specified and that the film-screen combination selected is the one listed by the technique chart. Having done this, the radiographer can proceed with the patient examination.

The procedure is simple. The problem is that patients are not "average". Most patients vary from the average in size, muscle tonus, or pathology present. These variations must be considered, and any necessary adjustments in exposure factors must be made before the radiation exposure.

The technique chart is established as a guide to exposure factors that will yield radiographs consistent with the radiographic density and contrast levels generally required within a particular radiology department. The *radiologist* may review the initial radiographs of a patient and request another image with either more or less contrast than that in the image produced. The radiographer must then adjust the given exposure factors to achieve a radiographic image with the requested change in contrast. The information the radiographer needs in order to do this is discussed in this and subsequent chapters.

Good radiographs are difficult to produce every time, because the exposure conditions change with each patient, part, projection, radiographic unit, and pathology. The radiographer adapts for the new exposure conditions each time a *requisition* for a radiologic consultation is received.

UNIV. OF ALABAMA RADIOLOGY PROG.   ROOM 213B   SEPTEMBER 4▼1990

CHEST-RIBS

CHEST PA GRID   72 "
CM	16	18	20	22	24	26	28	30	32	34	36	38	40
KV	110	110	110	110	110	110	110	110	110	110	110	110	110
MAS	0.45	0.6	0.8	1.4	1.7	2.2	3.5	4.5	5.7	7.6	10.2	11.9	15.4

CHEST LAT.GRID   72 "
CM	24	26	28	30	32	34	36	38	40	42	44	46	48
KV	110	110	110	110	110	110	110	110	110	110	110	110	110
MAS	2.6	2.9	3.5	4.5	5.7	7.6	10.2	12	15	20	31	37	51

CHEST PA NON GRID   72 "
CM	16	18	20	22	24	26	29	30	32	34	36	38	40
KV	90	90	90	90	90	90	90	90	90	90	90	90	90
MAS	0.66	0.89	1.1	1.7	2.2	2.9	3.3	3.9	4.4	5.6	8.9	10.9	13.3

CHEST LAT NON GRID   72 "
CM	24	26	28	30	32	34	36	38	40	42	44	46	48
KV	90	90	90	90	90	90	90	90	90	90	90	90	90
MAS	2.9	3.1	3.87	5.64	6.04	7.65	10.9	13.7	17.3	23.4	33	42.7	58.4

RIBS UPPER AP   40 " BUCKY- FOR LOWER RIB USE ABD. TECH.
CM	10	12	14	16	18	20	22	24	26	28	30	32	34
KV	70	70	70	70	70	70	70	70	70	70	70	70	70
MAS	3.7	5.5	7.3	9.0	13.2	18.5	20	24	26	33	37	42	51

ABDOMEN

ABDOMEN   40 "   BUCKY
CM	16	18	20	22	24	26	28	30	32	34	36	38	40
KV	70	70	70	70	70	70	80	80	80	80	80	80	80
MAS	18	28	40	57	82	106	81	122	138	179	203	264	325

UGI BE   40 "   SINGLE CONTRAST 110   KV MASx 0.9
CM	16	18	20	22	24	26	28	30	32	34	36	38	40
KV	90	90	90	90	90	90	90	90	90	90	90	90	90
MAS	4.6	7.4	11.1	14.8	20.3	25	36	50	64	84	100	139	167

PELVIMETRY   40 "   BUCKY
CM	24	26	28	30	32	34	36	38	40	42
KV	120	120	120	120	120	120	120	120	120	120
MAS	13	15	18	20	23	26	29	39	47	59

EXTREMITY

SHOULDER AP   40 "   BUCKY
CM	8	9	10	11	12	13	14	15	16	17	18	19	20
KV	70	70	70	70	70	70	70	70	70	70	70	70	70
MAS	6	7	9	10	11	13	15	18	20	25	28	30	36

SHOULDER TRANSTHORACIC   40 "   GRID
CM	16	18	20	22	24	26	28	30	32	34	36	38	40
KV	90	90	90	90	90	90	90	90	90	90	90	90	90
MAS	8	11	15	16	22	25	28	35	40	47	59	75	94

PELVIS & FEMUR   40 "   BUCKY
CM	14	16	18	20	22	24	26	28	30	32	34
KV	70	70	70	70	70	70	70	80	80	80	80
MAS	11	16	24	33	49	57	69	45	49	65	98

KNEE AP & LAT   40 "   BUCKY
CM	8	9	10	11	12	13	14	15	16
KV	70	70	70	70	70	70	70	70	70
MAS	4	5	6	7	9	10	11	13	15

EXTREMITIES DETAIL SCREENS   40 " TABLE TOP DETAIL FACTOR = 3.99
CM	2	3	4	5	6	7	8	9	10	11	12	13	14
KV	58	58	58	60	60	63	66	70	70	70	70	70	70
MAS	3.1	3.6	4.1	5.1	5.1	5.4	5.5	5.1	6.2	7.3	8.5	9.0	10.1

EXTREMITIES REGULAR SCREENS   40 " TABLE TOP
CM	2	3	4	5	6	7	8	9	10	11	12	13	14
KV	58	58	58	58	60	63	66	70	70	70	70	70	70
MAS	0.77	0.91	1.02	1.28	1.28	1.35	1.37	1.28	1.56	1.84	2.13	2.27	2.53

MA STATION CONVERSION FACTORS
MA STATION 100 200 300
FACTOR   1 0.97 1.07

SKULL-SPINE

SKULL AP   40 "   BUCKY
CM	18	19	20	21	22	FOR LAT. USE 70 KV
KV	80	80	80	80	80	FOR TOWNES USE 86 KV
MAS	11	15	16	17	18	

C-SPINE LAT.   72 "   GRID
CM	5	6	7	8	9	10	11	12	13	14	15	16
KV	70	70	70	70	70	70	70	70	70	70	70	70
MAS	10	11	13	20	24	29	33	41	49	57	65	73

C-SPINE AP   40 "   BUCKY
CM	5	6	7	8	9	10	11	12	13	14	15	16
KV	70	70	70	70	70	70	70	70	70	70	70	70
MAS	3.7	4.4	5.4	6.5	7.6	8.6	10.9	13.2	14.5	15.8	19.8	21.1

T-SPINE AP   40 "   BUCKY
CM	16	18	20	22	24	26	28	30	32	34	36	38	40	42
KV	75	75	75	75	75	75	75	75	75	75	75	75	75	75
MAS	6	11	15	21	31	39	60	91	102	120	145	205	229	241

T-SPINE LAT   40 "   BUCKY
CM	18	20	22	24	26	28	30	32	34	36	38	40	42	44
KV	85	85	85	85	85	85	85	85	85	85	85	85	85	85
MAS	6	7	8	9	12	14	17	19	26	31	38	48	72	84

L-SPINE AP   40 "   BUCKY
CM	16	18	20	22	24	26	28	30	32	34	36	38	40	42
KV	75	75	75	75	75	75	85	85	85	85	85	85	85	85
MAS	20	32	43	63	91	117	90	135	153	180	216	306	342	360

L-SPINE LAT.   40 "   BUCKY
CM	20	22	24	26	28	30	32	34	36	38	40	42	44
KV	90	90	90	90	90	90	90	90	90	90	90	90	90
MAS	25	30	33	42	50	60	67	92	108	133	167	251	292

PEDIATRICS

SKULL CHILD   40 "   BUCKY
CM	7	9	11	13	15	17
KV	70	70	70	70	70	
MAS	1.6	2.4	3.3	5	12	18

CHEST CHILD PA & LAT   72 "   NON GRID
CM	6	7	8	9	10	11	12	13	14	15	16	18
KV	60	60	60	60	60	60	60	60	60	60	60	60
MAS	3.1	3.4	3.8	4.4	4.6	4.8	5.5	5.8	6.0	6.2	6.9	8.5

RIBS UPPER CHILD   40 "   BUCKY
CM	6	7	8	9	10	11	12	13	USE ABDOMEN TECH.
KV	60	60	60	60	60	60	60	60	
MAS	1.1	1.6	1.8	2.1	3.6	3.9	4.8	5.3	FOR LOWER RIBS

T-SPINE CHILD AP   40 "   BUCKY
CM	4	5	6	7	8	9	10	11	12	13
KV	70	70	70	70	70	70	70	70	70	
MAS	1.8	2.3	3.0	3.6	4.2	4.7	5.8	7.0	7.8	9.5

T-SPINE CHILD LAT.   40 "   BUCKY
CM	10	11	12	13	14	15	16	17	18	19	20	21
KV	60	60	60	60	60	60	60	60	60	60	60	60
MAS	8	10	12	14	17	18	20	21	23	25	29	32

L-SPINE CHILD AP   40 "   BUCKY
CM	5	6	7	8	9	10	11	12	13	14
KV	70	70	70	70	70	70	70	70	70	70
MAS	1.2	1.5	2.0	2.4	2.9	3.3	4.1	4.9	6.5	7.3

L-SPINE CHILD LAT.   40 "   BUCKY
CM	6	8	10	12	14	16	18	20
KV	80	80	80	80	80	80	80	80
MAS	2.4	4.3	5.7	8.6	11.2	14.5	15.8	19.8

ABDOMEN CHILD AP   40 "   BUCKY
CM	5	6	7	8	9	10	11	12	13	14	15	16
KV	70	70	70	70	70	70	70	70	70	70	70	70
MAS	1.2	1.6	2.0	2.4	2.8	3.3	4.1	4.9	6.2	6.9	10.0	12.1

UGI BE CHILD   40 "   SINGLE CONTRAST 110   KV MASx 0.9
CM	5	6	7	8	9	10
KV	90	90	90	90	90	90
MAS	0.64	0.82	1.02	1.25	1.38	1.66

DD	DM	TD	TM	BD	BM	CF	DF
1.4	6.6	1.4	1.6	1.1	5.0	1.2	4.0

ALWAYS USE PROPER COLLIMATION AND PATIENT SHIELDING
SCREEN ALL FEMALE PATIENTS FOR PREGNANCY

FIGURE 11–4. Exposure technique chart. Exposure factors and conditions for radiography of the entire body. Chart is subdivided into groupings (Chest-Ribs, Abdomen, Extremities, Skull-Spine, and Pediatrics) of related parts. (From Support Plus: Computed Exposure Guides. University of Alabama Radiography Program, Birmingham, AL, 1990.)

ABDOMEN							40 "		BUCKY					
CM	16	18	20	22	24	26	28	30	32	34	36	38	40
KV	70	70	70	70	70	70	80	80	80	80	80	80	80
MAS	18	28	40	57	82	106	81	122	138	179	203	264	325

UGI BE					40 "		SINGLE	CONTRAST	110		KV	MASx	0.9
CM	16	18	20	22	24	26	28	30	32	34	36	38	40
KV	90	90	90	90	90	90	90	90	90	90	90	90	90
MAS	4.6	7.4	11.1	14.8	20.3	25	36	50	64	84	100	139	167

PELVIMETRY							40 "		BUCKY	
CM	24	26	28	30	32	34	36	38	40	42
KV	120	120	120	120	120	120	120	120	120	120
MAS	13	15	18	20	23	26	29	39	47	59

FIGURE 11–5. Exposure technique chart: abdomen section. Isolation of the abdomen section of the exposure technique chart. (From Support Plus: Computed Exposure Guides. University of Alabama Radiography Program, Birmingham, AL, 1990.)

ABDOMEN			
CM	16	18	20
KV	70	70	70
MAS	18	28	40

UGI BE			
CM	16	18	20
KV	90	90	90
MAS	4.6	7.4	11.1

PELVIMETRY			
CM	24	26	28
KV	120	120	120
MAS	13	15	18

FIGURE 11–6. Exposure technique chart: examinations. Lists the examinations included in the abdomen section. (From Support Plus: Computed Exposure Guides. University of Alabama Radiography Program, Birmingham, AL, 1990.)

The general factors the radiographer should know about each patient before performing a radiographic examination should appear on the radiographic requisition. This should include patient identification information and the patient's clinical history, current chief complaint, and known physical condition. A sample requisition is shown in Figure 11–8. If the information does not appear on the requisition, the radiographer must determine these factors from the patient. This material assists the radiographer to demonstrate the presence or absence of the suspected pathology or condition in the radiographic image and is necessary for an accurate interpretation of the image by the physician-radiologist.

IMAGE QUALITIES

What is a good radiographic image? What qualities are expected to be present in the image? First, the image of a specific part must appear in an appropriate relationship to other parts on the image receptor. To accomplish this, the radiographer must have an accurate knowledge of human structure and function. Ideally, the plane of the anatomical part should be parallel with that of the imaging surface and should be recorded by a beam whose central ray is perpendicular

to both. This precaution minimizes distortion of the object in the image. If these conditions cannot be achieved, the radiographer must use his or her knowledge of recording radiographic images and decide how best to demonstrate the anatomical part. Second, there must be sufficient radiographic density and contrast to enable the viewer to see maximum *detail* (i.e., recorded detail of small as well as large structures) of the part. Figure 11–9 depicts a quality image and some of the problems experienced in radiography. The images illustrate what occurs when those problems exist. A comparison with similarities found in photographic images can also be made.

Radiographic Density

Radiographic density refers to the overall darkness or blackness of the image when viewed on a normal illuminator (view box). The requirements of a good radiographic image include minimal distortion of the body part for a specific radiographic projection and

ABDOMEN							40 "		BUCKY					
CM	16	18	20	22	24	26	28	30	32	34	36	38	40
KV	70	70	70	70	70	70	80	80	80	80	80	80	80
MAS	18	28	40	57	82	106	81	122	138	179	203	264	325

FIGURE 11–7. Exposure technique chart: exposure factors. Exposure factors for specific measurements of a part of the abdomen. (From Support Plus: Computed Exposure Guides. University of Alabama Radiography Program, Birmingham, AL, 1990.)

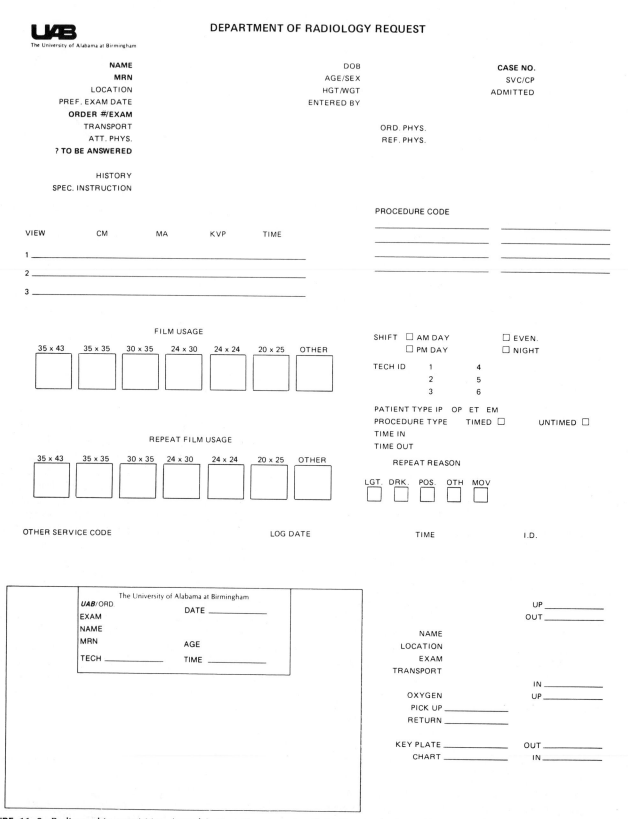

FIGURE 11–8. Radiographic requisition (sample). Form to request radiologic consultation. Titles of blanks indicate information to be entered. A multipurpose form; the upper section conveys patient demographic information, examination requested, and reason; the midsection provides for information from radiology department personnel during the course of the procedure; the lower section provides both the means of transferring information to each film emulsion of the procedure (at *left*) and details for in-patient escort to the radiology department and return to the patient's room. The back of the form has a blanket authorization form to be signed by the patient. (From University of Alabama Hospitals, Birmingham, Department of Radiology referral form.)

sufficient *contrast* to reveal each tissue density within the part. To produce a good radiograph, the radiographer must achieve a quality image while delivering the smallest possible x-radiation exposure to the patient. The radiographer must carefully consider the exposure factors for producing an image before using them. "Scout films," or *preliminary radiographs,* should never be performed merely to gain information about the accuracy of exposure factors. They should be used only to gain specific medical information.

Radiation emerging from the patient after it has passed around and through a patient body part produces *background* and image *density.* The radiation that emerges from the patient and produces image density is called *exit radiation* and is depicted in the Figure 11-10 diagram. Exit radiation is the result of passage of the primary x-ray beam through a patient part. Because of absorption by the body tissues, this emergent beam varies in x-ray distribution. The variation occurs because some of the tissue densities of the body part totally absorb x-rays, some interact with the x-rays to produce *secondary radiation,* and some allow the *primary radiation* to pass through with little or no interaction. If x-radiation is intercepted by a sensitive surface as it emerges from the part, it is converted into an image. The sensitive surface may be a film emulsion or the phosphor layer of an intensifying or fluoroscopic screen (Chapter 13).

In conventional radiography, the emerging beam is usually intercepted by the phosphor layer of an intensifying screen. This screen converts the x-ray energy to light energy and transfers the resulting light image to the emulsion of a film as seen in Figure 11-11. The light ionizes the silver halide crystals of the emulsion to form an image called the *latent image.* This latent image cannot be seen under normal viewing conditions until the film has been chemically processed to reduce the ionized silver salts to black metallic silver. It is the black metallic silver configuration in the emulsion that is referred to as a radiograph. The black metallic silver constitutes the radiographic density of the image.

As mentioned earlier, the primary beam from the x-ray tube is altered as it passes through the patient part. Some of the beam is totally absorbed by the thicker, denser portion of the body part. Little or no *primary radiation* reaches the film behind that part, resulting in a clear, or bright area in the processed image. Other x-rays in the beam area partially absorbed and produce *secondary radiation,* which can also affect the film emulsion. The amount of x-radiation getting through each tissue in the body part depends on the thickness, the atomic number, and the electron density of that tissue, and the kVp used to produce the x-ray beam. The image of the thicker parts is light gray, representing a small amount of black metallic silver in the film emulsion. Thinner parts allow more x-radiation to reach the film emulsion behind them and appear as darker shades of gray. It is this difference in shades of radiographic density within the image that constitutes the image quality known as *radiographic contrast.* Radiographic contrast allows anatomical parts to be distinguished from each other in the image (see Figs. 11-3 and 11-15).

Radiographic Contrast

Radiographic contrast permits visualization of details of the various structures in the body part. Four natural, basic body densities can easily be demonstrated in a radiographic image. These densities involve bone, muscle or fluid, adipose tissue, and gases. In some references, muscle, fluid, and adipose tissues are considered as one because of their extremely similar x-ray absorption characteristics. A fourth possible density included by the latter authors is metal, which is not a natural component of the body.

The first set of tissue densities previously named are components of most human body parts and exist in varying concentrations or thicknesses. In most body parts, one tissue density is superimposed by overlying and underlying tissues with different densities. Therefore, each area in the image varies in effective or average tissue density and x-radiation absorption characteristics as illustrated in Figure 11-12. It is evident that each structure in the body has varying x-ray penetrability characteristics. Radiographic contrast depends on these tissue characteristics, the energy of the applied x-rays, and other factors that can be standardized. This is evident in images of Figure 11-13.

Film Contrast

Radiographic contrast in an image can be separated into two general categories, *subject contrast* and *film contrast.* Film contrast refers to the capabilities of an individual film to permit the production of image contrast. Each film or batch of films has its own contrast, based on the manufacture and processing factors used. The manufacture of each film or film type is strictly standardized and must meet strict quality control standards of the manufacturer. The other factor that affects film contrast is the *chemical development* process. This includes the processing techniques used, chemical characteristics of the processing solutions, and the physical characteristics of the process (time in each solution, temperature of each solution, pH of fixer and developing solution, and so on). In medical radiology departments, the film type or types used, processing techniques, and processing chemistry are standardized for the entire radiology department or for specific department areas. Consistency of radiographic *image contrast* relies on these factors being standardized and remaining constant within each department or area.

Subject Contrast

Subject contrast is the part of image contrast that depends upon penetration of the body part by the x-ray beam, as demonstrated in Figure 11-14*B* (also see Figure 11-15). The penetration of an anatomical part depends on thickness of the part, electron density of the tissue, and the applied x-ray energy.

Four terms are used to differentiate the types of subject contrast. These terms include *long-scale contrast, short-scale contrast, high contrast,* and *low contrast.* The terms related to scale refer to the number of distinctly different densities (i.e., shades of gray) within

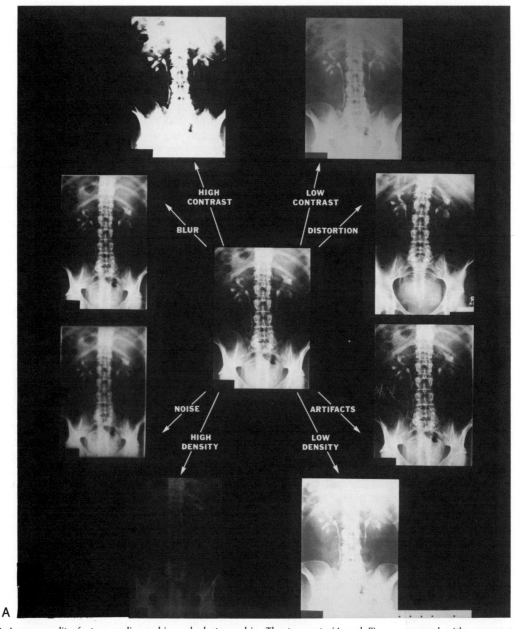

FIGURE 11–9. Image quality factors: radiographic and photographic. The two sets (*A* and *B*) are arranged with respect to specific, listed image quality factors. The central image in each set is considered a good-quality image. The surrounding images represent specific degradations of the center image caused by changes in identified quality factors. (From the ACR Learning File, American College of Radiology Institute.)

Figure continued

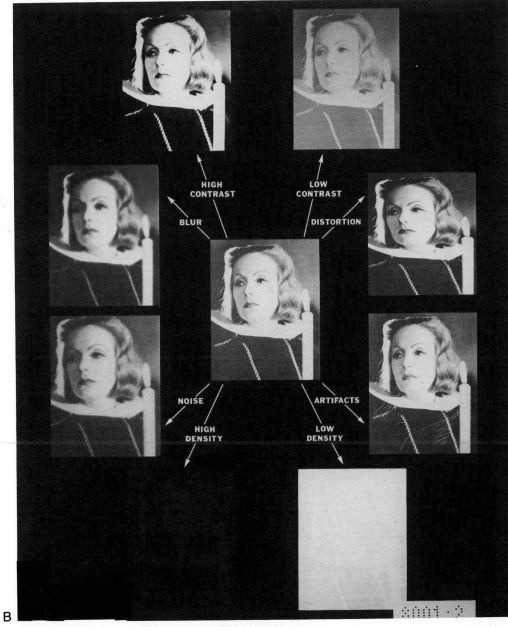

B

FIGURE 11–9. *Continued.*

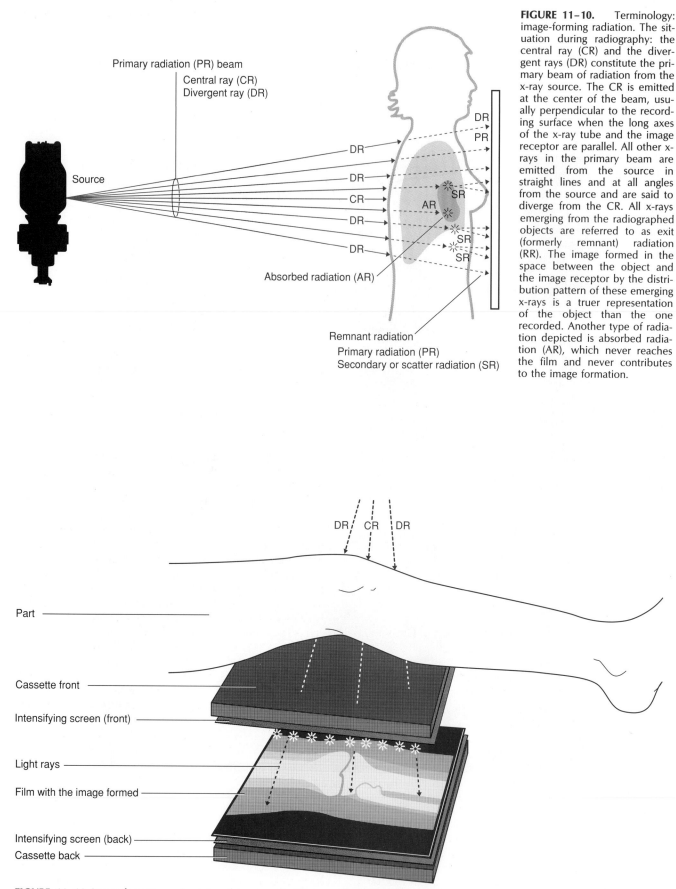

FIGURE 11-10. Terminology: image-forming radiation. The situation during radiography: the central ray (CR) and the divergent rays (DR) constitute the primary beam of radiation from the x-ray source. The CR is emitted at the center of the beam, usually perpendicular to the recording surface when the long axes of the x-ray tube and the image receptor are parallel. All other x-rays in the primary beam are emitted from the source in straight lines and at all angles from the source and are said to diverge from the CR. All x-rays emerging from the radiographed objects are referred to as exit (formerly remnant) radiation (RR). The image formed in the space between the object and the image receptor by the distribution pattern of these emerging x-rays is a truer representation of the object than the one recorded. Another type of radiation depicted is absorbed radiation (AR), which never reaches the film and never contributes to the image formation.

FIGURE 11-11. Image formation using intensifying screens. The x-ray beam (width, DR to DR) passes through the anatomical part and the cassette front. The intensifying screen on the inside surface of the cassette front emits a light pattern equivalent to the pattern of x-ray intensities that passed through the object (knee). This light pattern is transferred to the sensitive crystals of the film. When the film is chemically processed, the light pattern becomes visible (as demonstrated). The image is shown removed to a significant distance from the front screen in order to illustrate the light emitted from the latter. The intensifying screen attached to the back of the cassette has been sketched in correct relation to the overlying film.

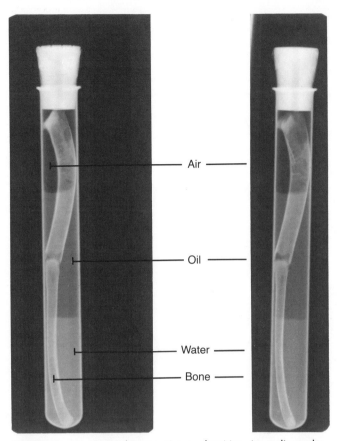

FIGURE 11–12. Basic human tissue densities in radiography. Images are of a test tube containing layers of air (upper layer), oil (middle layer), representing adipose tissue; water (lower layer), representing most muscle tissue. A small dry bone was immersed in these. The radiographic density for each tissue is as follows: air, 1.72; oil, 1.30; water, 1.07. Bone measured in the bone marrow area varies in each layer: bone with air, 1.13; bone with oil, 1.04; and bone with water, 0.84.

tinct density shades to demonstrate a satisfactory scale of contrast. The difference between adjacent densities that must be present to be considered distinct is 0.2 (determined with *densitometer* readings). The discussion of scales of contrast does not refer to a value of density difference except to establish a value setting limits for visibility when counting the number of density shades.

Density values determined by a densitometer are logarithmic values. In order to determine the equivalent increase or decrease in exposure between two or more areas, the antilog of the difference in density values of the two areas must be recognized. A 0.3-change in *density value* (densitometer measure) is equivalent to multiplying the mAs by 2. The density in this case has changed one hundred percent, or doubled. A densitometer reading that differs from an adjacent one by 0.1 varies from the adjacent density by approximately 26%. This means that the second density is approximately 1.26 times greater than the first, lesser one. This number indicates that the exposure to the film at the location of the second density is 1.26 times that received at the area of the first. Thus if the *intensity* (MR) of exposure to the film was 100 mR at point one, exposure at point two would be 126 mR. There is a direct relationship between intensity and film density.

A 26% difference in radiographic density is within the range of percentage difference usually listed as visually detectable (25% to 35% difference in density). The range of density values corresponding to the 25% to 35% range of difference in density may vary from 0.097 to 0.131. The adjacent densities that vary by these values in an image of a penetrometer (Fig. 11–15) are easily seen. In an anatomical image they may be difficult to recognize and distinguish from each other. A 0.2 difference in density value determined by using densitometer readings is approximately equivalent to a 58% exposure change from one area of the film when compared with an adjacent area. Parts that display this difference should be evident on a visual scan of the image in which the 0.2 differences in density value are found next to each other. If parts with these density values are separated by parts with density values of 0.1 to 0.2, even their value differences are not as easily recognized. Readers are invited to try this (see Fig. 11–23).

The contrast scales (long, short) and the degree of contrast (low, high) depend on penetration of the individual parts depicted in a radiographed area. The brightness or grayness of an image depends on the overall radiographic density of the image. This overall image density can be produced in a number of ways, but the preferable way is by primary radiation emerging from the part after penetrating it. Bright images are often produced by insufficient exposure (mAs or kVp) factors to provide the needed radiographic density. Gray, hazy images often have too much overall radiographic density, which results from the use of excessive exposure factors for the part or from some type of fog, as demonstrated in Figures 11–14B, 11–15, or 11–16.

an image. The last two terms refer to the difference or, more correctly, the percentage of difference between adjacent density shades (gray areas). Many radiography practitioners, when referring to images, use the term *low contrast* as if it is synonymous with *long scale* of contrast. They also use *high contrast* synonymously with *short scale* of contrast. Although the terms are synonymous in many cases, such references are erroneous. To add to the confusion, many practitioners consider all bright images as high contrast with a short scale of contrast. To these persons, an overall gray image has low contrast and a long scale of contrast.

One reference (Phillips, 1987) seems to recommend that such terms be eliminated when speaking of radiographic quality and does recommend assignment of specific numbers to a satisfactory scale of contrast: specifically, an image of a distal extremity must possess four or more distinct density shades to exhibit a satisfactory scale of contrast. The same reference states, an image of the torso or one produced using a Bucky grid exposure technique must possess six or more dis-

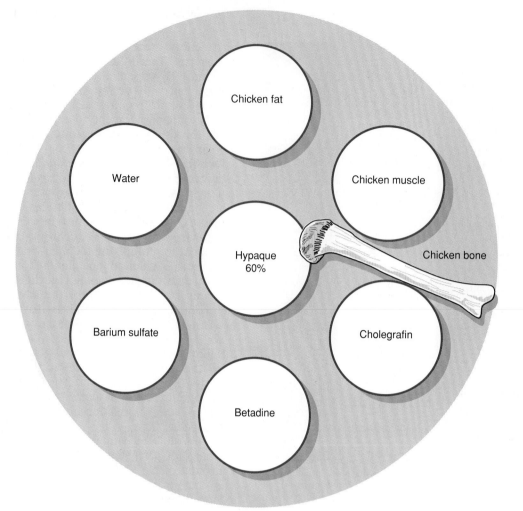

A

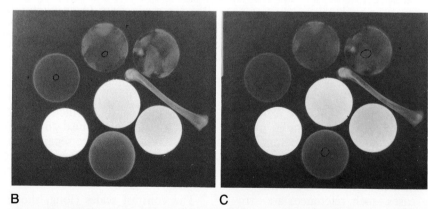

B   C

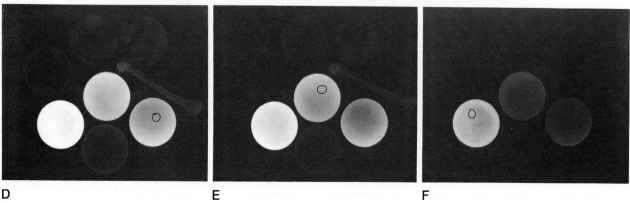

D   E   F

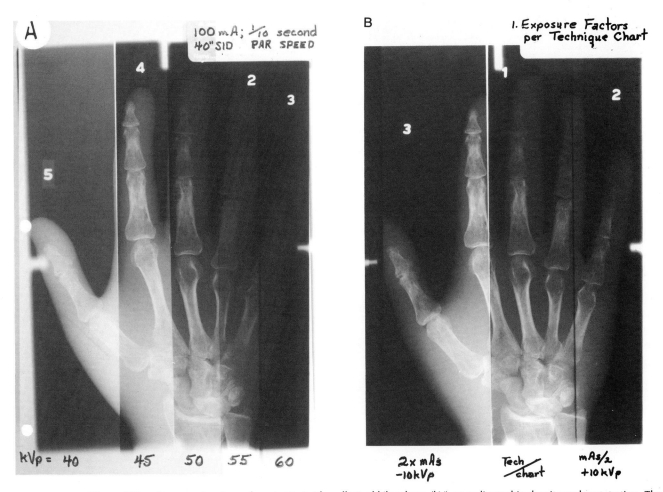

FIGURE 11-14. Effect of kilovoltage on density and contrast. *A,* The effect of kilovoltage (kV) on radiographic density and penetration. The peak kilovoltage (kVp) was increased from 40 to 60 in increments of 5. As the kVp increased, the radiographic density of the image increased. The bright images seen at 40 and 45 kVp begin to disappear or to become gray as the kVp increases. This indicates that these parts have been penetrated more than in earlier exposures. *B,* The effect of kVp on radiographic contrast. A lower kVp (radiation field 3 of the image) with a sufficient density demonstrates a greater difference between the shades of gray in the image (higher contrast). The higher kVp (radiation field 2) with the lower mAs demonstrates outlines of all the parts, but they are less distinct, because the differences between the adjacent densities has been reduced (lower contrast).

FIGURE 11-13. Absorption of radiation: tissue types and contrast media. Materials radiographed were 10 ml each of diatrizoate meglumine (Hypaque) 60%, cholegrafin (a lesser concentrate of iodinated contrast material), water, povidone-iodine (Betadine), and barium sulfate; a 2-cm layer each of uncooked chicken fat and uncooked chicken muscle; and 1 chicken bone (not dry). Materials radiographed, except for the chicken bone, were placed in 3-oz paper cups. Various exposures were used to determine the kilovoltage level needed to bring each of the materials to the same density value. The same milliampereseconds (mAs), source-image distance (SID), screen-film speed, and processing were used for all exposures. The radiographic density value sought for each material was 0.88 ± 0.05. *A* is a diagram of the arrangement of the materials radiographed.

In *B* (71 kVp), an equal density (0.88) was found for water and chicken fat. Betadine had a lower density but was within the limiting criterion. Muscle had a density value just outside the limit. *C* (74 kVp), density value of muscle was 0.89 and of bone, 0.83. *D* (97 kVp), the next material to exhibit a density value near 0.88 was cholegrafin (0.89). *E,* Hypaque 60% reached a density value of 0.82 at 105 kVp. *F,* Barium sulfate's density value at 140 kVp was 0.88, the same density value as water and chicken fat exhibited in *B.*

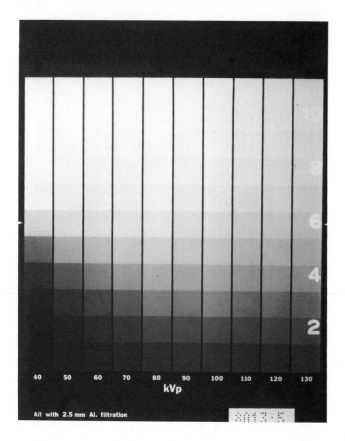

FIGURE 11–15. Effect of kilovoltage on radiographic contrast. The image of the penetrometer portrays the effect of kilovoltage on radiographic contrast. The kilovoltages ranged from a kilovoltage peak (kVp) of 40 through 130 kVp. Step 6 of the penetrometer is of approximately the same density value at all exposures. Study the image with regard to the number of distinct density shades visible at each kVp used; compare findings. This image helps clarify occurrences in Figure 11–16. (From the ACR Learning File, American College of Radiology Institute.)

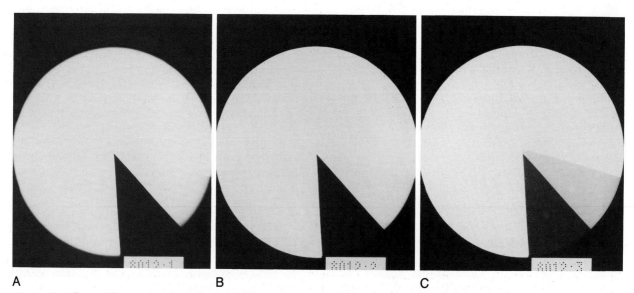

A   B   C

FIGURE 11–16. Effect of large area contrast on visibility of small objects. *A* through *C,* Three images of a circular penetrometer with decreasing area contrast. *A,* Highest area contrast; with normal illumination, only 1 lesion is seen. *B,* Less area contrast; with normal illumination, 2 lesions are seen. *C,* Least area contrast; with normal illumination, 4 lesions can be seen. It can be concluded from these images that radiographic images with a high area contrast demonstrate fewer small densities. When the area contrast is decreased those densities become visible. (From the ACR Learning File, American College of Radiology Institute.)

Fogging of the image can be traced to a number of other sources. These sources include

- Concentration or temperature of the processing chemicals is too high, especially the *developer* solution
- The storage area for unexposed film is at a temperature that is too high (over 75°F) or at an excessive *humidity* (over 60%)
- *Safelights* are mounted too close to the work surface in the darkroom, where film is loaded into cassettes
- Safelight bulbs are of a higher wattage than that specified for the particular film type in use
- Too many safelights are used in the darkroom
- The *safelight filter* is not the type recommended for use with the particular film type, or there may be a light leak around the filter or through a crack in the filter
- "White" light is leaking into the darkroom
- The grid ratio for the kVp level used to penetrate the tissue density or volume of the part is not correct, resulting in excessive *scatter radiation* reaching the film
- The area covered by the primary x-ray beam is larger than necessary to record the image of the part, producing excessive scatter radiation that reaches the film

Subject contrast varies with each patient. For each patient the radiographer is required to determine the variations in exposure factors and to make the appropriate technical adjustments. To do this, the radiographer must consider part thickness, tissue densities involved, various tissues that normally overlie (superimpose) each other in the projection to be performed, pathology (present or suspected) and its effect on the tissue in which it exists, and the devices available for producing the most shades of density with the greatest difference between the adjacent densities. After considering the type of film-screen combinations available and the characteristics of the available x-ray equipment, there are three basic questions to which the radiographer must determine the answers. These are

1. What is the normal anatomy of this part and how is it structured?
2. What imaging devices and exposure factors should be used to produce the best radiograph of this part under normal conditions?
3. What about this radiographic procedure differs from normal exposure conditions, and what must be done to compensate for the differences identified?

The radiographer must determine the correct answers to these questions to produce a satisfactory image. The radiographic density must provide sufficient density differences (contrast) between adjacent structures to demonstrate clearly defined images of each structural entity. To be a good radiograph, the image must demonstrate the structures of the part clearly (see Fig. 11–2).

Radiographic Detail

The clarity and sharpness of individual body structures in the image of the part are referred to as *radiographic detail*. Other words used in connection with this radiographic quality include image sharpness and resolution (differentiation of one structure from another). Radiographic detail has two important components—production and visibility.

Production of radiographic detail depends on a number of geometric factors, including those introduced by the materials used to produce the image, the size of the source of x-radiation, and motion of the body part. Visibility depends on the photographic properties of the image, radiographic contrast, and radiographic density. These subjects are addressed in much of this chapter. The geometric production of image sharpness and the use of devices to enhance visibility are discussed in a later chapter.

Radiographic Distortion

Another property of radiographs is distortion, which is usually undesirable in a radiographic image. *Distortion* is literally defined as *misrepresentation* and may be applied to the size or the shape of the object in the image.

Shape Distortion

Misrepresentation of shape is sometimes called true distortion or simply distortion. This usually describes an undesirable characteristic of the object in the image. It is caused by angulation of one or more of the three major elements of a radiographic exposure in relation to the other two. To avoid distortion, the plane of the anatomical part must be parallel to the plane of the image receptor, and the beam's central ray must be centered and perpendicular to both of these. If any one is positioned at an angle to the other two, the result is a *foreshortening* of one section and an *elongation* of another section of a body part in the image, as illustrated in Figure 11–17. If a part appears to be shorter in its image than it actually is, it is said to be foreshortened. If, however, the image appears to be longer than the part's actual length, it is elongated.

In some radiographic projections, distortion is deliberately introduced. This is done to remove the superimposition on a specific body part of primary interest by another part of equal or greater tissue density. Distortion is also chosen when it is necessary to place the plane of a particular structure that lies in an oblique plane in the body parallel to the plane of the image receptor or perpendicular to the x-ray beam. In either case, distortion of the other structures in the part is acceptable if the structure of primary interest is clearly visible, as in Figure 11–18.

Distortion is a natural part of every radiograph of a large area, such as the abdomen or pelvis, when lower *source-image distances* (SIDs) of 36 to 44 inches are

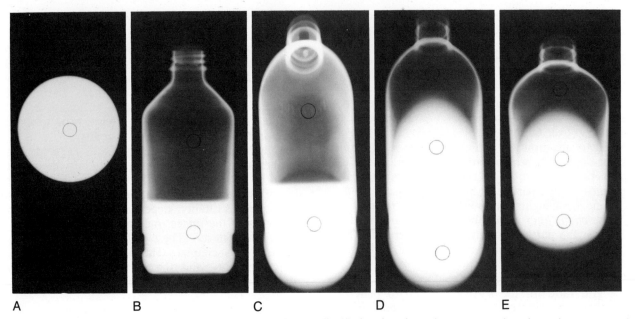

A   B   C   D   E

FIGURE 11-17. Radiographic distortion. Images are of a bottle partially filled with iodinated contrast media. These demonstrate what misrepresentations of the object in the image can occur in given instances. The relationship of the central beam, image receptor, and the part are given for each image. *A,* Long axis of the part and the central ray are coincident with each other and perpendicular to the plane of the film. *B,* Long axis of the part and plane of the film are parallel; the central ray is perpendicular to both. *C,* Long axis of the part and plane of the film are parallel and are at a 45° angle with the horizontal plane; the central ray is at the midpoint in a horizontal direction. *D,* Long axis of the part and plane of the film are parallel and at a 45° angle with the horizontal plane; the central ray is at the midpoint in a vertical direction. *E,* Long axis of the part is at a 45° angle to the horizontal plane, plane of the film is horizontal, and the central ray is directed vertically. (From the University of Alabama at Birmingham Radiographer Program Teaching file.)

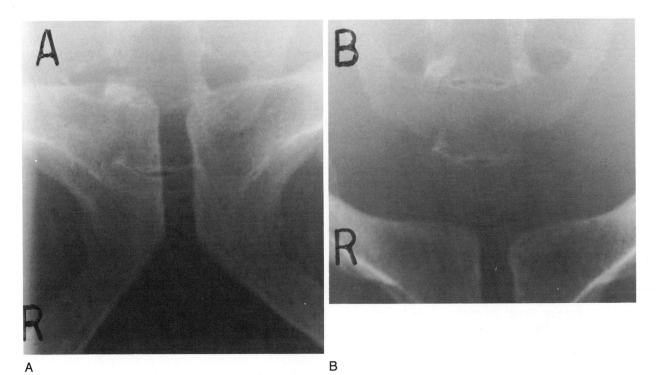

A   B

FIGURE 11-18. Purposeful radiographic distortion. Images of the coccyx. *A,* Performed with the central ray perpendicular to the film through the coccyx. The coccyx is superimposed on the pubic bones and is foreshortened or "stacked" in this projection. *B,* The central ray is directed perpendicular to the plane of the coccyx (at a caudal angle of slightly more than the average number of degrees listed by most positioning books because of the shape of the phantom pelvis). The right-side marker was on the initial exposure and was used as the reference for the "R", which was inked onto each image.

used. This distortion cannot be avoided. It occurs at the edges of the image, laterally and at both ends. These are the portions produced by the divergent rays of the primary x-ray beam.

Size Distortion

Misrepresentation of object size in the image occurs in every radiograph as slight magnification. Generally, the radiographer makes an effort to reduce this to a minimum or an acceptably low level.

Magnification of the object in the radiographic image often occurs because the exposure factors or conditions that must exist to minimize it cannot be achieved. These factors include

- Inability to place the anatomical part as near the recording surface as possible
- Inability to achieve the SID necessary for the exposure
- Condition of the patient does not permit the exposure conditions necessary
- Physical environment in which radiography is being performed does not permit achievement of exposure factors or conditions necessary

In radiography of specific structures or conditions, *magnification* can be used in order to enhance visualization of the part. This is particularly true for parts that are small or difficult to visualize in a routine radiograph of the area in which the part is located. In order to accomplish this the ratio of the SID to the *source-object distance* (SOD) is decreased. Usually, this is done by increasing the distance between the object and the film (OID) and using the same distance between the tube anode and the film (SID). A radiograph produced in this manner is called a macroradiograph.

The magnification causes some blurring of image sharpness and requires the use of specific factors or devices not considered for routine radiography to control this loss of recorded detail (Fig. 11–19).

PRIMARY EXPOSURE FACTORS IN RADIOGRAPHY

Several secondary exposure factors affect the appearance of the radiographic image. These are generally used to refine the appearance of the image and are discussed in later chapters. It is important that the primary factors be correct before the secondary ones are considered. No adjustment of secondary factors will compensate for the use of incorrect primary exposure factors in radiography. The primary factors have been identified as kilovoltage (kVp), amperage or milliamperage (mA), exposure time (seconds or milliseconds), and source-image distance (SID); also source-receptor distance (SRD), source-image receptor distance (SIRD), tube-film distance (TFD), anode-film distance (AFD), and focal-film distance (FFD).

Kilovoltage

Kilovoltage (kV) is the term used most often when referring to the energy to produce x-rays for diagnostic imaging. It is explained in the radiographic physics chapters (Chaps 1 to 4) that the term actually refers to the *peak kilovoltage* (kVp) required to supply the effective kilovoltage necessary to produce the x-rays to penetrate a body part and to provide an adequate ra-

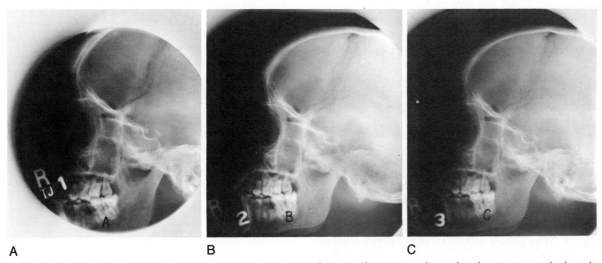

| A | B | C |

FIGURE 11–19. Radiographic changes with source-image distance (SID) changes. Changes in radiographic density occurred when the SID moved from 40 inches (A) to 72 inches (B). Exposure factors were compensated for the SID change. C involves adjustment in exposure factors to lengthen the scale of radiographic contrast that existed in B. Image B or C is acceptable. Between A (40 inches SID) and B (72 inches SID), there is change in the degree of magnification in the image. B presents a more accurate measurement of the parts of interest. For example, an anteroposterior oblique diameter of the sphenoid sinus in A is 4 cm, whereas in B the same diameter measures 3.6 cm. This represents a 10% change in magnification.

diographic density in the image. A large voltage (in the thousands) is required to produce diagnostically useful x-rays, hence the use of the term *kilovolts* or *kilovoltage*. Therefore, the radiographer refers to 80 kV or 80 kVp, instead of 80,000 volts as a requirement for exposure.

The kVp used to produce an image depends on a number of factors. However, before these factors are considered, the penetration of the part must be assured. The part and its physical characteristics determine the minimum kVp needed to penetrate it.

The minimum kVp selected for a specific exposure is determined by the thickness of the part, tissue types and densities within the part, and the equipment that will produce the exposure. Other factors of exposure that may effect changes in the kilovoltage selected include beam restriction, use of a grid (if applicable), contrast and density level preference of the radiologist, screen-film combinations available for use, probability of part motion, and use of contrast material. The minimum kVp needed to penetrate any part is usually found by using the exposure technique chart or by measuring the thickness of the part through the path of the central ray, multiplying that centimeter measurement by 2 and adding some constant factor. The rule of thumb for determining the minimum kVp, which has been followed for years, is 2 times the measurement in centimeters of the body part plus 30 for single-phase (1ϕ) equipment and then 2 times the measurement in centimeters plus 25 for three-phase (3ϕ) equipment. The rule gives consideration to the thickness of the part and the difference in equipment. If minimum kilovoltage is used, the exposure relies primarily on milliamperage and exposure time to provide the proper radiographic density of the image.

Most modern diagnostic radiology departments do not use minimum kVp levels for radiography. Higher kilovoltages are employed to reduce the absorbed dose of radiation to the patient. In many such cases, the part is measured, and the formula is used with a constant of a higher value added to determine the kVp required. A lower mAs value is used in conjunction with the higher kilovoltage. The scale of radiographic contrast is increased, and the difference between the adjacent densities (subject contrast) is reduced while maintaining the same average radiographic density of the image. This is demonstrated in Figure 11–14*B*; see also Figure 11–23.

Kilovoltages listed in technique charts have been established for use with persons in whom the tissues constituting each part are normal in type and distribution. Exposure technique charts do not generally list minimum kVp levels. All elements the radiology department considers important in the formulation of correct exposure factors for a body part except individual patient characteristics are considered when establishing the technique chart. With many *pathologies* and the variations in patients, there may be a need to adjust one or more of the primary factors to obtain a good diagnostic image of a specific body part for each patient examined.

Adjustment of Exposure Factors

Note. Although it is uncommon to provide a radiograph of a pregnant patient, an emergency situation may necessitate such a study. In that case, the radiographer must adjust exposure factors to reduce radiation exposure to the fetus and take into account the presence of excess fluid and other factors that affect image quality. The following example is considered for the purpose of illustrating important points that must be reviewed before such an examination.

Remember, there are questions the radiographer needs to answer before proceeding with any radiographic study. Each patient is different and should receive individual consideration for examination. The intent of the next few paragraphs is to illustrate the process, using a patient who is pregnant.

The normal anatomy of the abdomen is superiorly limited by the diaphragm and inferiorly by the pelvis. Between these two limits there are many tissues and electron densities, anatomical parts, and part thicknesses. A radiograph of the abdomen should have a longer scale of radiographic contrast to demonstrate all the variant tissue densities in the abdominal cavity. The kVp required is in the middle- to high-kV range. The exact kVp depends on the screen-film combination to be used. Bony structures must be well demonstrated. These include the spine from approximately the ninth or tenth thoracic vertebra through the tip of the coccyx, the lower ribs, and the bones of the pelvis to the upper anterior margins of the pubic rami. Soft tissue shadows of the lower border of the liver, kidneys, and psoas muscles should also be demonstrated.

The imaging devices and exposure conditions yielding the best demonstration of the structures in the normal abdomen include a lower mAs and a higher kVp than the radiographer would use to demonstrate the bony structures alone. To relax the abdominal muscles and to allow maximum separation of the abdominal contents and better radiographic demonstration, the exposure should be made at the end of suspended full exhalation. It is usually adequate to use those exposure factors and conditions identified by the technique chart for a recumbent abdomen.

A woman six months pregnant enters the department with a radiographic requisition for an AP projection of the abdomen. Because the patient is pregnant, the radiologist is notified of the ordered examination. The radiologist determines that there is a medical need for the projection. He does this either from the pertinent history included on the requisition form or by consultation with the referring physician. The radiologist notifies the radiographer to proceed with the examination.

In this case, let us assume the following conditions exist:

- The radiographic machine available for use has a 1ϕ generator
- The patient's abdomen measures 30 cm for the AP projection

- The exposure technique for an AP projection of the abdomen found on the technique chart is

    Bucky/grid = 12:1   mAs = 140
    kVp = 80   SID = 40 inches
    S/F speed = 400

This patient differs from the average patient; she is pregnant. This means there is excess fluid (amniotic fluid surrounding the fetus) in the abdomen that must be penetrated, the radiation dosage absorbed by the fetus should be kept as low as possible, and there is a possibility of blurring of the image caused by motion of mother or the fetus. More kVp is needed to penetrate the excess fluid. The radiation used should not easily be absorbed by the fetus. To accomplish this, the radiographer should avoid any addition of mAs and if possible, should reduce that factor. As to the hazard of blurring the image because of motion, the mother's motion can usually be controlled by clearly explaining the need for carefully following breathing instructions and controlling any motion. Another problem is fetal movement, which occurs in response to certain stimuli, and effort must be directed toward avoiding such movement.

Each of these problems is confronted separately.

- What is the probability of fetal motion at the time required by the exposure factors listed by the technique chart?

    If the probability is low, the radiographer may choose to use exposure factors from the technique chart adjusted only for increased fluid content of abdomen. This is not the preferred choice of exposure factors, because the absorbed radiation dosage will be higher than if adjustments are made in the exposure factors.

    If the probability is high and the patient's suspected condition requires relatively high radiographic contrast, fetal motion can be controlled by decreasing the exposure time as much as possible and altering the breathing instructions to the patient. The exposure change is accomplished by using the largest mA available coupled with the smallest unit of time consistent with the accuracy limitations of the exposure times for Bucky (grid) exposures. The product must be equal to the mAs value required. In the case cited, the product of the mA and exposure time must equal 140 mAs (the mAs value required by the technique chart).

    Breathing instructions normally given for abdominal AP projections are to request that the patient suspend breathing at the end of full exhalation. However, these breathing instructions will result in diminished oxygen content of blood circulated from mother to fetus, and the response will be fetal movement. The normal breathing instructions should be altered by having the patient inhale deeply approximately three times immediately before suspending respiration at full exhalation for the exposure. This method increases the oxygen content of the mother's circulating blood, which gradually de-

creases to a normal level as the exposure occurs. The probability of fetal motion during the exposure is reduced.

- Will the condition be demonstrated with the use of a longer-scale contrast and less difference between densities? The radiographer's answer to this question depends on the need for the examination.

    If the condition cannot be demonstrated by using a longer-contrast scale, the radiographer may use exposure factors from the technique chart adjusted only for penetration of the increased fluid content of the abdomen. This should provide an image with the desired contrast scale.

    If the condition can be well demonstrated with a longer-contrast scale, adjust exposure factors from the technique chart to provide high kVp and correspondingly smaller mAs values to maintain a proper density level within the finished image. This type of exposure technique provides a much smaller radiation exposure dose to the patient and fetus.

    If the radiography department performs AP projections of the abdomen of *gravid* females (e.g., recumbent abdomen, pelvimetry) often, the technique chart may list exposure techniques for the pregnant patient as a separate procedure from the AP abdomen of a *nongravid* patient (see Fig. 11–5).

    Exposure factors for pelvimetry are more common. If any of these are not listed, the base-line exposure technique given for nongravid patients must be used and exposure factors must be altered.

- What exposure factors are present on the room's exposure technique chart?

    The exposure factor choices that so far have been presented are

    a. Use exposure factors for an abdominal radiograph of a pregnant patient, if listed on chart
    or
    b. Use exposure factors for pelvimetry if listed on the technique chart
    or
    c. Use exposure factors for an abdominal radiograph of a nongravid patient listed on chart and adjust for extra fluid in the abdominal cavity
    or
    d. Alter exposure factors for an abdominal radiograph of a nongravid patient to reduce dosage to area, patient, and fetus (high kVp and low mAs, using a very short exposure time)

This makes the final choice much like that in a multiple-choice question. Choice *a* is obviously preferable if available on the chart; *b* would be the second preference; *c* is the least preferable choice in most cases; and *d* would be next best if neither *a* nor *b* is available.

Source-Image Distance

In radiology departments, the SID is generally standardized for each anatomical part. The distance between the source and the image receptor should be checked for accuracy each time a different procedure is performed. The standard SID value must be assured if the projection requires angulation of the central ray to avoid any variations in density of the images produced. The *inverse square law* of radiation intensity (i.e., $I_1d_1^2 = I_2d_2^2$) dictates that a change in the SID has a marked effect on radiographic density (see Fig. 11–19). Compensating changes in the exposure factors must be made for the change in the SID if a satisfactory image is to be obtained.

The standard SID value for each part is based on many exposure variables. The acceptable image size of the object (magnification) and the machine's generator capacity are of utmost importance.

The effect on radiographic density must be compensated when an SID change is requested or is necessitated by exposure conditions. For example, if the technique chart lists 36 inches as a standard SID for a particular part and radiographs must be made at 72 inches SID, either the mAs or the kVp must be increased for the exposure, as demonstrated by images in Figure 11–19. The amount of increase in mAs would be four times the value listed on the technique chart. To accomplish this one could

- Increase the mAs by a factor of 4, or
- Increase the mAs by a factor of 2 and increase kVp by 15% (recall that a 15% increase in kVp has the effect of doubling mAs), or
- Let the original mAs remain unchanged, and increase the kVp by approximately 32% (i.e., increase kVp by 15% twice)

Note: Rules for calculations used in the last two options are discussed in Compensating Exposure Factors later in this chapter.

In other circumstances, if the SID must be decreased from 36 to 30 inches, the result is that mAs or kVp must be reduced to provide the proper density of the image. Either the mAs can be reduced to 69% of its former value, or the kVp can be reduced by approximately 15%. Given this choice, it is preferable to reduce the mAs to approximately half the original value required and to retain the original kVp value. This

exposure will maintain a lower radiation dosage to the patient. If the original kVp level is relatively low, a reduction in kVp may result in insufficient penetration of the part (see Fig. 11–3*kB*).

The SID is seldom reduced to solve ordinary density problems in radiography, although it can be done in some cases. The reason is that a slight reduction in SID creates a significant change in the ratio between it and the SOD, because the ratio is decreased. This may significantly decrease the image sharpness (the magnification of the object in the image is increased). This is illustrated in Figure 11–20.

Two instances in which the SID may require reduction to achieve the needed radiographic density are these:

1. When using a low-intensity unit to radiograph a dense part of an extremely large patient. The best way to approach the problem of a low-capacity radiographic unit is to use one with a higher capacity. If this option is not available, the radiographer should use a shorter SID, which is found by making the necessary calculations based on the relationship of the mAs and SID required for imaging. The use of a shorter than normal SID should be entered on the patient's requisition to notify the radiologist who interprets the image.
2. When it is impossible to obtain the correct SID because of physical limitations (traction devices, bed height, etc.) in mobile (portable, bedside) radiography. In this case, the mAs must be reduced to a value that will result in the prescribed density levels for the image with as little radiation absorbed by the patient as possible. Again, the specific mAs for the exposure can be obtained by using the relationship of mAs and SID for imaging given later in this chapter.

In radiographic imaging, the kVp must first penetrate the part. The minimal kVp required to penetrate a part can be reliably calculated by using the rule of thumb of doubling the thickness of the body part in centimeters and adding a constant factor. The constant factor may vary, based on the equipment 1ϕ or 3ϕ generator) or the image contrast required in a specific department.

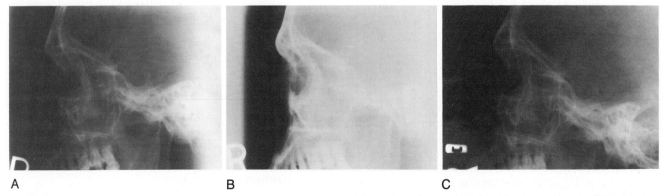

FIGURE 11–20. Source-image distance (SID) and radiographic density. Three images illustrate the effect of SID on radiographic density and a change of exposure factors to compensate for the density loss caused by increasing the SID. Image *A*, SID is 36 inches—adequate image of the sella turcica. Image *B*, SID is 72 inches—insufficient radiographic density. Image *C*, SID is 72 inches. The mAs was increased to four times the original value in Image *A*—the radiographic density is again adequate.

The rule of thumb for calculation of minimal kVp to penetrate a part based on machine generator is

$$2 \times \text{cm thickness} + 25 \ (3\phi \text{ equipment}) = \text{kVp}$$

$$2 \times \text{cm thickness} + 30 \ (1\phi \text{ equipment}) = \text{kVp}$$

Variance in the constant value added to account for the machine generator is a direct function of the average energy of wavelengths produced—that is, using an exposure with a kVp of 100, the average energy level of the photons produced with 1ϕ generation is 70.7% of the kVp; with 3ϕ, six-pulse generation, the average energy level is about 96% of the kVp. The percentage of the peak kilovoltage with 3ϕ, twelve-pulse generation is slightly higher than with 6-pulse generation as demonstrated by Figure 11–21.

The 3ϕ, six-pulse equipment was an interim development that has relinquished its brief period of popularity to 3ϕ, twelve-pulse and high-frequency generators. The use of 3ϕ equipment raised the efficiency of the beam to exceed that obtained with a 1ϕ unit by a factor of approximately 2. Therefore, the mAs, especially the exposure time, for a 3ϕ equipment exposure at a given kVp can be reduced to half or less than half that used with 1ϕ equipment (Fig. 11–22). This decreased exposure time reduces the probability of lack of recorded detail caused by patient motion. The use of 3ϕ equipment provides a higher tube capacity, increased efficiency of the image-producing beam, and an increased x-ray tube life. These factors are important for high-energy exposures, serial filming, the economy of the radiology department, and radiographic quality.

Compensating Exposure Factors

After determining the minimal kilovoltage required to penetrate the part and the mAs needed to provide sufficient image density, the radiographer can manipulate the values to produce the scale of image contrast preferred by a particular radiologist or radiology department. To accomplish this, the radiographer needs a thorough understanding of the interrelationship of kVp and mAs. The kVp primarily determines the image contrast and contrast scale. The mAs, which has a predictable effect on radiographic density, can be used to control that quality.

The starting point for radiography has been defined as the minimum kVp needed to penetrate the body part combined with an mAs to provide sufficient density for an image of the part. The usual dilemma presented to the radiographer is to provide a radiographic image with a longer scale of contrast, a decreased contrast in the radiographic image, and less absorbed radiation dose to the patient. To do this requires manipulation of the exposure factors and usually consists of increasing the kVp by 15% to lengthen the contrast scale and lower the subject contrast. A 15% increase in kVp means the amount of radiation absorbed by the patient is decreased and radiographic

density is increased by about two times the original density. The increased radiographic density caused by the kVp increase can be compensated for by applying this rule:

> For a specific radiographic density, to decrease the mAs by half, increase the kVp by 15%.

In this application, when the kVp is increased by 15%, logically it is necessary to reduce the original mAs to half of its original value to maintain the original radiographic density of the image. This rule can continue to be used until the proper radiographic contrast is achieved, which should be accomplished using a phantom segment rather than a patient or an actual radiographic exposure of any person.

Converting an Exposure to Produce a Longer Scale of Radiographic Contrast

)))))) EXAMPLE

The hip of a phantom segment measures 17 cm in the AP projection. This radiograph is performed at 40 inches SID, using Bucky exposure technique factors. The Bucky grid in the room has a grid ratio of 12:1. The x-ray generator in the room is a 1ϕ type. At the minimum kilovoltage, 40 mAs is required to provide the proper radiographic density in the image of the hip (Fig. 11–23A).

Step 1. The minimum kVp to penetrate part is calculated as shown:

$$kVp_1 = (2 \times 17 \text{ cm}) + 30$$
$$kVp_1 = 34 + 30$$
$$kVp_1 = 64 \text{ kVp} \qquad mAs_1 = 40$$

Step 2. Increase the kVp to obtain a longer scale of contrast (Fig 11–23B)

Increase kVp by 15%	and	Reduce mAs to one-half
$kVp_2 = 64 \text{ kVp}_1 + 15\%(\text{kVp}_1)$		
$kVp_2 = 64 + 0.15(64)$		$mAs_2 = 1/2 \times mAs_1$
$kVp_2 = 64 + 9.6$		$mAs_2 = 1/2 \times 40$
$kVp_2 = 73.6 \text{ or } 74 \text{ kVp}$		$mAs_2 = 20$

View the radiograph produced with the film quality–control person. If further lengthening of the radiographic contrast scale is needed, apply the same rule again (Step 3).

Step 3. Repeat Step 2. Use Step 2 exposure factors as a base from which to work to make this conversion (Fig. 11–23C).

$kVp_3 = kVp_2 + 15\%(kVp_2)$	
$kVp_3 = 74 + 0.15(74)$	$mAs_3 = 0.5 \times mAs_2$
$kVp_3 = 74 + 11.1$	$mAs_3 = 0.5 \times 20$
$kVp_3 = 85.1 \text{ or } 85 \text{ kVp}$	$mAs_3 = 10$

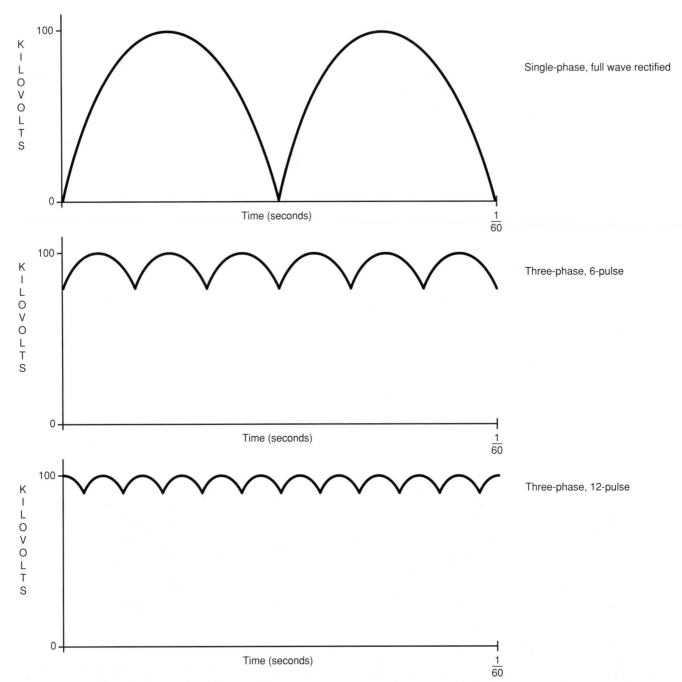

FIGURE 11–21. Effective radiographic voltage: current dependency. Three graphic representations of the electrical current supply for the production of x-rays. In the graphs, the voltage in each case is 100 kVp and the time represented for each is 1/60 second. If 100 kVp is selected for use, the effective voltage that produces an image is approximately 70.7% of the range between the minimum kV and the maximum kVp. For a fully rectified, single-phase current, this would yield 70.7 kV. Three-phase, 6-pulse current is said to have a minimum kilovoltage value that is approximately 13.5% below the peak kilovoltage. The effective voltage with this current would be ~96 kV. With three-phase, 12-pulse current, the minimum kilovoltage is approximately 3.4% below the peak kilovoltage. The effective voltage for a radiographic exposure with this type of current is ~99 kV. It is easily deduced that the radiation producing the image is more penetrating and that less total radiation is necessary to record the image. This circumstance has led to the reduction of exposure times used with this type of equipment.

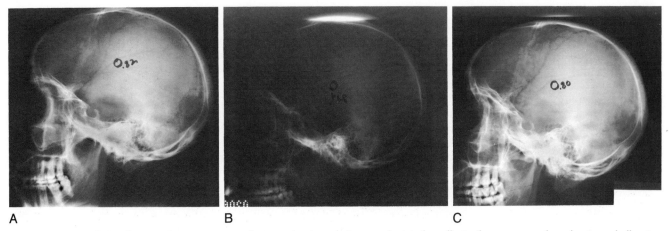

FIGURE 11–22. Effect of type of current generation on the image. Images depict the effect of exposures of a phantom skull using single-phase and three-phase current. *A*, Exposure using 70 kVp, 60 mAs, Par speed screen–film combination and a single-phase radiographic unit. The density value in the marked circle on the image was 0.82. *B*, Identical exposure factors were used with a three-phase current. The recorded density value in the same area of the skull was 2.14. *C*, Exposure factors were altered to use only 21 mAs with the other factors used in *A* and the three-phase current. A density value of 0.88 in the same area of the skull was achieved by reducing the exposure time to approximately one third of its value in *A*.

View this radiograph with the film quality–control person. Continue to repeat steps until the desired contrast scale is achieved. In each succeeding step, use the exposure factors from the previous step. Never make another radiograph without first viewing the one previously exposed with the film quality–control person. When the desired result is reached, stop the process.

Remember: The usual procedure is to solve this problem with a phantom segment before radiographing an actual patient, using the exposure factors thus determined.

Minor Changes in Exposure Factors

At some point during exposure factor adjustment, it may be noticed that the contrast is higher than desired, but a further increase in kVp by 15% will result in a loss of visible detail because of the lowered image contrast. An increase in the kVp by 5% with an accompanying 30% decrease in mAs may be used. If at any point a slight change in contrast is needed and a visible change in radiographic density is also needed, increase the kVp by 5% and allow the mAs to remain as it is. However, if the contrast is what you want and the

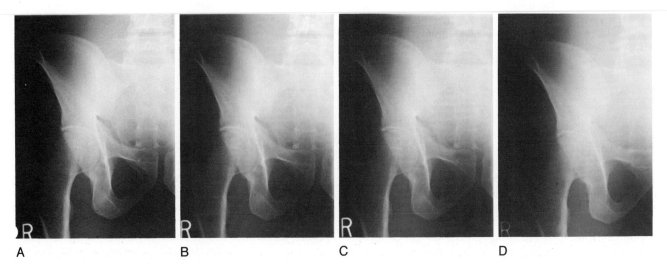

FIGURE 11–23. Exposure factors balanced for radiographic density. *A*, Exposure used 64 kVp, 40 mAs, and a source-image distance of 40 inches; the image is generally acceptable, but the greater trochanter is not well demonstrated. *B*, The mAs was halved and the kVp was increased by 15% to reduce the exposure to the patient in the gonadal region, and to lengthen the scale of contrast. The image contrast is lower; the greater trochanter remains poorly demonstrated. *C*, The same procedure, halving the mAs and increasing the kVp by 15%, was followed. The greater trochanter was again too dense; also the trabecular markings are less obvious. *D*, mAs was decreased by 30% and the kVp was increased by 5%. Neither the outline of femoral head nor the greater trochanter is as clear. This is not an acceptable image; the contrast scale is too long to reveal the smaller fine lines of the object in the image. The only instance in which this image might be acceptable is if there were no other images with which to compare it.

radiographic density needs reduction, leave the kVp as it is and reduce the mAs by 30% (Figs. 11–23D and 11–24).

Images should be studied carefully to determine the need to lower radiographic contrast further or to increase or decrease the radiographic density visibly, not necessarily doubling or halving it. If the latter situation is applicable, increase or decrease the mAs as appropriate for the density needed. The change in mAs should be about 30%. *Important:* Critically re-examine the resultant image each time a change of exposure factors is made.

Since radiographic contrast makes detail visible, it is imperative to produce the proper contrast scale and to maximize differences (contrast) between adjacent densities. An image of good radiographic quality should reveal all the different tissue densities represented in the part (see Fig. 11–3).

Tissues vary in absorption of x-radiation as a result of tissue thickness, tissue type, average atomic number of tissues, tissue density, and the x-ray energies used to record the image. The *penetrability* characteristics of various tissues are discussed in Chapters 8 and 14.

KILOVOLTAGE

X-ray energies are defined by the kVp level used to produce them. At a low kVp, photoelectric absorption of x-rays predominates. As the kVp increases, the percentage of the occurrence of Compton interaction of x-rays in the tissues increases. A characteristic of photoelectric interaction with tissue is that all of these low–energy x-ray photons are totally absorbed. This type of interaction produces the contrast between the tissues in the image of the part. Compton interactions of x-ray photons occur at all levels of exposure, becoming predominant with increasing kilovoltage levels in diagnostic radiography. This interaction produces secondary radiation (i.e., scatter) capable of affecting the film emulsion and does not necessarily contribute to image quality. Because the direction by which the secondary radiation approaches the film cannot be predetermined or directed, it creates a gray haze (fog) over the image and obscures detail (Fig. 11–25). Methods used to reduce the production of secondary radiation or to prevent its interaction with the film emulsion, thus enhancing the visibility of detail, are discussed in a later chapter.

It should be obvious that reduction of secondary radiation to the film can be accomplished by using lower kilovoltage values. It is also evident that lowering the kVp can create a situation in which not all of the tissues in a part are penetrated and therefore are not demonstrated in the image. Also, the part exposed will absorb more radiation. Both of these occurrences should be avoided.

Milliampere-Seconds

Milliamperage (mA) is the measure of the number of electrons flowing between the tube electrodes within a specific unit of time. The exposure time is the total length of time the electron stream flows through the x-ray tube to produce x-rays. Together the mA and exposure time compose the milliampere-seconds (mAs) for an x-ray exposure. This quantity designates the total number of electrons flowing through the tube during a radiographic exposure. The mAs signifies the total quantity of x-rays available for exposure with no inference as to their energy.

Mathematically, mA is inversely proportional to the exposure time for a given radiographic exposure or density. For example, 200 mA used with 0.5 second gives 100 mAs, as does 100 mA with 1 second, 400 mA with 0.25 second, and so forth. Theoretically, the quantity of x-rays is the same for each of these exposures if the machine is accurately calibrated. Illustrations of this theory appear in Figure 11–26.

The mA established at the control panel determines the filament current, which generates heat in the filament. The amount of heat generated determines the number of electrons freed at the filament. This number in turn forms the tube's *cathode* (electron) *stream* (tube current) when a potential difference is applied across the terminals of the x-ray tube.

Use of 100 mA produces a specific number of electrons in a single unit of time. If the mA is doubled, that is, increased to 200 mA, twice the number of electrons will be released in the same time unit. If the mA remains at a value of 100 but the exposure time unit is doubled, the total number of electrons produced while the current flows through the x-ray tube is doubled. In either instance, you have doubled the mAs and produced an increase (by a factor of 2) in the number of electrons entering into the production of x-rays.

As the mAs is increased, the number of electrons increases. At a given kVp, no matter what mAs is used, a given proportion of electrons receives the same energy while others acquire other energies. This accounts for the heterogeneous nature of the x-ray beam. Electrons of various energies produce x-rays with differing wavelengths and frequencies and therefore with a diversity of penetrating abilities. Remember, kVp value defines minimum wavelength ($\lambda_{min} = 12.4/kVp$) only. The number of electrons in the tube current is affected, but the count is unpredictable. The energy supplied to the x-ray tube generally reaches the tube in impulses (bursts), since the electrical supply is rectified alternating current, either 1ϕ or 3ϕ.

The development of 3ϕ equipment did not greatly affect the efficiency of the conversion of electron energy to x-rays. The same percentage of the electron energy is converted to heat, not to x-rays. It has, however, permitted the reduction of the exposure times required for specific densities on radiographs, because more impulses are produced per second in the x-ray tube operation and the average penetrating ability has increased.

The 3ϕ unit increased the average energy of the beam. This can be deduced from the graphic representations in Figure 11–21. This type of tube current produces a more uniform x-ray beam (i.e., a beam

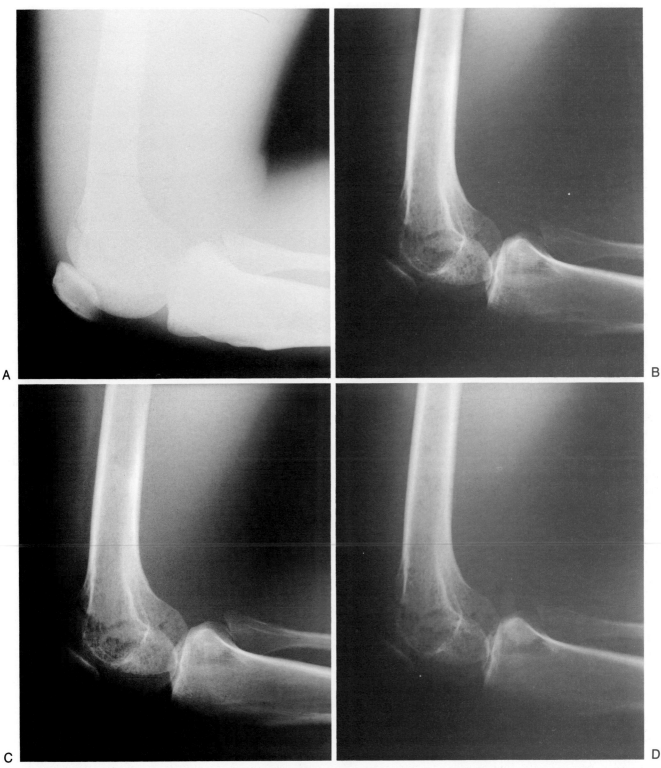

FIGURE 11-24. Milliampereseconds (mAs) and peak kilovoltage (kVp) changes in radiographic exposure. The objects are the knee phantom. The knee is rotated anteriorly and the lower extremity is not parallel with the film surface in all of the images. Positioning is not good. *A* (80 mAs, 40 kVp), Part is not penetrated; details other than the patella are not visible. Only 6 or 7 density shades can be distinguished in the penetrometer's image. *B* (20 mAS, 60 kVp), Eight or 9 distinct density shades are visible in the image of the penetrometer. The patella is too dense to be clearly visible. The lower femur in the image is penetrated. C (10 mAs, 70 kVp), Nine or 10 distinct density shades can be observed in the penetrometer's image. The patella can be seen better than in *B*. *D* (2.5 mAs, 90 kVp), The number of distinct shades of density in the penetrometer image has decreased to 6 or 7. Only the posterior surface of the patella can be distinguished in this image. The inferior end of the femur fades into the background density. *B* and *C* may be acceptable in cases with no other film for comparison. *C* is the best overall image.

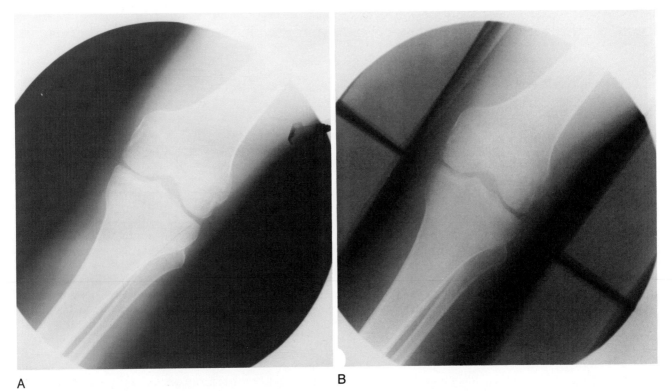

FIGURE 11–25. Scattered radiation: effect on image contrast. *A,* A knee (phantom) radiographed using a non–grid exposure technique. *B,* Radiographed under the same conditions as *A,* but additionally, paraffin blocks, equal in thickness to the knee, were placed against each side of the knee. This placed more material in the irradiated area and increased the volume of material to interact with the primary beam. More scatter radiation was produced in *B.* The knee image became gray and hazy. In *A* much less scatter radiation was produced because there was less "tissue" to interact with the primary beam.

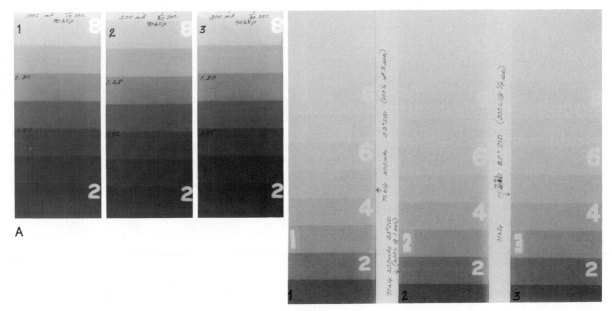

FIGURE 11–26. Reciprocity law and radiographic density. Two films, each with 3 penetrometer images. *Set A,* All images were exposed using 10 mA, 70 kVp, 40-inch source-image distance, and Par speed screens. Values of mA were 100 *(A1),* 200 *(A2),* and 300 *(A3).* The average density value of step 6 of the penetrometer in images *A1, A2,* and *A3* is 1.29 ± 0.01. In step 4 of the penetrometer in these same three images, the density values are 1.87 *(A1),* 1.82 *(A2),* and 1.85 *(A3). Set B,* All images were exposed using 200 mAs, 70 kVp, the source-image distance (SID) was adjusted to avoid unnecessary tube leading (the mAs was adjusted to compensate for the SID changed). These were nonscreen exposures: *B1* used 100 mA, *B2* used 200 mA, and *B3* used 300 mA.

with relatively the same wavelengths represented at all times). The exposure time can be reduced to a value of two thirds to one half of that required with a 1ϕ unit: and the same image density is radiographically represented.

mAs-Density Relationship

> If the kVp is sufficient to penetrate the part, the radiographic density is directly proportional to the mAs used for the exposure.

This means that if the image demonstrates a part that is penetrated but the radiographic density is not adequate to visualize the part well, the radiographic density can be doubled by multiplying the mAs by a factor of 2.

Rules of radiographic exposure concerning mAs can be stated as guides for radiographers in their manipulation of exposure techniques. These are given in the following paragraphs.

mA-Exposure Time Relationship

> To produce a specific radiographic density, mA is inversely proportional to time.

For example, 10 mAs can be derived by using 10 mA and 1 second, 100 mA and 1/10 second, 300 mA and 1/30 second, 600 mA and 1/60 second, and so on. If radiographic units are properly calibrated, each mA-time combination that yields the same product (mAs) should provide the same number of electrons to produce x-rays. Ultimately the same radiographic density is obtained, as illustrated in Figure 11–26.

mAs-SID Relationship

> The mAs required to produce a specific density on a radiograph is directly proportional to the square of the SID used to make the exposure.

Technique charts for exposure techniques are formulated using specific SIDs. If the SID used is not the one specified by the technique chart, the mAs must be adjusted, using the preceding rule—that is, if the distance is greater than that specified on the chart, the value of the mAs factor must be increased. If the SID is less than that listed on the chart, the mAs must be decreased.

The formula for calculating this conversion has several forms. These are as follows:

$$\frac{mAs_1}{mAs_2} = \frac{D_1{}^2}{D_2{}^2}$$

mAs_1 = value from technique chart

mAs_2 = value to be found

D_1 = SID from technique chart

D_2 = SID to be used

Probably the simplest method for calculating the mAs needed is to use the short formula:

$$mAs_2 = \left(\frac{D_2{}^2}{D_1{}^2}\right) \times mAs_1, \quad \text{or} \quad mAs_2 = \left(\frac{D_2}{D_1}\right)^2 \times mAs_1$$

Generally, the short formula allows the radiographer to quickly calculate the needed mAs, because the extremely large numbers with the original formula are not necessarily involved. This is true because (D_2/D_1) can often be reduced to smaller fractions (1/2, 1/3, 1/4, etc.) or whole numbers (2, 3, 4, etc.). These numbers can be dealt with more easily than the original distance values. For example, 1/2 can represent 36 inches/72 inches. One half squared is equal to 1/4, whereas 36/72 squared is equal to 1296/5184. Such large numbers normally require the use of a calculator.

The rule applies because at a given mAs, a specific number of x-rays are produced as required. They are produced at all angles from the target and all are moving in straight lines (Fig. 11–27). Those that emerge from the tube do so in a rectangular or a circular, cone-shaped configuration.

In the diagram, note the length differences along an imaginary line between ends of the outer divergent x-rays at 72 inches SID and an imaginary line between those same x-rays at 36 inches SID. Obviously, the rays are dispersed over a larger area as the distance from the anode (source) increases. Imagine this dispersal occurring over an area having two dimensions —length and width for rectangular fields and for circular fields, diameter and circumference. It becomes obvious that less radiation interacts with a single unit area of the film as the SID increases.

In production of radiographs, the density for a specific part must remain at the same value; therefore, the number of x-rays per unit area of film emulsion must remain at a given level. To maintain this level, the mAs is usually increased, using the formula given here. To increase the kVp would change the penetration of the part and would alter the image contrast.

When manipulating exposure techniques, remember that to be visually detected, for an overall change in radiographic density a change in mAs of about 30% or slightly more or a change in the kVp of approximately 5% is usually required. If the SID stated on the technique chart has a value near the SID used, it may not be necessary to alter the mAs or the kVp. The change in exposure factors may not be needed, but the radiographer does need to make that determination through careful consideration of the exposure conditions.

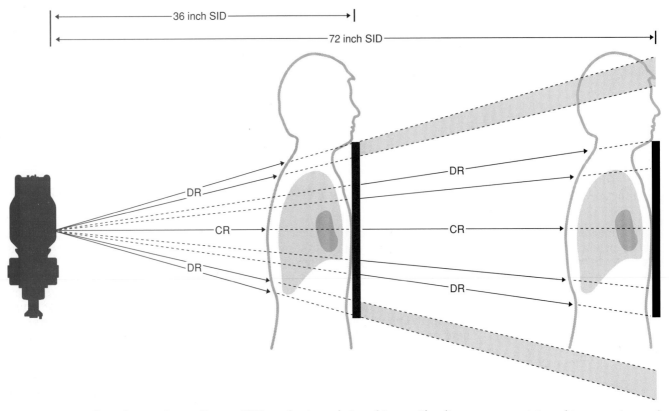

FIGURE 11–27. Effect of source-image distance (SID) on density and size of image. The diagram, representative of two superimposed radiographic situations, illustrates that the rays forming the image at a 36-inch SID are projected to cover an area 17 inches long by 14 inches wide and spread to cover an area 34 inches by 28 inches at 72-inch SID. The rays that form the image at the 36-inch SID diverge at a large angle from the central ray, creating distortion in the image of the object radiographed. The area covered is four times greater at 72 inches than at 36 inches. If the radiation that records the image at a 36-inch SID is spread over the area at a 72-inch SID, about one fourth of the radiation strikes each square inch of an image receptor system. This decreases the recorded radiographic density. At 72 inches, restoration of the radiographic density to its intensity at 36 inches requires an increase in the source intensity by a factor of four. Second, the image of the object formed at the 72-inch SID is on the same size film and is recorded with rays that form a smaller angle with the central ray–that is, they are closer to parallel with the central ray. There will be less distortion in the image, especially at the periphery of the image and of structures at some distance from the image receptor.

Chapter Summary/ Important Concepts

Radiographic images are formed when x-rays produced by an x-ray tube penetrate a body part to varying degrees and then interact with an image receptor such as a piece of radiographic film.

A good quality diagnostic radiograph is one that demonstrates the largest number of shades of gray that exist within the body part, with the greatest difference between the adjacent areas of radiographic density in the image.

When low-energy x-ray photons are used to produce a radiograph, there is
a. less penetration resulting in increased radiation absorption within the tissue

b. the need for more photons (i.e., mAs must be increased) to obtain sufficient radiographic density
c. increased radiographic contrast

When higher-energy photons are used, there is
a. greater penetration and less radiation absorbed within the tissue
b. no need for higher numbers of photons to obtain the desired radiographic density, since more photons reach the film (i.e., mAs can be decreased)
c. less radiographic contrast

The use of extremely low-energy photons or excessively high-energy photons is not recommended in the production of medical radiographs.

Technique charts provide the radiographer with an appropriate set of technical factors (i.e., kVp, mA, exposure time, distances) that should be used with the normal patient of average size in order to produce a diagnostic radiograph; technique charts are formulated for specific radiographic units.

Diagnostic medical radiographs should always contain sufficient radiographic density (i.e., darkening of the film), minimal distortion, sufficient contrast, and maximum radiographic detail (image sharpness).

Contrast permits the visualization of detail in a radiographic image; it depends on both the capability of an individual film to display differences in image density (film contrast) and differences in levels of density produced by the degree of penetration of the body part by the x-ray beam (subject contrast).

When preparing to make a radiographic exposure, the medical radiographer must consider (1) the body part thickness, (2) tissue densities involved, (3) tissues that may overlie each other in the projection desired, (4) the effect of suspected or known pathology, and (5) the equipment available that will produce the widest range of densities and the greatest contrast within the image.

Radiographic *detail* refers to the clarity and sharpness of individual body structures within a radiographic image. This characteristic may also be referred to as sharpness or resolution. Detail within a radiographic image is affected by both the production factors (e.g., geometric factors, materials used to produce the image, size of radiation source) and their visibility (i.e., photographic properties of the image, radiographic contrast and radiographic density).

Distortion in a radiographic image refers to misrepresentation of an object's size or shape. Misrepresentation of shape, or "true distortion," can be avoided by assuring that the plane of the object being radiographed is parallel to the plane of the image receptor (e.g., the film). In addition, the beam's central ray must be centered and perpendicular to both of these planes. In certain cases, distortion may be deliberately introduced to produce a better view of a structure of interest.

Misrepresentation of object size, or size distortion, generally occurs as a magnification of the radiographed structure; in certain cases, this can be helpful in viewing small body structures or structures difficult to visualize.

Magnification can be accomplished by decreasing the SID:SOD ratio. The radiograph obtained under these conditions is referred to as a macroradiograph.

The primary exposure factors in medical radiography are (1) kVp, (2) mA, (3) exposure time, and (4) the SID. The proper combination of technical factors for the average patient are formulated and grouped into technique charts. Technical factors may need to be adjusted as a result of pathologies or variations in body structure.

---

kVp determines the maximum energy of the x-rays produced and therefore their penetrating power. A rule of thumb for calculation of the minimal kVp to penetrate a body part is

$$2 \times (\text{cm thickness}) + 30 = kVp_{min} \qquad (1\phi \text{ units})$$

or

$$2 \times (\text{cm thickness}) + 25 = kVp_{min} \qquad (3\phi \text{ units})$$

kVp is also the prime determinate of image contrast and contrast scale.

---

mAs, the product of tube current and exposure time, is used to control the radiographic density of the image. Since the kVp determines penetrating ability, which in turn affects the number of x-rays reaching the image receptor, both kVp and mAs are used together to produce the required radiographic density. This interrelationship between kVp and mAs is indicated by the following practical rule:

For a specific radiographic density, an increase by 15% in the kVp should be followed by a 50% decrease in mAs

Other important relationships affecting the resulting radiographic density that were noted include

a. The radiographic density is directly proportional to the mAs used for the radiographic exposure
b. To produce a specific radiographic density (i.e., mAs), mA is inversely proportional to time
c. The mAs required for a specific radiographic density is directly proportional to the square of the SID used to make the exposure

---

When manipulating exposure factors, an approximate 30% change in mAs or an approximate 5% change in kVp is required to make a visible change in the radiographic density of an image.

After making adjustments in exposure factors, the radiographer must critically re-examine the resultant image before making additional adjustment exposures.

Important Terminology

Background Density. Blackening of an exposed and processed film in areas where no object part is interposed between the x-ray source and the film

Cathode Stream. Flow of electrons from the cathode to the anode of an x-ray tube during an exposure

Chemical Development. Process by which ionized silver halide crystals in a film emulsion are converted to black metallic silver and form an image of the object exposed to radiation

Constituent. Part of a whole

Contrast. In radiography the difference between adjacent shades of gray in an image

Contrast Scale. The number of visibly different shades of gray within the margins of an imaged part

Densitometer. Instrument used to determine the values of different densities within an image; values obtained are logarithms

Density. In radiographic imaging, the compactness of black metallic silver that determines the blackness of each area of the image

Density Value. Number denoting the relative amount of x-radiation absorbed by the sensitive film emulsion

Detail. Sharpness of fine-line structure produced within a radiographic image

Developer. Chemical that reduces ionized silver halide crystals to the black metallic silver that forms the radiographic image

Development. Process by which ionized silver halide crystals are converted (reduced) to black metallic silver

Distortion. Misrepresentation of the shape of the object in the radiographic image

Elongation. Form of distortion; the object appears longer than it actually is or longer in relation to other subjects in the image

Exposure Time. Length of time (seconds or fractions of seconds) that electrons flow through the x-ray tube and produce x-rays

Film Contrast. Inherent property of a film that allows specific differences in density because of manufacture of the x-ray film and the chemical development process used

Foreshortening. Form of distortion; the object appears shorter than it actually is or shorter in relation to other objects in the image

Gravid. Pregnant

High Contrast. A large difference between the adjacent densities within an image

Humidity. The relative percentage of moisture in the atmosphere compared with that present at saturation conditions

Image Contrast. Average difference between the various adjacent densities within an image

Increment. Step; a single definite number or quantity

Inverse Square Law (of radiation intensity). The amount of radiation received at a given point is inversely proportional to the square of the distance between the point and the radiation source

Ionizing Radiation. Electromagnetic energy form capable of producing positive and negative components (i.e., ion pairs) in the material through which it passes

Kilovolt, Kilovoltage (kV). 1000 volts; the usual unit of measure of the kinetic energy of the electrons flowing in the x-ray tube to produce x-rays

kV. Abbreviation for kilovoltage

kVp. Abbreviation for peak kilovoltage

Latent Image. Invisible image formed by ionized silver halide crystals produced by absorption of x-ray photons in the sensitive emulsion of a film after the x-ray photons have passed through an object

Long-Scale Contrast. Property of a radiographic image that possesses a large number of density shades

Low Contrast. Small difference between the adjacent densities within an image

Magnification. Misrepresentation of the size of the object in the image, making it appear larger in proportion to surrounding structures or larger than expected

Manifest Image. Visible image

mAs. Abbreviation for milliampere-second

Milliamperage (mA). The quantity of electrons flowing between the cathode and anode of an x-ray tube per second

Milliampere-Seconds (mAs). Value indicating the total quantity of electrons flowing through an x-ray tube during an x-ray exposure

Millisecond (ms). A unit of time equal to 1/1000 of a second

Misrepresentation of Shape. Distortion of the outline of an object in the image

Misrepresentation of Size. Area measurements of the image of a structure are not the same size as the actual structure; they are usually larger

Nongravid. Not pregnant

Pathology. Study of disease and disease processes

Patient Architecture. Form and build of the patient, includes muscle development; synonymous with *body habitus*

Patient Habitus. Form and build of the patient, includes muscle development

Peak Kilovoltage (kVp). Peak voltage of a voltage waveform that corresponds to the maximum energy of an electron in the electron stream producing x-rays; defines the minimum wavelength of the x-ray beam produced

Penetrability. Property of a material that indicates how easily something (in this case x-radiation) can pass through it

Preliminary Radiographs. Images made early in a radiographic procedure to visualize the anatomy of the body part before any changes in the procedure that will alter or obscure its visualization are made

Primary Radiation. X-radiation that is emitted from the x-ray tube

Radiation Intensity. The quantity of x-rays within a specified area

Radiograph. Image of an object produced by sending x-rays through it, recording the pattern of emerging radiant energy from it, and processing the image receptor (film)

Radiographer. One who produces radiographs

Radiographic Contrast. Difference between adjacent densities within the radiographic image

Radiographic Density. Overall blackening of the radiographic image

Radiographic Detail. Fine structural lines of parts in a radiographic image

Radiography. Production of an image by sending x-rays through an object and intercepting the energy

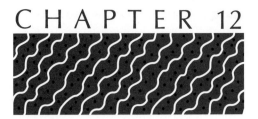

Geometrical Factors Affecting Image Quality

Janice D. Hall, M.A.Ed. R.T.(R)

Chapter Outline

Chapter Objectives

On completion of this chapter, the student should be able to

- Define basic radiographic terminology discussed in the chapter.
- Explain the difference between photographic and geometrical properties.
- Describe how penumbra affects detail of the radiographic image.
- Discuss focal spot size and explain how it can be manipulated to increase detail.
- Describe the situations in which the use of small and large focal spots is most beneficial.
- Explain the line-focus principle as it relates to radiographic detail.
- Explain how the anode heel effect is used to improve detail.
- Discuss the influence of source–image receptor distance (SID) and object-image receptor distance (OID) on radiographic sharpness.
- Explain and calculate the following formulas:
  - *magnification factor*
  - *percentage of magnification*
  - *geometric unsharpness*
- Discuss the two types of distortion as related to radiographic detail.
- Discuss the two major categories of motion unsharpness and explain how each affects radiographic detail.
- Discuss how exposure factors can be manipulated in order to maintain acceptable radiographic density and determine how each method affects detail of the image.
- Discuss screen unsharpness as it relates to radiographic detail.

OVERVIEW OF RADIOGRAPHIC QUALITY

Good radiographic quality is extremely important in that it provides the radiologist with the best image from which an accurate diagnosis can be obtained. In order to have good radiographic quality, there must be a proper balance between two properties. These two properties are referred to as photographic and geometric properties. To possess radiographic quality, the recorded image must achieve a proper balance of the best characteristics of both of these equally important properties.

The *photographic properties* refer to visibility of structural details on a radiographic image, whereas the *geometrical properties* refer to sharpness of structural details (Fig. 12–1). An image of radiographic quality must therefore possess a proper balance between visibility and sharpness of recorded detail on the image. It is important to recognize that the principles controlling geometrical properties are different from those controlling photographic properties.

Photographic Properties

Density and Contrast

Density and contrast are categorized as photographic properties. The photographic properties of density and contrast determine the wholeness of the radiographic image. *Density* refers to the overall blackness within the radiograph, whereas *contrast* refers to the ability to distinguish between density differences within the radiographic image. Chapter 11 discusses the photographic properties in detail. You may need to review that chapter if further understanding of these properties is needed. This chapter focuses on geometric properties and how they affect image quality. Remember, an image containing proper density and sufficient contrast is of little value unless the structural details are sharp.

Studying radiographic quality is learning to recognize and understand the effects of the multiple factors that influence the recording image. Radiographers have a number of factors, formulas, and techniques that can be manipulated in order to produce a desired effect. In order to manipulate these factors properly, radiographers must be able to understand the principles of the geometric and photographic properties so that manipulation and adjustment of exposure factors does not become a guessing game. To accomplish this, each of the major properties of the radiograph must be identified and examined. It is then necessary to differentiate among the principles that influence these properties, regardless of whether the influence is favorable or unfavorable to image quality. While examining these image properties and the multiple factors that influence them, notice that a change or manipulation of one exposure factor often results in a change of more than one property of the image. The radiographer's responsibility is to be aware of these multiple influences and to be able to determine whether the change is useful. It is obvious that a radiographer cannot perform a radiographic examination properly without a thorough understanding of the photographic and geometric properties of radiographic exposure and how to apply them. This is essential in the production of an image of high radiographic quality.

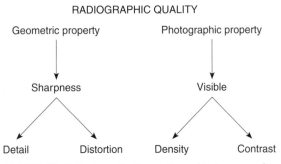

RADIOGRAPHIC QUALITY

Geometric property   Photographic property

Sharpness   Visible

Detail   Distortion   Density   Contrast

FIGURE 12–1. Factors affecting radiographic image quality.

GEOMETRICAL PROPERTIES

Detail and Distortion

Detail and *distortion* are geometric properties. Detail and distortion are inversely related; as detail increases, distortion decreases, and vice versa. Because the two are related in this manner, they must be discussed together. Detail can be defined as the visibility of fine lines or small structural edges on a radiograph. Other terms often used to describe the sharpness of the structural edges are *definition* and *resolution.* When structures have sharp borders and are clearly visible, there is good radiographic detail. The presence of borders or edges that are unsharp is known as *penumbra.* Excessive penumbra is undesirable to radiographic detail. Distortion refers to the misrepresentation of the true size and shape of an object in the radiographic image. Distortion greatly decreases radiographic detail. Keep in mind that not only is it necessary to have structures with sharp borders or edges, but these structures must also possess sufficient density differences for one structure to be easily distinguished from another. Therefore, in order to have good detail, the part must have been adequately penetrated by *kilovoltage* (kVp) and must possess an acceptable level of density, indicated by a proper balance between *milliamperage* (mA) and *exposure time* (seconds or milliseconds). kVp and mA are photographic properties and are not within the scope of this chapter; therefore, these factors are not discussed in further detail. If review of these important factors is needed, refer to Chapter 11.

Detail is primarily affected by the following geometrical factors:

- focal spot size
- source–image receptor distance (SID), also known as focal film distance (FFD) and target-film distance (TFD)
- object–image receptor distance (OID), also known as object-film distance (OFD)

Other factors that influence detail are *motion unsharpness* and screen unsharpness.

The geometric factors previously listed can be controlled to a certain degree by the radiographer in order to enhance the recorded detail on a radiograph. The *focal spot* size can be reduced to increase detail. The SID can be manipulated to enhance detail; as the SID is increased, the penumbra decreases, thereby increasing detail. Decreasing OID also increases detail by decreasing *penumbra* and *magnification.*

Focal Spot Size

Generally, each x-ray tube has two different focal spot sizes that can be selected by the operator. The choice of a large or small focal spot size should be determined by the specific application. The size of the

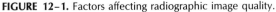

focal spot has a great influence on detail of the radiographic image. However, like many other factors in radiology, the specific choice of the *focal spot size* for a given examination involves a trade-off. Generally speaking, the larger the focal spot, the less radiographic detail present on the image. This is true because as the size of the focal spot increases, the area over which x-rays are produced also increases, resulting in penumbra on the radiographic image. Large focal spots are used for high-mA exposures that require a higher exposure load. This usually results in the use of 200 or higher mA.

The x-ray tubes most commonly available contain the following pairs of focal spots: 0.3 mm and 0.6 mm; 0.6 mm and 1.2 mm; and 1.0 mm and 2.0 mm. Large focal spots are usually available in 1.0 mm, 1.2 mm, 1.6 mm, or 2.0 mm, whereas small focal spots are available in 0.3 mm and 0.6 mm. Small focal spots are desired for detail work such as extremity radiography and magnification studies such as *angiography.* The criteria of acceptability of the focal spot depend on the application of the x-ray tube.

It would be an ideal situation if a point source of radiation could be produced. In this case, the x-rays would emerge from the x-ray tube at a single point. This point would always result in a sharp image with well-defined edges. Unfortunately, this is not true in the production of x-rays in the tube. The x-ray tube is an area source that generates x-rays over the entire focal area of the target; as a result, some degree of penumbra will always exist on the radiographic image (Fig. 12–2).

It is necessary to have some way of controlling the lack of sharpness produced from this area source. This control can be achieved by reducing the focal spot to the smallest possible size. Reducing the focal spot size decreases the area over which x-rays are produced, resulting in less penumbra on the image (Fig. 12–3).

Line-Focus Principle

Maximum definition can be obtained on a radiograph by the use of the *line-focus principle.* This principle states that at steeper or decreased target angles, the *effective focal spot* becomes smaller than the *actual focal spot* (Fig. 12–4). This principle allows a larger area of the target to be bombarded with electrons. It also increases the heat-loading capabilities of the x-ray tube thus preventing damage as a result of excessive heat. In addition, the steeper *target angle* increases resolution capabilities. The average target angle in the routine radiology department is approximately 17° from the vertical. However, one major disadvantage of the steeper target angle is that it limits the film size that can be used. This is due to the smaller area of coverage obtained with target angles steeper than 17°. Early steep-angle tubes with 10° targets were limited to field size coverage of 14 inches × 14 inches, with the x-ray tube 40 inches from the film. A 12° target angle will cover a 14-inch × 17-inch field size at the same distance as the 10° target angle. An option is to use a 10° target angle with a slight increase in distance (approximately 45 inches) from the x-ray tube to the film, resulting in a coverage of a 14-inch × 17-inch field size. Target angles steeper than 17° from the vertical are usually limited to special procedures radiography. Steep target angles greatly enhance detail; however, field size is limited.

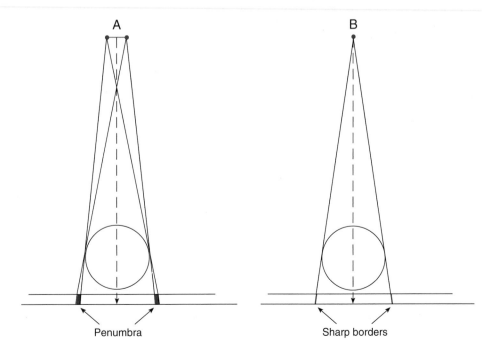

FIGURE 12–2. Area source *(A)* versus point source *(B).* Demonstration of how an area source of radiation produces an image with unsharp borders, known as penumbras, whereas a point source of radiation produces an image with sharply defined borders.

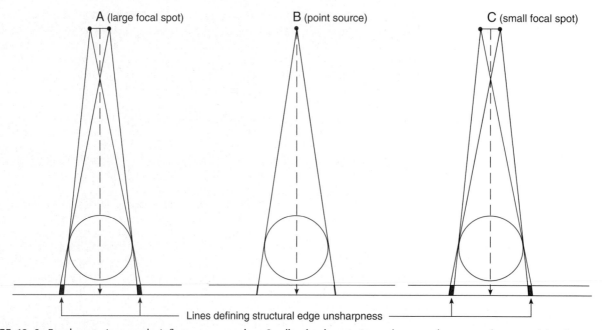

FIGURE 12–3. Focal spot size greatly influences penumbra. Smaller focal spot size reduces unsharpness of structural borders as noted when comparing A with C. Detail because of the effect of penumbra is decreased.

Anode Heel Effect

As target angle decreases, or steepens, what is known as the *anode heel effect* becomes more prominent. The target angle affects both the size of the focal spot produced and distribution of the intensity of x-rays within the beam. The anode heel effect is discussed here in relationship to radiographic detail. The heel effect is a variation in intensity of x-ray output along the longitudinal axis of the tube (depending on the angle of x-ray emission from the focal spot). The intensity diminishes fairly rapidly from the central ray toward the anode side of the x-ray beam. On the cathode side of

the beam, intensity increases over that of the central ray and then slightly diminishes. In other words, the anode heel effect is the result of decreased x-ray intensity at the anode end of the tube. It is a consequence of the line-focus principle. X-rays that are emitted toward the anode end of the x-ray tube must go through a thicker portion of the target material. Some of the x-rays are absorbed by the target material, resulting in decreased intensity at the anode end of the tube. The anode actually serves as its own filter. The anode end of the tube provides more visible detail because the size of the focal spot is smaller (Fig. 12–5).

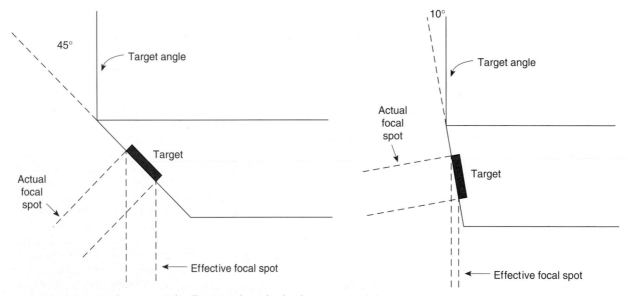

FIGURE 12–4. Line-focus principle, illustrating how the focal spot size and the projected field size vary with the target angle.

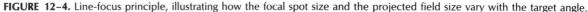

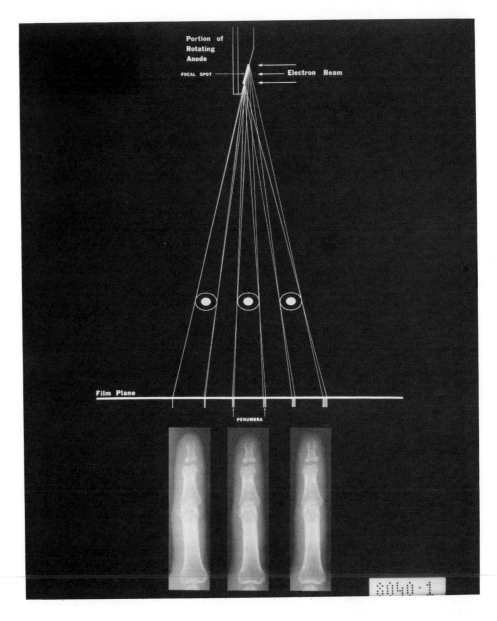

FIGURE 12–5. Three radiographic images of the third digit of a hand phantom show the effect of the focal spot size variation at the anode end of the x-ray tube. Greater detail is noted on the digit that is placed toward the anode position of the x-ray tube. (Courtesy of the ACR Learning File, Principles of Imaging, Sequence 140.)

The variation in intensity can be significant in some cases. Heel effect is more pronounced with steep target angles, short SID, and large field sizes with little or no collimation. The heel effect should be considered when radiographing body parts of varying thickness such as the thoracic spine. The thinner cervical area of the thoracic spine should receive less intense radiation from the anode portion of the beam, whereas the thicker chest area should be exposed to the more intense radiation from the cathode portion of the beam. This arrangement will result in a more even density throughout the image, thus increasing detail in the overall radiographic image (Fig. 12–6).

Source–Image Receptor Distance

Radiographic image sharpness can be influenced by the *source–image receptor distance* (SID), also known as *focal film distance* (FFD) and *target-film distance* (TFD). The SID can be defined as the distance between the source (x-ray tube) and the image receptor (radiographic film cassette). The conditions necessary for demonstrating maximum detail and minimum penumbra are use of a small focal spot, most reasonable maximum SID, and a short object-image receptor distance (OID). The OID can be defined as the distance between the object being radiographed and the radiographic film cassette. OID plays a crucial role in radiographic detail; however, before investigating its influence let us look further at the SID. Increasing SID enhances detail if all exposure factors are properly manipulated. However, the major disadvantage in maximizing SID is the increase in radiation exposure to the patient. As SID is increased, additional radiation is necessary in order to obtain a radiographic image of acceptable quality. As SID increases, radiographic exposure factors must be increased, resulting in more

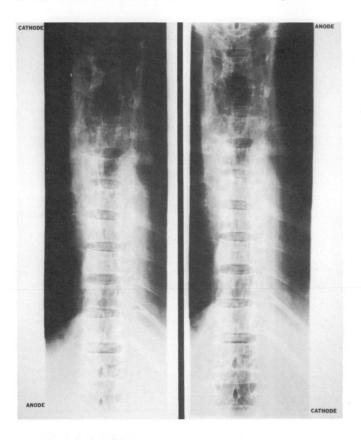

FIGURE 12-6. The anode heel effect is demonstrated in the radiographic image of the thoracic spine on the right. In cases in which the heel effect is expected to be a significant factor, the tube should be oriented with the anode over the upper thoracic spine and the cathode over the lower thoracic spine, where the thicker and denser body structures will receive greater exposure.

radiation exposure to the patient. According to the *inverse square law,* the intensity of radiation is inversely proportional to the square of the distance from the source of radiation. The intensity of radiation decreases at a longer SID; therefore, in order to maintain adequate radiation intensity, exposure factors must be increased, resulting in more patient exposure to radiation. At a set OID, increasing SID results in less magnification of image (Fig. 12–7). Some routine procedures such as radiography of the chest area have a routine SID of 72 inches in order to decrease magnification of the heart (Fig. 12–8*A,B*).

Except for rare cases, very little is gained from an increase in SID beyond 72 inches. Although 72 inches gives better radiographic detail, the overall increase in patient radiation exposure is too great to justify using this SID on a routine basis for every radiographic procedure.

With shorter SID, detail can be lessened because of magnification. Generally speaking, magnification occurs as SID decreases. Let us look again at the inverse square law in relation to a short SID. Radiation intensity is greater at a shorter SID because the source of radiation (x-ray tube) is closer to the object being radiographed. Therefore, more radiation exposure is delivered to the patient. Clearly, there must be an es-

tablished SID in order to obtain proper detail without subjecting the patient to excessive radiation. This is the reason SID is standardized at approximately 40 inches for the majority of routine radiographic procedures.

Ideal conditions for demonstrating maximum detail and minimizing unsharpness involve the use of a small focal spot, a long SID, and a short OID. Of course, for various reasons, these conditions cannot always be obtained. The use of a small focal spot may be disadvan-

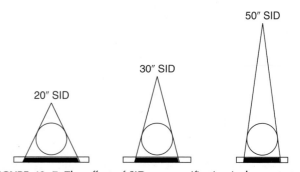

FIGURE 12-7. The effect of SID on magnification is demonstrated. Note on the diagrams that as source-to-image distance (SID) is increased, the degree of magnification decreases, and as SID is decreased, magnification increases.

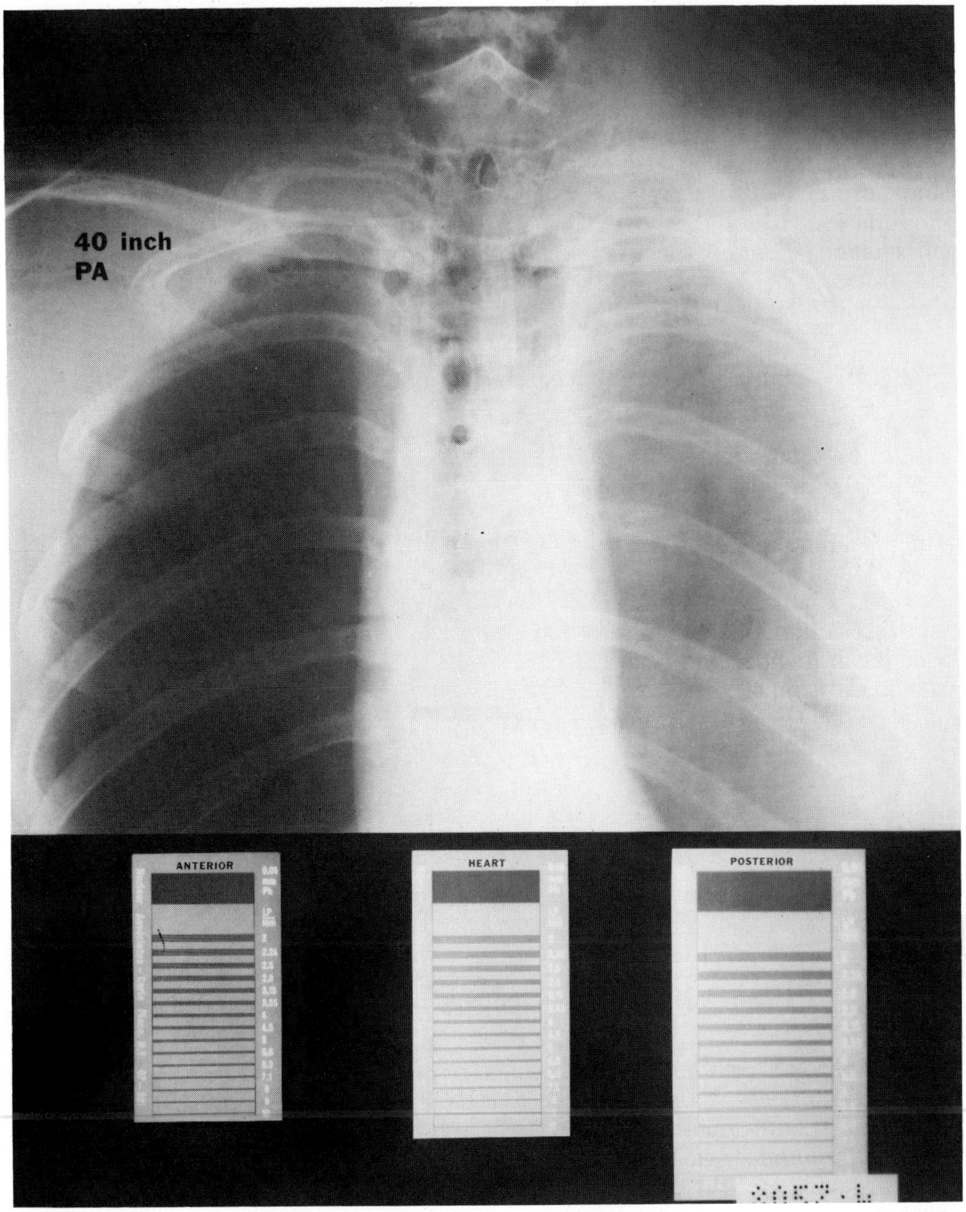

FIGURE 12-8. The effect of source-to-image distance (SID) on magnification and detail is noted on the PA projections of the chest phantom. Radiographic image made at an SID of 40 inches, *A*, shows more magnification of the heart compared with image made at an SID of 72 inches. *Figure continues.*

A

tageous, because it requires a long exposure time, since a smaller mA station is necessary. In turn, this increases the chance of patient movement or breathing during radiographic exposure. Increasing SID can enhance detail; however, more radiation will be delivered to the patient, since an increase in exposure factors is required.

It is important for the radiographer to realize that all three geometric factors—focal spot, SID, and OID—influencing geometric sharpness must be considered as combined interrelated factors in their effect on detail of the radiographic image. The radiographer can often use one or more of these factors to increase detail and sharpness. SID is the least critical of the geometric factors influencing sharpness, since it is a factor that is seldom changed. It would be necessary to make considerable adjustments in the SID in order to produce a visible change in radiographic detail. For this reason, a change in SID is not practical in most instances.

Object–Image Receptor Distance

OID has the greatest effect on radiographic detail of any of the three geometric factors. Increases in OID automatically increase magnification of the image.

Magnification

Magnification is a normal occurrence on most radiographs. The amount of magnification is determined by how the SID and OID are manipulated. As stated earlier, SID should be standardized at the longest possible distance. Whether the SID is long or short, it is

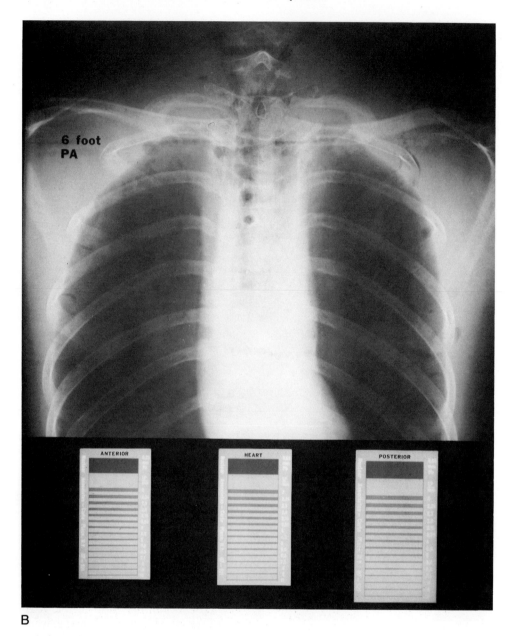

**6 foot
PA**

ANTERIOR

HEART

POSTERIOR

B

FIGURE 12–8 *Continued. B.* Overall radiographic detail is greater at 72 inches as noted when comparing the test patterns that were included on both radiographs. (Courtesy of ACR Learning File, Principles of Imaging, Sequence 157.)

absolutely necessary that the OID is kept to a minimum to control magnification of the image. It is extremely important to have the object being radiographed as close to the image receptor as possible. Unfortunately, some degree of OID is present with practically all images. In some instances, because of the position of the patient or specific structures being examined, it may be impossible to reduce OID.

When *table-top examinations* are performed, it is easier to maintain minimum OID since the object is placed directly on the film cassette. However, because of the thickness of some parts being radiographed, the use of a *Bucky grid* is necessary. Any time that an examination using a Bucky grid is performed, the OID slightly increases. Any object or anatomy that cannot be placed directly on the image receptor is magnified. Even small changes in OID can have a great effect on magnification and decrease radiographic detail (Fig 12–9*A,B*).

To determine how much magnification is present, the actual size of the object being radiographed must be compared with the size of the object on the image. Geometric factors are measurable, and the degree of magnification, or *magnification factor,* can be calculated with the following equations.

$$\text{Magnification} = \frac{\text{image width}}{\text{object width}}$$

Another way to state this formula is

$$\text{Magnification} = \frac{\text{SID}}{\text{*SOD}}$$

The *percentage of magnification* can be determined by subtracting object width from image width and divid-

---

* SOD (source–object receptor distance) = SID − OID.

FIGURE 12–9. Radiographs demonstrating the effects of object-image receptor distance (OID) on detail. Image *A* was taken with the object placed directly on the cassette. Image *B* was taken with the object placed 4 inches from cassette. Note the difference in magnification on image *B*. Also note how the radiographic detail is decreased in image *B*. The edges of the object on *A* are much sharper than on *B*.

ing by object width. The results are multiplied by 100. The formula is

$$\text{Percentage of magnification} = \frac{\text{IW} - \text{OW}}{\text{OW}} \times 100$$

Another way to state the same formula is as follows:

$$\text{Percentage of magnification} = \frac{\text{SID} - \text{SOD}}{\text{SOD}} \times 100$$

As demonstrated in Figure 12–10, the larger the OID, the greater is the penumbra, resulting in a decrease in overall radiographic detail.

In the routine of a radiology department, a radiographer may encounter many forms of radiographic unsharpness. In most cases, image unsharpness can be controlled by various methods, and image quality can remain high. Image distortion occurs on every radiograph to some extent; however, in most cases, the degree of image distortion can be controlled. Two types of distortion may occur on a radiograph. The radiographed image can possess varying degrees of size and shape distortion that the radiographer may or may not want. However, size and shape distortion are often used to the radiographer's advantage, so that a distorted image does not always result in an unacceptable radiograph.

Distortion

Size distortion is the misrepresentation of the actual size of the object that has been radiographed. The more common term used to describe this type of distortion is magnification. Recall that the magnification of a radiographed object can result from decreased SID or increased OID. The degree of magnification is greater as a result of an increased OID, whereas a decrease in SID has only a minimal effect on the magnification of the radiographed object. Size distortion can be used advantageously in many radiographic procedures. In angiographic procedures, the radiologist prefers a magnified image to increase the visibility of opacified vessels that are often extremely small. An increased OID is used to accomplish the desired level of magnification. The degree of magnification must be limited and a very small focal spot must be used so that there is no loss in detail, thereby decreasing the diagnostic qualities of the radiograph (Fig. 12–11).

Shape distortion is the misrepresentation of the actual shape of the radiographed image. The recorded image can be either *foreshortened* or *elongated,* depending on the position of the part, film, or central ray when the radiograph was obtained (Fig. 12–12). An image that possesses undesired shape distortion is usually the result of inadequate preparation by the radiographer. Shape distortion can be created in many ways. First, if an object to be radiographed is not parallel with the image receptor, the object will possess unwanted shape distortion (Fig. 12–13).

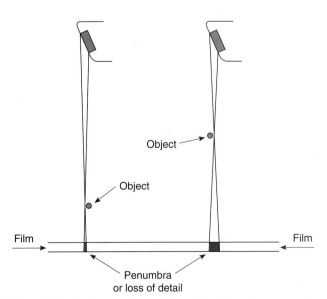

FIGURE 12–10. Diagram demonstrating how object-image receptor distance (OID) affects detail. An increase in OID increases penumbra.

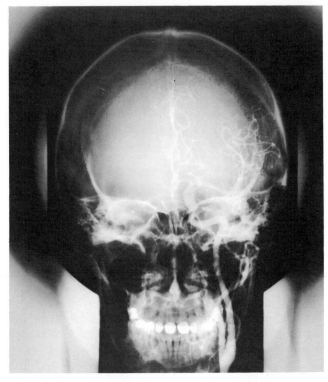

FIGURE 12-11. Cerebral arteriogram illustrating magnification radiography with the use of a 0.3-mm focal spot to maintain maximum radiographic detail.

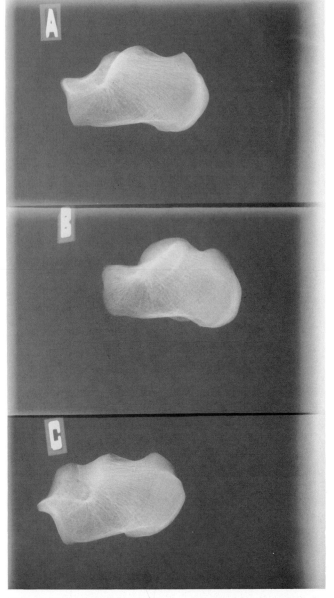

FIGURE 12-13. Distortional effect produced when the part to be examined is not properly aligned with the film. A dry bone is used for each image. *A,* The bone is parallel to the film. *B,* The anterior part of the bone is raised approximately 30°. *C,* The posterior part of the bone is raised approximately 30°. Note the foreshortening of image *B* and the elongation of image *C* compared with image *A.*

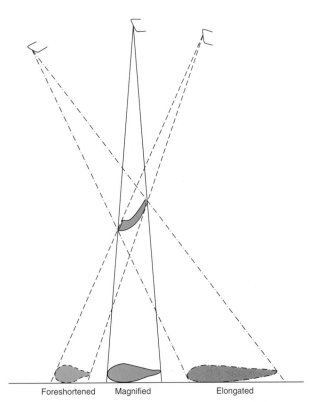

Foreshortened   Magnified   Elongated

FIGURE 12-12. Distortion resulting from the improper tube, object, and film alignment.

Shape distortion can also occur when the central ray of the primary beam is not placed over the center of the object as indicated in Figure 12-14. This distortion is most obvious when radiographing long bones.

The previously described forms of shape distortion are not useful. However, the shape distortion created by deliberate angulation of the central ray can be used advantageously in various radiographic procedures. The ability to avoid superimposition of anatomical parts is one reason for use of angulation of the central ray. For example, a special projection of the clavicle can avoid superimposition of structures that lie superior to the clavicle. As demonstrated, this projection straightens the natural curve of the clavicle, giving the physician a two-dimensional view of this bone. A fracture of the clavicle can also be visualized more effectively in this projection, as demonstrated by the radiographs of the clavicle (Fig. 12–15).

In most cases, image distortion is undesirable. In order to avoid any unwanted distortion, a thorough knowledge of what contributes to image distortion is a necessity for every radiographer. This knowledge is also necessary so that the radiographer can use image distortion advantageously.

As seen, manipulation of the geometric factors is not a simple task; rather, it involves a complex technical procedure. The radiographer must consider the multiple effects that the different geometric factors have on overall radiographic detail and must choose the changes that are most beneficial and least detrimental to the quality of the image.

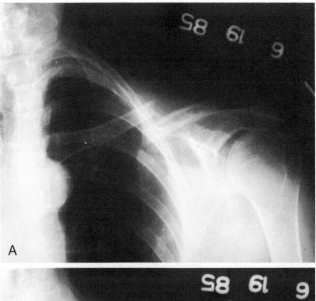
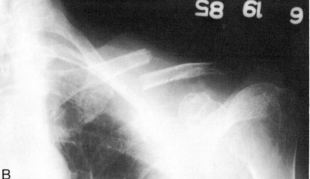

FIGURE 12–15. *A,* AP projection of the clavicle is demonstrated. *B,* An axial projection of the clavicle with cephalic angulation of the central ray. The fracture of the clavicle is seen much more effectively on the axial projection.

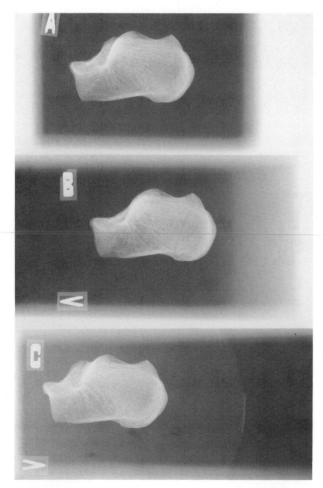

FIGURE 12–14. Distortion resulting from improper alignment of the central ray and the object to be examined. The part is parallel to the film on all images. The central ray is perpendicular on all images. *A,* The central ray is directed to the midpoint of the bone. *B,* The central ray is off-centered 6 inches to the left of the bone. *C,* The central ray is off-centered 6 inches to the right of the bone. Note the elongation of image *B* and the foreshortening of image *C* compared with image *A.*

■
EVALUATION OF RADIOGRAPHIC DETAIL

The factors contributing to geometric unsharpness are all measurable; therefore, the degree of unsharpness can be determined, measured, and expressed.

Recorded detail on the radiograph can be accurately evaluated by geometric methods. *Resolution* can be determined by the number of *line pairs* per millimeter that the imaging system is capable of recording. A line pair refers to a line and space. The human eye can detect lack of sharpness in a radiograph when the distinct lines of structural detail are wider than 0.2 mm (5 lines/mm). When the width of the recorded line pair measures above 0.2 mm, the level of unsharpness that exists is unacceptable. A count of 5 line pairs per millimeter means that there are five lines and five spaces per millimeter. Each line and each space is 0.1 mm wide, thus making each line pair 0.2 mm wide.

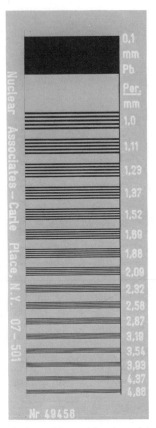

FIGURE 12-16. Resolution grid capable of resolving up to 10 line pairs per millimeter.

Resolution of the image can easily be identified by testing the image with a device known as a *resolution grid* capable of resolving up to ten line pairs per millimeter (Fig. 12-16).

Following is the formula used to determine the amount of geometric unsharpness present within a recorded radiographic image:

$$\text{Geometric unsharpness} = \frac{\text{Focal Spot Size} \times \text{OID}}{\text{Source-Object Receptor Distance (SOD)}}$$

MOTION UNSHARPNESS

Another factor that greatly contributes to lack of image sharpness is motion. It is the most important cause of image unsharpness. No matter how carefully the radiographer manipulates the geometric factors discussed earlier, if motion occurs, severe radiographic unsharpness will occur. *Motion unsharpness* can partially be controlled by using the smallest possible exposure time and obtaining maximum cooperation from the patient. These measures will prevent or limit patient movement and breathing during the radiographic procedure and will result in a sharper image.

Voluntary Motion

Motion can be categorized as voluntary and involuntary. *Voluntary motion* refers to a motion that can usually be controlled with a conscious effort. Most patients can cooperate and remain motionless in order to maintain a radiographic position. However, motion is most likely to become a problem when infants and children, the elderly, or injured patients are radiographed. Voluntary motion can usually be controlled with proper explanation and comfort to the patient along with use of *immobilization devices*. With patients such as children and infants, the exposure factors can be manipulated in order to obtain the shortest possible exposure time. Figure 12-17 demonstrates a radiograph of a patient who sneezed during the exposure. The overall quality of the radiograph is extremely poor because of the loss of detail. Sneezing is an example of voluntary motion that can be controlled. This type of situation does not often occur; however, taking a repeat radiograph with assurance from the patient that the "sneezing urge" is under control will greatly improve radiographic detail.

Involuntary Motion

For the control of unsharpness, involuntary motion must be given entirely different consideration. *Involuntary motion* occurs as a result of physiological activities of the systems of the body. The heartbeat is an exam-

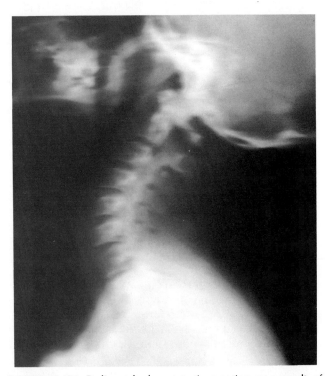

FIGURE 12-17. Radiograph demonstrating motion as a result of the patient's sneezing during exposure. The overall blurred appearance obscures radiographic detail.

ple of involuntary motion. The length of exposure time is the primary consideration with this type of motion. Short exposure time is essential in controlling involuntary motion due to the heartbeat or rhythmic action of other organs—*peristalsis,* for example. A reduction in exposure time can be accomplished by manipulating specific exposure factors such as mA and time or kVp and mAs relationships. A reduction in exposure time can also be achieved by substituting different imaging systems such as fast film–screen speed relationships. The major factor of radiographic quality affected by these adjustments is the radiographic density of the image. It is crucial that the overall acceptable level of density be maintained. Therefore, before adjustments are made, each area to be manipulated must be evaluated as to its influence on density in order to select relationships that will maintain overall proper radiographic density while achieving the desired reduction in time of exposure.

It also is important to remember that manipulation of exposure time in order to eliminate motion can affect radiographic detail as well as density. For this reason, to prevent an appreciable loss in radiographic detail, it is necessary to evaluate carefully each adjustment and to determine its effect on overall image sharpness.

Four means of maintaining sufficient radiographic density while reducing exposure time can be used. The methods are considered separately to determine how each affects radiographic detail.

1. Milliamperage-time relationship. This method should be considered first when attempting to control motion. It is fairly easy to maintain required radiographic density without affecting overall radiographic quality in most cases as long as a small focal spot is used. The problem arises when a higher mA is necessary in order to achieve the desired exposure time. In this instance, a large focal spot must be used, and as a result, radiographic detail will be lessened.
2. Faster intensifying-screen speed. This method can also be used to control motion unsharpness. It is usually the second alternative when the mA-time relationship is not workable. The faster *intensifying screens* allow the use of a shorter exposure time, thereby controlling motion during the radiographic procedure. The drawback is that it results in a loss of radiographic detail. Generally speaking, the faster the speed of the intensifying screen, the less the detail demonstrated on the image. The amount of loss depends on the screen-film combination used and their resolution properties.
3. kVp/mAs relationship. This method is another that can be used to aid in control of motion unsharpness. It is not the ideal method; although radiographic density can be maintained at a satisfactory level, the contrast is changed, thereby affecting the visibility of detail. This happens because the kVp must be increased for use of a lower mAs, which in turn allows the employment of a shorter exposure time. Since kVp controls the contrast, a higher kVp

produces more scatter radiation on the image, thus decreasing overall detail.
4. Source–image receptor distance (SID). This method should be used as a last alternative when other methods have failed to control motion unsharpness. The inverse square law can be used to maintain the proper density level with a decrease in SID; however, radiographic detail will be sacrificed. This method results in an increase in geometric unsharpness because of magnification of the object to be radiographed. However, if evaluation of the radiographic image determines that motion unsharpness is the contributing factor to the poor quality of the image, it may be necessary to use all means, including reducing SID, in order to improve the image. This may be the only alternative in eliminating the cause of the unacceptable radiograph in order to obtain a *diagnostic* if not *optimal image* for the radiologist. The radiographer must always keep in mind that patient motion is the single greatest factor resulting in radiographic unsharpness.

SCREEN UNSHARPNESS

Intensifying screens used in radiography are available in a variety of different speeds. The more efficient a screen, the less radiation intensity is required to produce a certain amount of film density. Knowing the speed of the intensifying screen enables the radiographer to select proper exposure factors, or maintain a desired radiographic density. Many of the factors related to the speed of the intensifying screen are inherent in the screen as produced by the manufacturer. The major factors influencing the speed of the intensifying screen are

- Use of different phosphor materials
- Size of the crystal of the phosphor
- Thickness of the phosphor layer
- Reflection of the phosphor layer backing material

Except for motion, the use of intensifying screens is the most significant factor contributing to image unsharpness (Fig. 12–18).

Intensifying screens depend on crystals of chemical phosphors with the property of fluorescence. Phosphor crystal size is a significant factor in both speed and resolution of the screen. As the phosphor crystal size becomes larger, the speed of the screen increases, and the resolution capability decreases. Another intrinsic factor affecting the speed and resolution of the screen is the thickness of the active layer of the screen. The active layer consists of phosphor crystals embedded in a binding material and bonded to a film backing. A larger number of phosphor crystals available to react to the x-ray beam results in greater speed of the intensifying screen. It can be concluded that an inverse relationship exists between screen speed and resolution. As the speed of the screen increases, the detail-recording capability of the screen and the radiographic quality of

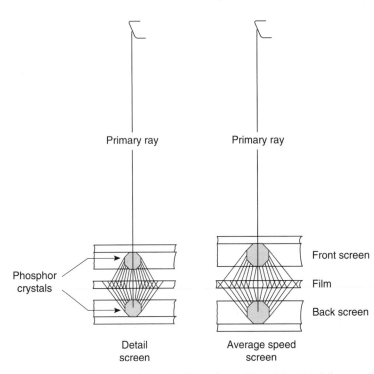

Primary ray

Primary ray

Phosphor crystals

Front screen

Film

Back screen

Detail screen

Average speed screen

Phosphor crystal size: significant factor determining detail loss

FIGURE 12-18. Diagram illustrating the major factor influencing the speed of an intensifying screen. Except for motion, use of an intensifying screen is the most significant factor contributing to image unsharpness.

the image decrease. Rapid imaging systems accomplish their goals by increasing the speed capability and achieve exposure reduction at the expense of decreasing the image resolution capability. High-speed, low-resolution systems are useful when radiation dose must be low and exposure time extremely short. Low-speed screens provide the best radiographic detail; however, when applied to general routine radiography, medium-speed systems produce sufficient resolution with an acceptable radiation dose and offer the best compromise in many situations.

Film-Screen Contact

It is essential that the film be in uniformly close contact with the screens. *Poor film-screen contact* decreases image sharpness in the areas in which the film and screen are not in proper contact with each other. In areas where there is a space between the screen and the film, light from the screen has to travel farther before reaching the film than in areas where the screen is in close contact with the film. The farther the light has to travel, the more it spreads laterally. This sideways spreading of the light tends to blur the image and make it less sharp. An image that has been carefully made, with consideration given to patient motion, focal spot size, SID, and screen speed, can be quickly ruined by blurring from poor film-screen contact (Fig. 12–19).

Poor film-screen contact can be due to many factors such as the following:

● Air trapped between screen and film. This problem was more common before the development of cas-

settes designed with curved front and back panels. Before cassette design was improved, pockets of air were often trapped between the screen and film as the cassette was closed. This trapped air resulted in poor film-screen contact. With the curved cassette, air is forced out as the cassette is closed, thus decreasing the possibility of poor film-screen contact.

● Foreign material on the screen. This circumstance is most likely to occur from a darkroom error when the cassette is loaded or unloaded. Any foreign material trapped between the screen and film can result in improper contact between screen and film. Keeping the darkroom work area and the screens clean is a necessity for this reason.

● Damaged cassettes and latches. Cassettes should periodically be inspected and replaced if necessary to prevent use of a damaged cassette. Cassettes should not be dropped or handled roughly. Dents or lack of alignment of the front and back will surely affect contact between the screen and film. Worn or torn felt around the edges of the cassette can also result in light leak and poor film-screen contact; therefore, the felt should be replaced if faulty. A regular schedule for checking to prevent poor film-screen contact should be a part of the quality control of the radiology department. It can be done simply by radiographing each cassette with a *wire mesh screen* on it (Fig. 12–20).

View the radiograph from a distance of at least 3 ft. Any areas of poor film-screen contact will appear as dark regions on the radiograph. The dark areas will also appear blurred.

Motion unsharpness appears as an overall blurred image, whereas poor film-screen contact is evident by

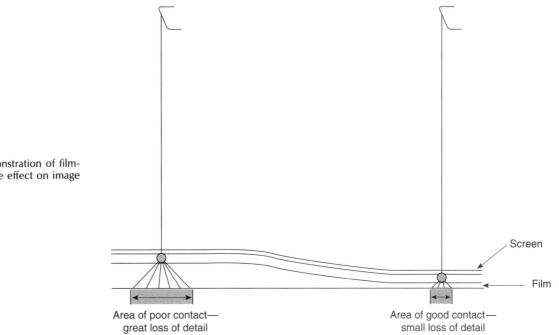

FIGURE 12–19. Demonstration of film-screen contact and the effect on image sharpness.

Screen

Film

Area of poor contact—
great loss of detail

Area of good contact—
small loss of detail

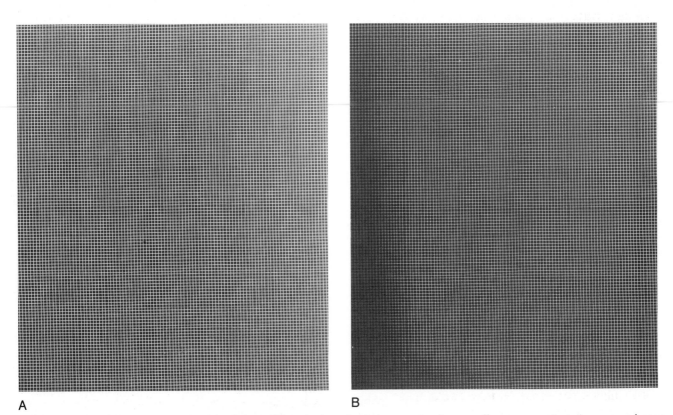

A

B

FIGURE 12–20. Wire mesh screens that have been radiographed to check the cassettes for poor film-screen contact. Any areas of poor film-screen contact appear as dark and blurred regions on the radiograph. *A* demonstrates good film-screen contact. *B* demonstrates poor film-screen contact as shown by the localized blurring in the dark regions.

localized blurring. Poor film-screen contact can have disastrous results on the image by producing a significant loss of detail. It is necessary that unsharpness caused by poor film-screen contact be eliminated from the radiographic image.

▰▰▰ Chapter Summary/ Important Concepts

Photographic properties refer to the visibility of detail, whereas geometric properties relate to the sharpness of detail. For good radiographic quality, there must be a proper balance between photographic and geometric properties.

Density and contrast are categorized as photographic properties, whereas detail and distortion are designated geometric properties. An image containing proper density and contrast is of little value if structural details are recorded as unsharp.

Detail and distortion are inversely related; as detail increases, distortion decreases, and vice versa.

In order to obtain clear detail, the part being radiographed must be properly penetrated by kVp and must possess sufficient density, indicated by proper balance between mA and exposure time.

Detail is primarily affected by geometric factors such as focal spot size, SID, and OID. Other factors that influence detail are motion unsharpness and screen unsharpness.

X-ray tubes are supplied with large and small focal spots. The size of the focal spot has a great influence on radiographic detail. Generally speaking, the smaller the focal spot, the greater the radiographic detail present on the image.

Large focal spots are usually available in 1.0, 1.2, 1.6, 2.0, or 3.0 mm, whereas small focal spots are available in 0.3 mm and 0.6 mm.

The x-ray tube is an area, not a point, source; therefore, using the smallest possible focal spot size should always be encouraged.

The line-focus principle increases resolution capability by use of steep target angles that in turn reduce the size of the effective focal spot. Steep target angles greatly enhance detail; however, field size is limited.

With steep target angles, the anode heel effect becomes more prominent. The heel effect is the result of decreased x-ray intensity at the anode end of the tube.

The anode heel effect is more pronounced with steep target angles, short SID, and large field sizes with little or no collimation.

The anode heel effect should be used with radiographic procedures such as those of the thoracic spine, which varies in thickness from the proximal to distal end.

Conditions necessary for demonstrating maximum detail and minimum unsharpness include the use of a small focal spot, maximum SID, and a short OID.

The radiographer must realize that all geometric factors influencing unsharpness must be considered as combined, interrelated factors in their effects on detail of the image.

Among the geometric factors, OID has the greatest effect on detail. Increases in OID automatically increase magnification of the image. It is extremely important to have the OID as short as possible for radiographic procedures.

The radiographic image can possess varying degrees of size and shape distortion.

Size distortion, the misrepresentation of the actual size of the radiographic object, is commonly known as magnification.

Shape distortion is the misrepresentation of the actual shape of the object in the radiographic image. Distortion can result in either foreshortening or elongation of the recorded image. Shape distortion can occur if the object being radiographed is not placed parallel to the image receptor. It also occurs when the central ray of the primary beam is not placed over the center of the object being radiographed.

Shape distortion can be used advantageously in various radiographic procedures to overcome superimposition of anatomical parts.

All geometric factors contributing to geometric unsharpness are measurable, and the degree of unsharpness can be determined, measured, and expressed.

Motion is the single most common cause of image unsharpness. It can largely be controlled by using the smallest possible exposure time and obtaining maximum cooperation from the patient.

▓▓ Review Questions

1. Identify and discuss the factors referred to as photographic properties and geometric properties.
2. Describe the significance of recorded structural details and sharpness as related to radiographic quality.
3. Describe a method you would use to control motion of a pediatric patient who cannot hold still for an abdominal radiographic examination.
4. Describe the influence SID manipulations have on radiographic detail and distortion.
5. Define image resolution, and describe how it is identified and measured.
6. Write the formula for determining the size distortion in a radiographic image.
7. Write the formula for determining the percentage of magnification produced in a radiographic image.
8. Explain how increasing the SID can lead to motion unsharpness.
9. Describe the influence of screen speed on radiographic detail.
10. Does an image possessing a proper balance of geometric properties of detail and distortion automatically ensure that you have produced a film that is of good radiographic quality? Explain your answer.
11. An object that is to be radiographed is located 10 inches above the film. The SID is 40 inches, and the diameter of the object is 12 inches. What is the magnification factor? What is the percentage of magnification?

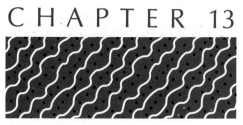

CHAPTER 13

Improving Image Quality

Marian P. Hattaway, B.S., R.T.(R.)

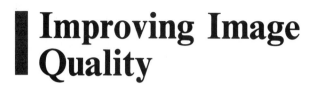

Chapter Objectives

On completion of this chapter, you should be able to

■ Identify by name the effects of an x-ray production feature and the use of identified accessory devices on the quality of the radiographic image.

■ Describe the effects of each of the following on the quality of the radiographic image:
  • *anode heel*
  • *beam filter*
  • *compensating filter*
  • *beam restrictor (each type)*
  • *image receptors (and all types of screens)*
  • *grid (any type or ratio identified)*
  • *air gap*

■ Explain the general principles that justify the use of the anode heel effect for image formation.

■ Distinguish between the types of beam restrictors with regard to construction, advantages, and disadvantages.

■ Explain positive beam limitation.

■ Describe the formation of an image on a medical x-ray film when an intensifying screen is used.

■ Describe the quantity and distribution of light emitted by intensifying screens when x-ray photons strike them during the imaging process.

■ Explain the effect of kVp on the speed of intensifying screens.

■ Determine changes in exposure factors when given the original factors of exposure and the
  • *intensifying screen speed is changed*
  • *beam restrictor size is changed*
  • *grid ratio is changed*
  • *grid type is changed*

■ Determine the necessary changes in exposure factors to obtain specific air gaps for radiography of various parts.

■ Suggest the exposure factors and devices to produce a diagnostic image for identified parts, specifically requiring that the smallest amount of radiation exposure be delivered to the patient.

An image receptor, an anatomical part, and an x-ray source in the general relationship depicted in Figure 13–1 are required to produce a medical radiographic image. Proper use of x-ray production features and other devices are needed to produce quality radiographic images and to conform to the standards established for the diagnostic use of ionizing radiation. These features and devices are considered in the order in which they affect the exposure as the x-ray photons move to the image receptor (film).

Radiography

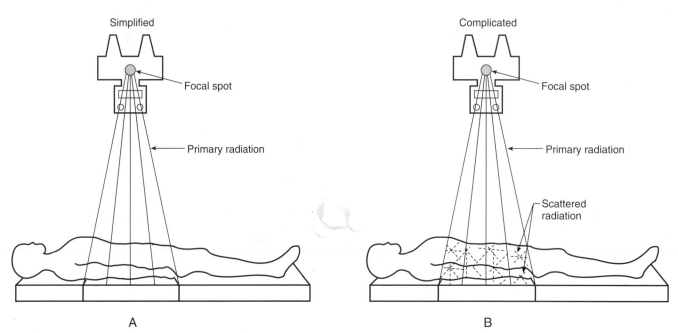

FIGURE 13–1. Situations in radiography. *A* represents the simplest form of radiography practiced today. X-rays are emitted from the focal spot of the anode, move through the air to the object (patient) and through the object to an image receptor. *B* represents a more complicated situation. In addition to the basics in *A*, secondary (scattered) radiation, which has an effect on the film emulsion, is being produced. (From Characteristics and Applications of X-Ray Grids, courtesy of Liebel-Flarsheim.)

ANODE HEEL EFFECT IN IMAGING

The origin of the x-ray beam is the focal spot of the x-ray tube. The size of the focal spot affects the formation of the image as discussed in Chapter 12. Besides the focal spot size, another feature occurring at the anode of the x-ray tube affects the x-ray beam and therefore the radiographic image. This feature is the anode heel phenomenon (see Chap. 6). The radiographic effect is a result of the variation of intensity of the x-ray beam along the longitudinal axis of the x-ray tube (anode to cathode). At the cathode, the intensity of the x-ray beam is higher than at the center of the tube and is much higher than at the anode. This phenomenon is referred to by radiographers as the *anode heel effect.*

The heel effect is most noticeable when large radiation fields are used at short source-image distances (SIDs). For example, when using a 14-inch × 17-inch radiation field lengthwise and a beam produced with a focal spot mounted at a 20° angle, the percentage of intensity for various SIDs at the respective ends of the tube are

| | Percentage of Intensity | |
SID (inches)	Anode end (%)	Cathode end (%)
25	31	95
30	56	102
36	~ 65	~ 103.5
40	73	105
60	85	104
72	~ 87.5	~ 103.5

If the central portion of the beam (the central ray) is considered as 100% intensity at 40 inches, along the 17-inch length of the film, the intensity varies 32% between the beam's cathode and anode ends. At a 72-inch SID, the variation is a total of 16%. If the SID is less than 40 inches—25 inches, for example—the intensities vary a total of approximately 64%. According to these numbers, the heel effect should be noticeable at a 40-inch SID, and evidence should become even more marked at shorter SIDs.

Modern x-ray tubes feature a more steeply angled anode. The anode heel effect is increased in the x-ray tube, although it is not as evident in the image. It exists sufficiently to use this fact to produce images with more uniform radiographic density of parts that vary in penetrability along their longitudinal axes. This use of the effect is accomplished by aligning the anatomical part with the long axis of the tube and placing the section of the anatomical part that is hardest to penetrate under the cathode end of the tube.

FILTRATION OF THE X-RAY BEAM

Once the x-ray beam leaves the anode and moves through the tube, the part of the beam that is directed toward the tube window exits from the tube. Some of the longer, less penetrating wavelengths are removed from the beam during its passage through the components and window of the tube. The glass envelope of the tube and its oil insulation are part of the *inherent filtration* in the x-ray beam.

The beam then passes through thin metal plates inserted in the tube housing below the exit window. This is the *added filtration* required to increase the average energy of the beam. A *filter* is the specific thickness of a given metal that will reduce the intensity of an x-ray beam to a specific level. In diagnostic radiology, the metal most commonly used is aluminum (Al). The amount of filtration is generally stated as mm of Al or mm of Al equivalent. This added filter removes the lower-energy photons in the beam that would otherwise be absorbed by the skin of the patient and are useless in the formation of the image. The amount of filtration in a beam is established by the National Council on Radiation Protection (NCRP) and is based on the energy levels used to produce the beam. The minimum *total filtration* (inherent plus added filtration) recommended by the NCRP is

Energy of Beam	Amount of Filtration
<50 kVp	0.5 mm Al
50–70 kVp	1.5 mm Al
>70 kVp	2.5 mm Al

The effect of filtration in the beam is to "harden" the beam by increasing its average energy. This also means the average wavelength is shorter and the average frequency is higher in the filtered beam. The x-rays that are more penetrating remain in the beam. More than 3 mm Al equivalent filtration contributes very little to the primary purpose of the filter (Fig. 13–2), that is, to reduce the radiation skin-dosage of the patient at the irradiated area. It does further reduce the average wavelength, ensuring to a degree the penetration of the anatomical part by the remaining x-rays and decreasing both the radiographic density and contrast (Fig. 13–3). To obtain the original radiographic density, the exposure (mAs or kVp) must be increased, adding radiation dose to the remaining skin dose to the patient. Exposure factors made necessary by the recommended beam filter appear in the factors listed on technique charts. These should not be altered unless the total amount of filtration is changed.

Additional filters may be used when imaging an anatomical part that varies noticeably in tissue density from one area to another as a way to enhance visibility of the entire structure without making additional exposures. These are called compensating filters. They function to prevent the total radiation used for the exposure from reaching the thinner, less dense areas of the anatomical parts being imaged.

Wedge filters are recommended for long parts that vary in thickness of tissue or tissue density along their longitudinal axes. An example is either a femoral arteriogram or an abdominal radiograph of a barrel-chested individual. In both cases, the superior areas are thick and require more radiation for radiographic demonstration. The inferior areas of the part are considerably thinner and easier to penetrate. To demonstrate these areas requires comparatively less radiation. Figure 13–4*A* is a diagram of the view of the flat surface and a cross-sectional view through the midline of this filter along its longitudinal axis.

A trough filter is used for chest radiography in many radiology departments. This filter is thicker at the lateral borders along its long axis. It is placed so that the thinner section covers the mediastinal area of the chest position and the thicker section the lung fields. This position allows the mediastinum to be imaged with increased density without overexposing the lung fields. Figure 13–4*B* depicts the flat surface and a cross-sectional view along the short axis of the trough filter.

Beam Restrictors and Their Uses

The x-ray beam passes through a *beam restrictor,* which usually changes the x-ray beam in two ways. Some of the beam emerging from the tube is eliminated in each case. The part that is occluded is a peripheral portion of the beam. When the perimeter is excluded, the shape of the beam quite often changes. If the aperture of the beam restrictor is circular, the beam is circular in shape, but its diameter (size) is reduced. If the aperture is rectangular, the beam shape becomes rectangular. A rectangular aperture reduces the area irradiated by the beam and assures that only the film will be exposed. The choice of beam shape should be based on the anatomical part to be radiographed—its size and shape and the extent of the surrounding area to be included in the radiation field.

A *beam restrictor* is used to reduce the beam so that the anatomical part to be radiographed is adequately exposed without exposing areas of the body outside the area of interest. This device eliminates unnecessary radiation exposure to body parts not shown in the radiographic image and eliminates scatter radiation produced in those body parts. Scatter radiation serves no useful purpose. It produces an overall gray haze called *fog* that covers the pertinent anatomy. This fog was depicted in Figure 11–25 (see Chap. 11).

Fog is detrimental to a radiograph. It increases overall radiographic density and obscures image sharpness, thus diminishing the diagnostic quality of the image. A secondary objective of beam restriction is to reduce fogging of the radiographic image. Decreasing the amount of irradiated tissue lessens the amount of radiographically effective secondary radiation. Doing this thins the overall radiographic density, effectively increases the radiographic contrast, and makes the recorded detail of the image more evident. Many references call this "enhancing *radiographic detail.*" The process does not increase *geometric detail* (i.e., production of image sharpness) but does augment *photographic detail* (i.e., the recognizability of image sharpness). Figure 13–5 offers radiographic proof.

Obviously, beam restriction reduces the amount of tissue irradiated and the whole body dosage to the patient. It also improves the radiographic quality of the image. This is especially true with modern exposure

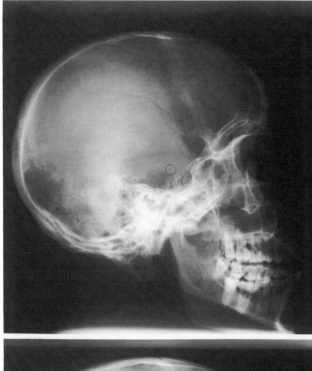

A

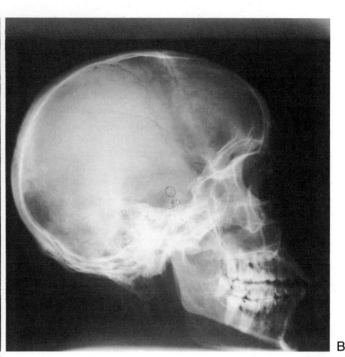

B

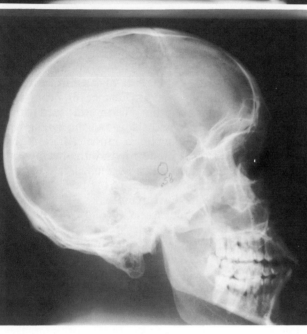

C

FIGURE 13-2. Effect of filtration in radiography. Three lateral projections of the skull (A through C), all exposed factors. The changes made between each projection were the mm of aluminum added as filtration, increased in increments of 2.0 mm. The differences in appearance are a loss in radiographic density and an apparent decrease in radiographic contrast as the filtration increases.

In A, density level obscures some of the thinner, peripheral structures of the head. There are three well-defined tissue density masses inside the image of the head; the largest is posterior to the mastoid air cells; two smaller masses appear immediately above it. B, Structures that were vague or obscured in A are revealed. The three masses remain visible and are outlined in B. The amount of aluminum filtration used here was 2.5 mm of aluminum as recommended for exposures above 70 kVp. In C, peripheral structures obscured in A are clearly visible, but the three internal masses in B have become progressively less distinct after A. The visibility gains and losses noted after A result from loss of density. (From the University of Alabama at Birmingham Radiographer Program Teaching File.)

techniques, which use higher average kilovoltages (kVp) than were possible a few years ago. These higher average kVp produce more radiographically effective scatter radiation; that is, if the same volumes of tissue irradiated with the new higher kVp are equal to those irradiated with the lower average kVp of 25 to 30 years ago, more scatter radiation will reach the film. The images in Figure 13-6 are examples of this.

At lower kVp exposures, very low-energy, secondary radiation is produced and is usually absorbed by the tissue. The patient dosage is increased over that received when higher kVp is used. At higher kVp levels, the secondary radiation is also produced but has the energy to reach the film and be photographically effec-

tive. This can easily be proved by the radiographs of the hand in Figure 13-7. Image A was produced by using 40 kVp and 5 mAs. One should note that this is the minimum kVp calculated to penetrate the hand. The image of the hand in B is produced with an exposure using 58 kVp and 0.833 mAs.

Fixed-Aperture Beam Restriction Devices

Various types of beam restrictors may be used. Examples of fixed-aperture beam restrictors are shown in Figure 13-8. One of the earliest was the *diaphragm,*

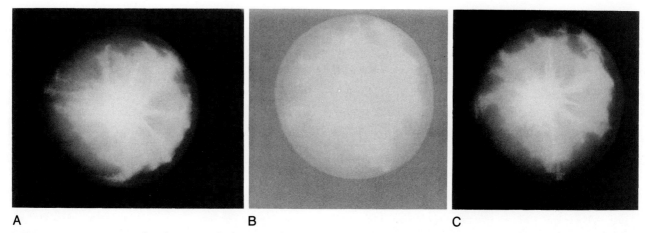

FIGURE 13-3. Compensation for changes in the amount of filtration. Three radiographs of an orange injected with an iodinated contrast material. A nonscreen exposure technique was made for each image. *A* (2.5 mm of aluminum [Al], 40 mAs, 80 kVp) is the standard image. The object is well penetrated, with sufficient density and contrast to visualize the section membranes, the pulp, and the distribution of the contrast material in the orange. *B* (5 mm of Al, 40 mAs, 80 kVp), Loss of density is significant; it is difficult to determine the correct orientation of the image. A large, irregular mass is revealed inside the orange outline. The sections cannot be differentiated, and the section membranes are not seen. The orange peel offers no differentiation from adjacent parts. *C* (5 mm of Al, 50 mAs, 82 kVp), With compensation the peel can be defined, as can the sections, pulp, section membranes (especially those that contrast material has reached), and the pattern of contrast material distribution is apparent. (From the University of Alabama at Birmingham, Radiographer Program Teaching File.)

consisting of a flat, radiopaque metal plate designed to be attached to the tube housing at its lower surface. There is an aperture or opening in this metal plate to allow part of the primary x-ray beam to pass through to reach the patient. The aperture may be round, rectangular, or any other shape. It is located directly beneath the site of the tube window. Diaphragms may be made commercially or by someone in the radiology department or hospital. When these devices are used for all radiographic examinations, a large number are required in each radiographic room for convenient exchange between examinations and adequate limitation of patient exposure. In addition to the inconvenience of changing them, secondary radiation produced at the aperture rim may reach and be absorbed by the patient. With higher energy radiation, this secondary radiation from the aperture rim may be radiographically effective. If this happens, the recorded detail of the image is decreased or obscured, and the image contrast is diminished by this radiation. Naturally, the overall

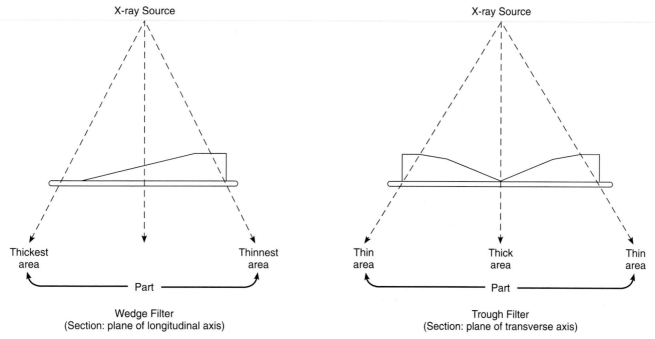

FIGURE 13-4. Compensating filters. Diagram of sectional planes through two different types of filters.

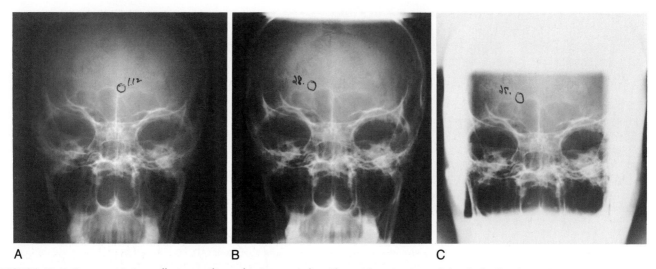

A   B   C

FIGURE 13–5. Beam restriction: effect on radiographic image quality. Three AP projections of the skull; all radiographed using 75 mAs, 75 kVp, and 40-inch source-image distance (SID). The decrease in image density from A (14- × 17-inch radiation field) through C (4.5- × 4.5-inch radiation field) is visibly detectable. The recorded detail of the image appears to be much increased in C. This can be attributed to the decrease in density and the increase in contrast as a result of the decrease in scatter radiation. The measured radiographic density value in A was 1.12; in B, 0.76; and in C, 0.67. (From University of Alabama at Birmingham Radiographer Program Teaching File.)

density of the radiograph is enhanced more than would be expected from the exposure factors.

The *cone* was the next beam restriction device to appear. *Flared cones* for large-area radiographs at shorter SIDs and *cylinder cones* for small areas were still commonly used in the 1950s. Cylinder cones were also used for large areas at greater SIDs.

In construction, the cone is effectively an extension of the aperture of a diaphragm. It consists of a base, a metal plate with an aperture (usually round), with

which the device is attached to the tube housing. From the metal plate, a sheet of metal forming a circular ring or, less commonly, a rectangle extends away from the tube. The distal end of the metal tube is larger than the aperture of the plate. It is designed to be effective in removing most of the secondary radiation produced at the rim of the aperture and a portion of the primary radiation coming from the tube.

This beam restrictor is more effective in limiting the size of the x-ray beam than was the diaphragm. How-

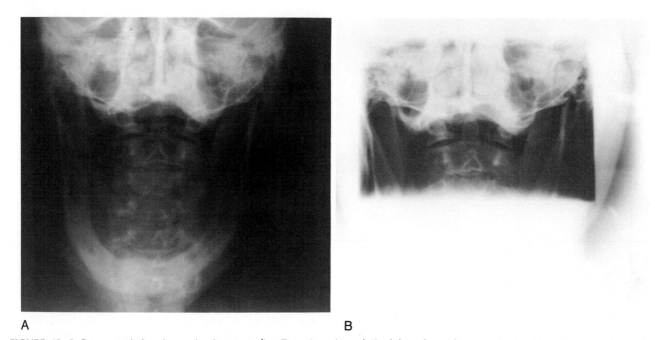

A   B

FIGURE 13–6. Beam restriction: improving image quality. Two views (A and B) of the odontoid process in the AP projection radiographed with 20 mAs, 82 kVp, 30-inch source-image distance (SID), and different radiation field sizes. In B (5.75 × 3.75 field size) structures of interest are seen much more clearly than in A (8 × 10 field size); the image density is diminished, and the radiographic contrast is increased. The image sharpness is markedly increased in B.

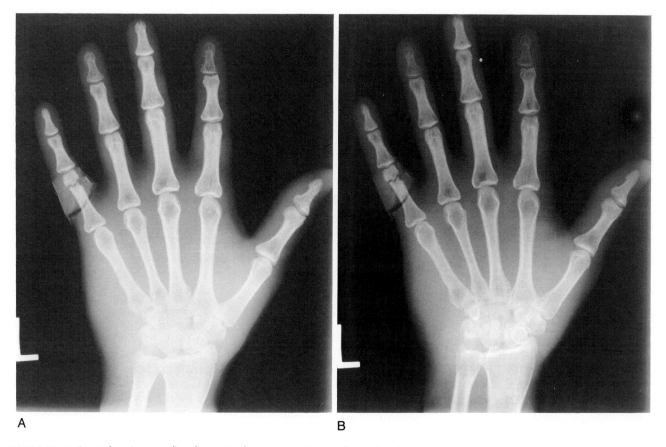

A   B

FIGURE 13-7. Secondary (scattered) radiation in thinner parts. Two radiographs of the hand. *A* was exposed using 5 mAs and 40 kVp; *B* was exposed using 0.83 mAs and 58 kVp. Densities between the images vary, although the mAs/kVp compensations to maintain identical radiographic densities were performed correctly. Densities were measured at an identical point on each image and *B* (density = 1.81) has a higher density value than *A* (density = 1.64). Some of the increased radiation density is caused by secondary radiation.

ever, the necessity of changing the size cone to properly radiate different sizes of body parts remained a problem. Cones are heavier than diaphragms, and the assortment of sizes needed routinely in a radiography department is only slightly fewer in number.

The cone that is best for limiting the beam size and eliminating secondary radiation is the *extension cylin-*

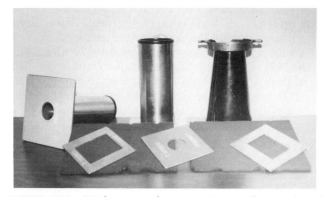

FIGURE 13-8. Fixed-aperture beam restrictors. Photographs of cones and diaphragms. Cylindrical cones of two sizes are shown, one lying on its side to show the aperture nearest the x-ray tube and base plate to which the cylinder is attached. The flare cone is an old one saved by the program for student demonstration. In the foreground of the photograph are three diaphragms. Two apertures are rectangular and one is circular.

der cone. The construction of this cone is similar to that of the cylinder cone except there is an outer-sleeve cylinder that can be released and moved to place the aperture of the beam restrictor closer to the area radiographed without reducing the SID. This device is particularly useful for radiography of smaller areas of thick, dense parts such as paranasal sinuses, gall bladders, and temporomandibular joints. It proved so useful in the past that it continues to be used with collimators.

Variable-Aperture Beam Restriction Devices

Collimators are the third type of beam restrictor to have been developed. They gained rapid popularity for several reasons that become evident in the discussion. A photograph of two of these devices appears in Figure 13-9. These devices are permanently mounted on the tube housing, and the radiation field size can be changed by adjusting a dial or a set of dials or levers located on the collimator. The first collimator this author used was a Viadex, which projected a round radiation field. There was a light localizer on the back side of the collimator that could be swung down into the radiation field. The light was used to center the radiation beam on the table, the anatomical part on the

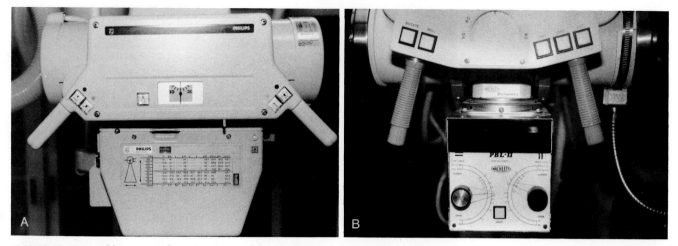

FIGURE 13–9. Variable-aperture beam restrictor. Photograph of two radiographic collimators illustrates available types. Note the features described in the text.

table, and the film on the body part and the radiation beam (central ray). There were some problems associated with this type of collimator. It projected a round field, meaning that a considerable amount of film was wasted (i.e., no image on part of it) or more of the body was irradiated than was necessary to produce the desired projected image.

Today, rectangular apertures for collimators are quite common modern radiographic equipment. These collimators are constructed with shutters for two sets of apertures, permitting adjustment of the aperture size. One set of shutters forms an aperture near the tube and consists of four adjustable shutters made of a radiopaque material. There are two longitudinal and two lateral shutters in each set. A second, more distally located aperture, is constructed like the one nearer the tube. The purpose of the second aperture is to reduce the secondary radiation from the first aperture to a minimum and to remove some of the periphery of the primary beam. The distal aperture is slightly larger than the proximal aperture. The size of the aperture is adjusted by using dials or levers on the collimator. A scale, located on the collimator on the operator side of the table, has indicators giving the usual field sizes at various SIDs. The scale is used to determine the appropriate size of radiation field for each radiographic exposure based on the size of the anatomical part, the film size, and the SID used.

This arrangement is obviously more convenient for the operator than changing diaphragms or cones for each exposure. The dual aperture of the collimator provides the best features of most beam restrictors. When an extension cylinder cone is needed for an exposure, many collimators are equipped for its attachment.

Two additional features of a collimator make the radiographer's job much easier. The first of these is the *light localizer,* a system composed of mirrors and a light bulb. These components are carefully arranged to project a visible light field that coincides with the invisible radiation field from the x-ray tube. The light field should be the same size and shape as the radiation field. The light-field size is adjusted simultaneously with that of the size of the radiation field.

The surface of the collimator away from the tube is open except for a transparent covering of glass or plastic. There are two crossed lines called cross hairs on this covering. The point where they cross indicates the position of the central ray of the x-ray beam. It is used to center the x-ray beam on the anatomical part or the table. Coincident with the laterally (side-to-side of the table) placed cross hair is usually a bright slit of light that projects past the edge of the radiographic table on the side nearest the operator. This can be used to center the midpoint of a film in the Bucky on the transverse level of the central ray or the central ray on the transverse level of the midpoint of the film.

The advantages of the collimator should be evident. To be used properly, the collimator should periodically be checked to assure that the light field does define the radiation field accurately. It must be determined that when using an SID of 40 inches, the light field is within 1.0 cm of the corresponding edge of the radiation field (equivalent to 2% of the SID used for the exposure) on all four sides of the field. The current minimal standards for accuracy are outlined in Title 21 of the Code of Federal Regulations (21 CFR, Part 800-1299). The length and width of the radiation field, as indicated by the light field, should be within 2% of the SID used with the field. If the mirrors or lightbulb forming the light field are improperly positioned, the accuracy standards have not been met.

Positive Beam Limitation

In 1974 the federal regulations were changed to specify that all fixed radiographic equipment incorporate a beam-limiting device that automatically limits the size of the radiation field to the size of the film used. This invention is called a *positive beam limitation device (PBL).* The size of the field is determined by sensors in the Bucky mechanism that detect the size of the cassette as it is locked into place in the Bucky tray. Furthermore, the radiation field size must be accurate to within 2% of the SID used for the exposure to meet the necessary radiation safety standards.

The x-ray beam emerges from the x-ray tube and passes through the collimator. It moves with negligible hindrance through the air of the room toward the patient. As the distance of the beam from the tube increases, the area of the beam increases and the intensity of the beam decreases (inverse square law). When the x-ray beam reaches the part of the patient to be radiographed, the body acts as a filter. It is a variable filter, dependent on the tissue content and thickness of the body part. Chapters 11 and 14 discuss exposure factors and their relationship to tissue types and thicknesses.

As a result of the interaction of the x-ray photons with the patient's body, secondary radiation is produced by two types of processes—photoelectric and Compton interactions. Classic scattering may occur to a negligible degree. The photoelectric interaction results in the production of both ion pairs and characteristic x-rays. Most are completely absorbed in the tissues of the body part. These usually do not have sufficient energy to affect the radiographic image. Because they do not, image contrast is attributed to this type interaction.

Above 100 keV, as the energy increases, the x-rays produce more and more secondary radiation that is radiographically effective (Compton interaction). For some thinner anatomical parts, this occurs at a lower-keV energy level, which means that there will be more fogging of the image, making its parts less distinguishable from each other. Every reasonable effort should be made to reduce this fogging.

Fogging of the radiograph produced by a body part is based on a number of factors. The first factor is the volume of tissue irradiated. The volume is determined by the area irradiated and its thickness. The area of the x-ray beam depends on the aperture of the beam restrictor and the SID at which the aperture is used. The thickness is the measurement in centimeters of the path of the central ray through the area irradiated. More secondary radiation is produced by an anatomical part that occupies a large area or is thick or dense. Less secondary radiation is produced in a small, thin body part. In the latter case, the beam restrictor is usually the device used to control fog.

The second fogging factor is the kVp used for the exposure. Lower kVp results in less fogging of the image but more patient absorbed radiation dose. Higher kVp usage produces a greater degree of image fogging, which may become objectionable unless a method is found to eliminate it or keep the secondary radiation fogging from reaching the film.

The third factor contributing to the fogging of an image is the tissue composing the area irradiated. Areas containing fluid-filled tissues or extremely dense tissues produce more secondary radiation, which fogs the film image, than do tissues that contain air. Much of this fog can be controlled by the proper use of beam restrictors.

Beam restrictors reduce the amount of total radiation reaching the film. The effect on the quality of the image is to decrease the overall density, increase the contrast between the structures depicted in the image, and enhance the recorded detail for visualization. These facts emphasize the need to reduce the useful beam to the minimum size for each exposure. In radiography, the intent is to produce images with the greatest contrast between adjacent structures of an anatomical part and to demonstrate as much recorded detail as possible.

Caution should be exercised when radiographing a small area within a large, dense mass of tissue. If the exposure technique for a large mass is the base exposure technique of the area, remember to replace radiographic density lost by the reduction of secondary radiation as a result of restricting the beam to a small area. This is done by increasing the primary radiation exposure. The amount by which it is increased depends on the amount of reduction in the tissue involved, the kVp level employed for a larger field, and the tissue type in the restricted field.

Some references list exposure technique conversions based on reduction of beam size by restrictors. The problem with this method is that exposure factor increases for the various areas of the body do not take into consideration the kVp level in use at a larger area or the type of tissue in a smaller area to be radiographed. When these are used without the other factor considerations, errors are made. If the small volume to be irradiated is surrounded by and contains air or air-filled tissue, the difference in exposure factors should be minor. If the area instead contains fluid or extremely dense tissue, the increase in exposure factors must be significant. The factor that also governs the amount of compensation for density is the kVp used. If exposure factors for a large area include a high kVp, their increase will be minor. Significant changes in exposure factors are required to compensate for density changes if the original kVp is low.

Every radiology department has specific recommendations for ways to compensate for a loss of radiographic density as a result of further restricting the x-ray beam. Most departments include this information in the exposure techniques for the more common radiographs of small areas such as lateral projections of the L5–S1 junction, paranasal sinuses, temporomandibular articulations, and so forth.

Image Receptors and Their Uses

The primary x-ray beam emerging from the beam restrictor moves through the air space between the tube and the patient. As it strikes and then moves through the patient, the primary beam undergoes several changes. Some of the x-rays in the beam pass through the body unaffected. Others are totally absorbed by the body tissue. Still others undergo changes as they move through the body. The radiation that emerges from the body part, known as exit *(remnant) radiation,* contains primary and secondary radiation.

This emergent radiation carries the most accurate imaging information about the internal structures of the body part. If the exposure is of a thin or small anatomical part, the part is in direct contact with the surface of the *film holder (cassette).* The exit radiation from the part goes directly to the image receptor in the cassette to record the information about the structures in a part.

A body part that is thick and dense requires the use of a *grid (Bucky)* to reduce the amount of secondary radiation in the exit radiation. In such cases, the part usually lies in contact with the grid surface or the radiographic table surface. The cassette is placed in the Bucky tray, which lies immediately below the table surface. Before the exit radiation from the part reaches the *image receptor* it must pass through the table top and parts of the Bucky mechanism. Both produce some secondary radiation that contributes to the exit radiation before it reaches the image receptor. This contribution adds radiation that may become part of the image but does not contribute to image quality. It may also obscure the information contained in the emerging radiation.

At the point the emergent beam leaves the patient, the information it contains is not evident. To become visually detectable, the information contained by the emerging radiation must be intercepted by a device called a receptor. In the simplest example of radiography, the next factor in the imaging process is the image receptor. The image receptor commonly consists of a fluoroscopic screen, a medical x-ray film, or a combination of an intensifying screen and a radiographic film. Fluoroscopic image formation and recording and imaging characteristics of medical x-ray film are discussed in other chapters.

Intensifying Screens

The most common image receptor used in radiography is the combination of an *intensifying screen* and medical x-ray film in a light-tight container called a *cassette.*

Intensifying screens and fluoroscopic screens are similar in their functional mechanics. Each emits visible light when x-ray energy strikes it. The pattern of light closely corresponds to the pattern of the x-rays. That is, where x-rays in larger concentration or of higher energy strike, a brighter portion of the pattern emerges. If the concentration is small or is composed of low-energy x-rays, only a small amount of light is emitted. Dark areas in the emitted light pattern are caused by few, if any, x-rays with low energies striking the screen at those points.

HISTORY

The intensifying screen was first designed by Edison, who used calcium tungstate as the phosphor. A *phosphor* is the crystalline form of a compound that can receive a higher energy (higher frequency, shorter wavelength) photon, absorb it, and emit a lower energy

(lower frequency, longer wavelength) photon. In this instance, the emitted energy is in the visible light spectrum. According to Edison's study of phosphors, there are 980 such compounds. He found calcium tungstate to be the most efficient in converting x-ray energy to the energy of visible light. Calcium tungstate crystals convert x-rays (0.01 Å to 0.05 Å) to ultraviolet-blue light (3500 Å to 4800 Å), which is more photographically effective than x-rays alone. The peak wavelength in this case is about 4300 Å and is visible as a violet color. The eye is not sensitive to this light level, but blue-sensitive film exhibits maximum sensitivity to it. An advantage of calcium tungstate crystals is that they stop emitting visible light instantaneously when the x-rays cease. In Edison's study, many of the other phosphor crystals continued to emit light after the x-rays ceased.

The first screens (1896 to the 1920s) had faults. As a result, they were used only for examinations in which the ability to intensify the density of the image was absolutely necessary. Faults included continued fluorescence after the radiation exposure ceased (referred to as screen lag), crystals that were not of uniform size and were not coated onto the base in uniformly thick layers, and screens that could not be cleaned without damaging the crystal layers. Any attempt to clean them caused a shifting in position or the removal of the phosphor crystals.

During the early 1920s the process of manufacturing screens was perfected to eliminate the earlier problems. That process and the rigid quality control of the process are still used today with some modifications.

SCREEN CONSTRUCTION

Intensifying screens are constructed by using a strong, slightly flexible base, first coated with an extremely thin layer of reflective material followed by a uniformly thick layer of phosphor crystals, and on the outside, a radiolucent protective layer. The crystals are suspended within a solution called a binder. This allows uniform distribution of the crystals for coating the base. The binder layer is then allowed to dry and harden on the surface of the base. After this an extremely thin coating is applied to protect the crystal layer from damage caused by normal use.

The *base layer* is a support for the other layers of the screen. It allows some flexibility in handling as the screen is placed inside a film holder. The base layer is permanently mounted with adhesive material on the front and back surfaces of the film holder. The *phosphor layer* is coated onto the base. It emits light energy in all directions when activated by x-ray energy (remnant and primary radiation). The *reflective layer,* located between the phosphor layer and the base, directs the light rays that strike it back toward the film. This layer effectively increases the speed of the screen by causing more light to reach the film, producing more radiographic density with less exposure than would otherwise be needed. Unfortunately, some loss of recorded detail in the image may be caused by the use of a reflective layer.

The *protective layer* coated on the surface of the phosphor layer is extremely thin and radiolucent. Its purpose is to protect the phosphor crystal layer against moisture, staining, and abrasion during both normal use and the cleaning procedures recommended by the manufacturer. However, it does not protect the phosphor layer against abrasive cleaning products and methods, metal objects or instruments, fingernails, or rough edges of film. Figure 13–10 is a diagram of screen construction.

Each film holder contains a set of two intensifying screens for most medical radiographic procedures. In some procedures—for example, mammography—only one screen is used. In this instance, a single-emulsion film is used. Double-emulsion films are used with the film holders that have two screens.

Screens are classified according to their speed. Speed has reference to the screen's absorption of incident x-rays and its efficiency in converting that x-ray energy into light energy. They are divided into two general groups, depending on the type phosphor used—regular or rare earth. *Regular* refers to calcium tungstate intensifying screens (slow, medium, and fast speed) and cadmium-lead sulfate (Du Pont's extra-fast phosphor). Rare earth screens refer to the more recently developed phosphors such as gadolinium oxysulfide and lanthanum oxybromide.

SCREENS: SPEED, CONTRAST, AND IMAGE SHARPNESS

The speed of any particular screen depends on a number of physical factors. Among the most important of these are

- The size of the phosphor crystal
- The thickness of the phosphor layer
- The presence of a coloring dye (may or may not be added to the binding material that holds the phosphor crystals)
- The presence of a reflective layer
- The kVp used for the radiation exposure
- The specific compound from which the phosphor crystal is made

As the size of the phosphor crystal increases, the phosphor emits more light for a given radiation exposure. The film has more light to absorb, but the light is spread over a larger area. The result in the radiographic image is greater overall radiographic density, higher radiographic contrast, and less image sharpness (recorded detail). This is obtained with smaller exposure factors and less absorbed radiation dosage to the patient. The images in Figure 13–11 demonstrate these radiographic results. Essentially the same thing occurs with an increase in the overall thickness of the phosphor layer.

Dyes are sometimes added to the phosphor binder to reduce the amount of light reaching the film emulsion from a distant point within the phosphor layer. This slows the speed of the screen, but the sharpness of the image (detail) is increased by the elimination of the diffuse light reaching the receptor. The purpose of adding the coloring to the intensifying screen is to increase the sharpness of the image.

If the screen manufacturer incorporates a reflective layer into the construction of the screen, more screen speed will be evident. The screen speed increases because more of the light rays produced in the phosphor layer are directed to the film. The reflection of these light rays increases the speed of the screen but degrades the image by causing a loss in the recorded detail of the image.

Intensifying screens vary in their response to light emission as the kVp levels vary for exposures. All intensifying screens respond less at lower than at higher kVp levels. The variance of rare earth screens is much greater at low kVp than that of the calcium tungstate screens. Rare earth screens demonstrate maximum speed at about 80 kVp and experience a reduction in response at lower and higher kilovoltages. The variation in screen speed is a problem only if less than 70 kVp is used. Calcium tungstate screens continue to increase in screen speed as the kVp increases, although only slight increases occur above 80 kVp.

As long as only one type of crystal phosphor, calcium tungstate, was used for the manufacture of most intensifying screens, the two physical properties of screens, namely, crystal size and thickness of phosphor layer, limited development of the technology of radiographic image production directed toward using a smaller amount of radiation while obtaining sharp, well-defined images.

Although calcium tungstate intensifying screens continue to be produced, the discovery and development of the rare earth phosphors has added information and other possibilities to this technology. These new compounds are called rare earths, not because they are scarce, but because they are difficult and expensive to separate from the earth and each other. The added information is related to the two physical properties of different phosphor compounds that may be used for intensifying screens. These properties are the absorption rate of the incident x-ray photon energy and the conversion efficiency of x-ray energy to light energy exhibited by each phosphor used.

In general, two types of phosphor crystals can be used in the phosphor layer if they are classified by the color of light emitted. One is a blue–violet light emitter; the type of crystal most often used as an example

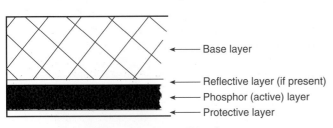

Film Surface of Intensifying Screen

FIGURE 13–10. Layers of the intensifying screen. A cross-section of an intensifying screen demonstrating the various layers that compose the screen.

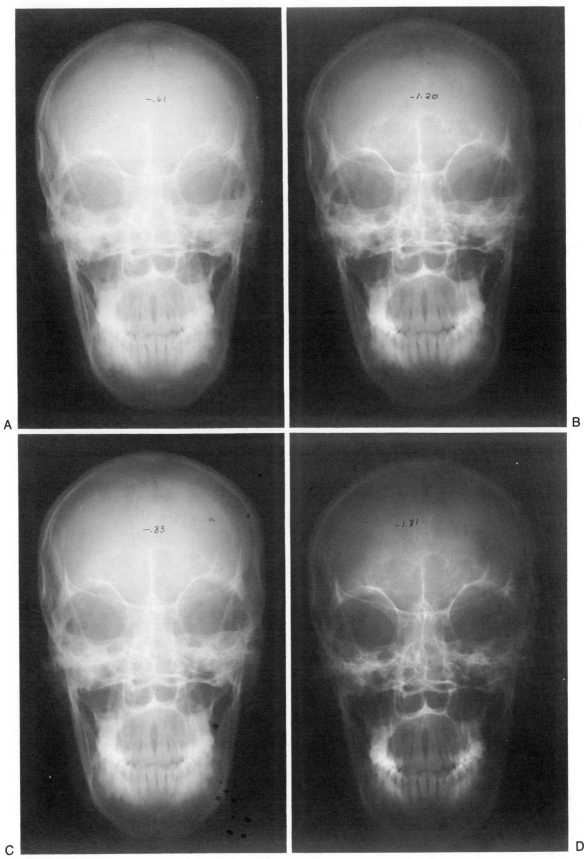

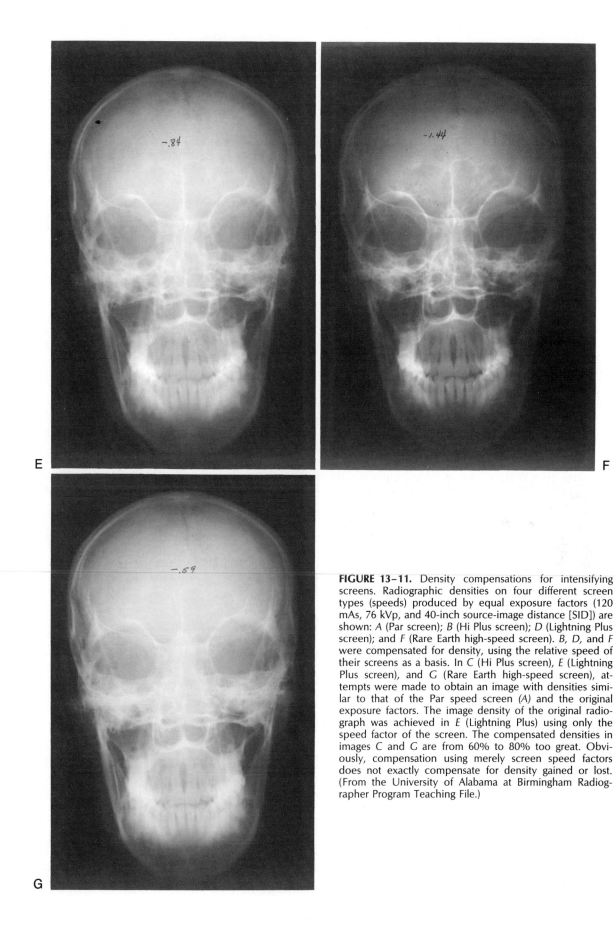

E

F

G

FIGURE 13–11. Density compensations for intensifying screens. Radiographic densities on four different screen types (speeds) produced by equal exposure factors (120 mAs, 76 kVp, and 40-inch source-image distance [SID]) are shown: *A* (Par screen); *B* (Hi Plus screen); *D* (Lightning Plus screen); and *F* (Rare Earth high-speed screen). *B, D,* and *F* were compensated for density, using the relative speed of their screens as a basis. In *C* (Hi Plus screen), *E* (Lightning Plus screen), and *G* (Rare Earth high-speed screen), attempts were made to obtain an image with densities similar to that of the Par speed screen *(A)* and the original exposure factors. The image density of the original radiograph was achieved in *E* (Lightning Plus) using only the speed factor of the screen. The compensated densities in images *C* and *G* are from 60% to 80% too great. Obviously, compensation using merely screen speed factors does not exactly compensate for density gained or lost. (From the University of Alabama at Birmingham Radiographer Program Teaching File.)

is calcium tungstate. The second type of crystal used is a green-light emitter.

Rare earth screens may emit blue, green, or ultraviolet-blue light. The color emitted depends on the activator used with the crystal compound. Activator compounds include thulium (blue) and terbium (green). The common rare earth phosphors are lanthanum oxybromide and gadolinium oxysulfide. Yttrium is not a rare earth but has properties similar to those of the rare earths. Screens using yttrium compound crystals are employed in much the same way as rare earth screens. Yttrium crystals exhibit a rather broadband emission spectrum—between 3370 Å and 4630 Å. Yttrium oxysulfide's spectral emission is within the sensitivity range of blue-sensitive film. The advantage of these yttrium phosphors is they can be used satisfactorily with blue-sensitive film. However, they exhibit more speed when used with green-sensitive film—especially true of yttrium oxysulfide with a terbium activator.

Screen speed primarily depends on two physical properties of the compounds used for the screen, their absorption of incident x-ray photons and their conversion efficiency. Absorption refers to the fraction of incident photons that interacts with the phosphor compared with the number that actually strikes the phosphor. The conversion efficiency is the efficiency with which the phosphor converts x-ray photon energy to light.

References list conversion efficiencies and percentages of absorption for the standard calcium tungstate phosphor and the various rare earth phosphors. To compare speeds of the calcium tungstate screens and the rare earth screens, the standard calcium tungstate phosphor is listed as having about a 5% conversion efficiency; the rare earth and yttrium phosphors, a conversion efficiency of about 20%. Calcium tungstate phosphors absorb approximately 20% of the x-ray photons in the beam, whereas the rare earth phosphors absorb about 60%.

A list of the general names of the screens, the phosphor compounds used in each, the color of the spectral emission, and the speed class of each screen appears in Table 13–1. This table is useful in determining the relative speed of each and making any corrections in exposure that are necessary when changing screen speeds. A screen is most effective when it is used with a film that is sensitive to the same wavelengths of energy that the screen emits. This is termed spectral matching of the screen and film. Some screen manufacturers combine a blue light–emitter phosphor with a green light–emitter phosphor. This combination provides a dual-light spectral emission. These screens can be used effectively with either blue-sensitive or green-sensitive film.

PHOTOSTIMULABLE PHOSPHORS

Digital imaging is the latest development of radiographic imaging; it uses a photostimulable phosphor. This phosphor is used in conventional x-ray exposures, and the crystals absorb some of the x-ray photons. The energies absorbed in high-energy traps are stored in the phosphor crystals and form the latent image. The screen is scanned by a laser beam, causing the energy traps to return to their original energy levels. A light image is emitted with this energy release. A photomultiplier tube views the light, and the output is an amplified analog image signal, which is sent to a computer. The computer converts the analog data to digital data and stores it. The computer can convert the stored digital image to an analog image and display it in one of the conventional forms. Note that no film is involved except possibly as a "hard copy" of the data stored in the computer.

In conventional high-contrast radiography, the range

Table 13–1: SPEED CLASS OF VARIOUS INTENSIFYING SCREENS

Manufacturer	Name	Phosphor	Spectral Emission	Film	Speed Class
Du Pont	Cronex Par Speed	$CaWO_4$	Blue	Cronex 4	100
	Cronex Hi Plus	$CaWO_4$	Blue	Cronex 4	250
	Cronex Quanta III	LaOBr:Tm	Blue	Cronex 4	800
	Cronex Quanta V	LaOBr:Tm and	Blue	Cronex 4	320
		Gd_2O_2S:Tb	Green	Cronex 8	400
	Quanta Detail	$YTaO_4$:Tm	Ultraviolet-blue	Cronex 4	100
	Quanta Fast Detail	$YTaO_4$:Nb	Ultraviolet-blue	Cronex 4	400
Kodak	X-Omatic Fine	$BaPbSO_4$ (yellow dye)	Blue	XRP	32
	X-Omatic Regular	$BaSrSO_4$:Eu (neutral dye)	Blue	XRP	200
	Lanex Fine	Gd_2O_2S:Tb (neutral dye)	Green	Ortho G	100
	Lanex Medium	Gd_2O_2S:Tb (yellow dye)	Green	Ortho G	250
	Lanex Regular	Gd_2O_2S:Tb	Green	Ortho G	400

Source: Christensen's Physics of Diagnostic Radiology, 4th ed. T. S. Curry III, J. E. Dowdey, and R. C. Murry, Jr. Philadelphia: Lea & Febiger, 1990. Reprinted with permission.
Note: Du Pont Cronex 4 is now largely replaced by Cronex 7 and Cronex 10, and Kodak Ortho G film by T-Mat G. The older films still accurately reflect relative intensifying screen speeds, which is the purpose of this table.

of exposure required to produce a black portion of the image is about 100 times that needed to produce a light gray image that can barely be detected. With this newer method, the exposure range between these two extremes is about 10,000 to 1. The effect of this wider latitude in exposure is that it allows a wider range of choice of the exposure factors kVp and mAs. The overall effect is a decrease of repeat exposures for the patient and an increase in the operational economy of the radiology department.

USE OF INTENSIFYING SCREEN IN PRACTICE

Several years ago, radiology departments standardized the speed of screens and film. As more and variable screen-film combinations with different speeds became available, decisions were made for different areas in a department to use specific speeds of screens. Hereafter, the simple term *screen speed* is used in discussion instead of *screen-film combination*. The decision for a particular screen speed depends on the needs of the radiographic examinations and patient conditions in each area, the degree of recorded detail required for certain examinations and the equipment available to perform radiographic procedures.

Patients who must have emergency procedures, special angiographic procedures, and mobile radiography are candidates for multiple radiographic exposures. These procedures need some degree of image sharpness, but emphasis generally is on the speed with which the procedure is completed, use of low-intensity

radiographic units, or reduced radiation dosage to the patient. The same is true for necessary radiographs of pregnant patients. Fast screen speeds (i.e., those yielding more radiographic density and contrast with a smaller exposure) are more necessary to the areas in radiography departments that examine these types of patients.

In other cases, such as mammography, emphasis is on image sharpness (i.e., radiographic detail). The radiation beam is restricted to the anatomical part to limit the radiographic dosage, and an extremely low range of kVp is used. Because of the emphasis on recorded detail, special screens were developed. Only one screen is mounted in a cassette. Macroradiography also requires an emphasis on image sharpness. These two specific areas of radiography use slower-speed screens, sometimes referred to as "detail" screens, as in Figure 13–12.

If cassettes from the different radiographic areas become mixed together, the radiographer should be aware of conversion factors necessary to adapt exposure techniques from one area for use in another area. These conversion factors are generally posted in the department and may be communicated to departmental technical personnel through an inservice meeting devoted to such operational changes.

Screens are ranked for "speed" with reference to the *intensification factor (IF)* of each. The intensification factor is the numerical ratio of the exposure (mAs) required to produce a specific radiographic density without using an intensifying screen to the mAs required to produce an identical radiographic density

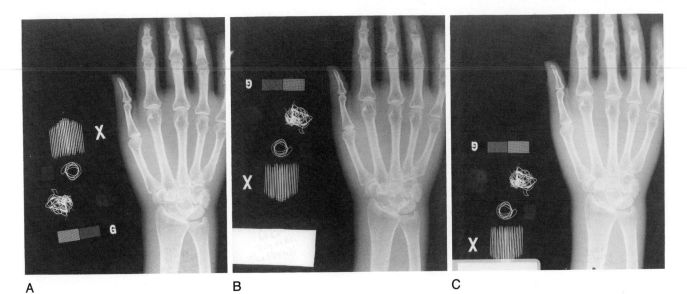

A   B   C

FIGURE 13–12. Intensifying screens: effect on radiographic detail. Three images to demonstrate radiographic detail. *B* (center): Various test objects that reveal fine-line structure. *B* is recorded using a nonscreen film holder (200 mAs and 60 kVp) that is noted for fine line structures in images. In *B* two structures in the test object reproduction reveal very little structural detail except for shape. *A* is recorded using an ultra-detail screen in the cassette (30 mAs, 50 kVp). In addition to the recorded detail of the original radiograph, steel wool is shown in the test object. Some detail is lost from the leaded markers. *C* is recorded using a Lanex Fine screen (40 mAs, 50 kVp). This image reveals fine-line details of one structure of the test object that was not revealed in *B* but loses some detail of the larger size mesh and reveals none in the smaller size mesh. Very good detail of most structures at much lower radiation doses is the advantage of these detail screens. *A* required about 2/25 of the mAs used in *B*. About 1/6 the radiation exposure was used for *C* as for *B*. This allows for reduction in exposure time and radiation dose in the patient, yet reveals much of the same image detail. (From the University of Alabama at Birmingham Radiographer Program Teaching File.)

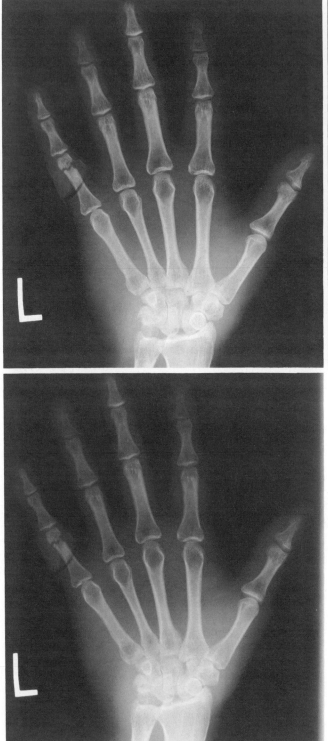

FIGURE 13–13. Screen conversion factor application. *A* was exposed using 6.67 mAs, 54 kVp, 40-inch source-image distance (SID) with 100-speed screens. *B* was exposed using the same exposure factors with 400-speed screens. This image is too dense. The speed factors were considered, and the image with 400-speed screens was repeated, using 1.67 mAs, 54 kVp, and 40-inch SID. There was a difference of 0.19 less in the average density of that film compared with *A*. Another radiograph was performed using 59 kVp (increased the kVp about 10%). In the final image, *C*, the average density values were compared and were only 0.01 less than that of *A*. (From the University of Alabama at Birmingham Radiographer Program Teaching File.)

using the screen being checked. If the IF equals 50 for one screen and 100 for another, the second screen is approximately twice the speed of the first one. This relationship implies that the second screen requires about one half the exposure of the first to obtain the same radiographic image density.

In the past, screens were named according to their relative speed. Such names as slow, average, fast, extra-fast, extra-extra-fast, detail, par, high-plus, lightning, lightning-plus, and so on, prevailed. More recently, the speeds of the various screens, rated by numbers relative to each other, have appeared on the outer surface of the back of the cassette. This practice has proved an effective guide for exposure factor conversion.

For example, a radiographer who returns to work to

find the usual par screen cassettes (100 speed) have been replaced with 400-speed screen cassettes must know how to adapt quickly. The exposure technique chart for new cassettes may not have been devised and posted. If the new cassette screen speed is 400, it is approximately four times faster than the par screen cassettes; therefore, the new exposure factor of mAs should be one fourth of the earlier ones. An example of this conversion is seen in Figure 13–13.

Film Holders (Cassettes)

The intensifying screens and the film are contained by a device designed to allow proper placement of the receptor for a radiographic exposure. This device is a *film holder,* commonly referred to as a cassette. A photograph of a selection of cassette types is in Figure 13–14.

The cassette is a thin, light-tight container for a film. It consists of two flat, normally inflexible surfaces (front and back) held together by a sturdy, rigid frame that encloses the edges of these flat structures.

The front of the cassette is composed of a material opaque to visible light but offering an insignificant resistance to the passage of x-rays. The opaqueness to light ensures that the film does not receive any light through the cassette front to contribute to the overall density of the processed film. The lack of resistance to x-rays means that an insignificant quantity of the exit radiation is absorbed before it reaches the film to form the image. One intensifying screen is mounted on the inside of this surface. If the set of screens for the cassette has two different phosphor-layer thicknesses, the thinner, slower one is attached to the front surface of the cassette.

The back surface of the cassette is composed of a sturdy, inflexible material. On the outside of this surface are devices that close the cassette securely and provide for normal handling of the film-filled cassette without any damage or light leak to the film. The components attached to the inside of the back surface differ, depending on the type of cassette. If the cassette is intended for use with automatic exposure devices, a

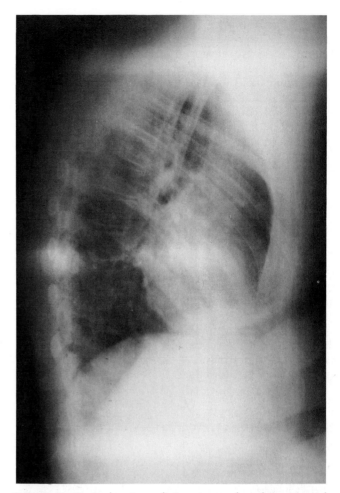

FIGURE 13–15. Backscatter radiation: image degradation. Lateral chest image. Radiograph demonstrates three horizontal bands of less density. These bands are images of the back of the film holders produced by scattered radiation from objects behind the film holder. (From the University of Alabama at Birmingham Radiographer Program Teaching File.)

resilient layer, either felt or a cushioned pad, is attached firmly to the inside of the back cover. If the cassette is not designed for use with an automatic exposure device, a thin lead foil sheet is interposed between the back and the resilient material. The purpose of the layer of lead foil in this instance is to prevent fogging of the image by backscatter radiation from structures behind the cassette. Examples of such backscatter image recording appear in Figure 13–15.

The second intensifying screen (the thickest, if the set has varying thicknesses of the phosphor layer) is mounted in the cassette, attached to the resilient layer with an adhesive material. The thicker screen is mounted on the back surface, since it will be further from the source of radiation when the cassette is correctly placed for an exposure. Some of the exit radiation is absorbed by the front screen and the film before it reaches the back screen. In this instance, the back screen is slightly faster than the front screen in order to compensate for the radiation absorbed by the front screen and to produce identical radiographic densities on both sides of the film.

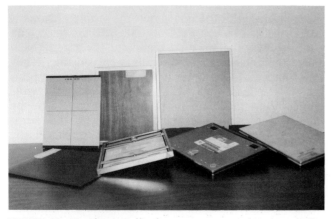

FIGURE 13–14. Photograph of an assortment of screened film holders and two nonscreened film holders.

The sturdy framework holds the other parts of the cassette in position. It also provides receptacles that permit a secure closing of the cassette and maintenance of light-tight conditions to protect the film while it is being handled. The closure of the cassette along with the resilient pad aids in maintenance of good screen-film contact for the production of the best recorded detail in the image. The contribution to blurring of the image of poor screen-film contact is discussed in Chapter 12.

Secondary, or scatter, radiation has been mentioned several times and has been discussed in relation to various devices used in radiography. It has become evident that this type of radiation should be reduced or eliminated from radiographic images. Higher kVp levels that produce more secondary radiation affecting the image have become the preferable technique for imaging anatomical parts. With the use of higher kVp and lower mAs values, the patient absorbs less ionizing radiation, and the contrast scale of the image is lengthened. Beam restriction can reduce the amount of secondary radiation by limiting the volume of tissue in which it can be produced. In many instances, with the use of beam restrictors there is less secondary radiation. However, with larger, thicker body parts, there is enough present to degrade the image.

Grids

In 1913 the stationary grid was invented by Gustaf Bucky. It consisted of a framework containing lead foil strips standing on edge, with the strip surfaces parallel to and equidistant from each other. These strips were also perpendicular to the surface of the film used to record the image. The lead strips were so thick that their broad shadows obscured image parts. The lead strips absorbed the radiation before it reached the image receptor. A diagram of a grid in cross section, showing the placement of the lead foil strips, appears in Figure 13–16.

In the 1920s Hollis Potter developed a mechanism for suspending the grid in a framework that allowed the grid to move between the patient and film during the exposure. This was known as the Potter-Bucky

diaphragm, commonly referred to as a *Bucky.* The motion of the grid eliminated the grid lines in the images. This created a problem, however, in that the overall image density was reduced from that obtained with the grid in a stationary position. To compensate, the exposure factors had to be increased. As a result of this increase, the patient absorbed even more radiation.

In the 1920s, most of the harmful effects of radiation dosage were not realized. There was little concern about the increased exposure, and the images did exhibit a uniform radiographic density.

The early Bucky movement mechanism involved piston action in an oil-filled cylinder. This allowed the grid to move slowly and smoothly in only one direction and over a distance of about 1 inch. Later grid movements involved an electronic motor–driven mechanism, but the principle of operation remained the same. Currently, the motion is continuous during the exposure. The total distance the grid moves is about the same.

With the exposure, the grid starts moving. At most points in its travel, the grid is not centered on the central ray. Rather, this centering occurs only when the midpoint of the grid passes directly under the point on which the central ray is centered. Because of this off-centering during most of the grid travel, the mechanism reduces the amount of primary radiation as well as the scatter radiation reaching the film during the rest of its operation. To replace this lost image density, exposure factors must be increased by approximately 10% to 15% more than that used for a stationary grid with the same characteristics.

A grid is the most effective way to remove secondary radiation from large radiographic fields. Primary radiation in the beam is directed along the same axis as the broad surfaces of the lead foil strips, passing readily through the interspaces between them to reach the film and record the image. Secondary radiation arises from many points in the irradiated tissue volume. It is *multidirectional,* and because of this, a large percentage is absorbed by the lead foil strips before it reaches the film, depicted in Figure 13–17. This is the means by which the scatter radiation is eliminated from the image. The overall gray haze that covers the film without the grid is greatly reduced, and the density differences produced in the image become visibly obvious.

The spaces between the lead foil strips are filled with a radiolucent material that maintains the space. Originally, the interspacing materials were organic. They could and did deteriorate with age, allowing the position of the lead strips to shift out of position while remaining in the main framework. The grid with the shifted lead strips became unusable as the strips shifted, varying the distances between them. Plastic and aluminum are used today as the interspacing material. These are structurally stronger and can be manufactured more precisely. With an aluminum interspacer, slightly more primary radiation is absorbed, requiring slightly higher exposures. Some say that aluminum interspacers, compared with other types of interspacers, require as much as a 20% increase in radia-

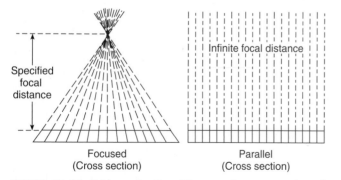

Specified focal distance

Infinite focal distance

Focused (Cross section)

Parallel (Cross section)

FIGURE 13–16. Grid construction. Diagram of a cross-section of grids. (From Characteristics and Applications of X-Ray Grids, courtesy of Liebel-Flarsheim.)

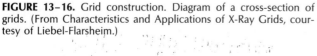

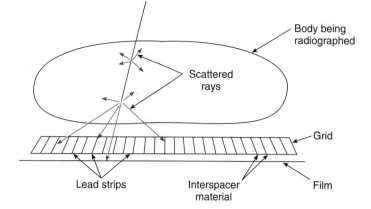

FIGURE 13-17. Action of a grid in stopping scattered radiation. (From Characteristics and Applications of X-Ray Grids, courtesy of Liebel-Flarsheim.)

tion exposure when lower kilovoltages are used. More secondary radiation is absorbed when aluminum interspaced grids are used. Figure 13–18 shows a table and a graph depicting the increase of radiation exposure needed at different kilovoltage levels when changing to grids with aluminum interspacers.

The amount of secondary radiation removed from the radiographic image is regarded as the *grid efficiency*. It is generally stated as a percentage cleanup, referring, of course, to the removal of secondary radiation. Grid efficiency depends on two physical characteristics, grid ratio and the line count, or *grid frequency*, which constitutes the *lead content* of the grid. Both characteristics are usually stated on the grid surface, specified by a label attached by the manufacturer.

Grid ratio is the relationship of the height of the lead strips to the distance between them. A wide assortment of linear grid ratios is available. Grid ratios are expressed as two numbers, as inferred by the

definition—for example, 5:1, 6:1, 8:1, 12:1, 16:1, 10:1, and even 32:1. The first five are in common use; 5:1 and 6:1 grid ratios are used in emergency rooms and mobile radiography and are efficient at kVp levels up to 80 kVp. The 8:1 grids efficiently remove scatter radiation produced by kilovoltages up to 100 kVp. Grid ratios of 12:1 and 16:1 are used for exposures above 100 kVp; the 16:1 grid has a higher cleanup efficiency, as does any larger grid ratio.

Higher grid ratios require higher exposure techniques. Radiographic density is decreased, and image contrast becomes higher as more scatter radiation is removed from the image. The effect of different grid ratios on the removal of scatter radiation is demonstrated by Figure 13–19.

The grid frequency is the line count, or number of lead strips, in a 1-inch or 1-cm wide area of the surface of the grid. As already stated, the grid ratio and the grid frequency determine the total amount of lead in

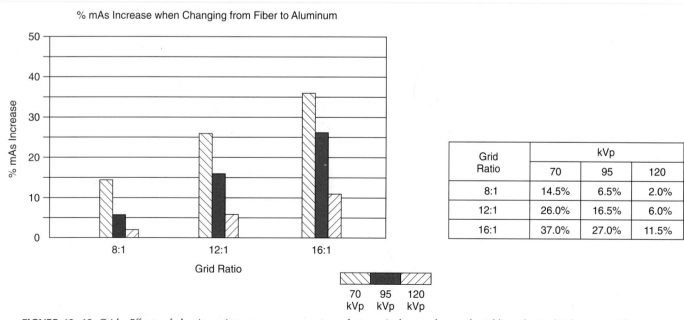

% mAs Increase when Changing from Fiber to Aluminum

Grid Ratio	kVp		
	70	95	120
8:1	14.5%	6.5%	2.0%
12:1	26.0%	16.5%	6.0%
16:1	37.0%	27.0%	11.5%

FIGURE 13-18. Grids: Effects of aluminum interspacers on exposure factors. A chart and a graph yielding identical information. Please note that the correction in percentage increase in mAs is for the aluminum interspacer and should be made after any compensation for the grid ratio has been done. (From Characteristics and Applications of X-Ray Grids, courtesy of Liebel-Flarsheim.)

Grid Ratio

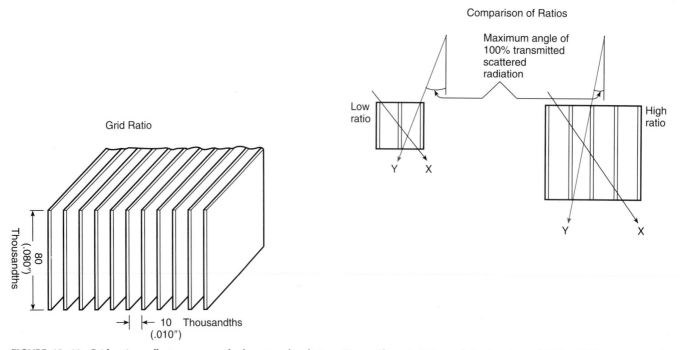

FIGURE 13–19. Grid ratios: effect on removal of scattered radiation. (From Characteristics and Applications of X-Ray Grids, courtesy of Liebel-Flarsheim.)

the grid (its lead content). The lead content of a grid is an indicator of its efficiency in the removal of secondary radiation before it reaches the film and affects the image.

There are two types of grids according to their construction, *linear* and *crossed* (crisscross). In the linear grid, the lead strips are arranged with their length coinciding with the long axis of the grid. This type may have its lead foil strips parallel with each other with the width of each foil strip perpendicular to the surface of the grid (known as a *parallel grid*), or the strips may be arranged with a slight incline toward the midline of the grid (known as a *focused grid*). The degree of angle is the same as that of the radii of a circular spoke pattern above the midpoint of the structure.

Linear parallel grids are best used with large SIDs or for small exposure areas. Large areas radiographed with short SIDs undergo a loss of density at the lateral borders of the image. This loss occurs because the angle of the x-rays striking the surface at the lateral edges are not parallel with the surfaces of the strips. As a result, some of the incoming radiation strikes the lead foil strips and is absorbed. Fewer primary x-rays reach the film at the lateral edges of the image.

The focused grid, illustrated in Figure 13–20, should ideally be used with the anode at a point in space called the *focal point* or, more accurately, the midpoint of the *convergent line*. This is a point or series of points at which the planes of all the lead strips would converge if extended into space above the grid surface. The central lead strip is perpendicular to the plane of the film. If its plane is extended to the focal point, that distance is the *focal length* or *grid radius*. Grid radius

is usually defined as the perpendicular distance from the focal point of the grid to its surface. This grid must be used with an SID equal to the grid radius to obtain the greatest benefit. The acceptable focal length for exposures with a specific linear focused grid is generally indicated by the manufacturer's label on the grid and is expressed as a focal range. The focal range is narrower for higher-ratio grids; lower-ratio grids have a wider focal range. It is important to have the imaginary convergent line toward the x-ray tube. This side of the grid should always be turned toward the x-ray

Cross Section of Focused Grid

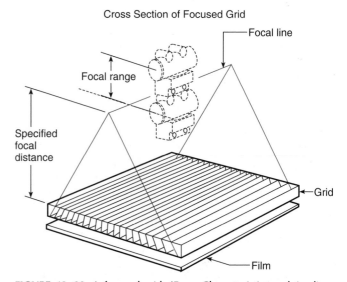

FIGURE 13–20. A focused grid. (From Characteristics and Applications of X-Ray Grids, courtesy of Liebel-Flarsheim.)

tube to avoid lateral grid "cutoff." The manufacturer uses the label *tube side of the grid* to avoid accidental misplacement.

Linear grids can be used for projections that require the x-ray beam to be angled. The x-ray beam must be angled on the long axis of the grid so that the central beam is linearly aligned with the lead strips of the grid.

Crisscross (or cross-hatch) grids may be parallel or focused. They are occasionally named for the shape of the figure formed in the image by the shadows of the grid strips— the *rhomboid grid,* for example. Crisscross grids are composed of two linear grids placed one on the other so that the lead strips of one are placed at an angle to those of the other. The latitude for use for crisscross grids is limited. The phrase *latitude for use* refers to the range at either extreme from the optimum measure that can be used to achieve an acceptable image. In this case, the term refers to the range of SID, the range of variance from center of the grid, or the range of central ray angulation from 90° with the grid surface. Conditions for the use of the crisscross grid include the anatomical part and central ray must be centered to the film. The central ray must be perpendicular to the surface of the grid. If the crisscross grid is of a parallel type, the field to be radiated must be small, or an exposure technique employing a large SID must be used. If a focused crisscross grid is used, the area may be larger, but the focal length is critical. The focused linear grid has a convergent line; the focused crisscross grid has a focal, or convergent, point. With the use of these grids, it is necessary to exercise great care in film placement and in x-ray beam centering and direction. Again, angulation of the x-ray beam produces a poor image. Examples of the problems occurring with the use of grids are depicted in Figure 13–21 and Figure 13–22.

Most commonly available crisscross grid ratios are 5:1, 6:1, or 8:1. A crisscross grid is efficient in cleanup of scatter radiation. As an example, a 5:1 crisscross grid is approximately as efficient as a 12:1 linear grid, whereas the efficiency rating of an 8:1 crisscross grid approximates that of a 16:1 linear grid when kilovoltages at or above 85 kVp are used. The special reason for use of a 5:1 crisscross instead of a 12:1 linear grid is that the radiation exposure required is approximately the same as with a 12:1 linear grid at medium to high kVp with about the same efficiency rating as the 12:1 grid in that range. Compare these grid ratios, using the bar graphs in Figure 13–23.

To evaluate grid performance, three methods are used. The first is primary transmission testing. *Primary transmission* is the measurement of the percentage of primary radiation transmitted through a grid. This method involves (1) narrowing the beam to a pencil-sized beam, (2) placing the phantom segment to be radiated at a large distance from the grid so that no scatter radiation reaches the grid, and (3) making two measurements: (a) one with the grid in place to determine intensity transmitted through the grid and (b) a second with the grid removed to determine beam intensity directed toward the grid from the phantom. The percentage of primary transmission can then be calculated using the formula

$$PT = \frac{I_a}{I_b} \times 100\%$$

where

$PT =$ percentage of primary radiation transmitted

$I_a =$ intensity of primary radiation transmitted by grid

$I_b =$ intensity of primary radiation directed to grid

The second method is to determine the *Bucky factor,* which is defined as the ratio of the incident radiation striking the grid to the transmitted radiation passing through the grid. It indicates absorption of both primary and secondary radiation by the grid. The Bucky factor is determined by using a large irradiated field and a thick phantom part. The radiation passing through the grid and the radiation incident on the grid are measured. The value of the Bucky factor is found by dividing the amount of incident radiation by the amount of transmitted radiation.

Such a determination reveals that high-ratio grids absorb more radiation than do low-ratio grids and that the Bucky factor varies with the energy of the x-ray beam. The low-ratio grids absorb less radiation from high-energy beams than do high-ratio grids. Radiographs demonstrating this appear in Figure 13–24.

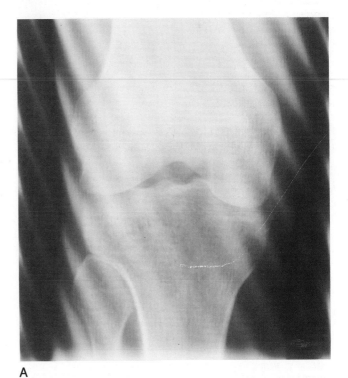

A

FIGURE 13–21. Grid placement errors that degrade the image. *A,* A "zebra" pattern in a radiograph of the knee. This was produced by using a 6:1 ratio grid cassette in the Bucky tray and angling the central ray cephalad about 10°.

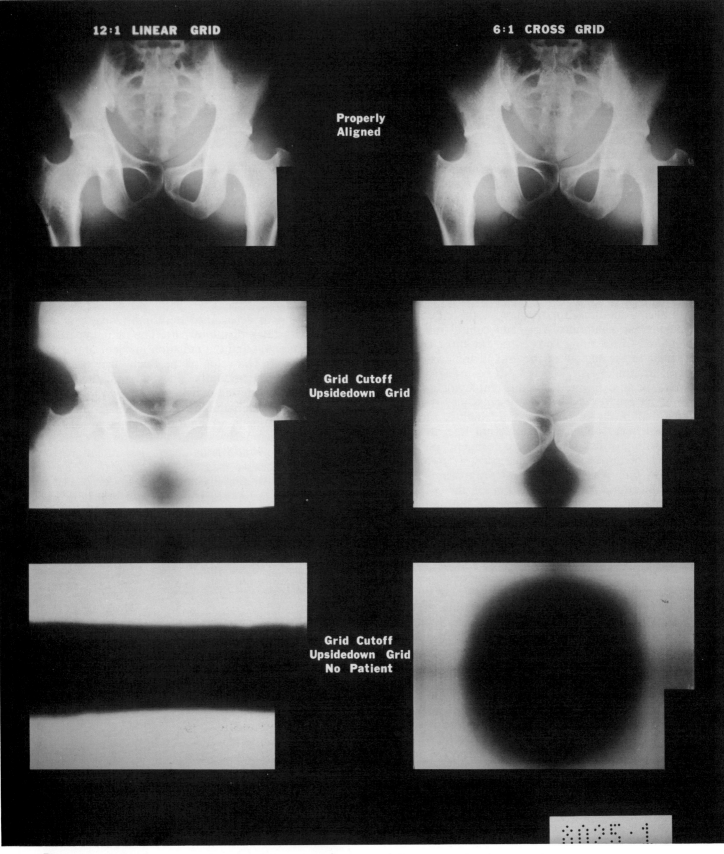

FIGURE 13–21. *Continued B*, Use and misuse of a 12:1 focused linear grid and a 6:1 focused crisscross grid. The labels on the six images in B are self-explanatory. (*B* is from the ACR Learning File, American College of Radiology Institute.)

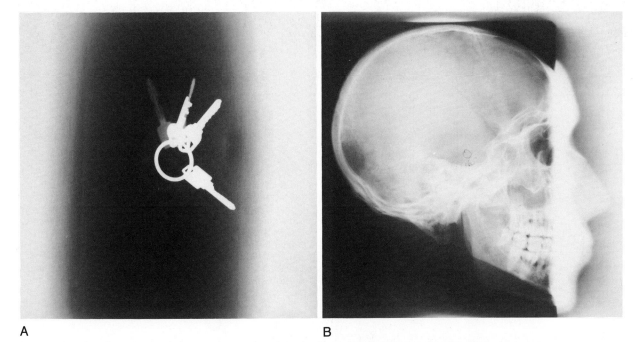

A   B

FIGURE 13–22. Tube placement and distance errors that degrade the image. *A,* Objects (keys) radiographed using a 12:1 focused grid with a focal range of 62 to 72 inches. *A* was exposed at a 30-inch source-image distance (SID) (near decentering). The radiographic density at the key ring is intense but rapidly fades with an increase in the number of grid lines visible before all the radiographic density is eliminated. *B,* A lateral projection of the head, using a 12:1 moving grid. The central ray is off-centered 2 inches toward the posterior surface of the head. Grid lines are visible in and anterior to the soft tissue of the facial bones. (From the University of Alabama at Birmingham Radiographer Program Teaching File).

From a practical standpoint, the Bucky factor reveals the factor by which the nongrid exposure is increased when a particular grid ratio is to be used for a radiographic exposure. High-ratio grids are desirable for improved film quality but are otherwise undesirable for two reasons: (1) greater exposure factors are required for high-ratio grids and (2) the patient receives a greater radiation dose when high-ratio grids are used.

The third method of evaluating a grid is by determining the *contrast improvement factor (CIF).* The contrast improvement factor is the ratio of radiographic contrast with a grid to radiographic contrast without a grid. The formula for calculating CIF is

$$CIF = \frac{\text{contrast with grid}}{\text{contrast without grid}}$$

which is a measure of the ability of a grid to improve contrast, its primary function.

The CIF depends on three factors in the exposure—kVp, size of the radiation field, and thickness of the anatomical part. The amount of scatter radiation produced by an exposure is determined by the same three factors.

Table 13–2 presents a table containing guidelines for selection of a grid for use in different radiographic situations. Figure 13–25 lists exposure factors for different grid ratios.

Some references recommend considering the use of a grid for any anatomical part measuring 10 cm or more unless the part is a chest. Other references favor a 12-cm measurement of an anatomical part as the point when the use of a grid should be considered. Because the amount of scatter radiation is the dominant factor to be considered, the use of a grid for an exposure should be considered at any centimeter measurement if one of the three factors that increase the production of secondary radiation is excessive. The three factors that result in an increase in secondary radiation are (1) volume of tissue irradiated, (2) density of the tissue, and (3) kVp needed to penetrate the part. If two of these factors are excessive, the use of a grid must be considered.

Air-Gap Technique

Several years ago, radiology departments began using air gaps, primarily for radiography of the chest. The object was to fully use the advantages of the longer scale of contrast obtained with high-kVp chest techniques without a grid and the exposure techniques required with it.

The purpose of the air gap is to reduce scattered radiation reaching the image from the anatomical part. Scatter and secondary radiation are produced in the patient's body as a result of high kVp (110 kVp and above); this radiation leaves the body in all directions.

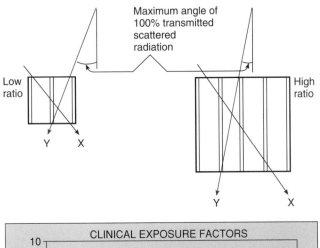

Comparison of Ratios

Maximum angle of 100% transmitted scattered radiation

Low ratio

High ratio

Y X

Y X

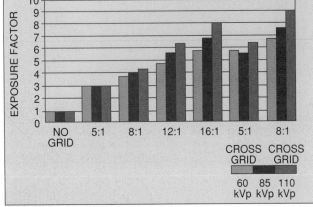

CLINICAL EXPOSURE FACTORS

EXPOSURE FACTOR

NO GRID   5:1   8:1   12:1   16:1   5:1   8:1

CROSS GRID   CROSS GRID

60 kVp   85 kVp   110 kVp

A

FIGURE 13–23. Grid efficiency. The diagrams show why higher ratio grids are more efficient in the removal of scattered radiation from an image than are lower ratio grids (A). B and C are radiographic demonstrations of this principle. An 8:1 ratio grid was used for B and a 16:1 ratio grid for C. Exposure for each was 15 mAs, 90 kVp, and 40-inch source-image distance (SID). The percentage of total scatter absorbed by each of these grids is cited as 82% (8:1), and 96% (16:1). (A is from Characteristics and Applications of X-Ray Grids, courtesy of Liebel-Flarsheim; B and C are from the University of Alabama at Birmingham Radiographer Program Teaching File.)

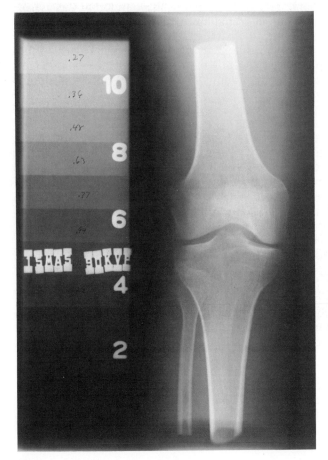

B

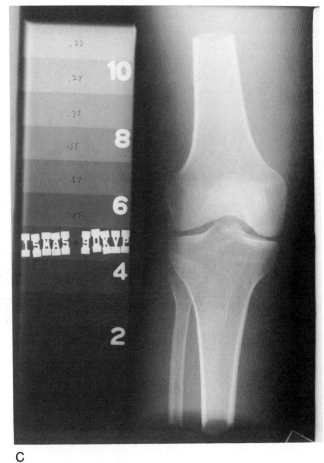

C

FIGURE 13–24. Scattered radiation cleanup: comparison of two grid ratios. Two radiographs of a large penetrometer. The left half of the cassette was covered by a 6:1 ratio, 85-line count focused grid; a 12:1 ratio, 85-line count focused grid covered the right half of the same cassette. The source-image distance (SID), 38 inches, was inside the focal range of both grids. A was exposed using 40 mAs and 60 kVp, whereas for B, 3.33 mAs and 105 kVp were used. The 6:1 grid (A) demonstrates a greater percentage of difference between densities; 9 distinct densities are clearly discernible. In the 12:1 grid (B), 8 distinct densities show a lower percentage of difference between the corresponding penetrometer steps. The 6:1 grid (A) is more dense overall. The number of discernible densities in B is eight. Here the 12:1 grid image reveals 9 distinct densities with much less variation in percentage difference between them at the thinner steps of the penetrometer. Visually, it appears the densities of the penetrometer steps in the 12:1 grid image in A and B correspond to the densities that are 1 step higher on the penetrometer in the 6:1 grid image. (From the University of Alabama at Birmingham Radiographer Program Teaching File.)

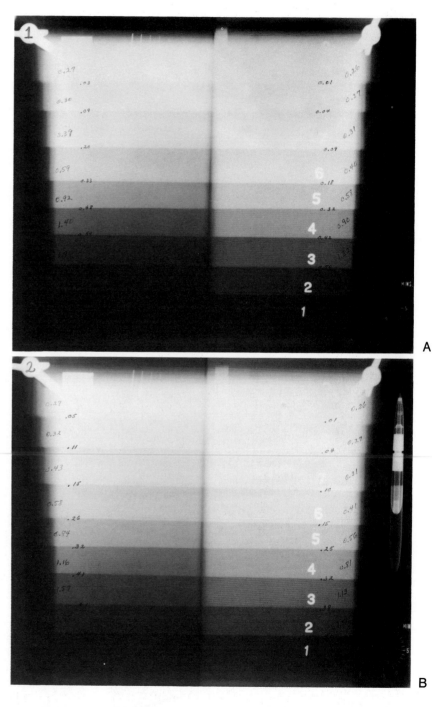

A

B

Table 13–2: GRID APPLICATION GUIDELINES

Type of Grid*	Cleanup	Positioning Latitude		Recommended to	Remarks
		Off-Center	Focal (Range)		
8:1 ratio, crisscross	Superlative	Very critical	Good	120 kVp	Not suited for tilted tube techniques
15:1 ratio, linear	Superlative	Very critical	Critical	Over 100 kVp	Extra care required for proper alignment Usually used in fixed mount
6:1 ratio, crisscross	Excellent	Critical	Very good	110 kVp	Not suitable for tilted tube techniques
12:1 ratio, linear	Excellent	Critical	Critical	110 kVp (also suitable for higher kVp)	Extra care required for proper alignment Usually used in fixed mount
5:1 ratio, crisscross	Very good	Critical	Excellent	100 kVp	Not suited for tilted tube techniques
10:1 ratio, linear	Very good	Fair	Fair	100 kVp	Reasonable care required for proper alignment
8:1 ratio, linear	Good	Good	Good	100 kVp	For general stationary grid use
6:1 ratio, linear	Moderate	Very good	Very good	80 kVp	Ideally suited for bedside radiography
5:1 ratio linear	Moderate	Very good	Very good	80 kVp	Ideally suited for bedside radiography

Source: Characteristics and Applications of X-Ray Grids. Courtesy of Liebel-Flarsheim.
* Grids are listed in descending order of cleanup effectiveness.

Exposure Factors for Grids

Grid Ratio	Exposure Factors					
	Experimental			Clinical		
	70kVp	95kVp	120kVp	60kVp	85kVp	110kVp
Non Grid	1	1	1	1	1	1
5:1 linear	3	3	3	3	3	3
8:1 linear	3.5	3.75	4	3.75	4	4.25
12:1 linear	4	4.25	5	4.75	5.5	6.25
16:1 linear	4.5	5	6	5.75	6.75	8
5:1 crossed	4.5	5	5.5	5.75	5.5	6.25
8:1 crossed	5	6	7	6.75	7.5	9

A

Comparison of Scatter Removal and Exposure Factors		
Grid Ratio	% of total scatter removed	Exposure factor
No Grid	—	1
5:1 grid	82%	3
8:1 grid	90%	4
12:1 grid	95.5%	5.5
16:1 grid	96%	6.7

B

FIGURE 13–25. Grid exposure factors. (From Characteristics and Applications of X-Ray Grids, courtesy of Liebel-Flarsheim.)

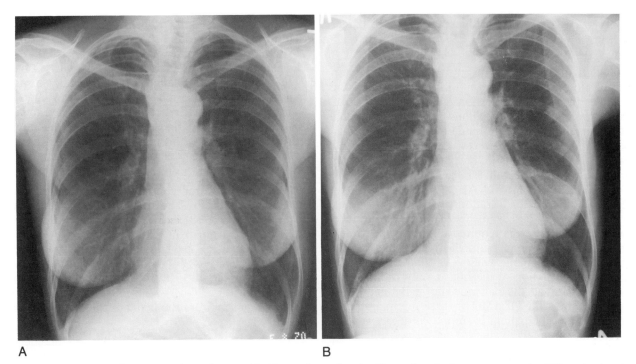

A   B

FIGURE 13–26. Air-gap technique: an alternative to grids. Two radiographs of a 20-cm chest in the posteroranterior (PA) projection. In *A*, 10 mAs, 80 kVp, 72-inch source-image distance (SID) and no object-image distance (OID) were used. In *B*, same exposure factors were used, but the anterior chest was 6 inches from the film surface and the SID was increased to 95 inches. The transverse diameter of the chest at the level of the 8th costovertebral articulation was 28 cm in *A* and 28.9 cm in *B*. The density loss in *B* is the result of reduced scattered radiation to the film plus the fact that the exposure factors did not compensate for the increased SID of 95 inches. (From the University of Alabama at Birmingham Radiographer Program Teaching File.)

The scatter radiation that affects the film usually originates in the adjacent superficial tissues. The air gap is most effective in removing scatter radiation when it arises close to the film.

As the distance between the object and the image receptor increases, the image sharpness deteriorates. To preserve image sharpness, the SID is usually increased from 6 ft to 10 ft.

The measure of air-gap width is analogous to grid ratio—that is, it is an indicator of the efficiency of scatter radiation cleanup. An air-gap ratio of 5:1 means that 5 scatter radiation photons reach the image receptor for every primary radiation photon. The ideal ratio would be 0:1, meaning that all of the photons reaching the film are primary photons.

Guidelines for the selection of an air-gap width include (1) a thicker anatomical part benefits from a greater air-gap width; (2) the first inch of an air gap improves contrast more than any subsequently added inch; in a multi-inch air gap, the contrast improves progressively less in the first inch, second inch, third inch, and so forth of the air gap; (3) recorded image detail sharpness deteriorates with an increasing width of the air gap unless the SID is increased to compensate for the magnification; (4) moving the patient away from the image receptor without increasing the SID moves the patient closer to the radiation source and increases his or her radiation dose.

Experience has shown that a 10-inch air gap, a 10-ft SID, and a beam energy level between 110 kVp and 150 kVp gives satisfactory results. Although this is not "best" for every patient measurement, it is satisfactory. Figure 13–26 presents a similar case. Because of the increased SID, the exposure factors must usually be increased. Even with this increase, the exposure to the patient is less (by about 23%) than it would be with the grid.

Chapter Summary/ Important Concepts

This chapter is devoted to factors that affect the primary beam from its production to the formation of the image. The anode heel effect is a variation in the intensity of the primary beam (quantity of x-rays) in the direction of the long axis of the tube. The intensity of the primary x-ray beam is greater at the cathode end of the beam as a result of this effect. This knowledge of the x-ray beam can be used to greatest advantage in radiography by placing the cathode end of the tube over the thickest or densest portion of the anatomical part to be radiographed. This practice is especially useful in radiography of parts that vary in thickness over a distance, such as the femur.

Filtration must be used in an x-ray beam used for diagnostic purposes. The total filtration of the beam includes the inherent filtration (composed of part of the x-ray tube and tube housing) and the added filtration (thin sheets of a metal inserted in the x-ray beam). The filters added to the diagnostic x-ray beam are usually made of aluminum (Al). The amount of both the inherent and the added filtration are stated in mm of Al or mm of Al equivalent. The amount of filtration of the x-ray beam is specified by and based on the kVp used to produce the beam. Filtration is required to absorb the lower-energy x-ray photons emitted by the tube before they reach the patient. These x-rays do not contribute to the formation of the image, only to radiation dose absorbed by the patient. The higher-energy x-rays remain in the beam to produce the image. The beam striking the patient is composed of x-rays with more uniform energy values.

The beam restrictor was developed to reduce the radiation absorbed by the patient. It does this by reducing the area of the radiation field. Less primary radiation strikes on the patient, and therefore less radiation is available for absorption.

The image benefits from reduction in radiation field size. Irradiation of the smaller area results in production of less radiographically effective secondary radiation, which produces unwanted radiographic density over the image. A decrease in the image density produces an effective increase in the radiographic contrast and improves the visibility of the recorded detail of the image.

There are two basic types of beam restrictors: fixed-aperture and variable-aperture. Fixed-aperture beam restrictors include diaphragms, cylinder cones, and extension cylinder cones. With these the effective beam restriction is accomplished by the aperture nearest the patient. The disadvantages of this type of beam restrictor are (1) the secondary radiation produced by the rim of the aperture, (2) the large number of devices required for each radiographic room to permit use of the required size of radiation field for each anatomical part size, and (3) the inconvenience of interchanging the beam restrictor for each different part size.

The variable-aperture beam restrictor is called a collimator. It contains two sets of leaded shutters. Each set is composed of four shutters, two that move longitudinally to determine the length of the radiation field and two that move laterally to determine its width. The aperture formed by the shutters is rectangular, the same shape as the image receptor. This type of beam restrictor became the type of

choice for several reasons: (1) the lower aperture eliminates from the beam the secondary radiation produced by the rim of the upper aperture; (2) the size of the aperture is easily adjusted without having to physically interchange it with a similar device of a different size; (3) it is equipped with a light localizer, a central ray indicator, and a method to center the central ray to the film; and (4) the rectangular shape of the radiation field coincides with the shape of the image receptor.

The light localizer consists of a system of mirrors and a light bulb. The light field projected demonstrates the size and shape of the radiation field if it is correctly aligned. Regulations require that the light field accurately outline the radiation field to within 2% of the SID used for an exposure. The size of the radiation field is controlled by the radiographer, using dials or levers in conjunction with scales that indicate the field sizes at specific SIDs.

In the interest of radiation protection practices for the general public, federal regulations require positive beam limitation (PBL) on all diagnostic radiographic machines manufactured after August 1974. PBL indicates that the mechanism for limiting the area irradiated is automated. The size of the beam is automatically limited to the size of the film. Further limitation can be obtained, but the area cannot be extended beyond the film size.

The primary x-ray beam leaves the beam restrictor and interacts with the tissues as it passes through the patient. The form of interaction depend on the density and electron density of the tissues in the irradiated area and the energy of the x-ray photons. Some photons are absorbed, some undergo changes in energy and direction, and others travel through the anatomical part unchanged. Those that undergo changes produce secondary, or scatter, radiation. If this radiation reaches the image receptor, it produces a haze over the entire image. This haze is unwanted density and is referred to as fog. With fog the radiographic density is increased, the visible image contrast decreases, and the recorded detail (image sharpness) is obscured. If fog is excessive, it must be reduced to an acceptable level. The beam restrictor reduces fog and is especially effective for small areas. For radiographs of a large area the beam size cannot be restricted very much or the part of interest cannot be completely visualized. Other means must be found to reduce the level of fog for radiography of large parts.

One method of reducing the secondary radiation fog is manipulation of the exposure technique. A lower kVp produces relatively less radiographically effective secondary radiation and requires more x-ray photons for the correct radiographic density. It also produces a beam composed of low-energy x-ray photons, which are more easily absorbed by the body tissues. Because of the greater x-ray photon absorption by the patient, this is not an acceptable means of reducing scatter radiation fog. The primary x-ray beam must provide the penetration (x-ray photon energy) to produce the preferred image contrast and as little radiation absorption by the patient as possible. The beam intensity (quantity of x-ray photons) must provide sufficient radiographic density in the image.

In the simplest form of radiography of an anatomical part, the part is placed against a light-tight film holder called a cassette. The cassette encloses two intensifying screens with a single medical x-ray film sandwiched between the phosphor surfaces of the screens. These intensifying screens increase the effect of x-radiation on the film's sensitive emulsion —that is, they produce more radiographic density in the image for the specific amount of x-radiation used.

The construction of an intensifying screen consists of a sturdy, slightly flexible base. A reflective layer may be included to redirect light rays emitted in the direction of the base toward the film surface of the screen. The phosphor layer (active layer) consists of the phosphor crystals embedded in a binder material. Finally, a very thin, radiolucent layer protects the phosphor layer from damage occurring with normal use.

Two types of phosphor crystals may be used in the phosphor layer. One is calcium tungstate (a blue–violet light emitter), and the second is rare earth crystals (green-light emitters).

Rare earth screens may emit green or ultraviolet-blue light. The color depends on the activator used with the crystal compound. Activator compounds include thulium (blue) and terbium (green). The rare earth phosphors are lanthanum oxybromides and gadolinium oxysulfides. Yttrium tantalate screens are used in much the same way as rare earth screens, because yttrium has properties similar to the rare earths. The advantage of the yttrium phosphors is they can be used satisfactorily with blue-sensitive film. However, the yttrium oxysulfide with a terbium activator exhibits more speed when used with a green-sensitive film.

Some screen manufacturers combine blue light–emitting phosphors with green light–emitting phosphors to provide a dual-spectrum light emission. Either blue-sensitive or green-sensitive film can be used with these screens.

Screen speed primarily depends on the size of the phosphor crystals, the thickness of the layer of phosphor crystals, and the two physical properties of the phosphor compounds used for the screen. The presence of a reflective layer in the screen construction contributes to the screen speed, as does the addition of coloring matter to the binder material in which the phosphor crystals are suspended.

The two physical properties of phosphor crystals are their absorption of the incident x-ray photons and the efficiency with which they convert x-ray energy to light energy. Standard calcium tungstate phosphors absorb about 20% of incident x-ray photons and have a 5% conversion efficiency; rare earth and yttrium phosphors absorb approximately 60% of incident x-ray photons and have a conversion efficiency of about 20%.

Development of photostimulable phosphors for radiographic use introduced the concept of "filmless" radiology departments. Information produced by the x-ray beam passing through the anatomical part is stored digitally by a computer for use in producing hard copies and possible additional manipulation. This type of imaging provides a wider exposure latitude for the technologist and patient and greater operational economy for the radiology department.

If the part is large, dense, or thick or if it contains an excess amount of fluid, a device to reduce the scatter radiation to the film is introduced into the beam of radiation. This device is a grid. The grid absorbs much of the scatter radiation in the exit radiation beam before it reaches the screen-film combination.

A grid is a series of lead foil strips in an orderly arrangement in a framework that holds the strips rigidly in place by means of interspacers in the framework between the lead foil strips. In early grids, the interspacers were composed of organic materials. In recent years a move toward grids with plastic or aluminum interspacers has occurred. These grids give more stability to the configuration of the lead foil strips, since neither of these materials deteriorates with age as did the organic material. Aluminum interspacers require some compensation in the exposure factors, especially at low-kVp exposures.

Grids are rated for their efficiency in removing scattered radiation from the image. The efficiency of a grid depends on its lead content. The total lead content of a grid is determined by the number of lead foil strips per linear unit of the width of the surface area (grid frequency, or line count per inch or centimeter) and the ratio of the height of the lead foil strips to the width of the interspacers between the strips (grid ratio). As the grid ratio increases, the lead content becomes greater, and the efficiency of removal of scatter radiation is enhanced. As more scatter radiation is removed, the radiographic density of the image is reduced, the image contrast increases, and image sharpness is heightened. In many cases, use of a grid requires an increase in the exposure factors to maintain an acceptable level of radiographic density in the image. The enhancement of exposure factors means an augmented radiation dose for the patient.

A negative factor of grid use is the appearance of grid lines in the image with the use of a stationary grid. Stationary grids, which are linear, may be parallel or focused. In parallel grids, the broad surfaces of the lead foil strips are parallel to and equidistant from each other. These grids can be used satisfactorily at greater SIDs or when radiographing small areas of the body. If they are used at shorter distances or in radiography of large areas there may be increasing grid cutoff toward the lateral areas of the anatomical part.

In focused grids, except for the perpendicular strip in the center of the grid, the broad surfaces of the lead foil strips are slightly inclined toward the midpoint of the grid. The planes of all the lead foil strips in the grid converge at a particular distance above the grid, forming a line of points called the convergent line of points. The midpoint of the line is often referred to as the convergent point or focal point of the grid. The perpendicular distance from this point to the grid surface is the focal length or grid radius of the grid. To use this particular grid type most efficiently, the anode of the tube should ideally be placed at this convergent point. The effect of the grid used in this manner, especially at shorter SIDs, removes the maximum amount of scattered radiation without producing objectionable images of lead foil strips in the image. There will always be some line images of the grid in the radiograph produced with a stationary grid.

Visible images of lead foil strips can be eliminated by using a moving grid (Bucky mechanism). The type of grid used in the moving grid mechanism is a focused grid. The motion eliminates images of the lead strips but removes more primary radiation. Therefore, the mAs should be increased slightly to compensate for the decreased overall image density caused by the use of a moving grid.

Another type of grid construction, the crossed (crisscross) grid, may also be used. A crossed grid is an assembly of two linear grids. The two linear grids are placed together with the lead foil strips of one at an angle to the lead foil strips of the other. The resulting grid efficiently removes scattered radiation. A pattern of lead foil images appears in the anatomic image. Use of this grid is more limited than is that of linear grids.

An alternative to the use of a grid that will also remove scatter radiation from the image is the air gap technique. This technique requires that the anatomical part be placed at a prescribed distance from the image receptor surface. This distance causes the image of the object to be magnified, and the exposure dose to the patient is increased if no other changes in the exposure conditions are made. Because of the magnification of the object in the image, the SID is lengthened to compensate. Increasing the SID reduces the exposure dosage to the patient and the radiation exposure to the image receptor. The resultant decrease in radiographic image density must be compensated by an increase in the exposure factors. To accomplish this, the increase in exposure factors depends on the kVp level in use, as it does when compensating for the loss of image density when a grid or beam restrictor is used.

Air gaps reduce the scattered radiation reaching the image receptor. The air gap provides sufficient space between object and image receptor for the scattered radiation from the object to miss the surface of the image receptor. The first inch of the air gap is the most effective in removing scatter radiation from the image. Subsequent inches of air gap are progressively less effective.

Important Terminology

Added Filtration. A specific thickness of a given material that is inserted into the x-ray beam between the source and the patient; usually attached at the tube housing, it reduces both the number of long wavelengths in the x-ray beam and the radiation absorbed by the patient.

Adhesive Layer. An extremely thin layer that allows the phosphor layer of the intensifying screen to adhere to the base of the screen

Anode Heel Effect. A variation in radiographic density along the long axis of a large film that corresponds with the anode heel phenomenon in the x-ray tube

Base Layer. Support structure for coating an intensifying screen with phosphor crystals

Beam Restrictor. Device used to limit the size of the field of irradiation for an exposure

Bucky. Mechanism that allows a grid to move smoothly between the object and the film during exposure so as to eliminate the appearance of grid lines from radiographic images

Bucky Factor. Ratio of the amount of x-radiation that strikes the tube surface of a grid to the amount of radiation emerging from the back of the grid surface; it is an indicator of the radiation absorbed by the grid

Cassette. A light-tight container for medical x-ray film

Collimator. Type of beam restrictor that allows the size of the irradiated field to be adjusted by changing the positions of two separate sets of shutters

Cone. A circular metallic structure (cylindrical or flared) mounted to a base; it restricts the size of the radiant beam at its distal opening.

Contrast Improvement Factor (CIF). Ratio of contrast with the use of a grid to contrast without the use of a grid; the value of the ratio depends on three factors that determine the amount of scatter radiation of an exposure: kVp, field size, and part thickness

Convergent Line. Line of points above the midline of a linear focused grid where the planes of the lead foil strips would meet (converge) if extended into space

Convergent Point. Point above the midline of a focused crossed grid where the two convergent lines of the two linear focused grids intersect.

Crossed Grid. Grid in which the lead strips are arranged so their projected images are at definite angles to each other; composed of two linear grids arranged so that the lead strips are at an angle to each other; a crisscross grid

Cylinder Cone. A circular cylindrical metallic structure mounted to a base with one of two openings; it restricts the size of the radiant beam at its distal opening

Diaphragm. A flat sheet of a radiopaque metal with an opening in it; mounted just beneath the x-ray tube, it limits the area of the radiant field to its aperture

Extension Cylinder Cone. A cylinder cone with an outer sleeve cylinder; has the same purpose as the cylinder cone but is more effective, because the distal opening can be extended nearer to the object and the film

Film Holder. A light-tight structure designed to hold an x-ray film during handling and radiation exposure

Filter. A sheet of metal, usually aluminum (Al) in diagnostic radiography; functions to remove low-energy photons from the primary beam

Flared Cone. Circular structure with two openings and a larger diameter at its distal end; mounted at one opening to a base just beneath the x-ray tube; restricts beam size at its distal opening

Focal Length. Perpendicular distance from the focal point of a focused grid to the surface of the grid; the source-image distance (SID) should be the same distance for the most efficient function of the grid

Focal Point. Same as convergent point except the name implies the focal area of the tube should be positioned at this point

Focused Grid. Grid with the center lead strip perpendicular to the surface of the grid and all other strips on either side inclined toward the midline of the grid

Fog. Overall haze of density on the radiographic image that is detrimental to image quality; unwanted density on a film

Geometric Detail. Fine structural lines of anatomical parts in an image produced by geometric factors (e.g., ratio of SID to object-film distance [OFD], speed of screen, phosphor size and thickness of phosphor layer, focal spot size); image sharpness

Grid. Device consisting of a rigid framework containing lead foil strips in a systematic arrangement (foil strips perpendicular to or at a slight angle with the grid surface, equidistant from each other); its purpose is to prevent secondary radiation from the object from reaching the film and fogging the image

Grid Efficiency. Percentage of secondary radiation absorbed by the grid and prevented from reaching the film; depends on the lead content of the grid

Grid Frequency. Number of lead foil strips within a given measure across the grid (e.g., line count = lines/inch or lines/cm)

Grid Radius. A feature of each grid, it is equal to the perpendicular distance to the grid surface from the point in space where the planes of the lead foil strips would converge if extended; the term is generally used with reference to a focused grid; for a parallel grid, the grid radius equals infinity

Grid Ratio. Usually expressed as two numbers (5:1, 8:1, 12:1, and so forth) that give the ratio of the height of the lead foil strips to the distance between the strips

Image Receptor. A sensitive surface that receives the emergent radiation from the body part and converts it to another form that can be made visible

Inherent Filtration. Removal of the long wavelengths in the x-ray beam by the materials composing the x-ray tube and tube housing; the amount is stated in mm of Al equivalent for each assembly.

Intensification Factor (IF). Ratio of the exposure needed to produce an image without the use of intensifying screens to the exposure needed to produce the same image with the use of intensifying screens

Intensifying Screen. Device with an active part composed of a phosphor layer that emits light when activated by x-rays; increases (intensifies) the effect of x-rays on the sensitive film emulsion

Lead Content. Amount of lead contained in a grid; depends on the grid frequency and grid ratio; value usually expressed as gm/cm^2.

Light Localizer. System of mirrors and a light that projects a light field the same shape and size as the field of radiation from an x-ray tube

Linear Grid. Grid in which the lead strips are arranged with the pattern of the grid lines in one direction, usually from one end to the other

Multidirectional. Having many paths at the same time

Parallel Grid. Grid in which the lead strips are arranged longitudinally and equidistant from each other at all points

PBL. Acronym for positive beam limitation

Phosphor. Compound that when activated by one

form of energy, emits another, lesser form of energy

Phosphor Layer. In intensifying screen construction, a coating of phosphor crystals on a support base permitting it to be handled and mounted in a cassette; the active layer of an intensifying screen

Photographic Detail. Fine structural lines of the image that are visible because of the density and contrast in the image

Positive Beam Limitation Device. Device in a Bucky mechanism that senses the size of the cassette in use and causes the collimator to automatically limit the size of the radiation field to the same area

Primary Transmission. In a discussion of grids, the amount of primary radiation traveling through the grid

Protective Layer. In intensifying screen construction, a thin, radioparent coating that prevents damage to the phosphor layer through normal use

Radiographic Detail. Fine line structure depicted in an image of an object; image detail

Reflective Layer. In intensifying screen construction, a thin layer between the base and the phosphor layer that redirects light coming to it back to the film

Remnant Exit Radiation. All forms of radiation emerging from the object to expose the film; consists of scatter and primary radiation

Rhomboid Grid. Crossed grid with the pattern of the linear grid lines forming equilateral figures, although the angle at which they intersect is not a right angle

Total Filtration. Total amount of material interposed in the x-ray beam that reduces the number of low-energy x-rays in the beam; equal to the sum of the inherent and added filtration; usually expressed as mm of Al or Al equivalent

Tube Side of Grid. Specific surface of a focused grid; the surface of a focused grid where the planes of the grid strips would converge if extended; usually labeled TUBE SIDE by the manufacturer to avoid confusion

Bibliography

Bushong, S.C. Radiologic Science for Technologists, 4th ed. St. Louis: C.V. Mosby, 1988.

Carlton, R.; McKenna-Adler, A. Principles of Radiographic Imaging: An Art and Science. Albany, NY: Delmar Publishers, 1992.

Carroll, Q.B. Fuch's Principles of Radiographic Exposure, Processing and Quality Control, 3rd ed. Springfield, IL: Charles C Thomas, 1985.

Characteristics and Applications of X-ray Grids. Cincinnati, Ohio: Liebel-Flarsheim, 1991.

Chesney, D.N.; Chesney, M.O. Radiographic Imaging, 4th ed. Boston: Blackwell Scientific Publishers, 1981.

Cullinan, A.M. Optimizing Radiographic Positioning. Philadelphia: J.B. Lippincott, 1992.

Cullinan, A.M. Producing Quality Radiographs. Philadelphia: J.B. Lippincott, 1987.

Curry T.S. III; Dowdey, J.E.; Murry, R.C., Jr. Christensen's Introduction to the Physics of Diagnostic Radiology, 4th ed. (1st, 2nd, 3rd, eds, 1972, 1978, 1984, respectively). Philadelphia: Lea and Febiger 1990.

DeVos, D. Basic Principles of Radiographic Exposure. Philadelphia: Lea & Febiger, 1990.

Donohue, D.P. An Analysis of Radiographic Quality: Lab Manual and Workbook, 2nd ed. Baltimore: University Park Press, 1984.

Fundamentals of Radiography. Rochester, NY: Eastman-Kodak Company, 1980.

Myers, P.A. Simplifying Radiographic Quality, 1972.

Phillips, M.L.W. Ensuring Image Quality, Assessing and Improving Radiographic Images. St. Louis: C.V. Mosby, 1987.

Seemann, H.E. Physical and Photographic Principles of Medical Radiography. New York: John Wiley & Sons, 1968.

Seeram, E. X-ray Imaging Equipment. Springfield, IL: Charles C Thomas, 1985.

Sprawls, P. Principles of Radiography for Technologists. Rockville, MD: Aspen Publishers, 1990.

Thompson, T.T. Cahoon's Formulating X-ray Technics, 9th ed. (and most previous editions by Cahoon.) Durham: Duke University Press, 1979.

Tortorici, M. Concepts of Medical Radiographic Imaging. Philadelphia: W.B. Saunders, 1992.

⚡ Review Questions

1. What is the anode heel effect?
2. What is the result of the anode heel effect in the radiographic image?
3. What is an x-ray beam filter?
4. What is the purpose of a filter in the x-ray beam?
5. How is the amount of filtration in the x-ray beam expressed? Why is it expressed in this way?
6. Define the following terms:
   a. added filtration
   b. inherent filtration
   c. total filtration
   d. compensating filter
7. What amount of total filtration is required in an x-ray beam produced by the following peak kilovoltages:
   a. below 50 kVp?
   b. between 50 and 70 kVp?
   c. above 70 kVp?
8. How does a filter accomplish its purpose?
9. What is the purpose of a beam restrictor?
10. Name and describe the various types of commercially available beam restrictors.
11. How does a beam restrictor accomplish its purpose?
12. What are the advantages and disadvantages of the listed beam restrictors?
    a. diaphragm
    b. cylinder cones
    c. extension cylinder cones
    d. collimators
13. What was the initial purpose for use of beam restrictors in radiography?
14. What is the effect of beam restriction in the radiographic image? Why does this occur?
15. In general, what changes should be made in exposure factors when
    a. increasing the beam restriction (decreasing size of radiation field)?
    b. decreasing the beam restriction (increasing size of radiation field)?
16. What is positive beam limitation (PBL)?
17. What is its purpose?
18. How is this purpose accomplished? To what circumstances of radiographic exposure does this not apply?
19. Describe the relation of screen speed to the following:
    a. radiographic density.
    b. radiographic contrast.
    c. the production of recorded detail.
    d. absorption of radiation.
    e. ability to convert x-ray photon energy to light energy
20. What is an intensifying screen?
21. What factors should be considered in radiography that
    a. produce scatter (secondary) radiation?
    b. reduce the production of scatter radiation?
22. What is "fog"?
23. List and define those things in common use and identified in this chapter that reduce the patient's radiation dose.
24. Differentiate between calcium tungstate intensifying screens and rare earth intensifying screens.
25. How do intensifying screens contribute to the reduction of the patient's radiation dose?
26. What is a grid? What is its purpose?
27. What is a Bucky mechanism? What is its purpose?
28. What is an air-gap exposure technique? What is its purpose?
29. What are the advantages and disadvantages of the air-gap exposure technique?
30. The exposure for an AP projection of a recumbent abdomen is listed on the technique chart as

80 mAs	3 mm of Al beam filter
80 kVp	100-speed screen-film combination
40-inch SID	collimation = 14-inch × 17-inch field
12:1 Bucky and grid	source current = 1φ generator

Using the exposure conversion factors given in this and previous chapters, convert the original exposure technique to use
   a. a 200-speed screen-film combination
   b. a 400-speed screen-film combination
   c. an 8:1 Bucky/grid
   d. a 12:1 stationary grid
   e. current source = 3φ generator
   f. 2.5 mm of Al beam filter
   g. 44-inch SID
   (Return to original exposure technique for each conversion.)
31. Using the information from this chapter and Chapters 11 and 12, make the calculations indicated in the following statements: The exposure factors listed by the technique chart for a PA projection of a chest that measures 28 cm in the anteroposterior direction are

30 mAs	3 mm Al beam filter
90 kVp	100-speed screen-film combination
72-inch SID	current source = 1φ generator
8:1 stationary grid	

   a. If an 8-inch air-gap exposure technique is used to radiograph this chest, what SID must be used to maintain the same degree of magnification of the part in the image as would be seen in a chest with the original exposure conditions?
   b. If the SID found in a is used, what mAs is required to maintain the image density of this radiograph?
   c. If the exposure factors in b are changed to a nongrid exposure, what are the new exposure factors?
   d. If the exposure factors in c are changed to use a 400-speed screen-film combination, what are the new exposure factors?

e. Working from the exposure factors in *d*, indicate the change to the exposure factors that would be used with a 3ϕ current source.

f. Working from the exposure factors in *e*, change to a high-kVp exposure technique (>110 kVp) if a high-kVp technique is not currently in the calculations.

g. List the exposure factors for this radiograph as they should appear on an exposure technique chart. (Use format given in introduction to question.)

h. Identify those factors in a radiography room and the requirements of a particular projection that may limit the use of the new exposure technique listed in *g*.

i. Identify any changes that could feasibly be made to achieve a nongrid, high-kVp exposure of this part using an air-gap exposure technique that would solve any limiting circumstances identified in *h*.

32. What effect does each listed factor have on the speed of intensifying screens?
    a. Size of the phosphor crystal
    b. Thickness of the phosphor crystal layer
    c. Dye added to the binder material in which the phosphor crystals are suspended
    d. Use of a reflective layer in construction of an intensifying screen
    e. kVp level used for radiographic exposures
    f. Type of phosphor crystal used in the intensifying screen

33. What is a photostimulable phosphor?

34. Discuss the purpose of the photostimulable phosphor and describe how it works in radiography. What is the anticipated impact of the phosphor on radiography, the radiography department, and the patient?

35. Is it really necessary to use a grid exposure technique when performing a lateral cervical spine at an SID of 72 inches? Explain your answer.

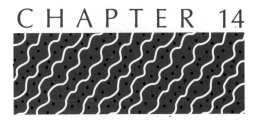

CHAPTER 14

The Effect of Patient Status on the Radiographic Image

Janice Hall M.A. Ed., R.T.(R.)

Chapter Objectives

On completion of this chapter, you should be able to

■ Define basic radiographic terminology discussed in the chapter.
■ Discuss the four general types of body habitus and how they affect the proper selection of exposure factors needed for optimal radiographic images.
■ Describe the four general classifications of human body tissue.
■ Explain why patients may have the same body measurements, yet require different exposure factors.
■ Briefly describe the composition of the body.
■ Differentiate between organic and inorganic substances in the human body.
■ Describe the process of attenuation in bone, air, and soft tissue.
■ Differentiate between negative and positive contrast media.
■ Define pathological conditions considered additive and those considered destructive.
■ List common disease processes affecting the radiographic image, and determine what changes in exposure factors are necessary.
■ Describe pathological conditions affecting the skeletal system and their radiographic manifestations.
■ Describe the two major pathological considerations related to the abdomen.

PHYSICAL CHANGES

The greatest variable the radiographer faces when performing a radiographic procedure is the patient. Before a patient is x-rayed, several factors must be taken into consideration. The physical characteristics and the area to be examined must be observed carefully. Clinical experience enables the radiographer to estimate the location of the organs according to body build of the patient. It is not so simple to evaluate x-ray absorption characteristics since they are unpredictable, thus sometimes making it difficult to estimate physical and pathological changes of body tissue. Small deviations from the normal tissue density or thickness can be overlooked, whereas compensation must be made for recognizable abnormal conditions of the body. Compensation can be accomplished by proper adjustment of selected exposure factors. First, how patient status is affected by physical changes within individual patients is considered. It must always be kept in mind that no two individuals are identical; therefore, body type or physique differs from person to person.

343

Body Habitus

The general form of the human body is known as *body habitus*. It determines the shape, size, location, muscle tone, and mobility of organs. It is important for the radiographer to have an understanding of body habitus types. The four general body types are (1) *sthenic*, (2) *hyposthenic*, (3) *hypersthenic*, and (4) *asthenic*. The organs most affected by variations in body habitus are the lungs, stomach, and gallbladder. The radiographer must be able to evaluate the patient accurately and thoroughly before the first exposure is made. The patient's overall physique and body mass should be noted. Through clinical experience and careful evaluation, a competent radiographer should develop expertise necessary to modify exposure factors according to individual physique and produce a diagnostic radiographic image.

Sthenic Body Type

The sthenic type body habitus makes up approximately 50% of the population. Persons with this physique are generally categorized as having an average type of body build. The word *sthenic* means strong or active; therefore, persons with this body habitus are generally physically fit, with good muscle tone and bone mass. The sthenic body habitus is a more slender version of the hypersthenic physique. The stomach is generally J-shaped and is located low in comparison with that of the hypersthenic build, and the gallbladder is less transverse. It lies halfway between the lateral wall of the abdomen and the midline of the body (Fig. 14–1). The sthenic body habitus is the basis for the established exposure factors. Exposure factors for all other physiques are modified from those for the sthenic body type.

Hyposthenic Body Type

The hyposthenic body habitus is slightly more slender than the sthenic. This type, which is a modification of the still more slender asthenic build, constitutes approximately 35% of the population. The stomach is J-shaped and elongated, extending somewhat below the iliac crest. The gallbladder is lower and

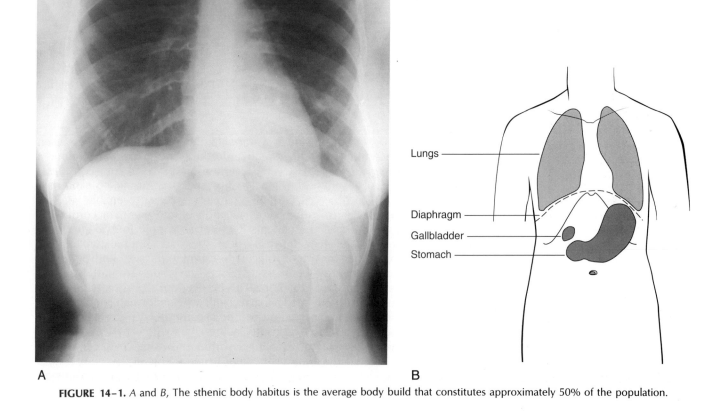

A   B

FIGURE 14–1. *A* and *B*, The sthenic body habitus is the average body build that constitutes approximately 50% of the population.

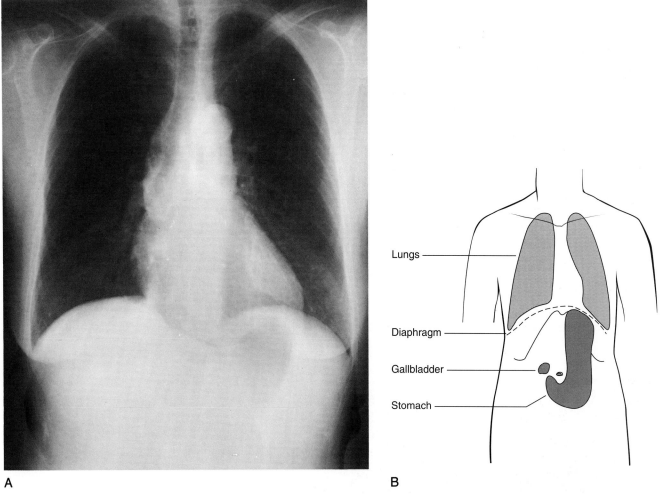

A   B

FIGURE 14–2. *A* and *B,* The hyposthenic body habitus, which includes approximately 35% of the population.

more toward the midline than that of the sthenic body habitus (Fig. 14–2). The primary distinction between the hyposthenic and asthenic types is not the size but the condition of the person's body. Whereas the asthenic patient is physically unfit and emaciated, usually as a result of pathology, the patient who is hyposthenic is usually healthy but thin and somewhat underweight for his or her height. Individuals of this body type are thin in comparison with the sthenic patient. Although the asthenic patient is usually advanced in age and frail, the hyposthenic patient is quite often young and strong despite being underweight. The hyposthenic body habitus requires less exposure factors than does the sthenic patient.

Hypersthenic Body Type

Persons with the hypersthenic habitus compose 5% of the population. Patients in this category have a massive or heavy body build. The chest and abdomen are broad from side to side and deep from front to back. The lungs are short and wide, lying on a transverse axis. The gallbladder is higher and lies farther to

the right in comparison with the sthenic body build. The stomach is also located high and in a transverse direction (Fig. 14–3). Persons with this body habitus are well padded with superfluous tissue and tend to become overweight.

Asthenic Body Type

Patients of the asthenic type are extremely slender and frail in appearance and oftentimes are advanced in age. These individuals are usually elderly. The bony structure of the body is small-framed. The lungs are long, and the apices extend quite a way above the clavicles. The heart is long and narrow with its long axis nearly vertical. The stomach and gallbladder are low and vertical and lie close to the midline of the body (Fig. 14–4). This body build usually possesses little muscle tone. The bones are prominent, especially in the area of the rib cage, shoulder, and pelvic girdles. Persons of this body type constitute only 10% of the population. Because of the size of these individuals, compared with the sthenic patient, a considerably smaller amount of radiation is needed to obtain a satisfactory radiographic image.

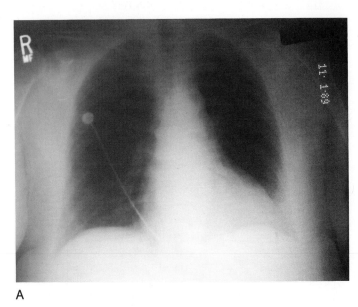

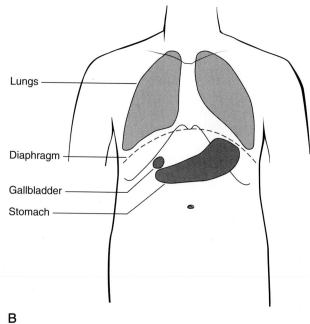

A

B

FIGURE 14-3. *A* and *B*, The hypersthenic body habitus; approximately 5% of the population is included in this group.

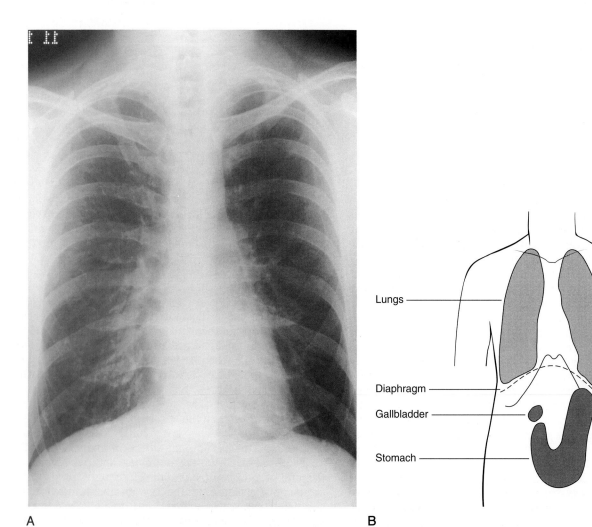

A

B

FIGURE 14-4. *A* and *B*, The asthenic body habitus, which represents about 10% of the population.

Classification of Tissue

Classification of tissue refers to the *radiolucency* and *radiopacity* of the various types of body tissue. The four general classifications of body tissue are listed as follows:

- *emaciated tissue*
- superfluous tissue
- muscle tissue
- normal tissue

The habitus of the body is usually an accurate guide to its relative tissue content. The asthenic body habitus is one with emaciated tissue, whereas the hypersthenic body build frequently has superfluous tissue. A sthenic, well-toned body habitus possesses muscle and normal tissues.

Generally, when attempting to determine exposure factors, patients can be categorized as having "easy" to penetrate, normal, or "hard" to penetrate tissue. Those patients with easy to penetrate tissue include the young, the elderly, the emaciated or underdeveloped, and those with *destructive pathology*. Normal tissues are those with the average thickness or development. Patients with hard to penetrate tissue are those possessing massive (heavy) or muscular body build and those with *additive pathology*.

To compensate for tissue differences in patients, divide them into three general groups, or classifications:

- Group 1 includes the small, emaciated, or thin patient (asthenic/hyposthenic habitus)
- Group 2 includes the normal or medium patient (sthenic habitus)
- Group 3 includes the large (obese) or muscular patient (hypersthenic habitus)

In classifications 1, 2, and 3, each patient requires adjustments in exposure factors because of tissue differences and body habitus. Group 1 requires a decrease in exposure factors compared with group 2. Group 3 requires an increase in exposure factors compared with group 2. If the same radiographic exposure factors (optimum kVp and same mAs) were used on all three groups of patients, group 1 would be overexposed, and group 3 would be underexposed.

Adjusting exposure factors would not be required if all individuals were of the same body structure and tissue consistency. We could measure all patients with calipers and have a standard exposure factor for all patients with the same measurements. Unfortunately, this is not the case. It is possible to have three different patients who have the same body measurements within the area of interest; yet, because of body structure, tissue consistency, or pathology, the use of different exposure factors may be necessary on each of these patients.

In radiography of the bones, several factors, such as *atrophy* of tissue due to age, disuse or pathology, must be considered. In chest radiography, the body habitus, age, consistency, and amount of tissue, along with the amount of air in the lungs, must be taken into account.

There is no simple, clear-cut route to obtaining *diagnostic* and *optimal images.* A competent radiographer takes all factors discussed thus far into consideration and weighs the available options that will yield the best radiographic results for each patient. It is most important to take time to evaluate patients individually for the best possible radiograph on each. No matter how accurate the technique chart, the radiographer must make the final adjustments necessary to yield a satisfactory image.

Composition of the Human Body

The body is composed of approximately 62% water, 15% fat, and 23% bone. By about age 17, approximately 40% of the total body weight is muscle. The human body consists of various organic and inorganic materials. Bone, soft tissue, and fat are the three major components in the composition of the body that account for most radiation absorption. Soft tissue and fat are organic substances, whereas inorganic substances are the major constituents of bone.

Organic and Inorganic Materials

Organic tissues contain a large amount of fluid and possess low x-ray absorption properties. Muscle tissue contains more fluid than fat, which explains why a body habitus that contains more muscle than fat requires a greater radiation exposure to adequately demonstrate the area of interest. Muscle tissue contains approximately 75% fluid, and fat contains approximately 20%. Patients who have excellent muscle tone and are extremely muscular pose a slight problem in obtaining high-quality images. The reason is that muscle tissue contains more fluid, making it more difficult to penetrate. To prevent underpenetration, an increase in kilovolt peak (kVp) is needed; however, this solution may result in excessive scatter radiation, thereby decreasing image quality. Lung tissue, on the other hand, contains a large amount of air, thus making it easier to penetrate. Hence lung tissue requires much less radiation exposure compared with muscle tissue.

Bone is by and large an inorganic substance that contains a smaller percentage of fluid compared with organic materials. The normal adult bony structure and cartilaginous skeleton constitutes approximately 23% of total body weight. Bone is the most dense tissue within the body; therefore, it absorbs a greater amount of radiation than any other tissue of the body.

Beam Attenuation Within the Body

The amount of *attenuation* is determined by the thickness of the part and type of material being irradiated. As the x-ray beam passes through the patient, it is attenuated, and a portion is completely absorbed by the body tissues. These areas of the radiograph appear least dense. Other portions of the beam pass through a body part with little or no attenuation; these areas appear as more dense on the radiographic image. The thicker body parts cause greater beam attenuation, whereas the thinner body parts result in less attenuation.

The type of absorber also affects attenuation. Materials with high atomic members attenuate a greater percentage of the beam compared with those materials having lower atomic numbers. Attenuation is influenced by the *density* of the absorbing material. Density is a way of describing how tightly the atoms of a given substance are packed together. The greater the density of a tissue, the greater its ability to absorb radiation. The beam is attenuated in varying amounts, depending on the thickness and density of the tissue being radiographed.

Bone

Bone is approximately twice as dense as soft tissue and absorbs about twice as many x-ray photons as a result of its density. The absorption can be attributed to the presence of calcium in the bone. Calcium has a higher atomic number than most materials found in the human body—approximately 20, whereas soft tissue has an atomic number of about 7.4.

Another consideration is the age of the patient. It is important that the choice of exposure factors for good bone radiography be adjusted according to age. With increasing age, the calcium deposits in the bones decrease, thus making them easier to penetrate. If exposure factors are not adjusted, the radiograph will have increased density. It is therefore necessary to decrease kVp in order to compensate for this loss of calcium.

In Figure 14–5 two radiographs demonstrate the effects of calcium on bone density. Radiograph *A* is of a young patient with good calcium deposits in bone. *B* is of an elderly patient and shows loss of calcium in the bone. Note the transparent appearance of the bone in *B*. Pathology also contributes to variations in bone absorption, and adjustments in exposure factors must

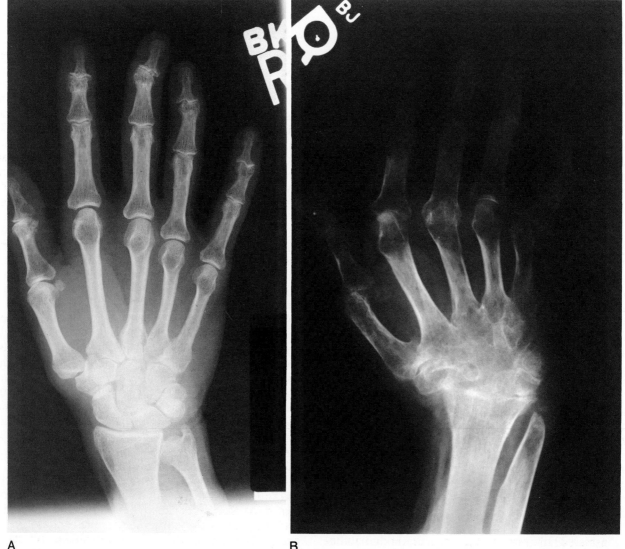

A   B

FIGURE 14–5. Effects of calcium on bone density. *A*, A 28-year-old patient with good calcium deposits in bone. *B*, A 72-year-old patient whose bones appear transparent as a result of loss of calcium. The radiographic appearance is also attributed to pathological changes caused by rheumatoid arthritis.

be made. Pathological changes are discussed in more detail later in this chapter.

Air

Air provides little interference with the passage of x-rays through a part. It has an atomic number of approximately 7.6, a higher atomic number than fat or muscle, but it has a significantly lower density than either of these. As a result, less attenuation of the beam occurs, because air absorbs fewer photons than other body substances. Air is easier to penetrate; therefore, significantly less radiation is required for radiography of the chest compared with that for abdominal studies.

Soft Tissue

Fat and muscle are two soft tissue structures. Muscle has a higher effective atomic number and a greater tissue density than fat; therefore, much more beam attenuation occurs in muscle than in fat. Muscle cells are more closely packed than fat cells. In comparison with fat, muscle has a higher water content. Large amounts of muscle tissue produce more scatter than an equal amount of fat. Fat absorbs fewer x-rays compared with muscle. As a result, radiographic density decreases with muscle, because it absorbs more photons than does fat.

It is the responsibility of the radiographer to evaluate the patient during the first few minutes of initial contact. Attention should be given to the body habitus, tissue composition, and possible pathology in order for the radiographer to decide on the best exposure factor adjustments necessary to achieve a diagnostic image.

Contrast Media

Contrast media are important diagnostic tools in radiologic procedures. Certain structures not readily demonstrated on standard radiographs because of their low *subject contrast* are better demonstrated radiographically with the use of contrast media. Subject contrast results from different absorption characteristics of the structures making up the part. Introduction of a contrast agent is used to alter the x-ray photon absorption of a structure in order to demonstrate it radiographically. The contrast agent must be of lesser or greater density than the walls of the organs it fills and also of surrounding structures. Contrast media constitute various nontoxic chemical preparations with high x-ray absorption properties. They are introduced into the body by ingestion or injection before radiography is performed. The medium may be a light substance such as air or gas or a dense substance such as barium sulfate or iodine. Contrast media can be categorized as (1) *positive contrast agents* and (2) *negative contrast agents*. Those that attenuate x-rays, resulting in a decreased density or lighter area on the radiograph, are known as positive contrast media, or agents. Contrast media that allow x-rays to penetrate through the part, resulting in increased density or darker areas

on the radiograph, are known as negative contrast media. Figure 14–6 demonstrates radiographic procedures using positive and negative contrast media.

Positive Contrast Agents

Many brands of positive contrast media exist. All are either iodine or barium elements bound to molecules with organic salts to render them nontoxic. These two elements are successful because of their high atomic numbers. The atomic number of iodine is 53 and that of barium 56. In order to convey the best information on a radiographic image, it is essential to be able to see through the positive contrast medium. In order to accomplish this, optimum kVp must be used with radiographic procedures requiring a contrast medium. Most iodine-based contrast agents give optimal opacification with kVp levels from 70 to 75. Barium-based contrast agents give optimal opacification with at least 100 kVp (except esophagrams and air-contrast studies, for which optimal kVp is at least 90). By using these kVp levels, the contrast media are penetrated and yield a more diagnostic result.

Negative Contrast Agents

Negative contrast agents are gaseous and include air, nitrous oxide, and carbon dioxide. The most common and readily available negative agent is normal room air. Air is useful because of its extremely low x-ray absorption properties. Negative contrast agents do not differ much in atomic number from soft tissue. The atomic number of air is 7.6 and that of soft tissue 7.4. Although the atomic numbers of air and soft tissue are similar, the physical densities of the two are different. The physical density of air is approximately 1/1000 that of soft tissue. This is why negative contrast agents are penetrated so easily by x-rays and result in a significantly darker area (increased density) on the radiographic image compared with the surrounding soft tissue.

Contrast Procedures Demonstration

Both negative and positive contrast agents are useful in demonstrating organs that could not otherwise be demonstrated radiographically. Several radiographic procedures are performed daily using contrast media. Figure 14–7A to C illustrates examples of common contrast procedures outlining various anatomical structures (Fig. 14–7). *A* demonstrates a radiographic procedure of the stomach known as an upper gastrointestinal (UGI) series. The contrast agents are ingested by mouth. This is a double-contrast study of the stomach using both positive and negative contrast media. The positive contrast agent is barium sulfate. The negative contrast agent is gas, used to distend the barium-coated stomach to better visualize it. *B* shows a radiographic study of the urinary bladder known as a cystogram. The examination is accomplished by direct instillation of iodinated contrast media into the bladder by a catheter. *C* depicts a renal arteriogram; this is a special radiologic procedure involving the study of

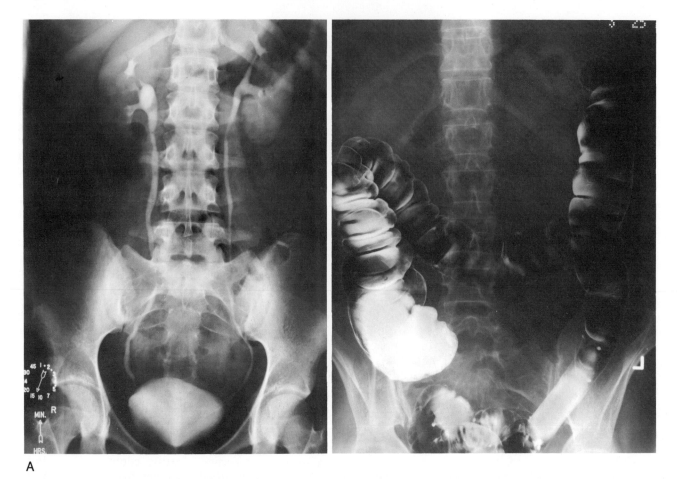

A

FIGURE 14–6. *A* demonstrates a radiographic procedure utilizing positive contrast media. Note the white appearance of the calyces of the kidneys, ureters, and bladder. This procedure is known as an intravenous pyelogram (IVP). *B* demonstrates barium enema with air contrast. Note the white appearance of the barium (positive media) and the dark appearance of the air (negative media).

the renal artery. A positive iodinated contrast medium is usually introduced into the renal artery by way of a catheter through a percutaneous puncture of the femoral artery.

PATHOLOGICAL CHANGES

Up to this point the patient has been considered in relation to physical changes. Here, the effects of pathology on patient status are considered. It is clear that each patient is unique and thus cannot be fitted into a mold. Patients not only have different tissue make-up but also many different pathological processes. These pathological conditions can affect the overall approach for obtaining an optimal image. Pathological conditions can be classified according to measures that must be taken with exposure factors in order to obtain diagnostic and optimal images. Earlier in the chapter, the concepts hard and easy to penetrate were briefly discussed in relation to differences in tissue composition. These features are now considered as they relate specifically to changes from pathology.

Hard Versus Easy to Penetrate

Pathology usually affects radiographic density in one of two ways: additive (hard to penetrate) or destructive (easy to penetrate). Additive pathology requires an increase in exposure factors, whereas destructive pathology requires a decrease in exposure factors. If factors of normal technique were used on either pathological condition, an unsatisfactory radiographic image would result. Since these variations in density deal with penetration and since penetration is controlled by kVp, the corrective change should preferably be made in kVp.

One cannot determine by looking at a patient the exact extent of the pathological process. When a patient is scheduled for radiological procedures, some type of clinical history should be available for the radiographer. Although the information provides assistance in choosing a proper technical factor, it does not totally prepare the radiographer. There is no clear-cut way to handle a patient's pathology from a radiographic standpoint. For instance, evaluation of exposure factors for a patient with a clinical history of *emphysema* is somewhat difficult. The first step is to know that this disease process is categorized as destructive pathology and to consider that a decrease in

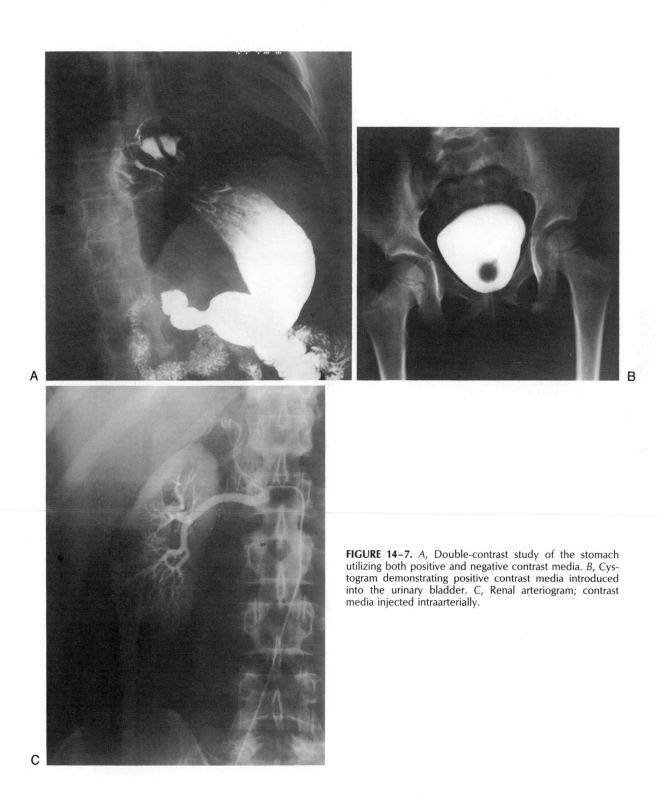

FIGURE 14–7. *A,* Double-contrast study of the stomach utilizing both positive and negative contrast media. *B,* Cystogram demonstrating positive contrast media introduced into the urinary bladder. *C,* Renal arteriogram; contrast media injected intraarterially.

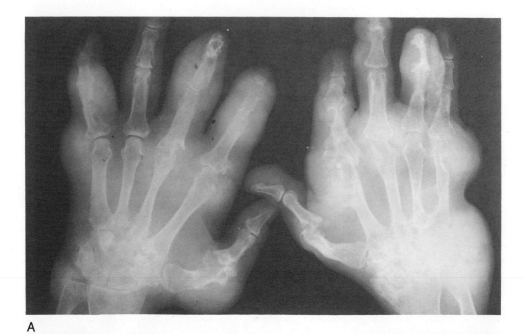

A

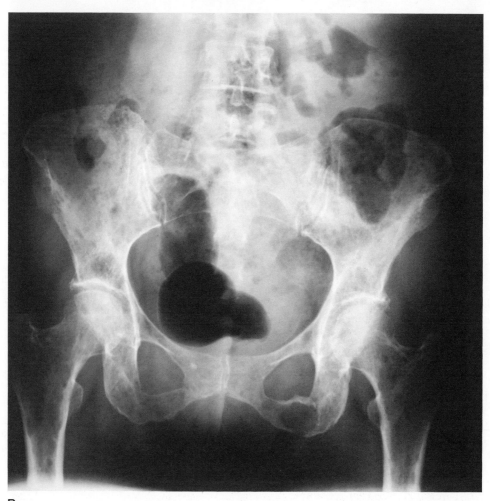

B

FIGURE 14–8. *A,* Osteolytic changes have resulted from bone destruction due to the disease process known as gout. Note the soft tissue swelling and bone destruction in the joints of both hands. *B,* Multiple myeloma produces osteolytic changes as a result of metastases. Radiolucent areas can be seen throughout the pelvis.

exposure factors *may* be necessary. The word *may* is emphasized because the course of action to be taken depends on the extent of this disease process. If emphysema is in an advanced stage, a decrease in exposure factors is necessary. If the process is in its early stage, compensation in exposure factors may not be required.

The stage of the disease process determines the amount of increase or decrease needed. In actuality, the change in exposure factors required for a particular disease process cannot be assigned a finite number. The most important concern for the radiographer is determining when the disease process requires an addition or reduction in exposure factors. Determining the extent to how exposure factors are manipulated improves with clinical experience. With more clinical expertise, the radiographer begins to learn the signs, or indicators, of certain diseases. For example, a patient with advanced-stage emphysema often breathes with a wheezing sound and has a barrel-shaped chest. Remember, the extent of the disease rather than its presence should regulate a change in exposure factors. One way to accurately determine technique changes for certain diseases of individual patients is to maintain individual patient files with exposures listed. This method is infrequently followed because it is time consuming and may be impractical in large radiology departments.

Disease Process in the Skeletal System

When dealing with pathology in the bony anatomy, the radiologist is concerned with whether there has been destruction or production of bone. *Osteolytic* changes require a decrease in exposure factors because of destruction of bone. Degenerative changes, bone tumors, disuse, and inflammatory changes may reduce the amount of calcium within a bone, resulting in an osteolytic condition. In some osteolytic changes, the radiographic manifestations appear as radiolucent areas within the bone substance. Examples of osteolytic changes are seen in Fig. 14–8*A* and *B*.

It is important to obtain high-contrast films so that the radiologist can detect early destructive changes that might not be seen with low-contrast films. This can be accomplished by using low kVp and detail screen-film combinations. *Osteoblastic* changes require an increase in exposure factors because of production of bone. These changes are seen radiographically as an increase in bone density resulting from new bone or cartilage formation. Osteoblastic lesions may require a large increase in kVp and a grid with a high ratio.

In general, most bone radiography requires short-scale contrast to provide maximum visibility of detail. The scale of contrast must be such that soft tissues and muscles are well demonstrated. Soft tissue swelling, calcifications, muscle wasting, and presence of gas in the soft tissue all are important radiographic findings (Fig. 14–9).

Disease Process in the Respiratory System

Detection of lung disease processes requires long-latitude films such as those obtained with high kVp. Most authorities agree that a minimum of 100 kVp should be used with the appropriate grid ratio for all adult chest radiography. Most pulmonary disease processes require standard exposure factors. If a decrease in density is necessary, this is best accomplished by decreasing milliampere-seconds (mAs) rather than kVp. Decreasing kVp affects overall radiographic contrast and tends to enhance the bony thorax, obscuring vascular details. A decrease in kVp could also result in underpenetration of the mediastinal structures. The radiologist wants to see through the disease process, which dictates what exposure factors are used. Figures 14–10 and 14–11 demonstrate pathological changes in the chest area.

Important Considerations Concerning the Abdomen

Two major conditions important to radiography of the abdomen are *ascites* and *bowel obstruction*. It is necessary to distinguish between these two in order to correctly modify exposure factors. The abdomen is distended in both cases, but the difference can usually be determined by palpation. If the distention feels like dough, it is likely to be due to accumulation of fluid (ascites). This condition requires an increase in exposure factors (usually kVp). Increases in kVp with the presence of fluid increases the production of scatter radiation, resulting in fog and reducing the overall

Table 14–1: DISEASE PROCESSES THAT AFFECT THE RADIOGRAPHIC IMAGE

Hard to Penetrate (Additive Pathology)	
Disease Process	*Common Location*
Aortic aneurysm	Chest/Abdomen
Atelectasis	Chest
Pleural effusion	Chest
Pneumonia	Chest
Enlarged heart	Chest
Ascites	Abdomen
Paget's disease	Skeleton
Osteoblastic metastases	Skeleton
Sclerosis	Skeleton
Cirrhosis	Abdomen
Easy to Penetrate (Destructive Pathology)	
Disease Process	*Common Location*
Active tuberculosis	Chest
Emphysema	Chest
Pneumothorax	Chest
Atrophy	Skeleton
Carcinoma	Skeleton
Degenerative arthritis	Skeleton
Osteoporosis	Skeleton
Bowel obstruction	Abdomen

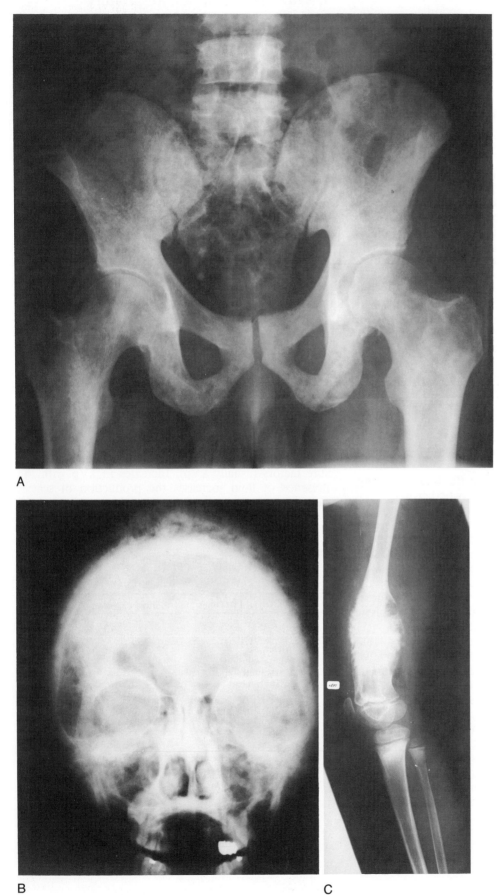

FIGURE 14–9. Osteoblastic changes are noted as a result of a pathological process known as Paget's disease. This process, also called osteitis deformans, is well demonstrated in the pelvis (A) and the head (B). The bones most commonly affected are those of the pelvis and skull. Various parts of the skull become soft and larger through a loss of calcium followed by a production of bone, and the skull eventually becomes lumpy and deformed as noted very well in B. C, Osteosarcoma of the femur; note the characteristic dense bone involving the area of the tumor. The patient had no sign of other bone metastases. (Courtesy of the ACR Learning File.)

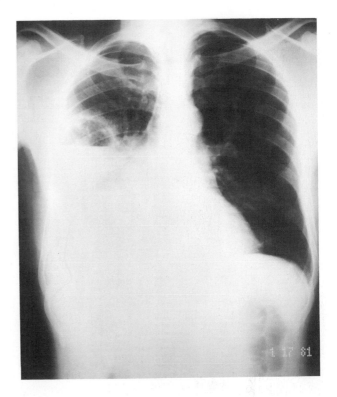

FIGURE 14–10. Posteroanterior (PA) chest radiograph demonstrating pathological changes due to pneumonia. Note the cloudy, white appearance of the involved area of the right lung. This condition requires an increase in exposure factors to compensate for the fluid or liquid matter in the lung.

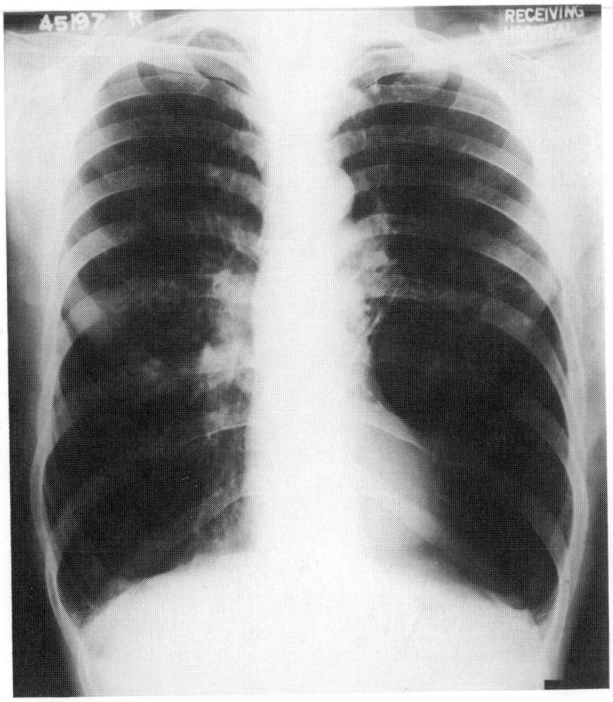

FIGURE 14–11. Posteroanterior (PA) radiograph of the chest demonstrating emphysema. Note the loss of pulmonary markings, particularly in the lower left lobe of the lung. Emphysema is characterized by air-filled expansion of the lungs.

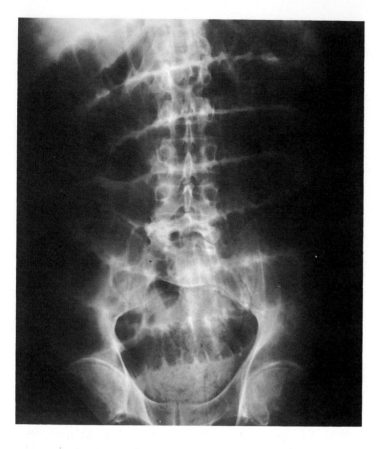

FIGURE 14–12. Radiograph of the abdomen demonstrating bowel obstruction of the small intestines. Note the increase in density due to the air in the small intestines.

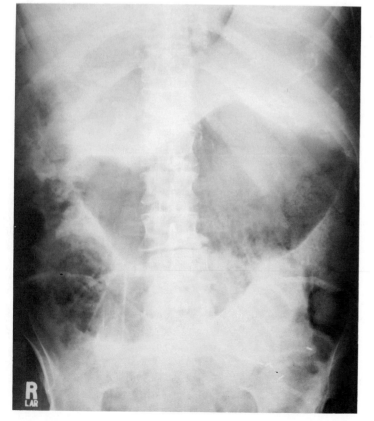

FIGURE 14–13. Radiograph showing an obstruction of the stomach. Air in the stomach also caused the density here.

image quality. A high-ratio grid can be used to improve contrast and detail.

If the abdomen is distended and feels taut, it may be due to air. Air distention of the abdomen due to bowel obstruction requires a decrease in exposure factors. Figures 14–12 and 14–13 illustrate radiographs with increased density due to obstruction.

As with other systems of the body, certain pathological conditions require changes in exposure factors.

Table 14–1 summarizes disease processes that can affect the radiographic image. The pathology is classified according to the needed change in exposure factors.

Chapter Summary/ Important Concepts

The patient is the greatest variable that the radiographer encounters when performing a radiographic procedure. X-ray absorption characteristics are unpredictable, making it difficult to estimate physical and pathological changes in body tissue.

Body habitus determines the shape, size, muscle tone, and mobility of organs. There are four general types of body habitus: sthenic, hypersthenic, hyposthenic, and asthenic.

Four general classifications of body tissue are
a. emaciated tissue
b. superfluous tissue
c. muscle tissue
d. normal tissue.

The body habitus is usually an accurate guide to its relative tissue content. Generally, patients can be categorized as easy to penetrate, normal, and hard to penetrate.

Since body structure and tissue consistency varies with each person, it is necessary to evaluate each patient individually and determine what exposure factors are necessary to obtain a diagnostic-quality image.

In bone radiography, factors such as atrophy of tissue because of age, disuse, or pathology must be taken into consideration.

In chest radiography, factors such as body habitus, tissue consistency and status, age of patient, and amount of air in the lungs must be considered.

It is important to take time to evaluate every patient individually to determine the best possible way to obtain a good radiograph.

The body is composed of various organic and inorganic materials. It consists of approximately 62% water, 15% fat, and 23% bone. By the age of 17 years, approximately 40% of the total body weight is muscle.

Organic tissues contain a large amount of fluid and have low–x-ray absorption properties. Inorganic tissues contain a much smaller percentage of fluid compared with organic material.

Attenuation is determined by the thickness of the part and the type of absorber being irradiated.

Bone is approximately twice as dense as soft tissue and will absorb about twice as many x-ray photons.

Calcium content in bones has a higher atomic number than most materials found in the body. Calcium content does however decrease with the age of the patient.

Air has a higher atomic number than fat or muscle but has a significantly lower tissue density; for this reason less attenuation of the beam occurs in tissues containing air.

Muscle cells are more closely packed than fat cells and have a much higher water content.

The introduction of contrast media aids in delineation of anatomical structures. Contrast media can be categorized as positive and negative contrast agents.

All positive contrast agents are either iodine or barium elements bound to molecules with organic salts to make them nontoxic. Negative contrast agents are gaseous, air being most commonly used. Air is useful because of its extremely low x-ray absorption properties. The physical density of air is approximately 1/1000 that of soft tissue.

Pathology usually affects radiographic density in one of two ways: it is either additive (hard to penetrate) or destructive (easy to penetrate).

Additive pathology requires an increase in exposure factors. Destructive pathology requires a decrease in exposure factors.

The extent of a disease rather than its presence should regulate change in exposure factors.

In pathology of the bone, the radiologist is concerned with whether there have been destructive changes (osteolytic) or productive changes (osteoblastic) of bone.

In general, bone radiography requires short-scale contrast to provide maximum visibility of detail. Contrast must be such that soft tissue and muscle are well demonstrated.

Long-latitude films are required in order to detect lung disease. The radiologist wants to see through the disease process, therefore dictating what exposure factors are to be used.

Ascites and bowel obstruction are the two major considerations in abdominal studies. Ascites requires an increase in exposure factors because of the accumulation of fluid. Bowel obstruction requires a decrease in exposure factors because of the excessive accumulation of gas in the abdominal cavity.

Important Terminology

Additive Pathology. Disease process causing increased density by production of bone

Ascites. Accumulation of fluid in the peritoneal cavity

Asthenic. A thin or emaciated body build person with flat, long thorax, accompanied by inferior muscular development

Atrophy. Wasting or reduction in size resulting from lack of nutrition of any part

Attenuation. Reduction in the total number of x-ray photons in a beam after passing through a given thickness of material

Body Habitus. General form of a human body

Bowel Obstruction. Blockage of the lumen of the large or small intestine

Density. Quantity of matter per unit of volume measured in kilograms per cubic meter

Destructive Pathology. Disease process causing decreased density by destruction of bone

Diagnostic Image. Radiographic image that conveys information necessary for the radiologist to make an accurate diagnosis

Emaciated. Wasted flesh; state of being excessively lean

Emphysema. A condition in which the alveoli of the lungs become distended or ruptured; usually the result of an interference with exhalation or loss of elasticity of the lungs

Hypersthenic. A massive or heavy physique with a broad chest and abdomen

Hyposthenic. A body habitus that is slightly more slender than the average body build

Negative Contrast Agent. A medium that allows x-rays to penetrate and results in a darker, more dense radiographic image

Optimal. The best or most desirable image; one that will yield the most information

Osteoblastic. Describes production of bone

Osteolytic. Describes destruction of bone

Positive Contrast Agent. A medium that attenuates x-rays and results in a low-density or clear area on a radiograph

Radiolucent. Partly or wholly permeable to x-rays

Radiopaque. Impenetrable to x-rays or other forms of ionizing radiation

Sthenic. A physique of average build that is active and strong

Subject Contrast. Degree of differential absorption resulting from varying absorptive characteristics of body tissue

Bibliography

Carlton, R.; Adler, A. Principles of Radiographic Imaging—An Art and a Science. New York: Delmar Publishers, 1992.

Carroll, Q.B. Fuchs's Principles of Radiographic Exposure, 4th ed. Springfield, IL: Charles C Thomas, 1990.

Cullinan, A.M. Optimizing Radiographic Positioning. Philadelphia: J.B. Lippincott, 1992.

Curry, T.S. III; Dowdy, J.E.; Murry, R.C., Jr. Christensen's Physics of Diagnostic Radiology, 4th ed. Philadelphia: Lea & Febiger, 1990.

Devos, D.C. Principles of Radiographic Exposure. Philadelphia: Lea & Febiger, 1990.

Donahue, D.P. An Analysis of Radiographic Quality, 2nd ed. Baltimore: University Park Press, 1984.

Eisenburg, R.L.; Dennis, C.A. Comprehensive Radiographic Pathology. St. Louis, C.V. Mosby, 1990.

Hiss, S. Understanding Radiography. Springfield, IL: Charles C Thomas, 1983.

Mace, J.D.; Kowalczyk, N.M. Radiographic Pathology for Technologists. St. Louis: C.V. Mosby, 1988.

Taber's Cyclopedic Medical Dictionary. Philadelphia: F.A. Davis, 1990.

Thompson, T.T. Cahoon's Formulating X-ray Techniques, 9th ed. Durham, NC: Duke University Press, 1979.

Review Questions

1. Explain the relationship between atomic number and attenuation.
2. How is attenuation affected by tissue density?
3. What are the differences in attenuation between fat, muscle, and air?
4. What elements compose the human body?
5. Explain the importance of being familiar with and understanding pathological conditions.
6. Describe the relationship between additive and destructive pathologies and state their effects on attenuation.
7. Why is it important for the radiographer to carefully evaluate each patient and to have a good clinical history for the patient?
8. Describe the effects of the following disease processes on the radiographic images:

   a. Paget's disease   c. ascites

   b. bowel obstruction   d. emphysema

9. Explain the best way to manipulate the exposure factors to obtain maximum detail when performing bone radiography.
10. List the four basic body builds and explain how they affect exposure factor selections.

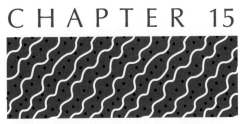

CHAPTER 15

Fluoroscopy: Viewing Motion with X-ray

Steven B. Dowd, Ed.D., R.T.(R.)

Chapter Outline

Chapter Objectives

On completion of this chapter, you should be able to

- Describe the historical development of fluoroscopy.
- Differentiate between fluoroscopy (dynamic radiography) and static radiography.
- List equipment contained within a fluoroscopic unit.
- Explain the function of equipment contained within a fluoroscopic unit.
- Differentiate between x-ray tubes and fluoroscopic tubes.
- Define *minification* and *flux gain.*
- Calculate total brightness gain.
- Describe how brightness of the fluoroscopic image can be controlled.
- Describe factors affecting quality of the fluoroscopic image: contrast, resolution, distortion, and quantum mottle.
- Describe the three types of fluoroscopic viewing systems.
- Evaluate the applicability of various recording systems for clinical use.
- Discuss the use of mobile fluoroscopic equipment.

HISTORY

Thomas Edison invented the fluoroscope in 1896, although Röntgen was the first to observe the fluoroscopic properties of the beam. Röntgen noticed that when bringing a piece of lead into an x-ray beam, the outline of his hand and the denser bones of the hand cast a shadow on a fluorescent object.

The use of the term *fluoroscopy* implies the use of a fluorescent screen; that is, a sheet of material that fluoresces, or emits light when struck by x-ray. Placing a patient between the x-ray source and the fluorescent screen provides a visible light image. The earliest fluoroscopes were hand-held in front of the patient and the tube. The next generation of fluoroscopes were mounted on a "C-arm" type of apparatus similar to today's fluoroscopes. Zinc cadmium sulfide, which emitted yellow-green light, was used for the fluorescent screen. Some of these units were totally unshielded, allowing the radiologist's face and eyes to receive the full beam. Later units were covered with lead glass to allow the radiologist to stare directly into the screen. An interesting contemporary side-note is that Siemens has developed a direct-view, panel-type image intensifier with, of course, no dose to the face of the viewer (Fig. 15–1).

These early fluoroscopic units allowed only one viewer to observe the image. The fluorescence produced by the screens was so faint that fluoroscopy had to be performed in a darkened room by a radiologist whose eyes had become adapted to the darkness. This was accomplished by having the radiologist wait in a darkened room for 20 to 30 minutes before the examination or by wearing red goggles in normal lighting conditions and was called dark adaptation.

Because the fluorescent image produced was so dim and faint, rod vision had to be used. Daylight (cone) vision is also known as photopic vision. Night (rod) vision is known as scotopic vision. The best visual acuity is provided by photopic vision. Photopic vision is about 10 times better than night vision.

The dilemma in providing an image bright enough for daylight vision is that an increase by a factor of about one thousand in the number of light photons produced by the screen is necessary. Initially, the only means of accomplishing this enhancement was by increasing the number of x-ray photons in the beam with a corresponding addition to patient dose. Therefore, raising the number of photons was not feasible. It was not possible to use daylight vision until the development of the image intensifier in the late 1940s. The intensifier enhances the brightness of the image an average of 5000 to 20,000 times, which also allows the use of cinefluorography, spot-film devices, and television monitors.

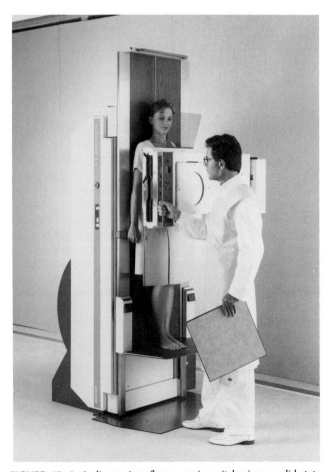

FIGURE 15-1. A direct view fluoroscopic unit having a solid-state panel type of image intensifier. (Courtesy of Siemens Medical Systems, Inc., Iselin, NJ.)

■ VISUAL PHYSIOLOGY

There are two different types of light receptors in the retina: rods and cones. Day vision, also called photopic, or cone, vision, is provided by the cones. Cones are densely concentrated in the fovea of the retina, with few found in the remainder of the retina. There is a high visual acuity for direct vision. Visual acuity refers to the ability of the eye to see two closely spaced structures as two separate entities rather than one. The cones found in the rest of the retina provide for daylight peripheral vision. Peripheral vision is that vision just outside of direct vision. The cones are almost blind to low levels of light.

Night vision is also called scotopic, or rod, vision. As there are no rods in the fovea, night vision is peripheral vision only. The eye is capable of adapting to low levels of light, forming the basis for dark adaptation discussed earlier in the chapter. The red goggles were worn by radiologists to further adapt their eyes to the dark by removing, for example, blue-green light, to which the rods are sensitive.

The cones have a visual acuity ten times greater than that of rods. This fact, which limited early fluoroscopic resolution in that the screen was capable of displaying more information than was observable by rod vision was always known to some extent. It was not, however, until a paper presented at the 1941 meeting of the Radiologic Society of North America indicated that normal reading conditions used light some 30,000 times brighter than fluoroscopy viewing conditions, that the magnitude of the problem was understood. The problem was solved some ten years later by the development of the image intensifier.

USES OF FLUOROSCOPY

Fluoroscopy is *dynamic radiography,* or radiography of motion. *Static,* or *plain-film, radiography* produces images of the body at one point in time. When organs are constantly moving (e.g., the heart) or when it is necessary to study motion in order to assess function (e.g., the esophagus), a plain-film does not provide enough information for proper diagnosis. The radiological tool to observe organs in motion is fluoroscopy. The use of fluoroscopy and static filming to study blood vessels is called *angiography.*

Fluoroscopy has a number of advantages, including speed and ease of use. Motion observed on fluoroscopy includes swallowing, breathing, and the opening and closing of heart valves. Also, the patient can be moved into various positions to best show specific abnormalities. With current technology, the only other means of providing information about moving structures is by exposing a series of radiographs in rapid succession. Such a method is used in conjunction with fluoroscopy during cardiac catheterization, called *cinefluoroscopy*. However, there are a variety of drawbacks to this method used alone:

- The time delay between serially exposed films may be too long to provide complete information (that is, something could be missed that was observable only between exposures)
- Film(s) must be processed before they can be viewed
- Unless many exposures are taken in rapid succession (30 per second or faster), the finished image exhibits flicker

Since fluoroscopy usually involves diagnosis, the primary function of the radiographer is to serve as a physician's assistant during fluoroscopy. Radiographers may use fluoroscopy under the supervision of a physician for static (spot-filming) purposes. It is not appropriate to use fluoroscopy as a localizing device before positioning the patient for regular radiographs. The extra dose to the patient far exceeds that of the normal repeat rate for films.

One important role of the radiographer during fluoroscopy is the setting and resetting of the timer used to indicate the length of total fluoroscopic exposure. It is also called the 5-minute timer, because these timers allow for a maximum setting of 5 minutes. Many state regulations mandate the use of these timers.

When five minutes have been exceeded, the timer must be reset as needed during fluoroscopy of a patient and must be reset before each patient. Some facilities require that the amount of exposure time be recorded for each patient. Five minutes of exposure time is a recommended maximum exposure time; this, of course, varies with the patient. There is no mandated maximum exposure time.

EQUIPMENT

The x-ray tube and image receptor of a fluoroscopy unit are mounted on a C-arm to maintain alignment of the tube and film. A C-arm allows the image recep-

tor to be raised and lowered while the tube remains in one set position. This set-up permits the bare essentials of fluoroscopy—an x-ray tube, a patient suspended in the middle, and a screen (Fig. 15–2).

Modern fluoroscopic equipment also contains devices that

- Provide for the making of individual radiographs known as *spot-films,* or cineradiographs, as needed
- Include or allow for added shielding needed for radiation protection
- Allow for special positioning such as upright, semi-upright, and Trendelenburg (head lower than feet) through the use of a table that can be angled up or down

The equipment suspended over the table is enclosed in a carriage. This contains either the image-intensification tube (making it an under-table unit) or the x-ray tube, if it is an over-table unit. Most stationary fluoroscopic equipment contains the x-ray tube under the table. The carriage also contains controls for the power drive, brightness, spot-film selection, tube shuttering, spot films/ciné camera, and the video input tube.

X-ray Tubes

The main difference between fluoroscopic tubes and diagnostic tubes is that fluoroscopy operates with tube currents ranging only from 0.5 mA to 5.0 mA, usually 1 to 3 mA. This is sometimes confusing when "fluoro mA" is often set on the machine at 200 mA or 300 mA. Actually, this latter number refers to the mA used for static spot filming, and is not the actual fluoroscopic mA that is discussed in this chapter.

The x-ray tube is fixed horizontally into position to keep the source–object distance to not less than 38 cm (~15 inches) on stationary fluoroscopes. This limit is not less than 30 cm (~12 inches) on mobile fluoroscopes.

Provision can be made (Code of Federal Regulations, 21 CFR 1020.32) for operation at shorter source-skin distances for specific surgical applications that would be prohibited at the previously indicated source-skin distances, but the shorter distance may not be less than 20 cm (~8 inches). These limits maintain a constant source-object distance. The source–image

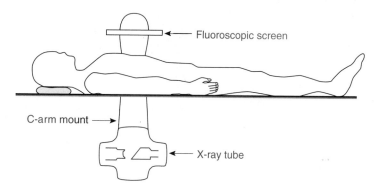

FIGURE 15–2. The essential components of a fluoroscopic unit.

Fluoroscopic screen

C-arm mount

X-ray tube

receptor distance is variable, and geometric magnification can be changed to a certain extent by moving the carriage closer to or further from the patient.

Image Intensification Tubes

The purpose of an *image intensification tube* is to amplify electronically the brightness of an image. A typical image intensifier is shown in Figure 15–3. When the primary beam exits the patient, it strikes the input screen of the image intensifier tube. The image intensifier is a vacuum tube with both a cathode and an anode. The fluorescent screen absorbs x-ray photons and emits light photons. These light photons strike the tube cathode (a photocathode) that is in direct contact with the input screen to prevent divergence of the light beam. The photocathode absorbs light photons and emits electrons. These electrons are accelerated from the cathode toward the anode by a potential difference between cathode and anode. Electrostatic lenses accelerate and focus the electrons on the small output screen. The increased brightness of the image is a result of this acceleration and focusing.

The output screen absorbs electrons, which are converted into light photons. The image may then be viewed or sent to a video system for further processing.

Input Screen

The input screen consists of a 0.1- to 0.2-mm layer of sodium-activated cesium iodide (CsI) phosphor. It is coated on the concave surface of the image intensifier tube, which is glass, titanium, steel, or aluminum. The diameter ranges from 6 to 23 inches, with sizes of 5 to 14 inches common. The screen is concave to maintain a distance between each point on the input screen and a corresponding point on the output screen, thus minimizing distortion.

CsI phosphors are packed together tightly to ensure a good conversion efficiency of photons to light, also called *quantum yield*. CsI has a medium atomic number and provides the same improved absorption of x-ray photons as seen in rare earth intensifying screens used in static radiography. CsI also causes a decrease in patient dose and improves spatial resolution because of its high conversion efficiency. A 50-keV x-ray photon produces about 2000 light photons.

Photocathode

The input screen is coated with a thin protective coating to prevent chemical interaction with the photocathode (Fig. 15–3), since the two layers are in intimate contact. The cathode is usually a combination of

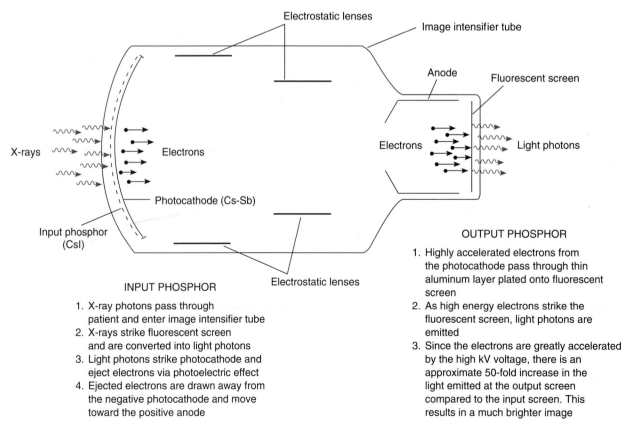

INPUT PHOSPHOR

1. X-ray photons pass through patient and enter image intensifier tube
2. X-rays strike fluorescent screen and are converted into light photons
3. Light photons strike photocathode and eject electrons via photoelectric effect
4. Ejected electrons are drawn away from the negative photocathode and move toward the positive anode

OUTPUT PHOSPHOR

1. Highly accelerated electrons from the photocathode pass through thin aluminum layer plated onto fluorescent screen
2. As high energy electrons strike the fluorescent screen, light photons are emitted
3. Since the electrons are greatly accelerated by the high kV voltage, there is an approximate 50-fold increase in the light emitted at the output screen compared to the input screen. This results in a much brighter image

FIGURE 15–3. Schematic drawing of an image intensifier tube.

antimony and cesium. These are photoemissive metals, meaning that they emit electrons in response to light. The photocathode is also called the photoemissive layer. The number of electrons emitted by the photocathode is directly proportional to the intensity of light emitted by the input screen.

Electrostatic Lenses

Electrostatic lenses are a series of positively charged electrodes within the glass envelope of the image intensifier tube. Each successive lens has a higher positive voltage than the preceding one. Electrons are attracted to the positively charged lenses, accelerating and focusing the electron stream. The electrons are influenced rather than captured by the lens as a result of the high acceleration and kinetic energy of the electrons. The image is reversed, turned right to left, and inverted. Multifield, or magnification, image intensifier tubes balance image size and quality. Larger modes are used to view larger anatomical areas. Image quality is better in smaller image modes.

The field size is changed by applying a higher or lower voltage to the electrostatic focusing lens. In a dual-field intensifier capable of 6- and 9-inch modes (Fig. 15–4), the voltage is increased in the 6-inch mode, focusing the electrons farther away from the output phosphor. In this mode, the optical system can see only the central part of the image derived from the central 6 inches of the input phosphor. This image is less minified, and therefore appears to be magnified on the monitor. When the unit is used in the 6-inch mode, exposure factors are automatically increased to compensate for decreased brightness from a decreased *minification gain*. Minification gain refers to the increase in brightness that results from making the image smaller (see the following section for a complete explanation of minification gain). One of the principal reasons that the image is brighter is its size reduction.

In the 9-inch mode, the voltage is decreased. The size of the output image changes; however, the physical size of the input and output phosphors does not change. This is illustrated in Figure 15–4.

Anode

To further attract electrons, the anode carries a positive charge, usually about 25 kV (25,000 volts). The anode sits inside the glass envelope, directly in front of the output screen. It contains a hole in the center that permits accelerated electrons to pass through the anode into the output screen.

Output Screen

The output screen is a silver (Ag)–activated glass fluorescent screen containing very small particles of zinc-cadmium sulfide phosphor (ZnS-CdS:Ag). Zinc-cadmium sulfide is used because the wavelength of the light generated matches film receptivity. This matching of wavelengths of light is known as *spectral matching*.

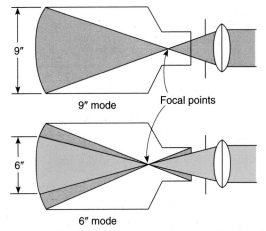

FIGURE 15–4. Dual-field image intensifier, 9-inch and 6-inch modes.

Electrons striking the screen are converted into light photons. In place of the glass fluorescent screen, newer intensifiers use a fiber optic disc. This eliminates the problem of isotropic or retrograde emission (in which light is also emitted back to the input screen) and also allows for efficient image transmittal over a distance without a loss in resolution. All output phosphors are coated with a thin plate of aluminum to help prevent retrograde emission of light to the photocathode.

REVIEW

The image intensification process is best remembered step-by-step (refer to Fig. 15–3):

1. An x-ray beam passes through the patient from the fluoroscopic tube and is attenuated.
2. The attenuated x-ray beam passes through the glass front of the image intensifier, striking the input phosphor. The crystals of CsI produce light proportional to the intensity of the beam.
3. The light photons strike the photocathode, which emits electrons proportional to the intensity of the emitted light.
4. The electrostatic lens focuses, accelerates, and inverts the electron stream.
5. The anode further attracts the electrons.
6. The output screen converts the electrons into light photons.

TOTAL BRIGHTNESS GAIN

Total brightness gain in an image is the product of two factors: a brightness gain resulting from minification of the image (minification gain) and a brightness gain due to conversion at the output screen of electrons to light *(flux gain)*. Minification gain occurs because the same number of electrons exist at the small output screen as were produced at the photocathode-input screen *interface*. The most common input screen sizes are 6 and 9 inches. Typically, the output screen has a diameter of 1 inch. Minification gain is the ratio of the area of the input to the output screen.

$$\text{Minification gain} = \left(\frac{\text{input screen diameter}}{\text{output screen diameter}}\right)^2$$

Thus with an input screen size of 6 inches and an output screen size of 1 inch, the brightness gain from minification of the image is calculated as follows:

$$\left(\frac{6}{1}\right)^2 = \frac{36}{1} = 36$$

With an input screen size of 9 inches and an output screen size of 1 inch

$$\left(\frac{9}{1}\right)^2 = \frac{81}{1} = 81$$

From these computations it can be seen that as the size of the input screen increases, brightness gain due to minification increases. With multifield image intensifiers capable of operating in several modes, it should be noted that the smaller the mode used, the less the minification. The term *mode* refers to the size of the field applied to the output phosphor. Thus smaller modes provide a larger image; however, exposure factors must be increased to compensate for the loss in brightness. In general, this is an inverse square relationship. To switch from a 9-inch to a 6-inch mode causes the automatic brightness control to double the dose rate. Switching from a 9-inch to a 4.5-inch mode requires an increase of four times the dose rate.

Flux gain is an increase in light photons resulting from the efficiency of the output screen. An output phosphor that produces 50 light photons for every electron that strikes it has a flux gain of 50 (Fig. 15–5). A decrease in image quality, similar to that exhibited by intensifying screens and caused by the penumbral effect of phosphor crystals, results from flux gain.

The trade-off is a brighter image using less x-ray photons.

Total brightness gain is a product of minification and flux gain. The formula is

$$\boxed{\text{Brightness gain} = \text{minification gain} \times \text{flux gain}}$$

To refer to the two image intensifiers with brightness gain due to minification of 36 and 81, assuming a flux gain of 50,

6 inches: $36 \times 50 = 1800$ total brightness gain

9 inches: $81 \times 50 = 4050$ total brightness gain

Brightness gain becomes less as screens age. Reduction can be as much as 10% per year. One way of checking this decrease is by comparing the dose required for automatic brightness-control operation to the dose that was required when the unit was new.

A second measure of brightness gain, recommended by the International Commission on Radiologic Units and Measurements (ICRU), is a *conversion factor.* This is a ratio of the luminance of the output phosphor to the input exposure rate. The conversion factor is about 1% of the brightness gain. Thus a brightness gain of 5000 is equivalent to a conversion factor of 50 $(5000 \times .01 = 50)$.

FLUOROSCOPIC GENERATORS

Brightness Control

Brightness can be controlled by adjusting fluoroscopic mA or kVp. The primary factor affecting the brightness of the fluoroscopic image is the size or den-

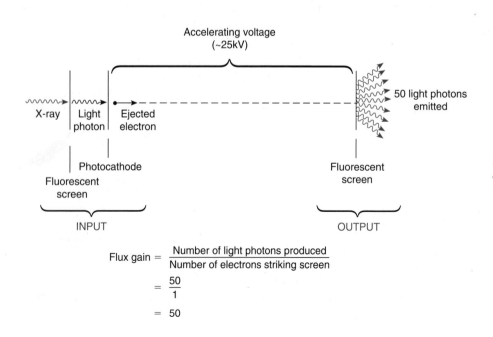

FIGURE 15–5. Interactions that occur at the input and output screens of an image intensifier tube.

sity of the anatomic part. This is due to the fact that an increase or decrease in size or density reduces or enhances, respectively, the number of photons that reach the input phosphor.

To maintain image brightness, usually either the number (mAs) or the energy (kVp) of photons must be adjusted for changes in part thickness or density. Older equipment often allows the operator to adjust mA or kVp to maintain optimum image brightness. Newer equipment uses photoelectric cells to measure the brightness of the output phosphor. This equipment adjusts the fluoroscopic kVp or mA in reference to a preset brightness level. The adjustment function goes by a variety of names: automatic brightness control, automatic brightness stabilization, automatic dose rate control, automatic exposure control, and automatic gain control.

KVp and mA affect the quality of the fluoroscopic image in much the same way they affect radiographic images. In general, a relatively high kVp and a low mA are preferred.

According to Krestel (1990), when the method used to maintain the image brightness of the monitor changes the intensity of radiation (mAs and kVp), it is called automatic dose rate control (ADC); when the video signal is adjusted, it is called automatic gain control (AGC); and when the sensitivity of the Vidicon (camera) plate is adjusted, it is called automatic brightness control (ABC).

IMAGE QUALITY

There are three fundamental descriptors for image quality: contrast, sharpness, and noise. Contrast, as in static radiography, is the relative difference in brightness between two adjacent regions of an image. Sharpness is the abruptness of margins separating contrasting regions and is a combination of resolution and distortion. Image noise is a combination of electronic noise (the video camera; this is described later) and quantum mottle. Contrast, sharpness, and noise are subtly interrelated and are also often related to radiation dose (i.e., diminishing quantum mottle with increased mAs increases patient dose).

Contrast

Image contrast is controlled through the amplitude of the video signal. In addition to scatter radiation and kVp, two factors diminish contrast in image intensifiers. These are (1) a lack of absorption of all photons and (2) light scatter leading to retrograde (backward) light flow. The input screen does not absorb all photons from the x-ray beam. Some x-ray photons transmit through the intensifier and are absorbed by the output screen. This transmittal increases illumination but does not contribute to the image. It can be considered a form of fog.

Light scatter (reflection and refraction) from the output screen also produces a form of fog by retrograde light flow. This light can pass back through the image tube, activating the photocathode (Fig. 15–6) and producing a fog that will reduce image contrast.

Contrast decreases at the edge of images. The brightest section of the image is at the center of the image. Contrast also diminishes with the age of the image intensifier.

Resolution

The factors affecting the geometry (resolution) of the image are the video monitor (the primary factor), minification gain, the electrostatic focal spot, the diameter of the input and output screens, object-to-image receptor distance (OID), and phosphor size and thickness. TV monitors can resolve 1 to 2 line pairs per millimeter (lp/mm); an optical mirror system is capable of resolving 3 lp/mm; a CsI image intensifier is capable of resolving 4 lp/mm; and magnification-multifield image intensifiers are capable of resolving up to 6 lp/mm in magnification mode. The more line pairs per millimeter the system is capable of resolving, the greater the resolution. If this concept is still unclear, review Chapter 10. The weakest link in the imaging chain in terms of resolution is the TV monitor.

Distortion

The primary influence on size distortion is OID in both static and dynamic radiographic systems.

Despite the concavity of the input screen, edge distortion at the output screen is not completely eliminated. The "pincushion" distortion and loss of brightness through vignetting (i.e., edge distortion, as shown in Fig. 15–7) that results is caused by the repulsion of electrons and the divergence of the primary beam from the focal spot of the x-ray tube. Distortion is minimized and contrast is improved at the center of the fluoroscopic image.

Quantum Mottle

Quantum mottle is a grainy or blotchy appearance caused by insufficient radiation to produce a uniform

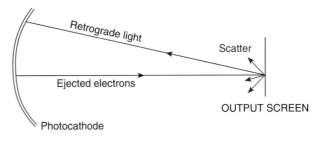

FIGURE 15–6. Light scatter resulting in retrograde light flow in the image intensifier tube.

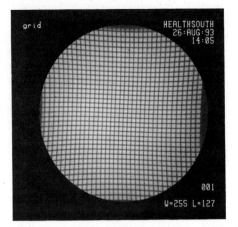

FIGURE 15–7. Test film of a wire screen from a 9-inch image intensifier illustrating the "pincushion" effect.

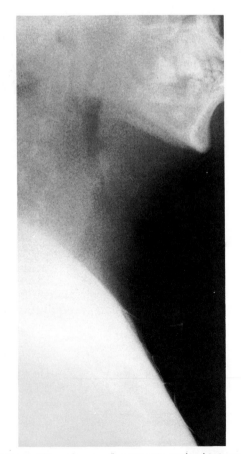

FIGURE 15–8. Although not a fluoroscopic study, this image of the cervical spine is an excellent example of quantum mottle and the resultant loss of image quality found with it. The mottled appearance is caused by the uneven distribution of light photons used to expose the film. (Courtesy of Robert Nelson, B.S., R.T.(R), University of Alabama Hospital.)

Table 15–1: FACTORS USED FOR ABDOMINAL FLUOROSCOPY AND SPOT FILMING OF A LARGE PATIENT

Technical Factor	Spot Film	Fluoroscopy
kVp	95	95
mA	150	3
Time (sec)	0.4	0.2
mAs	60	0.6
Ratio of number of photons based on mAs*	100	1

* That is, for every 100 photons produced at the spot film, only 1 is used to produce the equivalent fluoroscopic image.

image (Fig. 15–8). Since x-rays are emitted at random, variations in x-ray intensity are most evident when the fewest number of photons are used (low mAs values). Mottle is a problem in fluoroscopy because unit operation is based on the minimum number of photons required to activate the fluoroscopic screen through automatic brightness stabilization. This is illustrated in Table 15–1. It can be seen that compared with the spot-film radiograph, fluoroscopy of the same part begins with an "inferior" x-ray image that, as described earlier, must be intensified to be viewed.

Since the problem is an insufficient amount of radiation, the most common solution to mottle is to increase the fluoroscopic mA. However, increasing the efficiency of a variety of systems, including all of these: brightness gain, the conversion efficiency of the input screen, and the viewing system, helps to reduce quantum mottle. One means of reducing quantum mottle is through the high-level control (also called fluoro-boost, high contrast, image enhance, and low noise) option found in some units. This raises patient dose to levels higher than normally seen.

VIEWING SYSTEMS

The image produced at the output screen of the image intensifier tube is a much smaller, brighter image and as a result is difficult to view directly. Several methods have been developed to allow medical personnel to view and store the images produced. Today, video technology is commonly used in order to allow the images produced to be displayed on a video monitor, which allows ease in viewing. In order for this to occur, the image must first be transferred from the output screen of the image intensifier tube to the first stage of a television monitoring system such as a video camera.

Older image transfer systems used lenses and mirrors. These optical components were positioned such that the image produced at the output screen could be viewed either directly (Fig. 15–9A) or indirectly on a video monitor (Fig. 15–9B). Viewing the image directly, using the lens-mirror combination, was an adequate system but had disadvantages. Freedom of movement was extremely limited for the viewer and only one viewer could view the image at any one time. This was a severe limitation in training new medical personnel. For the radiographer, this meant that pathology as seen by the physician could not be ob-

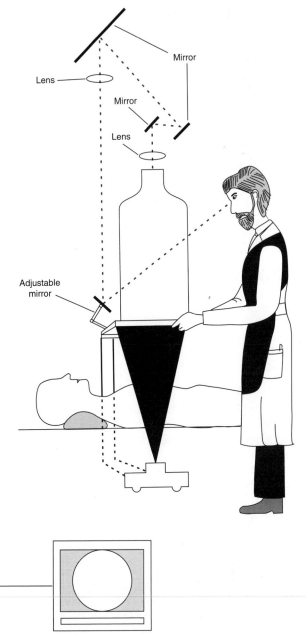

FIGURE 15–9. *A,* Mirror optics as used with an image intensifier tube.

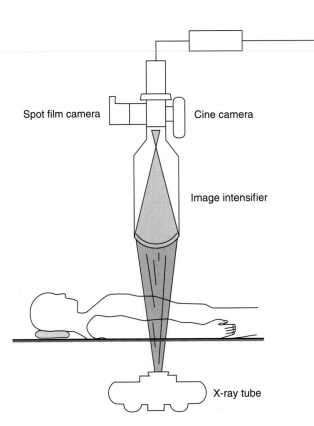

FIGURE 15–9 *Continued. B,* A fluoroscopic unit utilizing a video monitor display.

served. This made it difficult for the physician to indicate to the radiographer exactly what needed to be included on overhead (static) films.

Modern fluoroscopic units eliminated these problems by using a closed circuit television system through which to project the image. A lens-mirror arrangement was commonly used to bring the image to the video pick-up tube. This system had its limitations in that there were light losses in the transfer process. In today's modern fluoroscopic units, images are transferred with minimal loss of image brightness through the utilization of fiber optics. (*Fiber optics* refers to the transfer of light signals or images through light-conducting glass or plastic fibers).

The Video Display System

One major advantage of using the image intensifier is that it allows the transfer of the output image to a television monitor either by a lens system or fiber optics link. There are two essential components of a video display system: (1) a *video camera tube* and (2) a *video monitor.* A typical display system is illustrated in Figure 15–10.

The video camera tube, or pick-up tube, converts visual information, such as the image produced at the output screen of the image intensifier, into electrical signals. The most commonly used tubes in diagnostic imaging are the Vidicon and the Plumbicon. The choice of *video camera tube* depends on the specific application intended. Because of the characteristics of each tube, Vidicon cameras are well suited to imaging organs that are stationary, whereas the Plumbicon camera is better suited to imaging moving organs such as the heart.

The Vidicon tube, illustrated in Figure 15–11, converts the light image from the image intensifier into an electrical signal as the image of varying light intensity ejects electrons photoelectrically from the photoconductive layer of the tube. The number of electrons emitted is proportional to the intensity of the light striking the surface. Electrons accelerated from the cathode fill the electron deficiency at the surface. This event has the effect of discharging a capacitor, resulting in a current flow through a resistor, and in turn causing a varying voltage across the resistor. This varying voltage is referred to as the video signal. The signal consists of many individual pulses corresponding to

individual locations on the video tube target. These varying voltage pulses are later reassembled into a visible image by the video monitor.

Conventional video camera tubes have been replaced in many units by a solid-state component known as a charge-coupled device (CCD). This device is a semiconductor that has the ability to store charge in localized areas and later to transfer this charge to an appropriate display terminal. The advantage provided by solid-state technology is a unit that is smaller in size, lower in power consumption, lower in price, and has a longer life.

The final component in the video display system is the video *monitor.* It is the function of the monitor to convert the varying voltage from the Vidicon tube into a visible image. A video monitor consists of a picture tube, illustrated in Figure 15–12, and its associated electronics. A picture tube is a cathode-ray tube. It consists of an evacuated glass tube in which an electron gun is housed. The electron gun produces a stream of electrons that are accelerated toward a fluorescent screen located on the inside of the larger end of the tube. Focusing and deflecting coils around the neck of the tube keep the electron beam in exact synchrony with the Vidicon camera tube. Individual light and dark areas on the image screen are determined by regulating the number of electrons that strike the screen at specific points. This aspect of final image production is regulated by the control grid.

When individual light and dark areas are produced on the viewing screen to form the final image, on close inspection one can find hundreds of thousands of tiny dots of varying degrees of brightness. These dots are arranged in specific patterns along what are called horizontal scan lines. Typically, the United States commercial television systems and those employed in fluoroscopy use 525 horizontal scan lines. The electron gun of the picture tube creates an image as it sends out its pulsed stream of electrons in synchrony with the video signals from the Vidicon tube to strike the fluorescent screen within the picture tube. The electron gun within the picture tube scans from top to bottom in 1/60 second. Each scan is referred to as a field and contains 262 1/2 horizontal scan lines. A frame consists of two fields, or 525 horizontal scan lines, taking 1/30 second.

Although 30 scans per second is probably enough to eliminate flicker from the image, an interlace method (Fig. 15–13) of scanning is used to produce a better

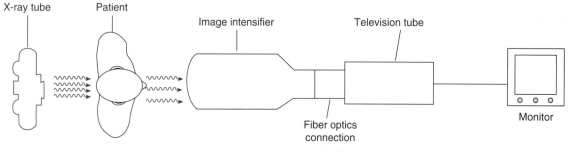

FIGURE 15–10. A typical video display system.

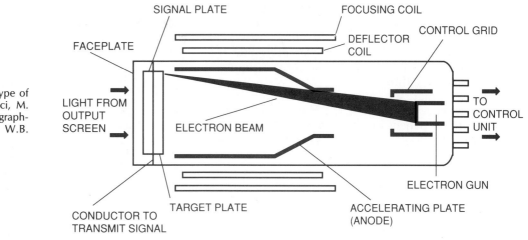

FIGURE 15–11. A Vidicon type of camera tube. (From Tortorici, M. Concepts in Medical Radiographic Imaging. Philadelphia, W.B. Saunders Company, 1992.)

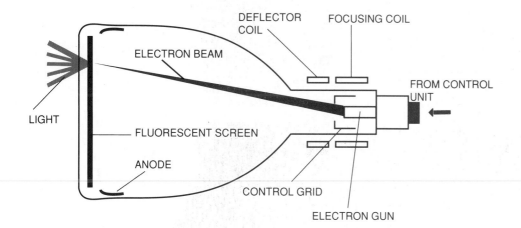

FIGURE 15–12. The picture tube of a video monitor (From Tortorici, M. Concepts in Medical Radiographic Imaging. Philadelphia, W.B. Saunders Company, 1992.)

FIGURE 15–13. Interlace method of scanning utilized in a video monitor picture tube.

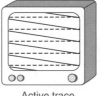
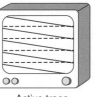

— Active trace   — Active trace   Video frame
--- Horizontal retrace   --- Horizontal retrace   525 lines, 1/30s

Field 1   Field 2
$262\frac{1}{2}$ lines, 1/60s $262\frac{1}{2}$ lines, 1/60s

image. The interlace method uses the first field to scan the even-numbered lines. A second field scans odd-numbered lines. This produces a new image every 1/60 second. Thus the first field scans alternating 262 1/2 lines in the first 1/60 second and the second, the next alternating 262 1/2 lines.

Advantages that the monitor possesses over the mirror viewing system include the possibility of many viewers, a lower patient dose, and increased brightness. However, it is more expensive and requires more space.

RECORDING THE IMAGE

Dynamic Systems

Cine Film Systems

Cinefluorography (a cine camera is a motion picture camera) uses a 16- to 35-mm movie camera to record the fluoroscopic image. The 35-mm format is usually preferred, because image quality is better, especially for cardiac angiography. However, patient dose is higher with the 35-mm format. Patient dose is greater with either format compared with regular fluoroscopy, because the short times used require higher milliamperages.

The cine camera is driven by an electronic synchronous motor. The number of frames per second is based on 60-Hz current and is normally divisible by 60. Common frame rates (framing frequencies) are 7.5, 15, 30, and 60 per second. Radiation dose increases with higher framing frequencies, since the x-ray tube makes an exposure with each frame. The beam is pulsed by using a grid-controlled x-ray tube. This tube is also called a triode tube because it has a third, intermittently negative electrode. When the third electrode (the grid) becomes negative, the electrons at the cathode remain at the cathode, and no x-rays are produced. When the grid is off, electrons can flow across the tube, and x-rays are produced.

A biplane cine system is illustrated in Figure 15–14. Biplane systems are used to image structures at a 90° angle (e.g., an AP and a lateral). This system uses an alternating pulse sequence—that is, when the film is being transported for camera A, the shutter is open on camera B. Ideally, a biplane system would not operate in this manner, because simultaneous images from each plane are preferred. However, scatter from one plane would degrade image quality in the other. Cine views acquired in each plane can be used to calculate the volume of the ventricle of the heart.

Videotape Recording

The use of television monitoring allows for recording the information from the television pick-up tube on magnetic media. This includes magnetic disk recorders, laser disk recorders, and multiformat cameras.

Videotape is one of the more common means of recording the fluoroscopic image on magnetic media. VHS (1/2 inch) and U-matic (3/4 inch) recorders are both used to record fluoroscopic images. Both video formats are available in cassettes and are used just as they are in a home video system. Videotape does not

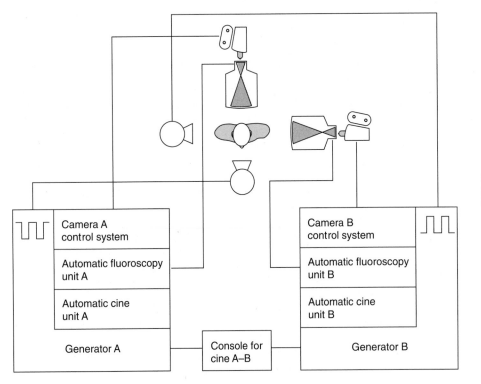

FIGURE 15–14. A biplane cine system. (Courtesy of Siemens Medical Systems, Inc., Iselin, NJ.)

normally exhibit high resolution, although expensive models capable of high resolution are available. It is easy to use, does not require film processing, and can provide instant playback by simply rewinding the tape. Perhaps most important, it does not provide additional dosage to the patient.

Spot-Filming (Static) Systems

Cassettes

For many years, the conventional means of recording images has been spot-film cassettes. They exhibit high image quality but also result in a relatively large patient dose. A delay of up to 2 seconds is also required before the cassette comes into place between the patient and image intensifier. The cassette is stored in a lead-lined compartment in the fluoroscopic carriage until the exposure is taken. When cassette films are taken, the tube must switch from fluoroscopic mA to radiographic mA.

Cassette spot films allow a variety of exposures. The entire film or a portion (1/2, 1/3, or 1/4) may be exposed. If the entire film is exposed, it is called a 1 on 1 setting, 1/2 is called 2 on 1, and so on. Because of their ease of use, low cost, and familiar format, spot films remain popular.

Spot-Film Cameras

Spot-film cameras (also called millimeter and photospot cameras) are similar to movie cameras. However, they expose only one frame when activated. The image, unlike those in spot-film cassettes, comes from the output phosphor of the image intensifier tube. This requires a lower dose, less heat-loading (as the mA remains on the low, fluoroscopic mA), and a shorter interruption of the examination. The only movement necessary before exposure is the beam splitting performed by the mirror.

A photospot camera consists of unexposed film on a storage film reel, a pull arm, an aperture, a take-up film reel (magazine) holding exposed film, and a shutter. Exposures are synchronized with the x-ray exposure. The larger the film, the better the film image quality. Both 105 mm (the largest) and 70 mm (the smallest) can expose up to 12 frames per second (Fig. 15-15).

Video Recorders

A magnetic disk recorder is similar to a videotape recorder but uses a hard magnetic disk. It also usually records single frames (Table 15-2). In playback mode, it displays the same image 30 times per second. A laser disk is similar to the magnetic disk, recording the image on a reflective metal disk sealed in plastic. Laser disks cannot be reused.

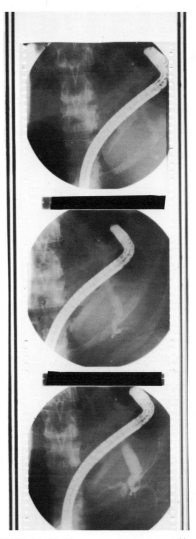

FIGURE 15-15. These are 105-mm spot films.

Digital Fluoroscopy

Digital, or computerized, fluoroscopy was developed in the late 1970s by Mistretta and colleagues at the University of Wisconsin (Fig. 15-16). Images produced statically by this device are called digital radiographs. They are light images of the output phosphor of the image intensifier. A video camera and a digital image processor are used to help obtain the image.

Variations in brightness of the output phosphor are *analog* in nature; that is, they occur as a range of theoretically infinite brightness levels. This image must be converted by an *analog-to-digital converter (ADC).* This data is then computer processed and stored in the digital image processor memory. When the data is to be viewed, it is retrieved and converted back to an analog image by a *digital-to-analog converter.* A film of the image can be made from the monitor, or the image can be recorded with a cine camera, providing a dynamic record.

Three basic types of studies are performed with digital fluoroscopy. The first, mask mode fluoroscopy, is

Table 15–2: COMPARISON OF RECORDING SYSTEMS

Factor	Spot Film	Photospot	Cine	Videotape/Disk
Quality	Excellent	Good	Good	Poor
Storage	Sheet	Sheet	Roll	Reel or disk
Patient dose	High	Low	Low	Low
Reusable	No	No	No	Yes (tape) No (disk)
Processor	Radiographic	Radiographic	Cine	None
Framing frequency	1/sec	12/sec	60/sec	60 rpm

Source: Adapted from Tortorici, M. Concepts in Medical Radiographic Imaging: Circuitry, Exposure, and Quality Control. Philadelphia: W. B. Saunders, 1992.

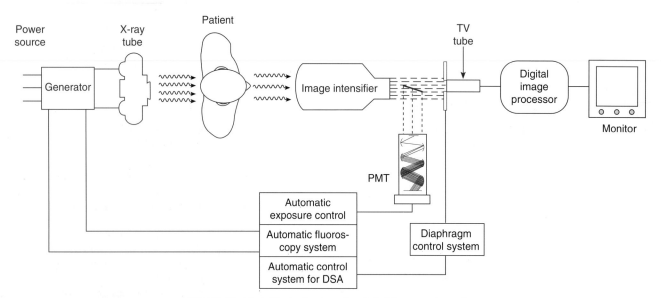

FIGURE 15–16. A block diagram of a digital fluoroscopy unit.

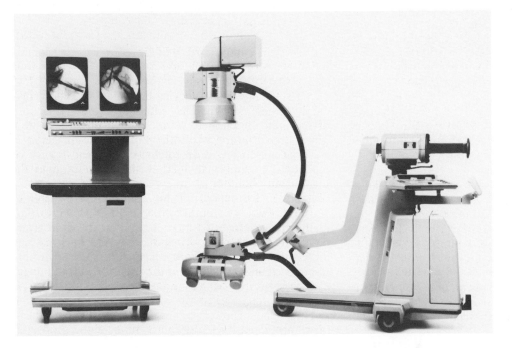

FIGURE 15–17. A mobile fluoroscopic unit. (Courtesy of OEC-Diasonics, Salt Lake City, UT.)

similar to film subtraction angiography with contrast media. The second is called K-edge fluoroscopy. It subtracts x-ray energies just above and just below the K-edge of a contrast medium. The third, time interval difference imaging, changes masks continually, giving information on changes in contrast media content in a structure over time.

Mobile Fluoroscopy

Mobile C-arm units can provide both static and dynamic images when connected to a video disc system (Fig. 15–17). Some units provide for modular upgrades that permit multiple uses, including keyboard entry of patient information, pulsed fluorography, and floppy disk storage.

▰▰ Chapter Summary/ Important Concepts

The use of the term *fluoroscopy* implies the use of a fluorescent screen. Fluoroscopy is dynamic radiography, or radiography of motion. Placing a patient between the x-ray source and the fluorescent screen provides a visible light image. The fluoroscope was invented by Edison. The development of the image intensifier provided for brighter images that could be viewed with daylight vision without increasing patient dose.

Step-by-step the image intensification process occurs as follows. First, the beam passes through the patient from the fluoroscopic tube and is attenuated. This beam then passes through the glass front of the image intensifier and strikes the input phosphor. Cesium iodide (CsI) crystals produce light proportional to the intensity of the beam. Light photons strike the photocathode, which in response emits electrons proportional to intensity of the light. The electrostatic lens focuses, accelerates, and inverts the electron stream. The anode further attracts the electrons. The output screen converts the electrons into light photons, which may then be viewed.

Total brightness gain in an image is the product of two factors: minification of the image (minification gain) and conversion at the output screen of electrons to light (flux gain). Minification gain occurs because the same number of electrons exist at the small output screen as were produced at the photocathode-input screen interface. As the size of the input screen increases, brightness gain due to minification increases. Flux gain is an increase in light photons resulting from efficiency of the output screen.

Image contrast is controlled through the amplitude of the video signal. The factors affecting the geometry (resolution) of the image are the video monitor (the primary factor), minification gain, electrostatic focal spot, the diameter of the input and output screens, OID, and phosphor size and thickness. The primary influence on size distortion is OID. The most common cure for quantum mottle is to increase the fluoro mA.

The image can be viewed through an optical mirror viewer or a video monitor. The image can be recorded through dynamic systems—cine film or videotape—and static systems—cassettes, spot-film (millimeter) cameras, and video disk recorders.

Digital fluoroscopy and mobile fluoroscopy are other methods of fluoroscopy. Today, many mobile systems can be modularized for specific uses.

Important Terminology

Analog. A continuous variable electronic signal

Analog-to-Digital Converter (ADC). Device that converts an analog signal into a digital signal

Angiography. Use of fluoroscopic and static imaging techniques to study blood vessels

Cinefluoroscopy. Production of motion images obtained by exposing a series of radiographs made in rapid succession

Conversion Factor. A second measure of brightness gain defined as the ratio of luminance of the output phosphor to the input exposure rate

Digital. Input that has a restricted number of discrete, or limited, values

Digital-to-Analog Converter (DAC). Device that converts digital signals into analog signals

Dynamic Radiography. Radiographic procedures that allow the visualization of motion

Fluoroscopy. Radiographic procedure used to study anatomical structure and function by observing, either directly or indirectly, dynamic images produced on a fluorescent screen

Flux Gain. Increase in output image brightness from an image intensifier tube expressed as the ratio of the number of light photons at the output screen to the number of light photons produced at the input phosphor

Image Intensification Tube. Major component of standard fluoroscopic equipment used to produce bright diagnostic images at low, fluoroscopic mA

Interface. A location or means of interaction between two points or systems

Minification Gain. The increase in output image brightness from an image intensifier tube that results from reduction in image size; expressed as the ratio of $(d_i/d_o)^2$

Monitor. Electronic component of a video display system that receives the video signal and again converts it into a visible image

Quantum Mottle. Grainy or blotchy appearance caused by insufficient radiation to produce a uniform image; refers to the fact that the image is intensified (converted to light and made brighter) rather than produced by using only radiation to produce an image

Quantum Yield. Measure of the efficiency of conversion of incoming x-ray photons to light photons

Spectral Matching. Producing equal wavelengths of light; usually refers to suiting the wavelength of light generated by a system with that required by an imaging system to produce the best or brightest image

Spot-Film (or Photospot) Camera. Camera mounted on the fluoroscopic tower that allows the output of the image intensifier tube to be recorded on film

Static (or Plain-Film) Radiography. Radiographic procedure that does not allow the visualization of motion

Total Brightness Gain. Minification gain multiplied by flux gain

Video Camera Tube. Electronic device used to convert a visible image into an electronic signal

Bibliography

Beck, T.J.; Galyer, B. Image quality and radiation levels in video-fluoroscopy for swallowing studies: A review. Dysphagia 5:118–128, 1990.

Bushong, S.C. Radiologic Science for Technologists, St. Louis, C.V. Mosby, 1988.

Cullinan, A.M. Producing Quality Radiographs. Philadelphia: J.B. Lippincott, 1987.

Curry, T.S. III; Dowdey, J.E.; Murry, R.C., Jr. Christensen's Physics of Diagnostic Radiology, 4th ed. Philadelphia: Lea & Febiger, 1990.

Dendy, P.P.; Heaton, B. Physics for Radiologists. Chicago: Year Book Medical Publishers, 1987.

Food and Drug Administration. Code of Federal Regulations. 21 CFR 1020.32. Washington, D.C., 1992.

Krestel, E. Imaging Systems for Medical Diagnostics. Munich: Siemens Aktiengesellschaft, 1990.

Snoeren, R.M., et al.: Solid-state image sensors in x-ray television. Med Mundi, 36:203–211, 1991.

Sprawls, P. Principles of Radiography for Technologists. Rockville, MD: Aspen, 1990.

Tortorici, M. Concepts in Medical Radiographic Imaging: Circuitry, Exposure, and Quality Control. Philadelphia: W.B. Saunders, 1992.

░░░ Review Questions

1. Electrons are accelerated and focused toward the output screen by the
   a. input screen
   b. photocathode
   c. electrostatic lenses
   d. photoemissive layer

2. Electrons are converted to light by the
   a. input screen
   b. photocathode
   c. electrostatic lenses
   d. output screen

3. As screens age, brightness gain decreases by as much as _____% per year.
   a. 10
   b. 20
   c. 30
   d. 40

4. When mAs and kVp are used to change image brightness, the function is named
   a. automatic brightness control
   b. automatic dose rate control
   c. automatic exposure control
   d. automatic gain control

5. The weakest link in the fluoroscopic imaging chain in terms of resolution is the
   a. image intensifier
   b. optical mirror system
   c. focal spot
   d. TV monitor

6. Common frame rates for cinefluorography include (1) 15, (2) 20, (3) 30, (4) 40.
   a. 1 and 2 only
   b. 1 and 3 only
   c. 1 and 4 only
   d. 1, 2, 3, 4

7. Disadvantages of cassette spot-filming include (1) relatively high patient dose, (2) delay for cassette to come into place, (3) unfamiliar format.
   a. 1 and 2 only
   b. 1 and 3 only
   c. 2 and 3 only
   d. 1, 2, and 3

8. Advantages of the photospot camera include (1) lower dose than with cassettes, (2) less heat-loading, (3) shorter interruption of the examination.
   a. 1 and 2 only
   b. 1 and 3 only
   c. 2 and 3 only
   d. 1, 2, and 3

9. Which of the following is a typical fluoroscopic mA?
   a. 2
   b. 20
   c. 200
   d. 2000

10. The primary factor affecting the brightness of the fluoroscopic image is
    a. mA
    b. kVp
    c. size or density of part
    d. gain

Exercises

1. Calculate minification gain with an output screen diameter of 1 inch and input screen sizes of
   a. 5 inches
   b. 10 inches
   c. 12 inches

2. Assuming a flux gain of 50, calculate total brightness gain for each of the above measurements.

3. Draw a block diagram of the image intensification process.

4. What are some of the names of methods used to maintain image brightness?

5. What factors affect resolution of the fluoroscopic image? Which of these is the primary factor?

6. Explain how the electron gun functions to remove flicker from the image.

7. Compare each of the static filming methods. What are the advantages and disadvantages of each method?

8. Compare each of the viewing systems. What are the advantages and disadvantages of each?

9. What is quantum mottle, and why is it a problem in fluoroscopy?

10. How do multifield (magnification) tubes operate?

Equipment and Accessory Malfunctions or Misapplications

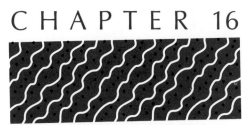

Charles Burns, M.S.P.H., R.T.(R.)
Steven B. Dowd, Ed.D., R.T.(R.)

Chapter Outline

Chapter Objectives

On completion of this chapter, you should be able to

- Determine likely causes of light, dark, low-contrast, and blurred images.
- Differentiate between underexposure, underdevelopment, underpenetration, overexposure, overdevelopment, and overpenetration as part of the trouble-shooting process.
- Describe or state the appearance of an image given a specific malfunction or error.
- State corrective actions for certain errors.

The production of high-quality radiographic images assumes that the correct *technical factors* were used and that the equipment used was operating properly. Failure of either of these conditions typically results in the production of a radiograph in which one or more of the image characteristics is substandard. The radiographer must be able to evaluate the film and if it is judged to be substandard determine the causes and take corrective action. Although only the radiologist can make patient diagnoses from a radiograph, the radiographer must make an initial determination of the acceptability of the radiograph to the physician prior to the diagnosis. This determination is referred to as film critique or radiographic film evaluation, which requires a knowledge of radiographic anatomy, positioning, imaging techniques, and radiographic pathology.

The process of radiographic film evaluation occurs as follows:

1. Visual evaluation of the image for acceptability
2. If the image is not acceptable, determination of the cause of the problem, such as
   a. Lack of clarity due to inappropriate density, contrast, recorded detail, or mottle
   b. A procedural problem in patient positioning or patient preparation
3. Once the problem has been identified, appropriate corrective action is taken, e.g.,
   a. Adjustment of technical factors
   b. Adjustment of positioning of the patient
   c. Correction of any equipment malfunction

This chapter addresses some of the most common problems encountered clinically, how they relate to the appearance of the radiographic image, and appropriate action that can be taken to correct the particular problem. Problems encountered may be attributed to equipment malfunctions or operator error. However, common problems with radiographic equipment and accessories that are caused by human error can only be reduced by careful attention to detail, proper orientation for new employees, and inservice education concerning all new equipment and accessories. Some of the problems encountered are true equipment failures and may occur infrequently. If such problems are repeated frequently, an equipment service call is warranted.

We now review some of the more common equipment-related problems in terms of their effects on resulting radiographs. The sources of these problems are explored along with a recommended course of action.

PROBLEM: NO EXPOSURE

Failure to get an exposure can represent a severe problem with the x-ray generator. Often however there are other more common causes. The following are more common causes of problems resulting in lack of exposure, based on analysis of service records.

No Power to Generator

Potential Problem Source. The unit is not turned on at the control panel or at the wall switch.

Remedy. Turn the unit on.

Potential Problem Source. The circuit breaker may be tripped.

Recommended Action. Reset the circuit breaker and turn on the generator. If the breaker opens again, notify supervisor or service before once more attempting to restore power.

Control Panel Settings or Switches Engaged

Potential Problem Source. One or more of the control panel controls are not set correctly. Many modern generators will not initiate an exposure if only one switch is improperly set. Examples are the failure to select the table or wall Bucky device or failure to turn on the automatic exposure control (AEC).

Recommended Action. Recheck all control panel switches to assure the correct position of each.

Automatic Collimator

If the unit is equipped with an automatic collimator, several situations can result in failure to initiate an exposure. In most of the situations, the interlocks do not allow prepping of the tube.

Potential Problem Source. The Bucky or cassette-holder tray is not pushed all the way in. The tray sensor connectors do not engage, the collimator does not sense that a cassette is in place, and the circuit does not allow prepping of the tube or an exposure.

Remedy. Push the tray in firmly to engage connector prongs.

Potential Problem Source. The tube crane or stand is not in the correct position to close the source-image distance (SID) sensor switch. Automatic collimators are designed to function only at certain SID positions. If the tube stand is in any other position, the circuit does not permit prepping of the tube or an exposure unless the collimator is switched to manual mode.

Remedy. Check the tube stand and adjust until the collimator ready light is on.

Potential Problem Source. Both radiographic table and upright cassette holder are engaged. The logic circuit in the automatic collimator cannot separate the signals. This occurrence does not allow preparation of the tube exposure.

Remedy. Disconnect the device not being used.

Rotor Operating But No Exposure

Potential Problem Source. The stator may not be operating or may not be bringing the rotor to the correct speed when the tube is prepared. If the rotor is not turning at the correct speed, the exposure is withheld.

Recommended Action. Listen to determine if the rotor is turning at all. If the speed is low, a service person will have to verify.

Potential Problem Source. The selected filament may be burned out.

Recommended Action. Switch to the other filament and make a test exposure.* Exposure on one filament and not the other indicates that a service call is necessary. The operational focal spot can usually be used within its limits until the service technician is on site.

Spot-Film Camera

Potential Problem Source. If the unit is an image-intensified fluoroscopy system equipped with a spot-film camera, exposures will not result if the film magazine is incorrectly mounted to the camera or if the film is loaded incorrectly into the magazine, so that the film does not advance.

---

* The term *test exposure* or *test film* in this chapter means an exposure using a phantom or a step-wedge, not the patient. In other cases, the problem is corrected, and a repeat exposure is made.

Recommended Action. Check to be sure that the film magazine is correctly mounted on the camera, the film is correctly loaded into the magazine, and the film is advanced. Most of these problems can be corrected by the careful attention to manipulation of the equipment and switches by the technologist. Occasionally, the preceding corrective actions do not resolve the problem. In this case, the supervisor or service engineer should be notified.

PROBLEM: INCORRECT RADIOGRAPHIC DENSITY

The first indicator of a technical problem is usually a radiograph with incorrect radiographic density. A complete discussion of the effect of technical factors on image density requires a careful examination of six terms:

Underexposure. Formation of too few latent image centers in the emulsion

Underdevelopment. An insufficient number of silver halide crystals are converted to metallic silver in the developer

Underpenetration. The kVp is too low to provide a sufficient number of photons at the receptor to produce the correct radiographic density

Overexposure. The formation of too many latent image centers in the emulsion

Overdevelopment. An excessive amount of silver halide crystals is converted to metallic silver in the developer

Overpenetration. The kVp is too high, producing an extremely large number of photons at the receptor

These terms can cause confusion for students because of their misuse. Visually, images that are *underexposed* and *underdeveloped* have similar appearance (Fig. 16–1). The background around the structure is gray. It is impossible visually to distinguish underexposure from underdevelopment. Overexposed images are often darker than overdeveloped images, and overdeveloped images have increased base fog.

Underpenetration is rare. For example, large numbers of abdominal radiographs are produced each day at kVp values as low as 60 kVp for intravenous urography. However, underpenetration can occur, usually from technical errors (Fig. 16–2). To determine if the image is underpenetrated, the kVp level must be known. Also, examine the background around the image of the part. If the background is black and the rest of the image is clear, underpenetration is likely.

In clinical practice, *overpenetration* should not exist. Technologist will not use a kVp that is too high, because they are aware of the effect of kVp on contrast. Most images classified as overpenetrated are really overexposed. They are best corrected by reducing mAs, not kVp. Correcting overly dense images by using mAs rather than kVp is also superior from a standpoint of protection from radiation.

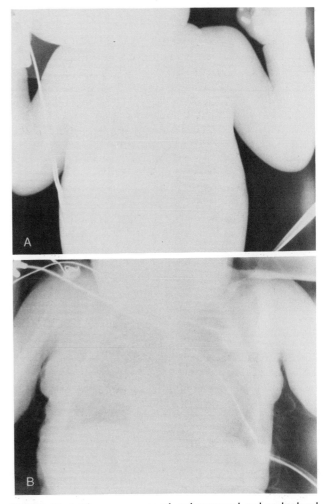

FIGURE 16–1. The appearance of underexposed and underdeveloped films is very similar. *A* is the result of underexposure resulting from low mAs. *B* is the result of underdevelopment caused by a low level of developer.

Some light and dark radiographs are the result of human errors in the use of the equipment or accessories. To troubleshoot the cause of inadequate images, a reliable technical factor chart must exist and must be used. Radiographic techniques are set for specific standard radiographic accessories. Correctly constructed, a technique chart usually varies the kVp or mAs as patient thickness changes. The following are common problems that are the result of misapplication of an accessory, the use of a technique intended for another situation, or an equipment failure. It is beyond the scope of this text or this chapter to completely address all problems. The outline format should improve decisionmaking when troubleshooting a particular problem.

Images With Insufficient Radiographic Density: Light Radiographs

Low-density, or light, images are the result of decreased response of the film during the formation of

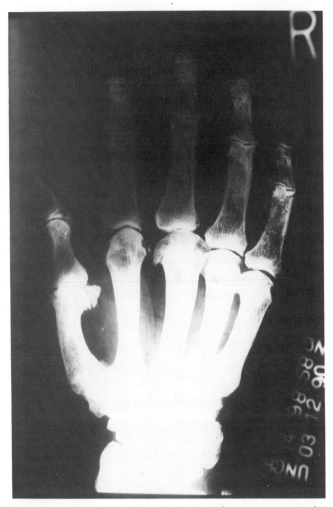

FIGURE 16–2. Underpenetration is rare. In this case, a new technologist performed a high-resolution hand image with the mammography unit, using 26 kVp rather than the normal 42 kVp. The image has the characteristic "underpenetrated" look with extremely high contrast; even thin parts (wrist) are clear.

the latent or manifest image and thus are either underexposed or underdeveloped.

Image Receptor Problems

Potential Problem Source. The cassette is used upside down with the back facing the tube. The back of the cassette is thicker than the front, normally containing a thin sheet of lead foil. The exposure to the screens and the film is reduced, producing a light image. The image shows the locks on the cassette back and often shows the small wrinkles in the lead foil (Fig. 16–3).

Remedy. Repeat the image with the tube side of the cassette facing the tube.

Potential Problem Source. The image receptor is slower than is specified by the technique. The screens are slower, the film is slower (it may be single- rather than dual-emulsion), or the film is not spectrally matched to light emission from the screens. The screen label is clear on the edge of the sheet of film, whereas the film type label is black (Fig. 16–4).

Remedy. If screen and film are mismatched, use the correct screen-film combination.

Potential Problem Source. In a small number of cases, it may be that the cassettes used have the same screens but their fronts have different attenuation characteristics. For example, carbon fiber and Kevlar cassette fronts for pediatric radiography are equivalent to less than 0.5 mm of aluminum (Al), whereas standard cassettes have fronts with 1.0 to 1.5 mm Al equivalents. If the technique is set for the low attenuation front and a cassette with a heavier front used, the image will be light.

Remedy. These problems generally are operator errors and administrative control problems. Facilities with different cassettes, screens, and film applications should have a clear method, such as color coding, for identifying each image receptor system.

Automatic Exposure Control

Automatic exposure control (AEC) systems are only as accurate as the settings made by service technicians and the technical factors selected by the radiographer. Modern AEC systems have relatively small detector fields, about the size of a credit card, and are extremely sensitive to alignment of the anatomy of interest over the active cell. The AEC is sensitive to accurate positioning by the technologist. Several problems can arise as a result of using AEC.

Potential Problem Source. The incorrect tube is selected for the exposure. This is not a common problem, since it can only occur in a radiographic room with two tubes in which one is dedicated to the upright cassette holder or to the table, and the upright, or chest, tube is selected when the patient is on the table. When the exposure is made, the back-up time buzzer sounds, but the patient and the cassette have not received any exposure and the image will be clear.

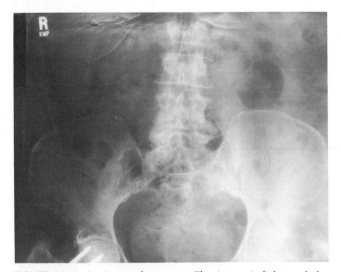

FIGURE 16–3. An inverted cassette. The image is light, and the wrinkles in the lead foil are clearly seen. In this particular image there is also grid cut-off, producing the uneven side-to-side density.

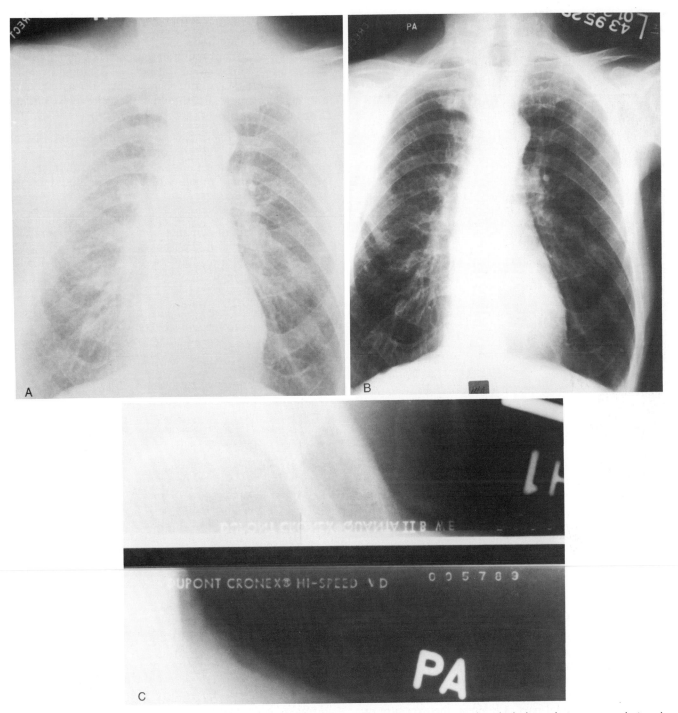

FIGURE 16–4. *A* was produced using a Du Pont Hi Speed screen rather than a Quanta II screen for which the techniques were designed. *B* is the repeat examination, using the same technique with the Quanta II screen. *C* is a close-up of the screen identification labels on the edge of each film. Be sure to read the edge of each image before repeating light or dark images.

Remedy. Repeat the exposure with the correct match of tube to receptor.

Potential Problem Source. The anatomical part is not centered over the active detector. The detector is exposed at a higher than normal exposure rate, and the exposure time terminates prematurely. A common example of this problem is an oblique projection of the lumbar spine, in which the spine is not centered on the active center chamber (Fig. 16–5).

Remedy. Repeat the examination, being careful to center the spine over the active chamber.

Potential Problem Source. The setting for the back-up time is too short. The exposure time reaches the back-up, the exposure terminates early, and the image is light (Fig. 16–6).

Recommended Action. The back-up time setting should be a time that is about 50% more than the technologist

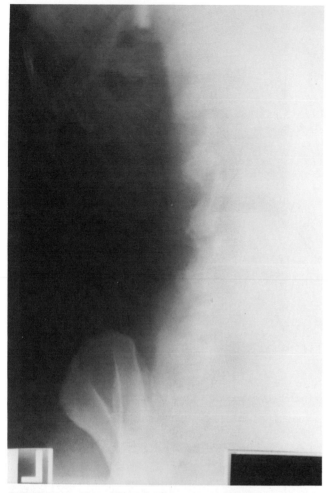

FIGURE 16–5. This oblique lumbar spine radiograph is not centered over the activated center chamber. The chamber is exposed at a higher rate, and the time is terminated early.

would use manually. Thus even when using automatic exposure control, the technologist must know the manual technique required for the exposure.

Potential Problem Source. The incorrect detector chamber is selected. For example, the technical factors were designed for the center chamber, but the lateral chamber or a combination of center and lateral chambers is selected. Since the outer chamber is not under the anatomical part of interest, the exposure rate to the detector is high, the exposure terminates prematurely, and the image is light.

Remedy. Repeat the examination, using the proper chamber.

Potential Problem Source. The density setting or chamber sensitivity selected is incorrect. The technical factors were designed for "(N)ormal" or zero (0) and the density is set on a negative (−) value. The exposure time terminates early, and the image is light.

Remedy. Reset the density or chamber sensitivity correctly, and repeat the exposure. These settings should always be checked before making an exposure.

X-ray Generator and X-ray Tube

Potential Problem Source. The timer circuit fails. The time terminates substantially earlier (>25%) than the set value. A smaller (<25%) change is not noticeable, since the exposure must change by at least 25% to produce an image density that is noticeably different from the normal or standard density.

Recommended Action. It is possible that only one timer station is faulty. Before committing the unit to an immediate service call, try an adjacent timer station with a test film. Problems of this type should be reported to the supervisor.

Potential Problem Source. One of the rectifier diodes is open or blown. In generators with mA compensators, the transformer is noisy (makes a "whoomp" sound) during the exposure, and an mA overload is likely. The overload light may come on, and the circuit breaker may trip.

Recommended Action. Report unusual sounds, situations, or odors to the supervisor.

Potential Problem Source. The generator control panel settings change without warning. The mA, time, or

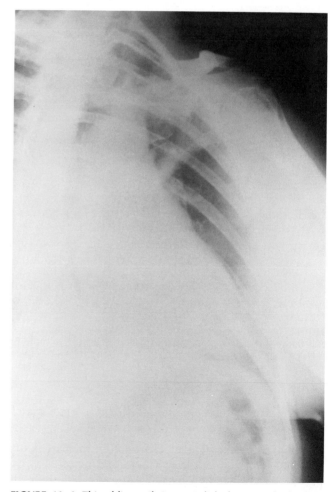

FIGURE 16–6. This oblique rib image is light because the back-up time was set at 0.1 sec, not the normal 0.5 sec. The exposure terminated at 0.1 sec when it should have gone to 0.3 sec.

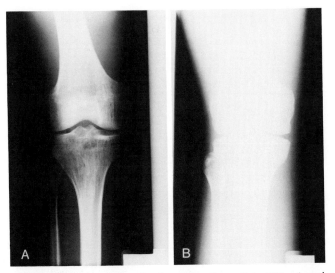

FIGURE 16-7. *A* is the result of resetting the unit to 150 mA and repeating the image. *B* is light because the generator switched the mA from 150 mA to 50 mA just before the exposure was made. Reconfirm control panel settings just before making the exposure. Once the rotor is started, the settings are not likely to change.

kVp changes without the technologist altering the technical settings. This situation is only likely with microprocessor controlled generators, in which the unexpected change in settings is due to static or power line disturbances (Fig. 16-7).

Recommended Action. Confirm generator settings just before making the exposure. If the unexpected changes occur frequently, notify the supervisor or the service engineer.

Potential Problem Source. A gassy tube, an arcing tube, or an arcing high-voltage cable may be present (Fig. 16-8). The exposure may be accompanied by a popping sound. Generator indicators act in unusual ways. The mA indicator may go to maximum value momentarily. Digital displays give unexpected values, usually accompanied with "error" messages.

Recommended Action. Notify your supervisor, service personnel, or both.

Potential Problem Source. There are "bad" or sticking contacts in mA control circuit: 100 mA at 0.4 sec, for example, is light.

Recommended Action. Try a different mA station, using the same mAs. Try 200 mA at 0.2 sec (which still gives 40 mAs) on a test film. Notify your supervisor, service personnel, or both.

Potential Problem Source. The mA is miscalibrated (filament current is low). The mA or kVp calibration is drifting.

Recommended Action. The calibration drift is a gradual process and should be detected by the quality control (QC) program. Notify service personnel.

Potential Problem Source. The filament selected for the exposure is malfunctioning.

Recommended Action. Try the other focal spot. Output can be low on the large filament but correct on the small one. Notify your supervisor or service personnel.

Potential Problem Source. Some evaporated tungsten from the filament or target may have been deposited over the tube window.

Recommended Action. This process is a gradual one and should be detected by the QC program. It will produce a reduced tube output and increased HVL. At extreme levels, the tungsten deposit will cause the tube current to arc to the housing. Notify your supervisor.

Darkroom and Processing

Potential Problem Source. There is a decrease in developer activity. The most likely causes are decreased developer temperature or under-replenishment. Other causes are developer contamination (low pH), improperly mixed developer (too much water added, specific gravity low), or the developer level is low because of a leak in the tanks, recirculation system, or replenisher system. The images not only are light, but are "flat," containing no black, only gray, in the image (Fig. 16-9).

Recommended Action. Notify the supervisor or the quality control technologist.

Potential Problem Source. A standby unit stops the processor with the film in fixer. The image will bleach out if the film stays in the fixer for several minutes.

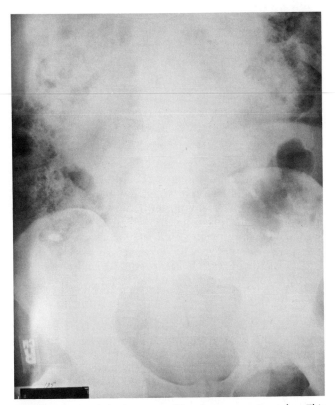

FIGURE 16-8. A light image resulting from an arcing tube. This was one of the first images exposed as the tube started to break down.

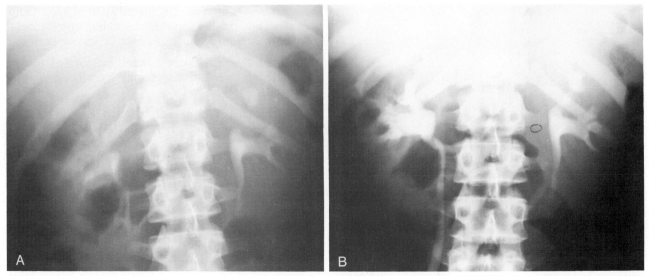

FIGURE 16–9. *A* and *B* were produced at the same technical parameters. However, *B* was processed in a different processor. The processor for image A contained only 3 inches of developer. The rest had drained out through an incompletely closed valve. Note that the image is slightly light and that there is substantial loss of contrast. The loss of contrast is caused by the reduced immersion time and the lack of activity of the hydroquinone. The phenidone had ample time to act, but phenidone does not produce high-contrast images.

Recommended Action. This problem can be avoided by confirming the count of films exiting the processor compared with the number entering it. If the count is low, activate the processor by pressing the standby switch. The films inside the processor will then exit the unit.

Ancillary Equipment

Potential Problem Source. The grid used is incorrect for the situation. The grid ratio is greater than the technique calls for, or the interspace material is aluminum when the technique is set for a fiber-interspaced grid.

Recommended Action. Check the grid used against the technique chart.

Potential Problem Source. There is grid cutoff as a result of focal range violation or centering error. If the central ray is not centered or perpendicular to the grid or if the FFD is larger or smaller than the focal range of the grid, excessive primary radiation will be absorbed, and the image will be light. Figure 16–10*A* is light with a gray background, exhibiting some vertical streaking. This is the result of using a 40-inch focused grid at 72 inches FFD. Figure 16–10*B* employed the correct 72-inch grid at 72 inches FFD.

Recommended Action. Check the alignment of the beam to the grid before the image is repeated.

Potential Problem Source. The beam size is inappropriate for the situation. The technical factors are designed for a larger beam size. A smaller beam size results in less scatter. Less scatter reaches the image receptor, and the image is light.

Remedy. Check the beam size from the technique chart.

Potential Problem Source. The total filtration in place is more than specified in the technique chart, which is a problem only when collimators with variable filtration, also called "dial-a-filter," are used. This type of collimator has a wheel with additional filtration that can be added to the standard filtration. The additional filtration is normally used when heavier filtration is needed for high-kVp radiography. If the filter wheel is left in the position for high-kVp imaging when using lower-kVp radiography, the filter will attenuate too much radiation. The image will be light, appearing underexposed, with lowered contrast.

Remedy. Check the position of the variable filter device before making an exposure.

Potential Problem Source. The focal film distance (FFD) is more than specified because of human error (Fig. 16–11) or an incorrect distance indicator. If the FFD violates the grid focal range the effect is amplified.

Remedy. Check to assure the correct FFD before the exposure. If distance indicator is in error, notify your supervisor.

Images With Excessive Radiographic Density: Dark Radiographs

Excessive density (dark images) is the result of increased response of the film during the formation of the latent or manifest image, and thus the film is either overexposed or overdeveloped.

Image Receptor Problems

Potential Problem Source. The image receptor is faster than specified by the technique. The screens are faster

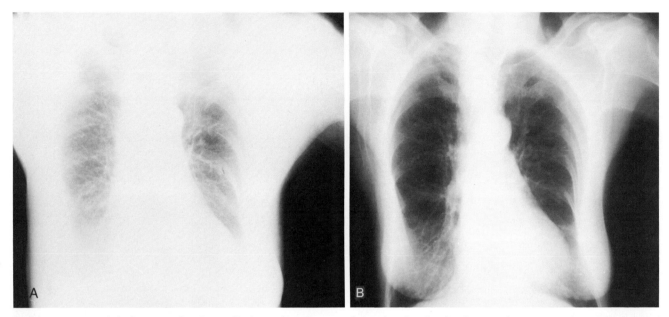

FIGURE 16–10. *A* is light because of grid cut-off. The grid in place is a focused grid with a focal range of 38 to 44 inches. With the focal film distance (FFD) at 72 inches for the chest, the amount of cut-off is substantial. Note the vertical streaking, or "corduroy effect," due to cut-off. *B* is a repeat, using the same technique but with the correct grid in place.

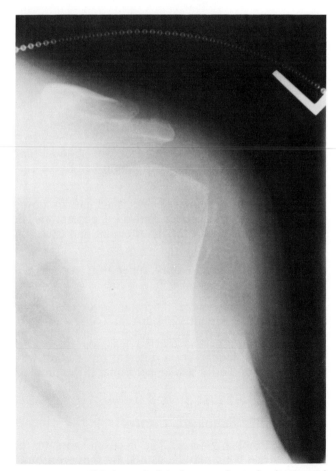

FIGURE 16–11. This image is light because the technologist used 40-inch technical factors at 72-inch FFD.

or the film is faster than specified. The screen label is clear on the edge of the sheet of film, whereas the label of the film type is black. Figure 16–12*A* was dark because the cassette was loaded with the faster Kodak RPS film used in pediatrics. Unfortunately, the technologist repeated the image as overpenetrated and decreased the kVp from 75 to 70. For Figure 16–12*B*, the correct GAF film was loaded by the darkroom technologist and is too light. Figure 16–12*C* is the edge of each image showing the type of film in black letters.

Remedy. Repeat the radiograph, using the correct image receptor.

Potential Problem Source. The cassettes that are used may have the same screens, but their fronts have different attenuation characteristics. If the technique is set for the standard aluminum-front cassette and a cassette with a low-attenuation front is used, the image will be dark.

Recommended Action. As discussed in the section on light radiographs, these problems are generally operator errors and administrative control problems.

X-ray Generator and X-ray Tube

Potential Problem Source. The timer circuit fails. The time terminates substantially later (>25%) than the set value. A smaller (<25%) change is not noticeable, since the exposure must change by at least 25% to produce an image density noticeably different from the normal or standard density. It is possible that only one timer setting is faulty.

Recommended Action. Before committing the unit to an immediate service call, try an adjacent timer setting.

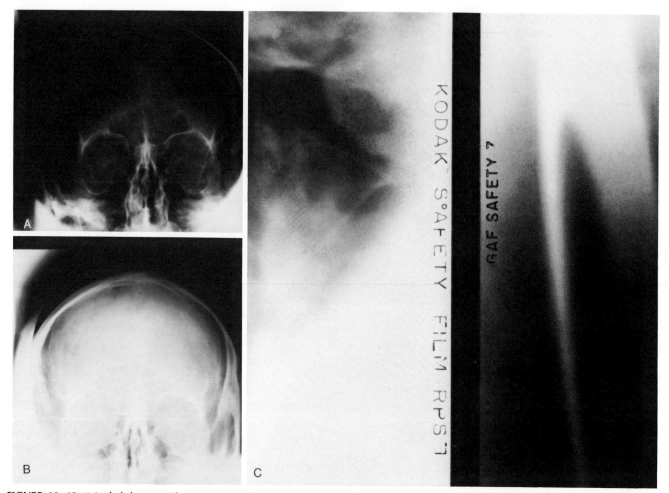

FIGURE 16–12. *A* is dark because the cassette was loaded with a faster film used for pediatric examinations. The technologist incorrectly decided that the image was overpenetrated at 75 kVp and reduced the kVp from 75 to 70 for the repeat exposure. *B* is the repeat. However, this cassette was correctly loaded with a slower GAF film. *C* is a close-up of the labels of the film types on the edge of the film.

Potential Problem Source. There is an unexpected change in generator control panel settings. The mA, time, or kVp changes without the technologist altering the technical settings. This situation is likely only with microprocessor-controlled generators. The unexpected change is due to static or power line disturbances.

Recommended Action. Confirm generator settings just before making the exposure. If the unexpected changes occur frequently, notify the supervisor or the service engineer.

Potential Problem Source. There are multiple (machine-gun) exposures before the technologist can release the exposure switch. The hand switch may be faulty; there may be a faulty relay or starting silicon-controlled rectifier (SCR). The Bucky may be misadjusted; the mechanism hits the exposure enable switch but not the stop switch. There is static noise or voltage spikes to the microprocessor.

Recommended Action. Notify supervisor, service personnel, or both.

Potential Problem Source. The calibration of the mA or kVp has drifted.

Remedy. Normally, these changes are gradual and should be detected by the QC program before the calibration change affects the image.

Potential Problem Source. There is an arc or power surge to the microprocessor-controlled generator. The surge can interfere with the timer circuit and cause the exposure to run long.

Recommended Action. Notify supervisor, service personnel, or both.

Potential Problem Source. There are poor contacts in the mA control circuit; 200 mA at 0.2 sec is good, whereas 100 mA at 0.4 sec is dark.

Recommended Action. Try a different mA station with the same mAs. Notify service personnel if the problem persists.

Automatic Exposure Control

Potential Problem Source. The exposure goes to the back-up time. This may be caused by the erroneously activating the upright AEC detector while the tube is aligned with the patient on the table. The activated detector does not receive any radiation exposure. The exposure will go to the back-up time, and the back-up warning buzzer will sound. The patient and the image receptor in the table are overexposed, and the image is dark.

Recommended Action. Carefully check chamber settings just before an exposure is made. This type of error is one of two primary reasons for setting the backup time to 50% above the expected exposure time. The second reason is to keep the patient dose low in case of phototimer malfunction.

Potential Problem Source. The AEC detector fails because of loss of high-voltage supply, loss of preamplifier circuit, or a short in the detector. The exposure will go to the back-up time, and the back-up warning buzzer will sound. The patient and the image receptor are overexposed, and the image is dark.

Recommended Action. Notify your supervisor and service personnel.

Potential Problem Source. The exposure time necessary to produce the proper density is shorter than the minimum response time (MRT). This is a problem with high-mA or kVp settings. Exceeding the MRT is responsible for dark images on thin body parts. Some older phototiming systems have an MRT of 20 msec (0.020 sec) or more.

Recommended Action. Know the MRT of each AEC system, and select an mA so that the exposure time termination by the AEC will be longer than the MRT of the unit.

Potential Problem Source. The incorrect detector chamber is selected. The technical factors are designed for one or both lateral cells. If, for example, the center chamber is selected, the time will run longer than desired.

Remedy. Check to assure that the correct detector chamber is selected for the technical factors used.

Potential Problem Source. An improper density setting is selected. If the technical factors were designed for "(N)ormal" or zero (0) and the density is set on positive (+) value, the time will run longer than desired.

Remedy. Check to assure proper density settings are selected.

Potential Problem Source. The settings were not adjusted to compensate for beam size. The technical factor settings were established during AEC calibration for a larger field (14 × 17 or 7 × 17) sizes. For example, assume that a smaller beam size (8 × 10) is used. This produces less scatter than the larger field. The detector is not properly exposed. The exposure time runs longer to compensate for loss of scatter. This can occur when using an AEC for lateral projections of the lumbar spine and the L5–S1 spot projections. Unless the radiographer corrects for the smaller beam size of the spot by using a negative (−) density setting, the spot will be darker than the lateral.

Remedy. Assure that AEC settings are adjusted to compensate for beam size.

Darkroom and Processing

Potential Problem Source. The developer activity is increased. The most likely causes are increased developer temperature or low bromide (Br⁻) ion concentration caused by the lack of "starter" or over-replenishment. The developer may be improperly mixed with insufficient water, resulting in an overactive developer with high specific gravity.

Recommended Action. The developer should be re-mixed.

Potential Problem Source. The films are fogged for one of the following reasons:

- White light leaks
- Safelight leak or safelight inappropriate for film type
- Film is past expiration date
- Film has been exposed to radiation or excessive heat.

Remedy. Take appropriate action in each of the preceding cases to remove the source of film fogging.

Ancillary Equipment

Potential Problem Source. The grid is inappropriate for the situation. The ratio is less than the technique calls for, or the interspace material is fiber when the technique is set for an aluminum-interspaced grid.

Remedy. Use the appropriate grid.

Potential Problem Source. There is no grid in the Bucky. During servicing the grid was inadvertently not installed.

Remedy. Re-install the appropriate grid in the Bucky.

Potential Problem Source. The Bucky grid does not move. The image is slightly darker than when the grid moves and grid lines are visible.

Recommended Action. Notify supervisor and service personnel.

Potential Problem Source. The beam size is inappropriate for the technique selected. The technical factors were designed for a small beam and a larger beam is used. The larger size produces more scatter, to which the image receptor responds, causing increased density.

Remedy. Use technical factors appropriate for the beam size.

Potential Problem Solving. The amount of filtration in place is less than that specified in technique chart. The filtration could have been left out following servicing of the collimator or tube head. Insufficient filtration is also a possibility if the unit is equipped with a collimator with variable filtration. If the filter wheel is left in the position for low-kVp when imaging with a higher-kVp, the filter will not attenuate sufficient low-energy radiation. The image will be dark.

Remedy. Check the position of the variable filter device.

Potential Problem Source. The FFD is less than specified because the distance indicator is incorrect. If the FFD violates the grid focal range, the effect may be negligible as a result of the canceling effect of the grid cutoff.

Remedy. If the distance indicator is found to be incorrect, notify your supervisor.

PROBLEM: UNSHARP IMAGES

The most common causes of image blur are motion and poor geometry. Most of these are discussed in Chapter 12.

Motion Blur

Potential Problem Source. The patient moves. This may be due to the patient's condition or communication problems between the technologist and the patient.

Remedy. If the problem is the patient's condition, then exposure time is reduced and the patient is immobilized. The most common methods of compensating for reduced exposure time are to increase mA, increase kVp, or increase receptor speed.

Potential Problem Source. The image receptor moves because of a mechanical problem in the Bucky tray.

Remedy. The Bucky frame is loose. The grid motion causes the tray holding the cassette to move during the exposure. Tighten the Bucky frame.

Potential Problem Source. In rare instances, the tube stand, or *tube crane,* will continue to move after being positioned by the technologist. The amount of movement may be extremely small and the technologist may not notice it. However, since the motion is so far from the receptor, even a small amount of motion is magnified at the level of the image receptor. The motion is normally caused by loosening of the mounts, worn bearings, or loosening of the overhead support. In addition to producing image blur, this condition is potentially dangerous—the tube mount could give way and fall on the patient.

Recommended Action. Notify your supervisor and service personnel.

Potential Problem Source. The focal spot may exhibit motion as a result of worn rotor bearings that cause the rotor to wobble during rotation. This makes the effective focal spot larger. It is not possible to distinguish focal spot motion from focal spot bloom with the test for focal spot size. In both cases the focal spot appears enlarged. However, the worn bearings are extremely noisy during the *tube preparation* cycle, as the

anode begins to rotate. This noise should be a clue to potential focal spot motion.

Recommended Action. Notify supervisor and service personnel.

Geometric Blur

Potential Problem Source. The focal spot size is larger than intended. The incorrect focal spot may have been selected. Also, the focal spot may have enlarged, or bloomed, as a result of aging or pitting of the anode surface. Focal spots normally enlarge with age; however, the blooming eventually produces a focal spot of unacceptable size.

Recommended Action. Check the focal spot selected. If correct, notify supervisor or quality control staff.

Potential Problem Source. The object-film distance (OFD) is sufficiently large to produce unacceptable blur.

Remedy. The effect of a large OFD can be overcome by decreasing focal spot size or increasing FFD. However, care must be taken that the corrective action does not cause an increase in exposure time sufficient to produce motion blur (see Chapter 12).

Image Receptor

Potential Problem Source. There is poor film-screen contact caused by a warped cassette frame or worn out backing foam or felt. Check with wire mesh test to confirm (see Chapter 17).

Remedy. Replace cassette.

Potential Problem Source. The image receptor is faster than desired. This is not likely to occur, since a faster image receptor also produces an extremely dark image.

Remedy. Use an image receptor of appropriate speed.

Pseudoblur

Potential Problem Source. A low-contrast (gray) image may appear unsharp because of the large edge gradient that occurs with low contrast.

Recommended Action. Evaluate the potential causes of blur before corrective action is taken. Pseudoblur refers to false blur in the image.

PROBLEM: LOW-CONTRAST IMAGES

Technical Factors

Potential Problem Source. The radiographic density is low. The lower density places the densities in the image on the area of the Hurtter and Driffield (H & D) curve, where the toe gradient causes a substantial decrease in contrast.

Remedy. Adjust technical factors to provide necessary radiographic density.

Potential Problem Source. The kVp is too high for the part or pathology, resulting in lowered subject contrast. The loss of contrast is due to reduced differential attenuation and increased percentage of scatter photons in the beam. Certain pathological conditions, such as osteoporosis, result in lower contrast.

Remedy. Lower the kVp to a more appropriate value.

Potential Problem Source. The grid contrast improvement factor is inadequate for the anatomical part and kVp. The grid lead content is low for the radiographic application. For example, a 8:1/103-line per inch grid would not be used for lateral lumbar spine radiographs. The grid only attenuates less than 80% of the scatter. The large volume of tissue irradiated generates substantial quantities of scatter, which the grid cannot absorb, resulting in low contrast. On the other hand, a 12:1 80-line per inch grid is able to absorb most of the scatter from a lateral lumbar spine exposure.

Remedy. Use an appropriate grid having sufficient lead content for the specific radiographic procedure.

Processing

Potential Problem Source. The developer activity is altered because

- The developer is exhausted because of under-replenishment
- The developer is oxidized
- The developer has been contaminated with fixer
- The developer temperature is lower than the standard
- The developer level in the processor tank is low as a result of a faulty valve (see Fig. 16–9A). With the lower level of chemistry, only the phenidone, which produces gray tones quickly, has an opportunity to function. The hydroquinone does not have time to develop the high-contrast image.
- The developer temperature is higher than the standard. The image is dark, and chemical fogging occurs.

Remedy. Take the appropriate corrective action to obtain proper developer activity.

Potential Problem Source. The fixer is exhausted or contaminated. The undeveloped silver halide is not cleared from the emulsion, and the image is "foggy."

Remedy. Notify your supervisor. Replace fixer.

Potential Problem Source. The standby unit stops the processor with the film in fixer; the image will "bleach out" in the concentrated fixer.

Recommended Action. Notify your supervisor and appropriate service personnel.

Image Receptor

Potential Problem Source. The base plus fog level of the film is increased by improper storage conditions or exposure to radiation or chemical fumes, or the film is outdated.

Remedy. Replace with fresh, uncontaminated film. Notify your supervisor of the problem.

Potential Problem Source. The screen is not spectrally matched to the film. Examples include using blue-sensitive film with green-emitting screens or green-sensitive film with blue-emitting screen with technique correction for speed (density) change. However, the speed correction will not correct for the loss of contrast.

Remedy. Use appropriately matched screen-film combinations.

Potential Problem Source. The cassette has a low-attenuation front. Plastic or Kevlar cassette fronts are designed for extremely low kVp. If used at higher kVp, significant amounts of scatter will enter receptor. This reduces contrast.

Remedy. Use the appropriate cassette for the kVp used.

PROBLEM: MISALIGNMENT OF PART AND IMAGE RECEPTOR

In some cases equipment-related problems can result in images in which the anatomy is not centered on the image receptor or is not correctly aligned with the receptor. The most common equipment related causes are listed.

Potential Problem Source. The Bucky tray is not pushed all the way in. This is usually a human error. However, it is possible that the Bucky tray rail is bent causing the tray to stop prematurely.

Remedy. Check to assure that the Bucky tray is completely pushed in and that the Bucky tray rail is not bent.

Potential Problem Source. The tube detent for centering on the table and Bucky is out of adjustment, and the central ray is not centered to the Bucky, table, and part.

Remedy. Check to assume that the central ray is properly centered.

Potential Problem Source. The tube may be rotated in the ring mount. This will cause the central ray to be angled, misaligning the part and the film. The angulation also produces grid cutoff.

Recommended Action. Notify your supervisor and appropriate service personnel.

Potential Problem Source. The cross-hair template on the collimator is out of position. The central ray does not correspond to the cross hair, leading to misalignment.

Recommended Action. Notify your supervisor and have cross-hair template adjusted.

Potential Problem Source. The collimator is not properly seated or is loose. The central ray is not correctly aligned.

Recommended Action. Notify your supervisor and have collimator adjusted, aligned, or both.

OTHER EQUIPMENT PROBLEMS

If at any time smoke comes from a piece of radiographic equipment, turn off the power immediately. Be sure to turn off the power switch on the generator control panel before turning off the wall panel switch. As soon as the power is off, remove the patient and notify the supervisor.

In case of a smell of burning rubber near the tube or high-tension cables, *do not touch the cables.* This may represent a malfunctioning high-tension cable arcing from core to shield. Turn off the power, remove the patient, and notify the supervisor.

Chapter Summary/ Important Concepts

Perhaps the most important characteristic of a technologist is the performance of radiography with precision and accuracy. This includes the ability to recognize equipment malfunctions and human errors that result in suboptimal images. By recognizing these problems the technologist can avoid unnecessary patient exposure caused by multiple repeat images, reduce the overall operating costs of the radiology department and improve patient care by minimizing the amount of time required to complete an examination. The following concepts include common problems and their causes.

If there is no exposure, possible causes include the following:
a. No power to generator
b. Control panel settings, switches are not engaged
c. Possible automatic collimator interlock problem
d. Stator failure or filament burned out
e. Possible spot-film camera problems

If incorrect radiographic density for
Light radiographs—possible problems include
a. Image receptor
b. Automatic exposure control
c. X-ray generator circuitry or tube
d. Darkroom
e. Ancillary equipment such as grids, collimators, filtration, or distance indicators

Dark radiographs—possible problems include
a. X-ray generator circuitry
b. Automatic exposure control
c. Image receptor
d. Darkroom and processing
e. Ancillary equipment such as grids, Bucky, collimators, or filtration

If images are unsharp or blurred, possible causes include
a. Motion of patient or equipment components
b. Geometric blur caused by focal spot "blooming" or inappropriate distance relationships
c. Problems with the image receptor
d. Pseudoblur due to low-contrast image

If images are low-contrast, possible causes include
a. Low radiographic density as a result of technical factors, or problems with the film processor or image receptor

If the anatomical part is not centered on the image receptor, possible cause includes
a. Central ray not centered on Bucky tray or film as a result of mechanical problems

Other serious equipment problems include
a. Smoke or sparks from equipment
b. Odor of burning rubber
c. Odor of hot metal or excessive heat from equipment

In order to properly analyze the cause of suboptimal images, it is mandatory that a baseline be established by the use of an accurate, updated technical factors chart. If the technical factors have worked reliably, then any deviation from the baseline is an indication that either a technical problem exists or a human error was made.

Although this section has not addressed every possible problem that can affect radiography, it should have established a pattern for logical decision making. Radiographers should be able to
a. Determine the problem with the radiograph
b. Determine the possible causes of the problem
c. Take appropriate action to correct the problem

Taking this specific course of action reduces patient and occupational radiation exposure by minimizing the number of necessary repeat films.

Important Terminology

Overdevelopment. Elevated image density caused by excessive conversion of exposed silver halide to metallic silver during chemical processing; the response of the film to a given exposure is exaggerated

Overexposure. Elevated image density caused by a high number of photons interacting with the film

Overpenetration. Elevated image density resulting from an excessively high beam energy (kVp); the image is also characterized by low-contrast and higher-fog levels; overpenetration is rare because one would not generally set the kVp at an excessively high level

Technical Parameters (Factors). Elements that affect exposure to the receptor or response of the receptor to the exposure; these include mAs, kVp, film-screen type, grid, and processing

Tube Crane. Mechanical support for the tube housing and collimator; the tube crane may be a ceiling, floor, or floor-to-ceiling mount

Tube Preparation. First stage of the exposure switch; the filament temperature is raised from standby to thermionic emission levels, the rotor is accelerated to the correct speed, and a space charge is established; the tube is ready to produce x-rays

Underdevelopment. Insufficient image density caused by inadequate conversion of exposed silver halide to metallic silver during chemical processing; the response of the film to a given exposure is diminished

Underexposure. Insufficient density as a result of a low number of photons interacting with the film

Underpenetration. Insufficient image density because of an excessively low beam energy (kVp); the image is also characterized by high contrast with areas that are completely "clear"; underpenetration is rare, because one would not normally set the kVp at an extremely low value

▰▰▰ Review Questions

1. What should you do if the circuit breaker trips after resetting?
2. The generator will not make an exposure. In fact, the rotor will not even start when the exposure switch is pressed to the preparation position. The power light is on, and all the control panel switches are in the correct position. List two reasons for the failure to make an exposure.
3. A light radiograph exhibits some small fine dark "wrinkles" on the image. What is the likely cause of the light image?
4. What causes underpenetration?
5. Describe the appearance of the screen identification on the radiograph.
6. An AP lumbar spine is being performed using an ion chamber AEC. Describe the image resulting from use of a lateral chamber rather than the center chamber.
7. One forgets to change the grid in the upright cassette holder from 40-inch to 72-inch focus for a chest radiograph. What will be the appearance of the radiograph?
8. The serviceman has just released the x-ray room to you after repairing the collimator. The first four images are dark. What is a likely cause of the dark images?
9. The normal density setting for an AEC timed AP lumbar spine is zero (0). The radiologist asks for a coned down spot of the L4–L5 junction. What will be the appearance of the radiograph if a 6- × 8-inch field is used to produce an image with a density setting of 0?
10. As you enter a radiographic room, you smell burning rubber and notice a thin wisp of smoke from the transformer vault. What are the first two things you should do?

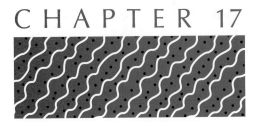

CHAPTER 17

Quality Control

Charles Burns, M.S.P.H., R.T.(R.)
Steven B. Dowd, Ed.D., R.T.(R.)

Chapter Outline

Chapter Objectives

On completion of this chapter, you should be able to

- Define quality assurance and quality control.
- Describe the roles of quality assurance and quality control in delivery of radiology service.
- State the basic differences between first-, second-, and third-level quality control testing procedures.
- List the primary reasons for implementing a quality control program.
- Describe the rationale for monitoring x-ray equipment performance.
- Describe the simple (routine) quality control monitoring tests for x-ray–producing equipment, processors, and ancillary equipment.
- Describe the quality control test procedures in which a dosimeter is used.
- Describe the quality control tests using specialized test equipment such as the kVp meter and star pattern.
- List the values that should be measured, recorded, or plotted for a processor QC program.
- List the monitored performance standards of an x-ray generator.
- Describe the basic goal of repeat analysis.

The process of producing a diagnostic radiographic image has multiple stages, as indicated in Figure 17–1. Any one of these may be a source of variability resulting in a suboptimal finished radiograph. Suboptimal radiographs require repeat examinations, resulting in increased radiation exposure and increased examination costs. Structured routine procedures are used to monitor and control these variables. These procedures make up part of a *quality assurance* program. *Quality control* (QC) in diagnostic radiology ranges from daily checks of the processor to semiannual or quarterly checks of equipment performance standards.

Evaluation of equipment performance standards can be done by physicists or service personnel. In many cases, routine quality control tests are performed by specially trained registered technologists named quality assurance or quality control technologists. In many instances, this role supplements their regular duties. See the boxed material for a description of some of the duties performed by a quality assurance and control technologist.

A quality control or quality assurance technologist is responsible for developing systems of quality assurance and control that conform to state and federal laws, to voluntary requirements for accreditation, and to requirements of third-party payers. This individual quite logically is also often responsible

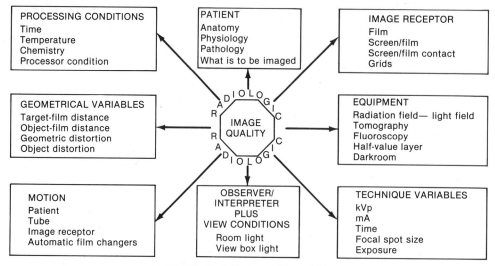

FIGURE 17-1. Radiographic variables.

for ensuring routine film quality by passing films, for routing patients for examinations, and for department inservice education. The purpose of QC testing is to document and maintain the consistency of x-ray equipment. QC tests provide a variety of data. Most of these are hints as to the potential for suboptimal performance.

QUALITY ASSURANCE AND QUALITY CONTROL

Quality assurance and *quality control* are terms that are often used interchangeably. Both terms refer to a process to improve the quality of radiology services delivered. The main difference between quality assurance and QC is the scope of their objectives. QC is one aspect of total quality assurance.

The Deming Management Method, for example, which has given rise to Quality Control Circles (QC) and Total Quality Management (TQM), views the input of the employee as important to improving the quality of a product. In radiology, the two products are quality patient care and diagnosis. Overall quality assurance in radiology consists of two factors: QC and quality patient care services. The radiographer provides patient care and produces the diagnostic film.

Radiographers must have a knowledge of equipment and the end-product sufficient to comment on potential problems. Although a staff radiographer may not perform quality assurance tests on a regular basis, a radiographer must have a knowledge of equipment that extends beyond a simple, "Something is wrong." Similarly, this individual must understand what goes into quality patient care beyond simply "being nice to the patient." As Deming has noted, quality is a never-ending process that is subject to ongoing improvement.

Quality Assurance

Quality assurance is an important factor in the accreditation process employed by the Joint Commission for Accreditation of Healthcare Organizations (JCAHO). Quality assurance is best carried out by a team. In the radiology department, this team consists of radiographers, administrators, radiologists, and other health care personnel.

Quality Control

The focus of this chapter is on QC tests, primarily those tests most commonly performed in radiology departments. QC is a series of activities or tests designed to monitor and maintain the stability of the technical elements in the imaging process. The end goal is the provision of satisfactory, dependable, and economical consumer service. Even the most expert technologist cannot compensate for erratic equipment. Variations in the *radiographic imaging chain* cause repeat radiographs, thus increasing both patient exposure and costs. A QC program is designed to ensure that the equipment is functioning consistently, leading to

- Improvement of image quality and consistency
- Reduction of repeat rates, examination costs, and patient exposure

QUALITY CONTROL TEST PROCEDURES

QC tests are a series of procedures to monitor the radiographic imaging process from its beginning (the

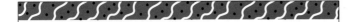

■ DUTIES OF A QUALITY ASSURANCE TECHNOLOGIST

The following are typical duties taken from the job description of a quality assurance technologist in a medium or large institution. This is adapted from job descriptions developed by the American Society of Radiologic Technologists (ASRT).

1. Tests new equipment and procedures.
2. Supervises care and maintenance of image receptors (film).*
3. Establishes quality control testing for generators, to include kVp evaluation, mA calibration, and mR and mAs evaluation and comparison.*
4. Monitors processor operation.*
5. Maintains processor log and control chart.*
6. Supervises care and maintenance of processors.*
7. Responsible for photographic quality control.*
8. Maintains silver reclamation equipment.*
9. Tests and evaluates screens, cassettes, and grids.*
10. Evaluates and maintains accessory equipment.
11. Constructs technique charts.
12. Determines the testing frequency and acceptability limits of quality control evaluations.
13. Prepares maintenance and replacement schedules.
14. Prepares test results and initiates corrective action.
15. Maintains quality control test equipment.
16. Recommends new equipment, modification of equipment, and new construction.
17. Conforms to all budgetary, regulatory, and voluntary accreditation standards.
18. Maintains communication with appropriate personnel to maintain quality control program.
19. Participates in and makes recommendations to the total quality management programs of the hospital and department.

x-ray tube and generator) to its end (the processor). QC testing performed on a regular basis may first indicate that a potential problem exists. QC tests are also used to identify the cause of an imaging problem.

The prescribed testing procedure for the radiology department is conducted in an organized and a methodical manner. Staff technologists may or may not participate in QC testing, especially the more complex procedures. However, all staff technologists need to participate in the QC program by reporting inconsist-

* All of these are described in this chapter.

ent radiographic images, equipment malfunction, or unusual noises and odors coming from the equipment. Many of these were described in Chapter 16. This reporting is consistent with a focus on overall quality assurance.

Levels of Testing

QC testing occurs at three levels, distinguished by the complexity of the procedure, its invasiveness, and the qualifications of the tester. First level tests are simple, noninvasive tests performed by technologists using inexpensive equipment. Examples include

- *Penetrometer (step-wedge)* tests for image consistency and mAs reciprocity. A simple tool, a step-wedge can provide information about film processor sensitometry, differences between screen-film combinations, differences between generators, and rough information about generator calibration
- The eight-cent test for x-ray beam–light beam (collimation) congruence
- Wire mesh images for film-screen contact

Second-level tests are more complex, noninvasive tests using more sophisticated equipment. This includes ion chambers, kVp meters, or special QC units such as the *N*oninvasive *E*valuation of *R*adiation *O*utput (NERO). Second-level testing is generally performed by a technologist trained in QC.

Third-level tests are complex, invasive equipment performance evaluations that involve some disassembly of the unit. Third-level tests are performed by engineers or physicists. The decision on testing levels and the selection of the QC test tools depends on many factors, including level of personnel availability at the facility, ease of use of the equipment, accuracy, and cost. A facility can start a basic QC program for less than $500 but may expend in excess of $10,000 for a more complex second- or third-level program.

This section discusses simple, first- and second-level QC tests, which may be performed by a technologist using QC test tools in a hospital or one-room clinic setting. Those wishing a more complete description of advanced second- and third-level QC programs are referred to the sources listed at the end of this chapter. These tests also usually require advanced training.

Basic Quality Control Testing

The simplest QC program requires a step-wedge and a simple metal thermometer (Fig. 17–2), a dedicated cassette (preferably one with 100-speed screens), identified as the QC cassette, eight pennies, and assorted lead markers. A mercury thermometer is not acceptable, since mercury can contaminate the processing tank. This is the type of program often seen in small, single-tube facilities such as small clinics and physician's offices.

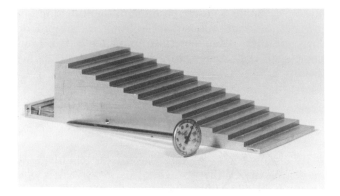

FIGURE 17-2. A simple aluminum step-wedge and metal probe thermometer used for first-level quality control.

Basic Penetrometer (Step-Wedge) Quality Control Check

The basic QC program begins with the establishment of a standard reference step-wedge (penetrometer) strip. After the processor is cleaned, filled with fresh and properly mixed chemicals, an image of the step-wedge is produced, using 70 to 80 kVp and an mAs sufficient to produce densities on the step-wedge from nearly clear at one end to black at the other (Fig. 17–3). The temperature of the developer is measured with the thermometer and recorded. The technical factors used to produce the step-wedge image are recorded, and the image is filed as a reference. This step-wedge image is reflective of both the processor and generator functions, since the step-wedge is produced by an x-ray exposure.

Each morning following the establishment of the standard reference, the step-wedge is radiographed at the same technical factors as the original standard. The resultant image is compared with the standard. If the wedge densities are off by more than one step, there is a problem with the radiographic imaging chain (Fig. 17–4).

If this is observed, the developer temperature should be checked first. Correct developer temperature does not rule out a processor malfunction. However, the most common processor problem is incorrect developer temperature. At this point, the cause of the incorrect density on the step-wedge is not known. If the problem is consistent, it can be compensated for until the cause of the problem can be determined.

It is most important to control the processor before beginning additional quality control tests.

Processor Quality Control

To more clearly define the causes of problems demonstrated with the simple, daily step-wedge QC test, a more extensive program of QC must be instituted. This program must begin with the processor, since many problems are processor-related. Many of the additional test procedures use film as a permanent recording medium. Processor quality control has four components:

1. Chemical activity
2. Cleaning
3. Maintenance
4. Monitoring

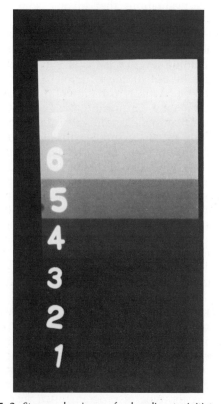

FIGURE 17-3. Step-wedge image for baseline to initiate a quality control program. This baseline image should be safely filed as the standard reference.

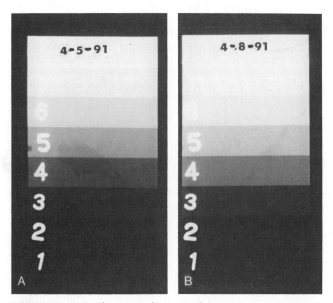

FIGURE 17-4. Quality control step-wedge image compared with the baseline. The most recent image is light by more than one step. This indicates some type of exposure or processing problem.

Chemical Activity

Chemical activity can be assured by accurate mixing of the chemical solutions and routine checking of replenishment rates and the chemical activity.

If the chemicals are mixed by hand, manufacturer's directions on the container must be followed exactly. If the chemicals are added with insufficient water, out of sequence, or without sufficient mixing, pH shock, precipitation, chemical layering, or other problems may result in inadequate chemical activity.

If a chemical mixer or premixed chemicals are used, the pH and specific gravity should periodically be tested to assure that the chemicals were mixed in the right proportions. A solution can exhibit correct pH and specific gravity but may be out of tolerance. This could be due to pH shock during mixing or some type of physical abuse to the chemistry such as freezing during transit or storage.

Use the processor manufacturer's guidelines for checking replenishment rates. Follow the chemistry and film manufacturers' recommendations for setting the rates and the total amount of chemistry added per film. Replenishment rates should be checked each time the processor is cleaned. A processor equipped with a replenishment indicator or rate gauge can routinely and visually be monitored as films are processed. Normally, replenishment rates are set using the 14-inch side of a 14- × 17-inch film as the norm. In order to maintain correct replenishment, follow the film-feed direction guide supplied with each processor.

Films fed into the processor in the wrong direction may produce under-replenishment or over-replenishment of chemicals. Under-replenishment allows the working chemicals to become depleted, resulting in loss of density and contrast. Over-replenishment wastes chemicals and may cause significant changes in contrast, especially with newer anticrossover film types.

Cleaning and Maintenance

Keeping the processor clean and performing simple preventive maintenance is the surest way to avoid processing artifacts and to reduce failure of the mechanical parts of the transport system. The initial step is to follow a routine procedure for start-up and shutdown of the processor.

1. We begin with the processor off. The top should be ajar to allow the developer and fixer fumes to escape without building up on the exposed rollers and gears. Turn on the water. If the unit has a mixing valve using hot and cold water, it is not necessary to allow the water to reach normal temperature before start-up cleaning.
2. Remove the top and crossover rollers, if they are removable. Rinse or wipe the crossover rollers to eliminate any chemical residues or emulsion build-up, turning the rollers by hand to clean all surfaces.
3. Observe the level of the developer and fixer, which should be within 1 mm of the top of the processing tank. If the level is low, activate the replenisher pump, or manually transfer replenisher from the

storage tank to the processor until sufficient chemical is added to fill the tank.

4. Turn on the processor, wipe all exposed rollers with a clean, damp cloth, being careful not to get the cloth caught in the rollers.
5. With the crossover removed, observe the rollers and gears for any hesitation or asymmetry of rotation. Check any exposed screws and roller tension springs for integrity. Tighten screws and replace broken tension springs when necessary.
6. Replace the crossover racks and the top. Check the incoming water temperature to be sure that it is within the manufacturer's suggested guidelines. This is usually 8 to 10° below the operating temperature of the developer. A processor can function acceptably if the water temperature is low. However, the developer heater must remain on to maintain the desired developer temperature. This significantly shortens the life of the heating element of the developer heater.
7. To shut down the processor at the end of the day, reverse the procedure. Remove the top and crossovers. Wipe down exposed rollers and crossovers. Ideally, the crossovers are removed and stored adjacent to the processor to minimize chemical fume encrustations. Turn off the processor. Turn off the water. Replace the top, leaving about 1½-inch gap for the chemical fumes to escape.

Following this simple 15- to 20-minute procedure adds years to the life of the processor and eliminates most processor transport artifacts.

Monitoring

The basic daily step-wedge procedure is expanded by using a *sensitometer* for processor monitoring. Use of a reliable, consistent exposure source (the sensitometer) in the test procedure for the processor attributes changes in the step-wedge or other simple QC procedures to equipment variation rather than the processor.

To initiate the processor control program, the processor is cleaned and filled with fresh, properly mixed chemicals. The developer is "seasoned" by adding the correct amount of starter solution and by processing eight to ten exposed, unprocessed sheets of scrap film.

Starter solution is stabilized potassium bromide. The replenisher solution mix contains no bromine (Br^-) ions. It is not necessary to replenish bromine, since the reduction of the silver bromide by the developer provides sufficient bromine ions to function as the restrainer. However, fresh chemicals must have bromine ions added before processing film to minimize *base plus fog*. Specific amounts of starter, usually about 100 ml per gallon of developer in the processor, are added to the developer, depending on the processor type and the manufacturer's recommendations.

Film strips cut from a specified box of film are exposed with the sensitometer and processed. The metal thermometer probe is used to measure the developer temperature. The average of these processed control strips becomes the standard reference (Fig. 17–5A). Without a *densitometer* to measure the film

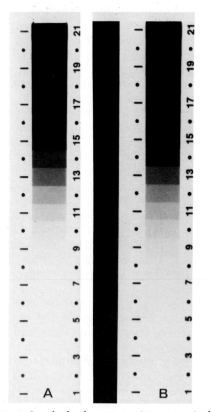

FIGURE 17–5. *A*, Standard reference sensitometer strip for processor. *B*, Sensitometer strip with increased density resulting from elevated developer temperature.

density values, subsequent strips can be compared only with the standard. The use of a densitometer is described in Chapter 10. If the new strip is "off" by one or more steps (Fig. 17–5*B*), a processor problem exists that requires correction.

The addition of a densitometer to the QC equipment allows accurate measurement of the sensitometric strip. Four density values are measured. These four values relate to the sensitometric evaluation measurements of speed, average gradient, and base plus fog. From the processed strip, three steps are identified (Fig. 17–6):

- S is the speed index step, which should have a density near 1.2 (1.0 above base plus fog)
- H is a high-density step, which should have a density near 2.2 (2.0 above base plus fog)
- L is a low-density step, which should have a density near 0.45 (0.25 above base plus fog).

H minus L is the contrast index. Base plus fog is measured in the clear area adjacent to the strip. These values are recorded in chart or graph form (Fig. 17–7) to monitor processor trends. These are known as trend charts and can indicate potential problems before they occur by showing movements toward unacceptable values.

The values from the sensitometric strip should fall within the standards recommended by the National Center for Devices and Radiological Health:

- Base plus fog: ±0.05
- Speed index: ±0.10
- Contrast index: ±0.10

Any values that fall outside the recommended variance require corrective action. A steady increase or decrease in the speed or contrast index, or an upward trend in base plus fog should receive attention before the values exceed allowable error.

Other Simple QC Test Procedures

Once the processor is being monitored in a QC program, other QC tests using film can be employed to monitor equipment function.

mAs Reciprocity

The step-wedge can also be used to perform a mAs *reciprocity* test. Theoretically, any combination of mA and time that produces the same mAs should produce the same exposure when all other variables are constant. This provides the same image density. The step-wedge and the QC cassette are used to produce three images of the wedge at three mA-time combinations —for example, 100 mA at 0.1 sec = 10 mAs; 200 mA at 0.05 sec = 10 mAs; 400 mA at 0.025 sec = 10 mAs.

All the step-wedge images should be the same density. Since all three step-wedge images are on the same

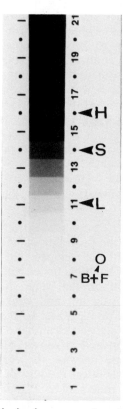

FIGURE 17–6. Standard reference sensitometer strip for processor quality control for use with densitometer. Specific steps to determine a contrast index are identified for reference as speed index, S; high, H; and low, L.

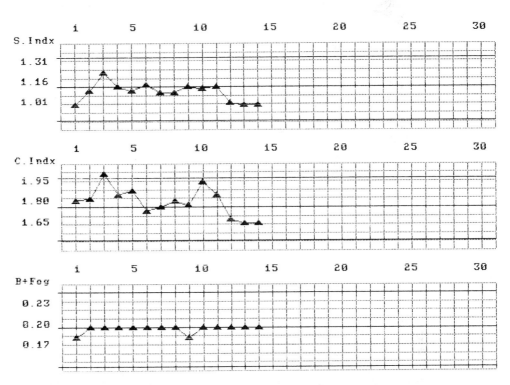

FIGURE 17–7. Trend chart plotting data from several weeks of sensitometric strips.

sheet of film, any differences are due to generator variation, not the processor. Small differences are normal. However, differences of more than one full step (Fig. 17–8) indicate a calibration problem.

X-ray Beam–Light Beam Congruence

To collimate tightly to the anatomy of interest, the area illuminated by the collimator light must coincide with the actual x-ray beam. The *congruence* of the x-ray beam and the projected collimator light beam is an extremely important factor in radiation protection and needs to be checked frequently.

One of the easiest QC tests to perform is the eight-cent test for x-ray beam–light beam congruence, or agreement. The x-ray beam–light beam congruence should be within 2% of the source-image distance (SID). For example, at a 40-inch SID, the x-ray–light beam congruence should be within 0.8 inch, or approximately the diameter of a penny.

To perform the eight-cent test, the SID, or focal film distance (FFD), is set at 40 inches. The collimator is adjusted to cover an area of about 8 × 10 inches on a 10- × 12-inch cassette. The eight pennies are arranged in the pattern shown in Figure 17–9. The pennies touch at the edge of the light beam, where the dark

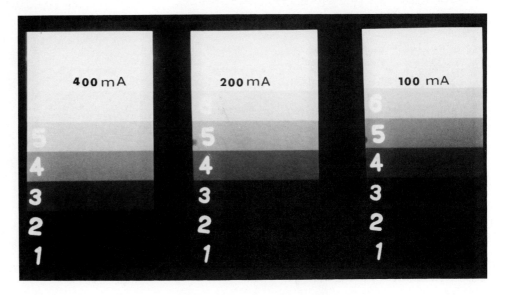

FIGURE 17–8. mAs reciprocity test using a quality control step-wedge.

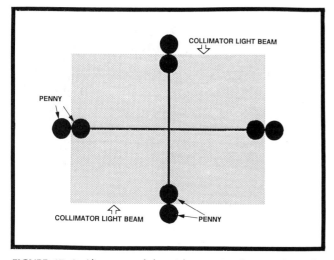

FIGURE 17–9. Alignment of the eight pennies, forming the eight-cent test tool.

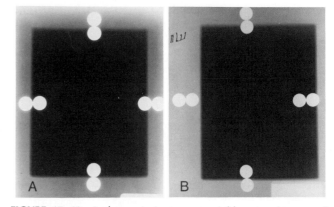

FIGURE 17–10. *A* demonstrates an acceptable x-ray beam and light congruence. *B* shows unacceptable alignment and collimator should be serviced immediately.

lines (cross hairs) intersect the edge of the light beam. A low-level x-ray exposure is made. The collimator is opened to cover the entire cassette, and a second exposure is made in order to visualize all the pennies. Proper *alignment* is evident when less than half a penny is included or excluded from the x-ray beam (Fig. 17–10*A*). If more than an extra half a penny is included in or excluded (Fig. 17–10*B*) from the original beam, the collimator is out of alignment.

X-ray Beam–Bucky Tray Alignment

The central ray of the x-ray beam must be aligned with the center of the cassette in the Bucky tray. This alignment can be checked by producing an image of a lead "o" placed 10 cm or so above the table top. Using the Bucky *centering detent locks,* align the central ray to the Bucky tray containing an 8- × 10-inch or 10- × 12-inch cassette. To aid in determining the direction of misalignment, place a metallic marker in the edge of beam, toward the Bucky tray handle. Align the lead "o" marker with the central ray cross hair. Make

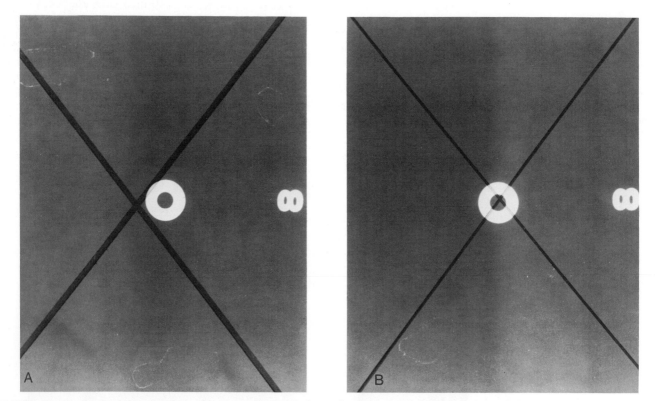

FIGURE 17–11. Check of the central ray alignment with the Bucky. *A* shows improper alignment of central ray and Bucky tray. Image *B* shows proper central ray–Bucky alignment.

an exposure sufficient to image the lead marker. Evaluate the alignment by marking an "x" on the film from corner to corner (Fig. 17–11). The "o" should be within 1 cm of the center of the film. If the alignment errors are greater than those stated, the collimator, tube mount, or centering detent lock must be adjusted.

Routine Physical or Visual Evaluations

The SID indicators and tube-angle indicators should also be evaluated for accuracy. The SID indicators are checked with a tape measure. Measure from the focal spot mark on the end cap of the metal tube housing to the table top and to the level of the Bucky tray. If the end cap does not have a focal spot mark, use a point about 2.5 cm from the bottom of the metal tube housing end cap as a reference point for the actual position of the focal spot. The distance indicators should be accurate within ±2% of the indicated value.

Check the angle indicators first by angling the tube in both directions to be sure that the indicators are not stuck. Then using a simple carpenter's level and a large plastic protractor, check the accuracy of the angle indicator.

ADVANCED GENERATOR AND X-RAY TUBE PERFORMANCE STANDARDS

With more sophisticated equipment, additional QC or performance tests of the generator and tube can be conducted. When a specific mA, kVp, or time value is set on the generator control panel, the generator should deliver those values with minimal variations. It is also important that the mA stations be linear to each other to achieve consistent image density using different combinations of mA and time for a specific mAs value.

Digital Dosimeter

One of the most common devices used for multiple QC test procedures is a dosimeter, or digital display ionization chamber (Fig. 17–12). Although these ion chamber dosimeters add to the cost of the QC program, the improved accuracy is worth the increased cost. Several tests of generator consistency and performance can be made with this unit using a single-equipment set-up when the distance is held constant. These tests include

1. mAs Reciprocity: The mAs and kVp are held constant, using different combinations of mA and time. The output (mR/mAs) should not vary more than 10%.
2. mA, or Time *Linearity*: With the kVp constant, either the mA *or* time is altered in multiples (2×,

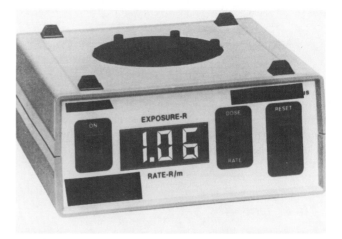

FIGURE 17–12. A simple ion chamber dosimeter for checking x-ray outputs.

4×, etc.). The output (mR) should be linear within 10% to the variable of mA or time being tested.
3. *Reproducibility.* The mA, time, and kVp are constant. The output should not vary by more than 10%.
4. kVp (*beam quality* test) using HVL.

Each set of data must be accurately gathered under precise conditions. The parameters such as kVp, mA, and time must be correctly set, with an exact alignment of the beam/ion chamber. Each of these tests is now described in greater detail.

mAs Reciprocity

Select at least three sets of exposure factors (mA × time) that produce the same mAs. Be sure to select combinations that represent mA and time values commonly used to produce images. Measure the exposure (mR) for each set of factors. Calculate the mR/mAs ratio for each exposure. Calculate the average value of the mR/mAs ratio. Determine the reciprocity variance by using the following formula:

$$\frac{\left(\dfrac{mR}{mAs_{max}} - \dfrac{mR}{mAs_{min}}\right)}{2} = \text{variance}$$
$$\overline{\text{Average } \dfrac{mR}{mAs}}$$

The variance should be less than 0.10.

))))) EXAMPLE

mA	sec	mAs	mR	mR/mAs
50	0.40	20	102	5.1
100	0.20	20	104	5.20
200	0.10	20	115	5.75
400	0.05	20	90	4.5

$$\text{Average } \frac{mR}{mAs} = 5.14 \qquad \frac{\dfrac{5.75 - 4.5}{2}}{5.14} \approx 0.121$$

This test indicates that the generator is not performing within allowable limits since the variance is greater than 0.10. However, since there are two variables, the error may be either mA or time related. Performing timer linearity and mA linearity tests with the same set-up will help determine the cause of poor performance.

Timer Linearity

Use the same time values as in the mAs reciprocity test. Keep the mA and kVp constant. The mA may be any value but should be one commonly used in clinical radiography. Measure the exposure (mR) for each set of factors. Calculate the mR/mAs for each exposure. Calculate the average mR/mAs. Determine the timer linearity variance by using the following formula:

$$\frac{\dfrac{\left(\dfrac{mR}{mAs_{\text{max}}} - \dfrac{mR}{mAs_{\text{min}}}\right)}{2}}{\text{Average } \dfrac{mR}{mAs}} = \text{variance}$$

The variance should be less than 0.10.

))))) EXAMPLE

mA	sec	mAs	mR	mR/mAs
100	0.40	40	201	5.0
100	0.20	20	106	5.30
100	0.10	10	51	5.10
100	0.05	5	24	4.8

$$\text{Average } \frac{mR}{mAs} = 5.05 \qquad \frac{\dfrac{5.30 - 4.8}{2}}{5.025} \approx .049$$

The time stations are well within allowable variance, since the value obtained is less than 0.10. Therefore, timer accuracy can probably be ruled out as the cause of the poor performance noted by the mAs reciprocity test. Thus the most likely cause is mA calibration. However, this should be confirmed with an evaluation of the mA linearity.

mA Linearity

Select one of the time values (this example uses 0.2 sec) from the mAs reciprocity test. Keep that time value and the kVp constant. Use the same mA values from the mAs reciprocity test. Measure the exposure (mR) for each set of factors. Calculate the mR/mAs

ratio for each exposure. Calculate the average mR/mAs. Determine the mA linearity variance by using the following formula:

$$\frac{\dfrac{\left(\dfrac{mR}{mAs_{\text{max}}} - \dfrac{mR}{mAs_{\text{min}}}\right)}{2}}{\text{Average } \dfrac{mR}{mAs}} = \text{variance}$$

The variance should be less than 0.10.

))))) EXAMPLE

mA	sec	mAs	mR	mR/mAs
50	0.20	10	50	5.0
100	0.20	20	105	5.25
200	0.20	40	228	5.70
400	0.20	80	362	4.525

$$\text{Average } \frac{mR}{mAs} = 5.12 \qquad \frac{\dfrac{5.70 - 4.525}{2}}{5.12} \cong 0.115$$

The resulting value of 0.115 indicates that the mA stations are not linear within acceptable limits. The normal response to this data would be to have a service engineer recalibrate the mA stations.

Reproducibility

The technologist also expects the same set of technical factors to produce the same exposure each time the set of factors is used. Many times a service engineer receives a request to correct "an erratic exposure" problem without any additional information.

Reproducibility is a test that can document a problem with erratic or inconsistent exposures. A set of exposure factors is selected. If a technologist indicates that certain technical factors are inconsistent, the set of factors should be the same as those used when the inconsistency occurred. For routine QC testing, the set of factors should be those used in clinical applications. Measure several exposures (mR) with the dosimeter.

At least three exposures must be made (some recommend five or ten). Five should be sufficient for QC, but more may be necessary to document a problem. If this test is performed to document a service request, it may be necessary to manipulate the mA, time, or kVp controls between exposures when the inconsistency is due to poor contact in one of the control relays or switches. Always make the exposures with the same technical values. Record the exposures and use the values in the following formula. The resulting variance should be less than 0.10.

$$\frac{mR_{\text{max}} - mR_{\text{min}}}{mR_{\text{max}} + mR_{\text{min}}} < 0.10$$

))))) EXAMPLE

100 mA, 0.1 sec, 80 kVp

Exposure #1	51 mR
Exposure #2	49 mR
Exposure #3	53 mR
Exposure #4	50 mR
Exposure #5	52 mR

$$\frac{53 - 49}{53 + 49} = \frac{4}{102} \cong 0.04$$

The data indicate this x-ray generator is consistent at the selected mA and time. This does not mean the generator is equally consistent at other mA or time settings.

Beam Quality

The consistency of the beam energy can be monitored by measurement of the half-value layer (HVL). The HVL can be used as a reference standard for kVp calibration or tube aging. Tube aging is a hardening of the beam as a result of tungsten deposits on the inside of the glass tube housing. For QC purposes, the HVL measured should not vary from its original value, established at the acceptance of the x-ray unit or at the start of the QC program.

The HVL is the thickness of any material that when placed in the x-ray beam, reduces the beam intensity to one half its original value. The HVL is dependent on the effective energy of the beam, which is primarily affected by the generator waveform, the total beam filtration, and the kVp. Thus the HVL provides information on the beam energy or quality that is more accurate and meaningful than the kVp. kVp indicates peak kilovoltage rather than the range of kilovoltages produced by the tube.

The HVL is used in a quality test to verify that the beam is sufficiently filtered to reduce the patient's exposure to low-energy radiation. The HVL is determined by constructing a plot of exposure (mR) compared with millimeters of aluminum *attenuator* plates added to the x-ray beam.

Set up the dosimeter, turn it on, and center the x-ray beam on the active portion of the ion chamber. Adjust the tube and the ion chamber so that the source-to-chamber distance is 60 to 80 cm. Carefully collimate the beam so that it is slightly larger than the ion chamber. Set an exposure technique—for example, 200 mA at 0.3 sec (60 mAs) and 80 kVp. Make an exposure using no attenuation plates to determine the initial radiation intensity (I_o).

Add aluminum plates between the collimator face and the ion chamber. Add the plates in sequence, placing 1.0, 2.0, 3.0, 4.0, 5.0, and 6.0 mm plates of aluminum in the beam. As each thickness of aluminum attenuator is added to the beam, measure the intensity with the aluminum plate in position. The tube, attenuator plate, and chamber alignment must stay constant during all measurements. Assemble the data by recording mR versus millimeters of aluminum added to the beam. Plot the data on semilog graph paper with millimeters Al on the X axis and mR on the Y axis (Fig. 17–13). Determine one half of the original intensity.

In Figure 17–13 the I_o is 200; one half of this is 100. Locate that value on the Y axis. Locate the intersection of that value with the curve resulting from the plot. Draw a vertical line from that point to the X axis. The value on the X axis is the HVL in millimeters for that x-ray unit at 80 kVp. In Figure 17–13, that line intersects the X axis at approximately 3.1 mm Al. For radiation protection regulations, the HVL must be >2.3 mm for an 80-kVp beam.

For QC monitoring, the determined value should remain nearly constant over time. If the HVL rises, this would indicate an increase in the actual kVp or tungsten deposits on the inside of the glass housing from vaporization of the target or filament. If the HVL decreases, this indicates a drop in the actual kVp.

The second HVL can also be determined. The second HVL is the fourth value layer (intersection of one fourth of the I_o on the curve), minus the first HVL. In Figure 17–13, one fourth of 200 is 50, and 50 mR intersects the curve at approximately 6.5 mm Al. The fourth value layer is approximately 6.5 mm Al, and the second HVL is 6.5 minus 3.1, or 3.4 mm Al.

By dividing the first HVL by the second HVL, the homogeneity coefficient is determined. It should be

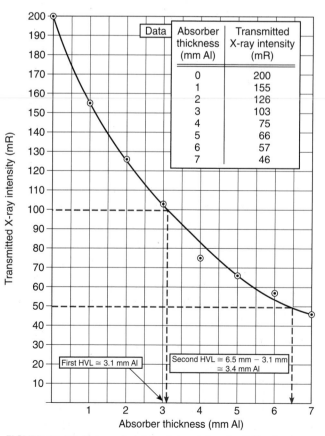

Data	Absorber thickness (mm Al)	Transmitted X-ray intensity (mR)
	0	200
	1	155
	2	126
	3	103
	4	75
	5	66
	6	57
	7	46

First HVL ≅ 3.1 mm Al

Second HVL ≅ 6.5 mm − 3.1 mm ≅ 3.4 mm Al

FIGURE 17–13. Data and plot for determining the half-value layer

less than 1.0. If the value is greater than one, the second HVL is smaller than the first HVL. This represents a significant problem with the equipment or the test methodology. Since each HVL removes photons of the lowest energies, each successive HVL should be larger than the previous HVL.

$$\text{Homogeneity coefficient} = \frac{\text{first } HVL}{\text{second } HVL}$$

))))))) EXAMPLE

From the data given in Figure 17–13, the homogeneity coefficient is

$$\text{Homogeneity coefficient} = \frac{\text{first } HVL}{\text{second } HVL}$$
$$= \frac{3.1 \text{ mm Al}}{3.4 \text{ mm Al}} \cong 0.91$$

Other Tests Performed by Dedicated Equipment

Kilovolt Peak

kVp calibration accuracy can be confirmed with a kVp test cassette (Ardran and Crooks cassette or Wisconsin test cassette). However, most QC programs have abandoned the kVp test cassette for more convenient, easy-to-use digital kVp test meters. kVp test meters are similar in size and shape to the QC dosimeter in Figure 17–14. The kVp test meter is placed on the radiographic table, and the x-ray beam is directed to the active area indicated on the top. The kVp meter is exposed, using kVp settings common to diagnostic radiography. The normal range is 50 to 140 kVp in 10- or 20-kVp increments. Follow the manufacturer's exposure recommendations to provide sufficient exposure to the meter for correct operation. The actual kVp measured by the meter is displayed. At least two readings should be made at each kVp evaluated. The kVp value displayed should be within ±5 kVp of the value set.

Timer Accuracy

Timer accuracy can be checked with one of several available test devices. If the generator is single-phase, a simple mechanical or manual spinning top can be used. The single-phase generator produces a pulsed x-ray beam with a period (dead time) between pulses when no x-rays are emitted from the tube head. The mechanical spinning top is placed on a cassette and is spun by hand. Before the top stops spinning, an exposure is made. The resulting image in Figure 17–15 shows a series of dots corresponding to the number of pulses of x-rays. A single-phase, half-wave rectified

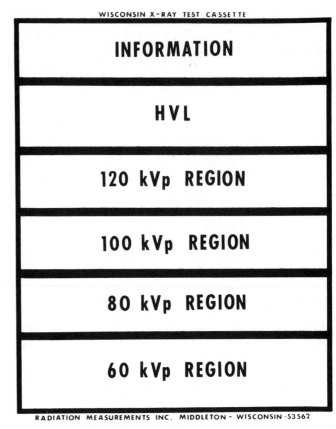

FIGURE 17–14. A kVp test cassette.

generator produces 60 pulses per second. A single-phase, full-wave rectified generator produces 120 pulses per second. The number of dots is divided by the number of expected pulses per second. The resulting value should correspond to the actual exposure time within ±5%.

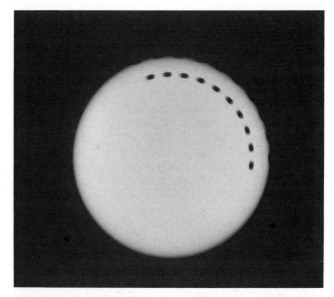

FIGURE 17–15. A manual spinning top image for a single-phase, full-wave rectified generator. The image shows ten dots, which would correspond to ten pulses of exposure.

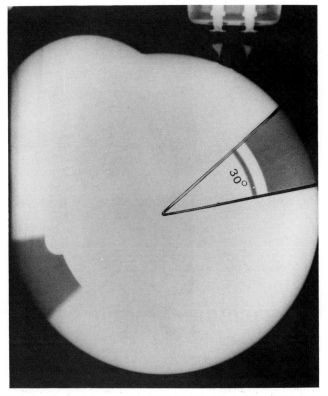

FIGURE 17–16. Motorized spinning top image. This 30° angle shows an actual exposure time of 0.083, or 1/12 sec.

For three-phase, or high-frequency, generators, which do not have dead time between pulses, a more sophisticated and expensive, motorized, synchronous spinning top, turning at one revolution per second may be used. The resulting image in Figure 17–16 demonstrates a solid arc of exposure without dots or pulses. The arc is measured with a simple protractor and divided by 360° to determine the actual exposure time in seconds.

Another timer test device, the digital timer test tool, shown in Figure 17–17, gives a direct readout of the actual exposure time. The digital timer test meter is

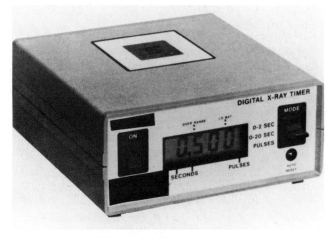

FIGURE 17–17. Digital timer test tool.

aligned with the central ray directed to an indicated area on the top of the meter. The SID is adjusted according to manufacturer's recommendations. The desired display mode of pulse, in seconds or milliseconds, is selected on the meter. The meter is exposed in a range of times commonly used in diagnostic radiography. It is especially important to check some of the extremely short exposure times because of the effect of a small error on the percentage of change from the original. The displayed values should be within ±5% of the timer settings. For example, a 0.003 sec error at 0.3 sec setting is not significant; however, if the selected time is 0.008 sec, a 0.003 sec error is excessive.

Focal-Spot Size

Only the pinhole camera can be considered 100% accurate in measurement of the focal spot. However, since the pinhole camera is difficult to use accurately and requires extremely high tube loading to achieve the pinhole images, an ongoing clinical QC program should evaluate the focal-spot size with a star pattern, such as shown in Figure 17–18, or similar QC device.

Focal spots "bloom", or become larger, as the tube ages. When the focal spot has reached an unacceptable size, the tube should be replaced because of increased geometric blur produced by the enlarged focal spot. It is difficult to determine how much enlargement is unacceptable. National Electrical Manufacturers Association (NEMA) standards for new tubes allow the focal spots to be 50% larger than the specified value. For example, a 0.6 mm focal spot may be as large as 0.9 mm and still be acceptable by NEMA standards. The amount of unacceptable focal-spot enlargement is usually a management decision. Management decides when focal-spot enlargement is unacceptable; there is no one set standard due to the wide variance allowed by NEMA.

The star-pattern test tool, when imaged correctly, utilizes the effect of geometric blurring on *resolving power* to determine the nominal size of the small and large focal spots. This procedure monitors any change in focal spot caused by blooming. The star pattern is used to evaluate focal-spot size because radiation from different sections of the focal spot produces areas of periodic blurring of the pattern, as a result of penumbra effects. Knowing the geometric factors and the width of the blurring on the image of the star permits calculation of the focal-spot size. This test provides accuracy similar to determinations with the pinhole camera.

Mount the star pattern on a radiolucent surface above a nonscreen image receptor, with one set of lines aligned with the anode-cathode axis. It is acceptable to tape the star pattern to the bottom of the collimator. Adjust the tube so that the star is about midway between the focal spot and the film (SID is about 24 inches). Adjust the beam so that the central ray is perpendicular to the center of the star pattern. Use the same mA station with the large and small focal spots.

Expose the film at 70 to 80 kVp with sufficient mAs to produce a suitable density. Process and check the

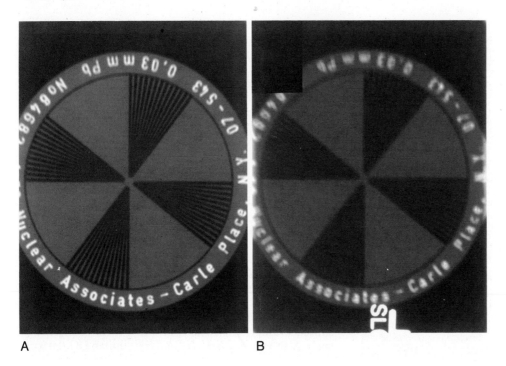

A   B

FIGURE 17–18. Star pattern image for measuring focal spot size, showing small (A) and large (B) focal spots.

image density. It should be about 1.3. Repeat the exposure if necessary. Determine the magnification by dividing the image diameter by the true diameter of the pattern. Scan the image of the star pattern to locate the blur, or zero-contrast band, a region with no contrast between the lines and spaces of the star, closest to the periphery. Mark the center of the blur band, and measure the transverse and anode-cathode diameters between the blur bands. If the blur band is too large for the pattern, decrease the magnification and repeat the exposure.

Calculate the focal spot size by the following formula:

$$\text{Focal-spot size (mm)} = \frac{N}{57.3} \times \frac{D}{(M-1)}$$

where:

N is the angle in degrees of the star pattern
D is the diameter of the zero-contrast region in mm
M is the magnification (i.e., size of the image divided by the size of the star-pattern disk)

Record the sizes for large and small focal spots. If the focal spot is more than 50% larger than desired, administration may elect to replace the tube.

QUALITY CONTROL ON ANCILLARY EQUIPMENT

The ancillary, or accessory, equipment, such as cassettes, screens, grids, illuminators, and protective apparel, should also be monitored on a routine basis.

Image Receptors

All image receptors (cassettes and intensifying screens) should routinely be checked for wear and mechanical damage. Each cassette should be inspected for wear, looseness, and light integrity. Cassettes with broken or loose latches, loose hinges, deteriorated light seals, or screen compression material should be replaced or repaired. Inspect the screens for wear, discoloration, abrasions, or stains.

Screen Cleaning

Clean screens on a periodic basis. The cleaning solution recommended by the screen manufacturer should be used. Be sure to use a soft, nonabrasive, lint-free cloth. Pour the screen cleaner onto the cloth, not directly onto the screen surface. Gently wipe the screen to remove dust and debris. Wipe off excessive cleaning solution and allow the screens to thoroughly air dry before reloading with film.

Screen-Film Contact

Periodically, each image receptor should be checked for screen-film contact by radiographing a wire-mesh test tool. Perform this test routinely, since the loss of contact can be gradual or subtle and difficult to detect from routine radiographs.

Expose all of the receptors on the radiographic table top. The wire mesh is placed in contact with the loaded image receptor on the table top. Use a technique that will produce a density near 1.5. Place the wire-mesh image on the viewbox and evaluate from 4 to 6 ft away. A wire-mesh image exhibiting good screen-film contact has a uniform density, as shown in Figure 17–19A, whereas an image exhibiting poor

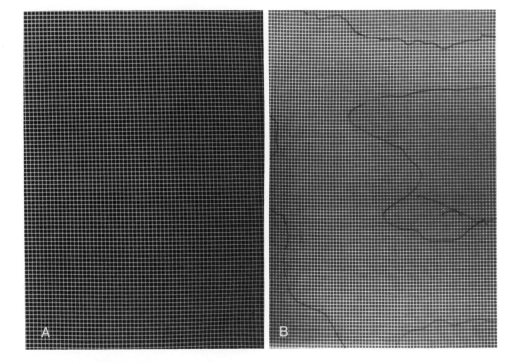

FIGURE 17–19. Wire mesh images to evaluate screen-film contact. *A,* Uniform density; good screen-film contact. *B,* Areas of poor screen-film contact are outlined in ink.

screen-film contact has areas that appear darker than the rest of the image (Fig. 17–19*B*). Good screen-film contact can sometimes be restored by replacing the foam or felt pressure pad under the screens. If the loss of contact is caused by a warped cassette frame, broken locks, or loose hinges, the cassette should be replaced or repaired. If the cassette is replaced, the screens can be removed and used in the new cassette, especially if they are less than three years old and in good condition.

Grids

Grids that are misaligned in the Bucky (grid cutoff) or stationary grids that have been damaged attenuate more of the primary beam. If the cutoff is not recognized, the resultant light radiographs cause the technologist to increase technical factors, resulting in higher patient exposure.

The following is a simple test to evaluate grid cutoff and to detect damaged grids. Place a homogeneous attenuator in the position normally occupied by the patient. The best attenuator is aluminum or plastic. However, a large flat container (>18 inches × 18 inches) filled with about 10 cm of water is usually easier to acquire. Place the phantom crosswise on the table or lengthwise on the stationary grid. If evaluating the Bucky-grid alignment, place the cassette in the Bucky drawer with the 17-inch dimension of the Bucky crosswise as for an AP projection of the pelvis. Use technical factors to produce a density of 1.3 to 1.5 in the center of the image.

A properly aligned, undamaged grid demonstrates a uniform density across the image. An uneven density indicates grid–central ray misalignment or grid damage and requires corrective action such as realignment of the beam or replacement of the grid.

Illuminators

Illuminator variation is probably the most overlooked aspect of radiographic quality control. An image may have perfect density on the illuminator by the processor but may appear dark on the illuminator that the radiologist is using. It is not uncommon for a radiologist to bring an image to the supervisor as too light or too dark. This can result from inconsistent illuminator densities or the acceptance level of the radiologist. Figure 17–20 shows how radiologists' concepts of image lightness or darkness must be considered by the technologist.

Illuminator intensity varies with the age of the bulb, the model or type of bulb, the color and thickness of the illuminator cover, and the cleanliness of the illuminator face. All bulbs in the illuminators must be the same model and from the same manufacturer; and they should be from the same production run. If one bulb in a panel of illuminators is replaced, all bulbs in the panel should be replaced to guarantee uniform illumination.

QC testing of illuminators is performed with a simple photographic light meter that can be purchased from a local camera store. The light meter is held at the same distance (2 to 3 ft) from each illuminator, and light readings are observed. If significant differences are noted, two actions are possible:

- Notify all members of the professional staff
- Act to correct the problem; however, replacement of a large number of bulbs in a large radiology facility would be extremely expensive

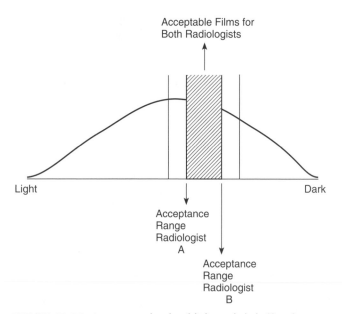

FIGURE 17-20. Acceptance levels of light and dark films by two radiologists and range of films are acceptable to both physicians. Radiologist A will accept lighter films, whereas Radiologist B prefers films that tend to be dark. Radiographers will probably need to produce films within a range acceptable to both radiologists.

Protective Apparel

Incorrect storage of protective lead aprons and gloves may lead to loss of protection because of cracks in one or more of the lead-vinyl layers. Periodically and before accepting new aprons, all protective apparel should be fluoroscoped or radiographed at 100 kVp to detect any loss of integrity. Some studies have indicated that 20% of new lead aprons and gloves may be defective. Cracks and other flaws should be reported to the radiation safety officer for corrective action, or in the case of new apparel, returned to the vendor.

REPEAT ANALYSIS

A *repeat film analysis,* also called a *reject film analysis,* is a systematic procedure of cataloging repeat films and determining the cause of repeats. Knowing the reason for repeats leads to solutions that will minimize the number of repeats, which in turn should lead to

- Improved departmental efficiency. Keeping the number of repeats low decreases the amount of time patients must spend undergoing procedures. This increases patient satisfaction and allows the department to x-ray more patients in the same period of time.
- Saving money through film, processing, and other costs. The estimated cost for a repeat film (this varies with silver costs, film size, cost of labor and so on) is $25 per film. An average of 20 repeats per day

costs a department, on average, $180,000 per year. That repeat rate could represent the cost of one room. Service costs now average $150 per hour; greater use of equipment means more service will be needed.
- Reduction of patient radiation exposure. For example, every time a repeat is needed on one view of a two-view series, radiation exposure is increased by about one third.

There are a variety of ways to conduct repeat analysis; these are not presented in detail here. What is most important is understanding the goal of a repeat analysis—to improve patient care.

Typically, a repeat analysis categorizes films according to the reasons they are repeated. These can include overexposure, underexposure, positioning, static, fog and motion—any reason that requires another film to ensure a diagnostic examination. Repeats are often collected by radiographic room, examination type, and, more rarely, technologist. One of the best uses of a repeat analysis is to determine areas for potential departmental inservice.

Consider the following data from one month in a four-room radiology department:

)))⟩⟩⟩) EXAMPLE

Reason for Repeat	Room 1 (%)	Room 2 (%)	Room 3 (%)	Room 4 %
Too Dark	35	30	35	35
Too Light	40	45	25	25
Centering	4	3	25	5
Positioning	20	18	7	29
Motion	1	4	8	6

A Pareto chart is commonly used in management to determine priority or frequent occurrences. A Pareto chart using these numbers can be found in Figure 17-21. This chart graphically shows the most common

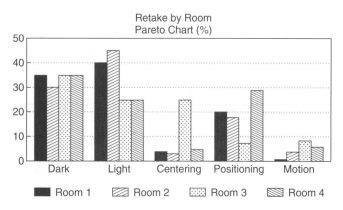

Series = Room number

FIGURE 17-21. Pareto chart graphically showing numerical values for repeats.

problems. A QC technologist can use these numbers to assist in determining the probable cause of mistakes. Questions asked should include

- Is the equipment at fault?
- Do certain technologists (e.g., new employees) show this trend?
- Is a department inservice necessary?

Note that Room 3 had a high percentage of repeats due to centering. A repeat analysis by examination type would be helpful in this case. Repeat analysis provides the quality assurance technologist with clues to performance. Actual determination of the cause of suboptimal films usually requires more "digging" on the part of the quality assurance technologist.

▓▓▓ Chapter Summary/ Important Concepts

Quality assurance refers to structured methods for monitoring and controlling variables in the clinical environment. Quality control (QC) is one aspect of total quality assurance. It usually refers to technical tests of imaging equipment. The three levels of QC tests are first, second, and third. The level of testing performed in a facility depends on the level of the facility and the training of technical personnel.

The most basic tests include daily penetrometer (step-wedge) checks; processor QC, to include chemical activity, cleaning, and maintenance, and monitoring; mAs reciprocity, using a step-wedge x-ray beam–light beam congruence; x-ray beam and Bucky tray alignment; and routine physical or visual evaluations.

Advanced generator tests and x-ray performance standards include the following tests performed with a digital dosimeter: mAs reciprocity, timer linearity, mA linearity, reproducibility, beam quality, and half-value layer tests. Other tests performed by dedicated equipment include tests using the digital kVp meter, tests for timer accuracy that use a manual or motorized spin top or a digital-timer test tool, and tests for focal-spot size using the pinhole camera or star test pattern.

Tests on ancillary equipment include image receptor tests and maintenance (cleaning screens and the wire mesh test), tests for grid cutoff and damage, illuminator tests, and tests of lead aprons and gloves.

Repeat analysis is a systematic procedure of cataloging repeat films and determining the cause of re-

peats. Knowing the reason for repeats lowers patient dose and decreases the cost of procedures.

Important Terminology

Alignment. The closeness of agreement between the center or edge of the x-ray beam and any piece of radiographic or QC equipment

Attenuator. Any object or material that reduces the intensity of an x-ray beam

Base Plus Fog. Inherent density of an unexposed, processed sheet of film as a result of the opacity of the base and spontaneously produced latent image as meant in the emulsion

Beam Quality. Energy of an x-ray beam

Centering Detent Lock. Mechanism that locks the x-ray tube in place with the Bucky; centers and aligns vertically the x-ray tube, film, and Bucky

Congruence. Closeness of agreement between the size and edge alignment of the x-ray beam and the collimator light field

Control Strip. Series of sequential densities or steps on a sheet of film that has been exposed by a sensitometer or by x-rays passing through a step-wedge

Densitometer. Device used to measure the photographic or optical density of film

Density or Optical Density. Measurement of the opacity of processed film owing to deposition of silver grains in the emulsion. Density = log opacity, or $\log_{10} (I_o/I_t)$, where

$$I_o = \text{incident light intensity}$$

$$I_t = \text{transmitted light intensity}$$

(See Chapter 10 for more details.)

Linearity. Ability of an x-ray system to produce exposures that have a linear relationship to the variable that has been altered, e.g., double the time, double the exposure; kVp cannot have linearity

Penetrometer (Step-Wedge). Device (usually of aluminum) consisting of a series of steps of increasing thickness; provides a measurement of x-ray beam quality and quantity when exposed on an x-ray film

Quality Assurance. Structured methods to monitor and control variables in the clinical environment

Quality Control (QC). One aspect of total quality assurance; usually refers to technical tests of imaging equipment

Radiographic Imaging Chain. Refers to all the components needed for a finished radiograph, from x-ray tube to processor

Reciprocity. Ability of an x-ray system to produce the same exposure for the same mAs regardless of the mA and time combination used

Reject or Repeat Film Analysis. Systematic evaluation of repeated radiographs to determine the cause of repeat exposure

Reproducibility. Ability of an x-ray system to produce

the same exposure from the same technical factors time after time

Resolving Power. Ability of an imaging chain to record small structures that are extremely close together

Sensitometer. Device used to provide a precise, consistent graduated step, light exposure to a sheet of film

Bibliography

Basic Quality Control in Diagnostic Radiology. American Association of Physicists in Medicine (AAPM) Report #4, 1978.

Burkhart, R.L. A Basic Quality Assurance Program for Small Diagnostic Radiology Facilities. Washington, DC: U.S. Dept. of Health, Education, and Welfare, U.S. Government Printing Office, 1983.

Burkhart, R.L. Checklist for Establishing a Diagnostic Radiology Quality Assurance Program. Washington, DC: U.S. Dept. of Health, Education, and Welfare, U.S. Government Printing Office, 1983.

Burkhart, R.L. Quality Assurance Programs for Diagnostic Radiology Facilities. Washington, DC: U.S. Dept. of Health, Education and Welfare, U.S. Government Printing Office, 1988.

Gray, J.E., Winkler, N.T., Stears, J., et al.: Quality Control in Diagnostic Imaging. Rockville, MD: Aspen Publishers, 1983.

McKinney, W.E.J. Radiographic Processing and Quality Control. Philadelphia: J.B. Lippincott, 1988.

Quality Assurance for Diagnostic Imaging. Report #99. Bethesda, MD. National Committee on Radiation Protection and Measurements (NCRP) Publications, 1988.

Walton M: The Deming Management Method. New York: Perigree Books, 1986.

⬛ Review Questions

1. Why are quality assurance and quality control programs important in a radiology facility?
2. What are the major differences between quality assurance and quality control?
3. What are the major components of processor quality control?
4. What values are taken from the processor quality control sensitometric strip?
5. What quality control tests should be routinely performed on x-ray equipment?

6. What is the primary function of the following tests?
   a. 8 cent
   b. mAs reciprocity
   c. star pattern
   d. wire mesh
7. What are the primary goals of a quality control program?
8. What type of quality control testing is normally *not* performed by technologists?
9. What type of test would detect the build-up of tungsten inside the glass housing of the tube?
10. A mechanical spinning top may be used to check the timers of _____ generators.

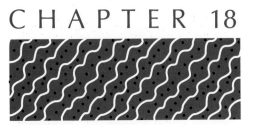

CHAPTER 18

General Radiation Biology

Alfred J. Lawson, Ph.D.
Steven B. Dowd, Ed.D., R.T.(R)

Chapter Outline

Chapter Objectives

On completion of this chapter, you should be able to

- Label the segments of the dividing cell cycle and their relative radiation sensitivity.
- Describe the collection of sciences used to ascertain the effects of radiation on living tissue.
- Explain the two mechanisms of radiation energy transfer to biological systems.
- Describe the result of radiation energy transfer to a cell's genetic material.
- Explain how DNA repair affects the results of radiation injury.
- Differentiate between dividing and nondividing cells in their response to radiation injury.
- Differentiate between direct and indirect damage.
- Identify the cellular conditions that modify the interaction of radiation with various components of the cell.
- Label and describe the principle components within a mammalian cell.
- Describe the concepts of LET, RBE, and OER and their interrelationship.
- Explain why the results of radiation damage are dependent on the division potential of cells irradiated.
- List the acute radiation syndromes.
- Describe the radiosensitivity of various organs.
- Differentiate between radiation injury to an adult and that to a fetus.
- Describe the differences between radiation damage of male and female reproductive organs.
- Describe the fetal effects of radiation before and after implantation of the fertilized ovum.
- Explain the association of sublethal radiation injury and carcinogenesis.
- Outline the time-related development of acute, delayed, and late radiation effects.

Radiation biology makes use of a collection of sciences, including biology, radiation physics, and epidemiology to ascertain the effects of radiation on living tissue. There are aspects of radiation biology that are well understood—primarily radiation physics-related topics—and those that are poorly understood, such as the long-term effects of low-level radiation on human beings. This is illustrated in Table 18–1.

A variety of factors affect radiation response. The following are discussed in this chapter:

- Mitotic rate
- Oxygen concentration
- Dose rate
- Radiation type
- Repair capability
- Radioprotective substances

Table 18–1: CONTINUUM OF RADIATION EFFECTS

Level of Understanding			
High	*Good*	*Medium*	*Poor**
Radiation production	Chemical effects	Single-cell effects	Cellular carcinogenesis
Dosimetry			Tissue-level effects
Atomic level interactions			Host effects
			Clinical cancer induction

* These are poorly understood because of confounding and synergistic effects that may not be due to radiation (e.g., combining smoking with radiation exposure).

Table 18–2: CELL COMPOUNDS

Components	Percent	Functions
H_2O	85%	Universal solvent; chemistry of water essential to organism survival
Protein	10%	Structural communication enzymes (facilitators)
CHO	1.5%	Energy storage; antigenic diversity
Lipids	2%	Energy stages; membranes
Minerals and miscellaneous	1.5%	Cofactors and stabilizers

This chapter concentrates on theoretical aspects of radiation biology. This leads into the next chapter, which discusses the clinical implications of radiation biology.

REVIEW OF CELL BIOLOGY

To understand the variable expression of radiation injury within a biologic cell system, a review of cell biology is valuable. Water constitutes approximately 85% of the cell. Distributed within this water is a variety of subcellular components which are composed of various combinations of proteins, carbohydrates, lipids, and nucleic acids. Table 18–2 summarizes the functions of these components. Each component provides a

wide variety of functions within a given cell. For example, lipids can be found within various cellular membranes, where they provide both structure and permeability barriers to random diffusion of molecules and may also function as a storage site for metabolic reserves (adipose tissue).

The schematic presentation of cellular structure in Figure 18–1 is a two-dimensional representation of a dynamic three-dimensional structure. The dynamic aspect of a single cell refers to the continuous replacement and turnover of subcellular components, the expression of cell function, as well as the capacity for cell division. Table 18–3 summarizes the location and function of the organelles (small organs) of the cell. The source of diversity in a cell is contained in the *deoxyribonucleic acid (DNA)* sequences within the cell nucleus. This genetic code provides the instructions for production of new subcellular components, as well as their assembly, utilization, and expression.

The ability of a cell to survive moment to moment is largely thought to be determined by the adequacy of

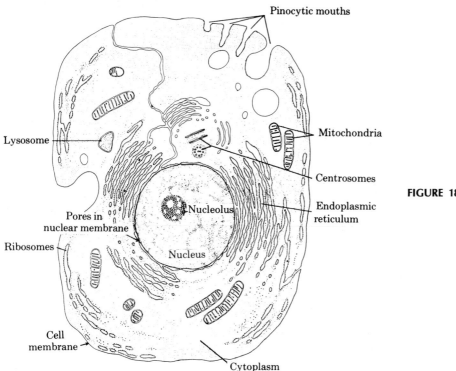

FIGURE 18–1. The cell.

Table 18-3: LOCATION AND FUNCTION OF CELLULAR ORGANELLES

Organelle	Function
Cytoplasm	
Cell membrane	Limiting structure; actively and passively regulates the flow of all substances in and out of the cell
Endoplasmic reticulum	
Granular	Protein synthesis
Agranular	Not well understood; may make substances other than proteins
Golgi bodies	Concentrate and package secretory products; carbohydrate synthesis and the binding of other organic compounds to proteins
Lysosomes	Contain enzymes capable of breaking down proteins and carbohydrates
Mitochondria	Source of energy provided through oxidation; also involved in protein synthesis and lipid metabolism
Ribosomes	Release protein in response to messenger-RNA
Nucleoplasm	
DNA	Directs cellular activity; also transmits genetic information
Chromosomes	Linear threads that contain DNA
Genes	Basic unit of heredity; located on chromosomes
Nuclear membrane	Prevents some materials from being exchanged between the cytoplasm and nucleus; allows others to pass
Nucleolus	Contains most of the RNA
RNA	Controls protein synthesis

the membrane barriers represented by the cell or plasma membrane. The selective permeability of membranes is maintained by the continuous metabolism of carbohydrates and the resulting production of high-energy phosphate compounds that serve as the energy source for most of the subcellular reactions.

In contrast to the acute survival of cells, the long-term survival of the cell is determined by the adequacy of the genetic material contained within the nucleus. Damage to the DNA may impair the cell's ability to provide the correct code for the assembly of required proteins and lipids to maintain long-term viability of a given cell. Additionally, alteration of the DNA may prohibit a given cell from undergoing division and may therefore deplete cell populations that are dependent on continuous cell replacement (such as cell types contained within the bone marrow, skin, and gastrointestinal tract).

Cell Cycle: Mitosis

The cell cycle has two phases. First, a mitotic phase, in which recognizable structures (chromosomes) appear within the nucleus and are distributed equally to the next generation of cells. Second, the time period between the end of *mitosis* and the initiation of the next mitosis is described as the interphase of the cell. Through the use of radioactive tracers in various subcellular components, interphase has been found to be composed of an active period of DNA synthesis described as the "S-phase." This discovery yielded two gaps in knowledge concerning the operations within the cell ongoing between the end of mitosis and the initiation of the synthetic phase and between the conclusion of the S-phase and the initiation of mitosis. These were titled "G-1" and "G-2."

Today it is commonly believed that cells not actively dividing reside within G-1 before beginning the next round of DNA synthesis. The length of G-1 is highly variable and may range from one to eight hours. The S-phase is characterized by the accumulation of DNA metabolites and the replication of the DNA by a process termed semiconservative replication. At the conclusion of the S-phase, complete chromosome duplication has occurred—that is, two complete and distinct copies of the normal genetic sequence are contained within the nucleus. The duration of the S-phase is approximately six to eight hours. During the G-2 phase of the cell cycle, cellular mechanisms are preparing for entry into mitosis and ultimate division of the cell. G-2 lasts approximately two to four hours.

Mitosis is composed of four distinct phases, which are described as follows (Fig. 18-2):

1. Prophase. Genetic material undergoes condensation, which gives rise to recognizable chromosomes; by late prophase, the nuclear membrane disappears; the chromosomes have a random orientation, and spindle fibers are formed.
2. Metaphase is identified by the alignment of chromosomes along the central axis of the cell. This is the phase of mitosis that is used to perform morphological assays for chromosome abnormalities.
3. Anaphase is characterized by the separation of the chromosomes and their movement toward opposite ends of the cell.
4. Telophase. The chromosomes become less distinct; the nuclear membrane is reconstructed. Mitosis is completed when the cell membrane partitions the original cell into two new cells.

Mitosis is the shortest phase of the cell cycle, requiring only 30 to 45 minutes for completion.

Cell Cycle: Meiosis

Meiosis (Fig. 18-3) is a type of cell division of germ cells (sperm or ova) in which two successive divisions of the nucleus produce cells that contain half the

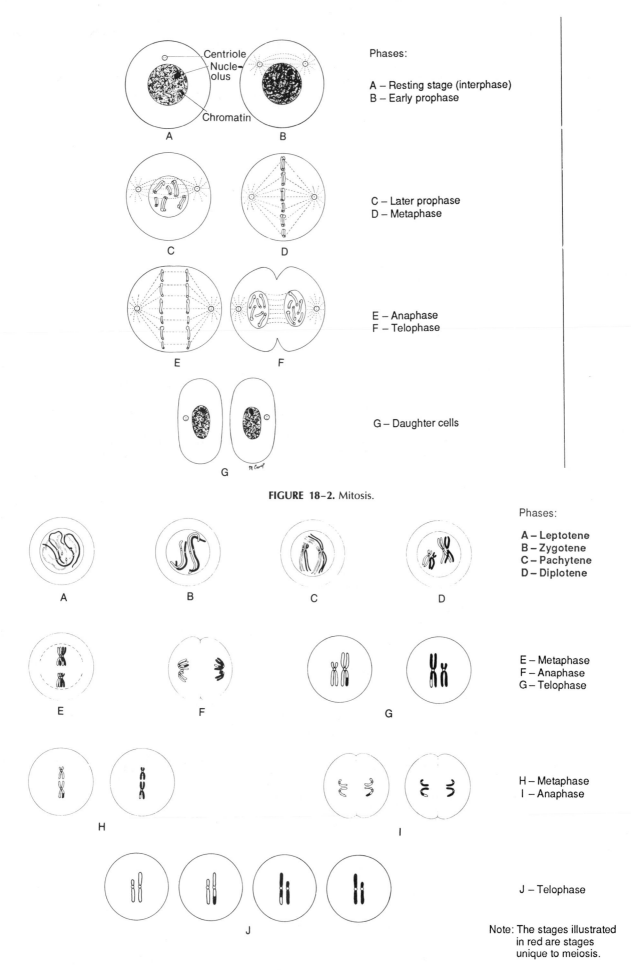

Phases:

A – Resting stage (interphase)
B – Early prophase

C – Later prophase
D – Metaphase

E – Anaphase
F – Telophase

G – Daughter cells

FIGURE 18-2. Mitosis.

Phases:

A – Leptotene
B – Zygotene
C – Pachytene
D – Diplotene

E – Metaphase
F – Anaphase
G – Telophase

H – Metaphase
I – Anaphase

J – Telophase

Note: The stages illustrated in red are stages unique to meiosis.

FIGURE 18-3. Meiosis.

number of chromosomes present in somatic cells. Thus the normal number of somatic chromosomes first is doubled to produce tetrads. Then a first division produces two cells with the normal diploid somatic number; these then divide again to produce cells with a haploid number.

DIRECT AND INDIRECT DAMAGE

Radiation exposure of cells may result in

- No damage
- Direct alteration of essential molecules within the cell
- Indirect alteration through the generation of free radicals resulting from the ionization of water (Fig. 18-4)

Within cells, DNA is the essential target molecule for the cells' long term survival. Damage sustained within DNA is thought to alter the genetic sequence and impair ongoing cellular functions and the ability to divide. More specifically, ionizations within DNA may result in either single- or double-strand breaks since DNA is a double-stranded helical molecule. Single-strand breaks can be quickly repaired and restored to the normal sequence. Misrepair of a single base leads to a *point mutation*. Point mutations are frequently undetectable and are largely considered to be sublethal alterations to the DNA. A double-strand break of the DNA represents an irreparable form of damage to the DNA and may induce a *frameshift mutation*. Frameshift mutations may alter the expression of a greater number of bases within the genetic sequence. Double-strand breaks may provide a greater opportunity to induce cell lethality. Direct damage of the DNA is a relatively low-probability event, since it is greatly outnumbered by other molecules within the cell, such as proteins, lipids, inorganic materials, and most importantly, water (Table 18-4 illustrates the relative density of DNA in relation to other cellular molecules).

X-rays represent a category of radiation that is char-

Table 18-4: RELATIVE DENSITY OF DNA IN RELATIONSHIP TO OTHER MOLECULES

Substance	Number of Molecules Per Molecule of DNA
DNA	1
RNA	4.4
Protein	700
Other organic	4000
Lipids	7000
Inorganic materials	7.0×10^4
Water	1.2×10^7

acterized by a low *linear energy transfer (LET)*. LET is a numerical value used to describe the quantity of energy deposited in a medium per unit of path length traveled. This is described in greater detail later in the chapter. Radiations interact within the absorber in a random fashion; therefore, they are most likely to interact with molecules present in the greatest concentration. As noted earlier, 85% of the cell consists of water molecules. The indirect pathway of damaging cells represents ionizations occurring within water that subsequently affect other molecules such as DNA.

Figure 18-5 indicates a diagrammatic relationship for the radiolysis of water. The hydroxyl *free radical* is thought to cause approximately two thirds of all radiation damage. Damage through the indirect pathway most likely achieves single-strand breaks of DNA because of the extremely low probability of free radical attack on the double-stranded DNA molecule at points immediately opposite one another.

Acute lethality to cells from extremely high doses of radiation (20,000 cGy*) is thought to represent disruption of membrane permeability barriers. This temporary disruption leads to a passive diffusion of calcium from the extracellular fluid into the cell. The increase of intracellular calcium disrupts a variety of metabolic events within the cell that may ultimately cause the death of that individual cell. The DNA, although damaged, may not be involved with the mechanism of acute cell death.

The ratio of direct to indirect damage may be modified by the type of radiation which is employed. The higher the LET, the greater the probability of direct

---

* The unit used throughout this chapter is the *centigray* (cGy), which is equivalent to the traditional unit of the rad. Units are discussed in greater detail in Chapter 20. The gray is equivalent to 100 rads.

$$HOH \longrightarrow HOH^+ + e^-$$
$$HOH + e^- \longrightarrow HOH^-$$
$$HOH^+ \longrightarrow H^+ + OH^-$$
(This causes about 2/3 of all biologic damage)

$$HOH \longrightarrow OH^- + H^-$$

The water molecules may then either recombine to form a normal water molecule, or they may chemically react to damage cellular macromolecules.

FIGURE 18-5. Radiolysis of water.

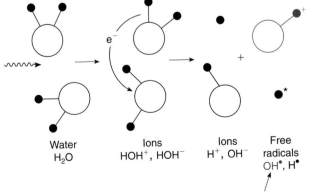

Water
H₂O

Ions
HOH⁺, HOH⁻

Ions
H⁺, OH⁻

Free radicals
OH•, H•

Note: This is the hydroxyl free radical, responsible for 2/3 of biologic damage.

FIGURE 18-4. Free radical formation.

damage and disruption of the DNA structure. The higher the total dose and dose rate, the greater the probability of acute cell death. Low-LET radiations may sterilize cells' ability to divide but may allow their continued metabolism for a given period of time—that is, the cells may morphologically look relatively normal, but reproductively they have been sterilized (mitotic death).

Cells that die before entry into the next mitotic phase are deemed to have died an interphase death. In general, mitotic death may occur at lower doses of radiation but it may require longer periods of time to be evident compared with interphase death. Interphase death requires high total doses of radiation, but the nature of the injury is seen within hours of the deposition of the radiation energy. The indirect pathway for damaging intracellular components can be modified by the addition of agents modifying reactions of the free radicals induced within the intracellular water. Compounds that minimize the transfer of damage from free radicals to essential cellular components can provide radiation protection. Such compounds are generally composed of *sulfhydryl* groups. They operate at multiple levels within the cellular physiology to minimize the amount of indirect damage sustained. One of the principal mechanisms that may either enhance free radical damage or minimize its effects comes from manipulation of the oxygen concentration.

Procedures that reduce the oxygen content provide radiation protection to the cell, whereas compounds that increase oxygen or mimic the presence of oxygen increase the cellular radiosensitivity.

FACTORS INFLUENCING RADIATION ENERGY TRANSFER

Ionizing radiations differ in terms of a variety of characteristics, including charge, mass, and energy. Concepts have been developed that permit the comparison of various radiations to induce a given endpoint, such as destruction of a certain percentage of cells or the amount of energy produced. Central to the understanding of radiation injury and modification of that injury is an understanding of three concepts. These are described in greater detail following.

Linear Energy Transfer

The LET of a given radiation describes the amount of energy transferred (absorbed) per unit of path length. LET is expressed in units of keV/μm. LET describes the average amount of energy transferred as radiation passes through an absorber. Because it is an average, it is important to stress that there are variations in energy deposition along that path. Some representative LETs are listed here.

Type of Radiation	LET in keV/μm
Diagnostic x-ray	3
10 MeV protons	4
5 MeV alpha particles	100
Heavy nuclei	1000

There are two broad categories of LET radiations—low and high (Fig. 18–6). Table 18–5 provides a comparison of low- and high-LET radiations and their characteristics. For the purposes of this discussion, low LET radiation can be summarized as being sparsely ionizing and having a random interaction potential along the path length of the radiation. Because of the low ionization potential, these radiations tend to have the capacity to travel great distances in air or tissue and clearly present an external hazard. Examples of low LET radiations are x-rays and gamma photons. Within biological systems, low-LET radiations are considered to exert their damage by the indirect pathway, the generation of free radicals, and single-strand breaks of the DNA. Since the lesions in the DNA are single-stranded, perfect repair is a highly likely outcome.

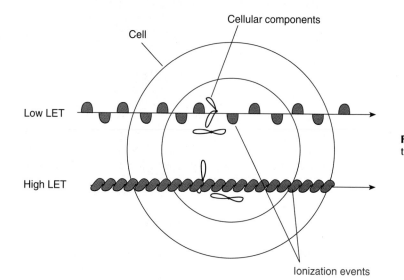

FIGURE 18–6. Illustration of high and low linear energy transfer (LET).

Table 18–5: COMPARISON OF LOW- AND HIGH-LET RADIATIONS

Low LET	High LET
<10 keV/μm	>10 keV/μm
Sparsely ionizing	Densely ionizing
Random interactions	Uniform energy deposition
Penetrating radiation	Superficial penetration
External radiation hazard	Internal radiation hazard
Indirect damage	Direct damage
Single-strand break	Double-strand break
Predominately perfect repair	Highly error prone
Point mutation	Frameshift mutation
Sublethal	More likely lethal
Dependent on oxygen concentration (maximum OER)	Independent of oxygen concentration (minimal OER)
Examples: x-ray photon	Fission fragments, charged particles

Therefore, low LET radiations are considered to induce sublethal alterations within the cell.

High LET radiations, in comparison, are densely ionizing and more uniform in distance between ionizations. Because of the increased density of ionization, high LET radiations tend to penetrate poorly and pose more internal risk than external hazard. Once internalized, the total path length of the radiation may be equal to only several cell thicknesses. Therefore, high LET radiations impart more energy to individual cells than the low LET radiation. Examples of high LET radiations are alpha particles, low-energy neutrons, and fission fragments.

Within the biological system, the transferred high LET radiation energy has an increased likelihood of double-stranded breaks in DNA, which are poorly repaired, and thereby provides an increased potential to induce a lethal alteration. For double-stranded DNA breaks, the complementary base section of the DNA is similarly damaged; therefore, the mechanisms of repair are much more highly error-prone and cell death is more likely.

Relative Biological Effectiveness

The second important concept that aids in categorizing various radiations is *relative biological effectiveness (RBE)* as shown in Table 18–6. Because of the

Table 18–6: RELATIVE BIOLOGICAL EFFECTIVENESS (RBE)

$$RBE = \frac{\text{standard radiation dose (cGy)}}{\text{test radiation dose (cGy)}}$$ Comparison made at the same end point

Also expressed as

$$RBE = \frac{\text{dose of 250 keV x-ray}}{\text{dose of test radiation}}$$ To achieve same effect or end point

RBE may vary by the end point selected as well as the assay used

variation in the rate of energy transfer, different LET radiations produce different degrees of the same biologic response. That is, equal doses of two different LET radiations do not necessarily yield the same biologic response.

The concept of RBE is defined as the comparison (ratio) of a dose of test radiation to elicit a given end point, such as killing ninety percent (90%) of the cells exposed to that amount of radiation and comparing that with the dose of radiation required to achieve the same biological end point when a standard radiation is used (e.g., a 250-kV x-ray). Using this definition of radiation interaction provides a *quality factor* for the conversion of delivered dose from various radiations to a different unit. This provides a more direct measure of the potential for that dose to cause injury. Previously, this quality factor would be used to convert a radiation absorbed dose (rad) to roentgen equivalents-man (rem). Today, it is more appropriate to say that it would be used to convert a dose measured in *grays* (Gy) into sieverts (Sv). The RBE of a given radiation provides a broad general statement of the potential of that radiation to cause biological injury. It is not sufficiently quantitative or exact, since the same radiation may have different rates of energy transfer to the medium, depending on where along the path length this energy transfer is measured, and it may also vary, based on the initial energy of a specific radiation.

Additionally, the RBE for a given radiation type may also vary, based on the biological end point used in the analyses. Therefore, it is important to stress that the concept of RBE provides only generalization as to the potential impact of a given radiation and does not necessarily describe the specific situation at hand.

Oxygen Enhancement Ratio

The final term that assists in the conceptualization of radiations and how they interact within a biological system is *oxygen enhancement ratio (OER)*. The OER is measured by comparison of the amount of cellular injury (e.g., lethality to cells) induced in the presence of oxygen with that in the absence of oxygen.

Those radiations, such as x-rays, that require well-oxygenated conditions to exert their greatest effects are said to have a high OER (i.e., OER equals 3.0). Other radiations, such as alpha particles, demonstrate an insensitivity to oxygen concentration, and the same radiation dose in the absence of oxygen induces the same level of effect as in the presence of oxygen (thus OER equals 1). The differential response between the absence and presence of oxygen to a given radiation is thought to represent the importance of oxygen in propagating free radical damage induced in the indirect pathway previously discussed.

Relationships Among the Three Factors

The interrelationship of these three parameters—LET, RBE, and OER—can be described as follows:

- As the LET of the radiation increases, particularly beyond 10 keV per micrometer, the RBE of the radiation dramatically increases
- Inversely, as the LET of the radiation increases beyond a value of 10 keV per micrometer, the importance of oxygen to maximum biological effect is dramatically decreased. Thus RBE and OER (in general) decrease.
- In terms of the effect of oxygen, in its increased presence the indirect effect is amplified, and the volume of action for low LET radiation is enlarged. The effective volume by action for high LET radiation remains unchanged, since maximum injury will have been inflicted by direct effect.

GENETIC EFFECTS

A *mutation* of DNA can be defined as a permanent change in the primary sequence of DNA bases that in turn provides an altered set of instructions for some cellular function. In classic genetics, a gene mutation is called a point mutation. Point mutations are not microscopically detectable but may result in an altered phenotype, such as sickle cell anemia. These result from the substitution of a single amino acid in the protein structure of a gene, which may arise from a single alteration along the sequence of DNA bases. Radiations can cause strand breakage of DNA, and if the exact original sequence of DNA bases is not restored leads to a mutation of the broken section of the DNA. The substitution, gain, or loss of one or more bases in the DNA molecule can cause such mutations. Point mutations may give rise to a nonsense or an inappropriate mis-sense codon, which will provide no useful information for that particular segment of DNA. That is, a change in a sequence is similar to a change in a word. "Rowd" is not identifiable as "word," and "w _ _ d" is similarly unintelligible.

Frameshift mutations result from the gain or loss of one or more DNA bases. Such a mutation can alter the interpretation of an extended length of DNA sequence and provides a greater probability for the induction of a detectable change.

Two researchers have provided us with the bulk of research on genetic effects. First, Muller's (1927) experiments with fruit flies *(Drosophila melanogaster)* led to a variety of conclusions:

1. There was no increase in the quality of mutations or the types of observed mutations. Instead, radiation was found to increase those types of mutations found spontaneously in nature.
2. Most mutations observed were recessive. Thus both parents had to carry the gene for the effect to be observed in the offspring.
3. No threshold was observed. Lethal mutations increased equally with equal increases in dose; thus the effects observed were linear and nonthreshold.
4. It did not matter whether one large dose or many small doses (fractionated) were given, so long as

the total amount of radiation was the same. This suggests that mutations were single-hit phenomena and were cumulative in nature.

A husband-wife team (Russell, 1963) experimented with millions of mice over a period of many years (known as the "megamouse" experiment). Their data differed from Muller's in that a dose-rate effect (number 4 above) was seen; a given dose extended over a long period of time showed fewer effects genetically than one large dose.

Cytogenetic Effects

It has been said that mutations currently alter the reproductive fitness or life span of 10% of the population. For some of these conditions the causal relationship is better established than for others. In other cases, radiation is suspected of causing these effects. From human studies (follow-ups) and animal experiments, data exist that show radiation can cause the following:

- Leukemia and other forms of neoplasm
- Altered sex ratios
- Increased spontaneous abortion or stillbirth
- Increased infant mortality
- Increased congenital effects
- Decreased life expectancy
- These dominant inheritable diseases:
    achondroplastic dwarfism
    polydactyly
    Huntington's chorea
- These recessive inheritable diseases:
    cystic fibrosis
    Tay-Sachs
    hemophilia
    albinism

Doubling Dose

From experiments the concept of a doubling dose has resulted. This is the dose of radiation that produces twice the frequency of genetic mutations as would have been observed without radiation. Mutations exist in nature with a certain frequency. One current estimate for spontaneous mutation is 6%, which corresponds well with the number of observed congenital abnormalities (4% to 6%). Of course, not all mutations can be detected, and some congenital abnormalities are not genetic in nature.

Muller's fruit fly studies and early reports on A-bomb survivors indicated that the doubling dose in humans was 20 to 200 cGy. Recently, figures from 50 to 250 cGy have been cited as the doubling dose in humans, based primarily on the megamouse experiments. It has also been estimated that the doubling dose in females is 40% or more above the male value. Whalen and Balter (1984) note, "Mother Nature thus seems to be protecting her own, since ovarian shielding during abdominal x-ray examinations is not usually feasible." It appears, based on the Russell experiments, that mutation rates are lower in females at low dose rates (compared with males), but higher than males at higher dose rates.

Genetically Significant Dose

The *genetically significant dose (GSD)* is an average calculated from actual gonadal doses received by the whole population. It takes into account the expected contribution of these individuals to children. It is assumed that this dose, if received by every member of the population, would have the identical genetic effect as the doses received by those individuals actually exposed to ionizing radiation.

The GSD concept assumes that the long-term effects of radiation can be averaged over a population. It is calculated by a complex statistical formula that looks at the average gonadal dose per examination, the number of persons receiving x-ray examinations, the total number of persons in the population, and the expected number of future children per person.

The validity of the concept of GSD is predicted mainly on the following points derived from experimental animals:

- Mutations produced in the precursor cells of ova and spermatozoa are cumulative. Therefore, the number of new, radiation-induced mutations that an individual will transmit to offspring depends on the amount of radiation the gonads have received from the individual's own conception until the time each of his or her offspring is conceived.
- Any dose of radiation, no matter how small, has a probability of producing a mutation, and the number of mutations produced bears a linear relationship to the absorbed dose.
- The genetic significance of new mutations within the population is determined by the total number transmitted, regardless of the number of mutations transmitted per individual. The potential impact on a population for genetic mutations is the same, whether one thousand persons are exposed to 0.02 cGy or one person receives 20 cGy.

Again, it must be clearly emphasized that GSD is not a measure of biological effect but is a means of estimating the genetic impact of low-level radiations on a population.

Although this would not be an accurate calculation of the GSD, the concept can be simplified as follows: If two individuals receive radiation of 100 mrad (0.100 cGy) and 50 mrad (0.050 cGy), and a third receives none, then the average to that small "population" of three people is 50 mrad (100 + 50 = 150; 150 ÷ 3 = 50). Of course, it takes many more people than that to make a population and this is also a much simpler averaging than the GSD. The future genetic effects to the population of three are based on a 50 mrad exposure, even though one received twice that amount and one individual received nothing.

CELLULAR RADIOSENSITIVITY

Radiosensitivity has largely been defined by the rate of response following radiation. The sooner a biologic response is observed following a given dose of radiation, the more sensitive the biologic parameter is thought to be. By 1906 various studies led to the conclusion that dividing cell populations were most likely to be affected by radiation exposure. Bergonié and Tribondeau (1906) elaborated three basic characteristics that identified cell populations as susceptible to radiation injury:

- Cells that were primitive in their degree of maturation
- Cells that were rapidly dividing at the time of irradiation
- Cells that had the potential to divide for extended periods of time

Cells exhibiting these traits appeared to be the most radiosensitive populations—that is, those that show the evidence of radiation damage soon after exposure.

In 1925 Ancel and Vitemberger proposed that the inherent susceptibility of any cell to radiation damage was the same, but the time to the appearance of radiation-induced damage differed among different cell types. Furthermore, their work suggested that the appearance of radiation damage was influenced by the conditions to which the cell was exposed, pre- and postradiation. These conditions relate primarily to the stresses on the cell. One of the most significant stresses it undergoes during its life span is the process of cellular division. The concept of cellular division relative to radiation exposure is useful in understanding the temporal development of radiation-induced injuries to biological tissues, organs, and organisms. That is, the stage of the cell cycle in which the cell currently resides influences potential radiation damage.

As a brief summary, cells that are actively dividing at the time of radiation show the evidence of radiation injury first and therefore are considered most sensitive to the actions of radiation. Those not dividing at the time of radiation but that will divide at some point after radiation exposure because of biological demands placed on them have a more intermediate degree of radiosensitivity. And finally, those cells that do not have to divide to carry out their normal function are least sensitive to the lethal actions of radiation. In conclusion, mitotic death occurs at lower doses of radiation than interphase death (susceptibility of the cell before entry into the next mitotic cycle).

During the 1950s and 1960s, techniques became available to grow and maintain cells within culture flasks *(in vitro)*. The capability to grow large populations of dividing cells led to the description of a number of variables that could affect division rates. The use of such techniques in conjunction with radiation exposure has indicated that the radiosensitivity of individual cells varies according to their position within the cell cycle.

The most radiosensitive phases of the cell cycle are considered to be mitosis and the transition from late G_1 into early S-phase (Table 18–7). The most radioresistant phase of the cell cycle appears to be mid-to-late S-phase. However, no definitive answer can be given as to why cells in mitosis are most radiosensitive.

A number of speculations have been substantiated with data to suggest that the physical nature of DNA as it exists during mitosis may make repair less likely. Therefore, damaged copies of the DNA may be transmitted to the next generation of cells without repair by the mechanisms operative at other phases during the cell cycle. DNA in cells that are in mid-to-late S-phase may, in fact, physically provide the greatest likelihood for DNA repair. In late S-phase, the DNA is uncoiled, synthetic enzymes are readily available, and the metabolites for DNA synthesis are also present, since the process of DNA synthesis is currently active. Under nonsynchronized conditions, when cells are irradiated, the response seen represents the combination of damage induced in all phases of the cell cycle and the extent and effectiveness of repair mechanisms. The overall effect is measured as a decrease in the number of cells reaching the next mitosis in comparison with the number that were expected from parallel conditions in which no radiation was employed.

In biological systems, cells of the same type can be found in organized patterns called tissues. All of these cells, although of the same cell type, may not have the same division potential. Recognition of these differing division potentials was the basis for Rubin and Casarett's (1968) classification of cells according to their relative radiosensitivities (Fig. 18–7). According to this classification system, cells that are permanently in a nondividing state—that is, fixed postmitotic (FPM) cells, are least sensitive to the actions of ionizing radiation. Cells composing this category are highly differentiated and specialized and are the result of previous cellular division. FPM cells may have either a long or a short life span. Examples of long-lived FPM cells are neurons and striated muscle. These cell types are the result of cellular divisions that ceased during either the fetal or neonatal period and presently have no capacity for replenishing their cell numbers.

Another subcategory of FPM cells has a relatively short life span as individual cell types. Examples in this category are granulocytes and erythrocytes in the blood and superficial mucosal cells of the alimentary tract and skin. The short-lived cell types result from

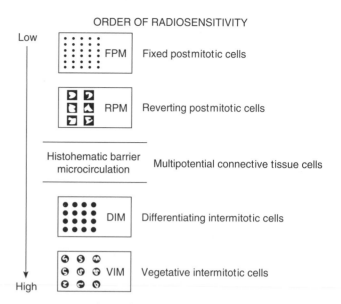

FIGURE 18–7. Rubin and Casarett's classification of cells according to radiosensitivity.

the process of continuous cell division from progenitor or *precursor* cells that differentiate, mature, and eventually transit into the FPM category. FPM cells are the most radioresistant and require tens of thousands of centigrays to induce interphase death.

A distinction must be made between long- and short-lived FPM cells, since doses far lower—in the tens to hundreds of centigrays—may affect the process of cellular division and maturation that gives rise to the short-lived elements. Cells in active cellular proliferation are found in the categories of vegetative intermitotic cells and differentiating intermitotic cells. Vegetative intermitotic cells divide infrequently, but because they are the most primitive cell type, death of one of these cells may represent the loss of hundreds of cells that would have resulted from its division. Vegetative intermitotic cells divide and become differentiating intermitotic cells. Differentiating intermitotic cells are the most rapidly dividing components in the tissue and are somewhat less sensitive than the vegetative intermitotic cell. They are relatively short-lived as individual cell types.

Differentiating intermitotic cells may divide only a limited number of times, and they differentiate between each division. With differentiation, they become more resistant. Therefore, differentiating intermitotic cells also represent a gradual transition from extremely sensitive to less sensitive as they complete the number of anticipated divisions and differentiate between each of them. The cumulative survival of these two categories of cells is responsible for the long-term survival and the function of a given cell renewal population.

Another category of cells is called reverting postmitotic cells. This category is described as possessing intermediate radiosensitivity. The cells do not divide regularly, but under appropriate stimulation they may revert to a proliferative phase to produce more cells of the same type. These cells are classically exemplified

Table 18–7: RADIOSENSITIVITY OF RAPIDLY AND SLOWLY DIVIDING CELLS

Radiosensitivity	Rapidly Dividing	Slowly Dividing
High	1. Mitosis	1. Mitosis
	2. Late G_1 to early S	2. Late G_1 to early S
	3. Late G_2	3. Late G_2
	4. Mid-to-late S	4. Early G_1
Low		5. Mid-to-late S

by hepatocytes (liver cells). However, they are part of a broad category of cells that includes many of the glandular tissue cells within the pancreas, adrenal, thyroid, parathyroid, and salivary and pituitary glands. Radiation injury of these cell types does occur, but they require weeks to months to show the evidence of that injury.

The remaining cell types constitute the multipotential connective tissue and vasculature found in various organs throughout the body. These cells divide regularly and sporadically in response to a variety of stimuli. They also have variable life spans that are longer than the dividing populations found in the differentiating and vegetative intermitotic cell category, but shorter than those found in the reverting postmitotic category. Examples of cells in this category are endothelial cells, active fibroblasts, and smooth muscle cells. Table 18–8 summarizes the classification of cells according to relative radiosensitivity.

RELATIVE ORGAN RADIOSENSITIVITY

Organs are combinations of various tissues organized into given structure and function relationships. They are composed of a *parenchyma* and a *stroma.* The parenchyma of an organ is the functional tissue. The stroma is a more broadly defined component of connective tissue and vasculature that supports the organ parenchyma in its structure and function.

The mechanisms of organ radiosensitivity can be subdivided into the responses of their individual components. In general, tissues and organs that contain radiosensitive cells are sensitive to radiation. Tissues and organs that contain radioresistant cells are resistant to radiation.

If an organ's function is highly dependent on the process of cellular proliferation, the evidence of radiation injury will be evident shortly after exposure as a loss of the dividing cell components. If the number of dividing cells is not restored, then the total number of cells decreases, which may affect function of that organ shortly after irradiation. The greater the number of dividing cells affected, the shorter the time until the injury is evident. Examples of organs that respond in this fashion are bone marrow, the gastrointestinal tract, the skin, and testes.

Functions of other organs are dominated to a greater degree by the integrity of the stromal elements. Examples of this type of organ are the lungs and kidneys, which depend on an intact microvasculature for their structure and function. In these organs, although equal doses of radiation will cause equal numbers of strand breaks in the DNA, the evidence of the injury is delayed.

In these cases, although cellular division occurs, it does so at a greatly reduced rate in comparison with bone marrow and the other organs in that category, previously mentioned. In fact, the initial histological presentation and clinical symptoms are relatively nonspecific. During the initial days and weeks postradiation, organs principally composed of dividing cell elements dominate the response to radiation, whereas organs composed of either slowly dividing or nondividing cells appear to be relatively unaffected by the same dose of radiation. However, with time as these slowly cycling cells begin to divide and replenish their numbers in the course of normal attrition, latent damage to DNA may impair their ability to divide sufficiently for normal cell replacement needs. The delay in the appearance of radiation damage is thought to be proportional to the number of cells in active cell division, as well as the rate at which the mature functional cells must be replaced. It is not uncommon that organ responses in this category may take up to six to nine months to show the evidence of radiation injury.

Essential to a discussion of radiation-induced injury to organs is an understanding of radiation effects on small blood vessels. Blood vessels have four basic structural components: endothelial lining cells, smooth muscle cells, elastic fibers, and connective tissue. Radiation-induced injury of small blood vessels following high doses of radiation can be seen as vacuolization

Table 18–8: RUBIN AND CASARETT'S CLASSIFICATION OF CELLS ACCORDING TO RELATIVE RADIOSENSITIVITY

Cell Type (Sensitivity)*	Characteristics	Examples
Fixed postmitotic (FPM)	Do not divide; highly differentiated, specialized cells	Long-lived neurons, short-lived erythrocytes
Reverting postmitotic (RPM)	Divide in response to specific stimuli; relatively long-lived; specialized	Hepatocytes, ductal cells, glandular cells
Histohematic connective tissue and vasculature (HHB)	Multipotential connective tissue cells; divide irregularly in response to variety of stimuli	Tissue fibroblasts Endothelial cells
Differentiating intermitotic (DIM)	Most rapidly dividing; short-lived as individual; limited division potential; differentiate between divisions	Blast cells of bone marrow (erythroblast, myeloblast, etc.) Proliferative zone in the intestinal crypts
Vegetative intermitotic (VIM)	Most primitive; divide periodically; differentiate into DIM or VIM	Stem cells

* Cells are listed in sequence from least to most sensitive.

and cellular swelling of endothelial and smooth muscle cells within the vessel wall. The combination of these two cellular alterations leads to a restriction of blood flow in the affected vessel, which can also increase the probability of focal tissue alterations and occlusion by blood clots. At lower doses of radiation, these same acute findings may be absent or difficult to demonstrate. As endothelial cells require replacement because of normal aging processes, the surrounding endothelial cells must divide to compensate for this degree of cell loss. As these endothelial cells begin active cell division, subtle sublethal changes may become apparent when they are unable to complete one or more mitotic divisions.

Frequently, enlarged atypical endothelial cells and thickening of the vessel wall caused by deposition of a hyalin-like material may lead to areas of altered vessel architecture. These changes may appear as greatly dilated blood vessels (telangiectasia or perivascular fibrosis). These changes, if they become widespread, can impair blood flow and nutrition of the surrounding cells within the organ. This impairs their function, which can lead to overt clinical failure of that organ.

Classically, this phenomenon is demonstrated following radiation of the spinal cord. Although the individual nerve fibers are nondividing, they still have a continuous need for oxygen and nutrients to maintain normal cellular function. As the surrounding vasculature becomes thickened, the delivery of oxygen and other nutrients is restricted. As the fuel for cellular metabolism is decreased, the ability to maintain a polarized membrane for the nerve fiber is diminished. This leads to reduced nerve conduction that may be evident as weakness in the lower extremities, sphincter muscle changes, tingling sensations within the fingers, and so on. This is all dependent on the spinal cord level at which the nerve fibers have been affected.

Radiation injury within the microvasculature and connective tissue of organs relates to the terminology used by Rubin and Casarett (1968) as the histohematic barrier (see Fig. 18–7). It is widely believed that damage within these compartments of cells in various organs, as well as damage to the parenchyma, gives rise to the late effects seen following therapeutic courses of radiation for cancer treatment.

Summary

The relative radiosensitivity of tissues and organs can be summarized as follows. Highly radiosensitive tissues and organs such as lymphoid tissue and bone marrow exhibit cytopenia and hypoplasia with a dose of 200 to 1000 cGy. Intermediately radiosensitive organs and tissues demonstrate effects with doses of 1000 to 5000 cGy. Examples of the latter include skin (erythema), cornea of the eye (cataracts), and the liver (ascites). Organs and tissues that are resistant to radiation such as muscle (potential effect: fibrosis), brain (necrosis), and spinal cord (transection), show effects at 5000 cGy or more.

TIME SEQUENCE OF RADIATION INJURY

In the preceding paragraphs, descriptions were given to illustrate the ways various cellular types such as differentiating intermitotic and FPM cells respond following irradiation. It is frequently helpful to envision the overall process in terms of a flow diagram (Fig. 18–8). This diagram illustrates the individual processes giving rise to measured responses. For example, following irradiation, several outcomes may be possible. If the radiation dose is very high, 20,000 cGy or more, then within minutes to hours, cellular changes such as swelling, indicating permeability changes in the membrane, may become evident. These changes may immediately give rise to ulceration and *necrosis* of the area. However, at far lower doses, these acute changes are not probable since insufficient damage is sustained by membranes of the individual cells. It is more likely that at lower doses, the first obvious outcome will be a reduction in the number of dividing cells. The reduction in mitotic activity is dose-dependent. Therefore, the appearance of parenchymal hypoplasia (decreased cell numbers) depends on the dose of radiation. The greater the dose, the shorter the time to hypoplasia and, conversely, the lower the dose, the longer the time until a hypoplasia develops. There may be complete recovery through regeneration of surviving cells in the area. The process may take days or weeks to be completed.

Although the parenchymal cell numbers may be restored, the vasculature and connective tissue damage may develop at a different rate and therefore may appear months following the exposure. The stromal effects of *telangiectasia,* vascular sclerosis, and fibrosis

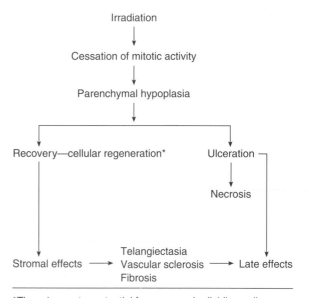

Irradiation
↓
Cessation of mitotic activity
↓
Parenchymal hypoplasia
↓
Recovery—cellular regeneration*   Ulceration
↓   ↓
                                        Necrosis
↓
Stromal effects → Telangiectasia
                   Vascular sclerosis → Late effects
                   Fibrosis

*There is greater potential for recovery in dividing cell populations.

FIGURE 18–8. Time-related sequence of radiation injury.

may give rise to ulceration and necrosis of the surrounding parenchyma at times long after the original irradiation and its acute affects are apparent. Therefore, it becomes important to consider that the presence or absence of radiation injury may be relative to the specific time of measurement.

EFFECTS OF SYSTEMIC IRRADIATION

The influences of dose and length of time after irradiation are dramatically illustrated when the systemic effects of whole body irradiation are studied. Classically, the effects of total body radiation are viewed within the concept of the lethal dose to 50% (LD 50) of the individuals exposed and the time period in which these deaths occurred. This gives rise to the concept of LD 50/60 for humans, which is considered to be 350 cGy. The 60 refers to the time in days. When studying total body effects of radiation, groups of symptoms that appear postradiation are collectively identified as a radiation syndrome. The radiation syndromes are named in accordance with the organ system attributed to the cause of death of the person. Figure 18-9 provides a categorization of the radiation syndromes. The conditions under which these syndromes are elicited are as follows:

- The radiation is deeply penetrating at a high dose
- The entire body volume is irradiated
- The radiation is delivered within minutes to hours

The first important generalization from these data should be that the higher the dose of radiation, the shorter the time of survival postradiation. The second is the clear distinction between induction of interphase death of cells beyond the thousands of centigrays range versus the impairment in cellular proliferation at lower doses. For example, at extremely high absorbed doses, molecular death results in minutes to hours. In this syndrome, molecular elements such as proteins, membranes, and so forth are altered by both direct and indirect damage that impair their normal function. Even nondividing cell components, such as nerves of the autonomic nervous system, may be damaged, giving rise to acute seizures or cardiac failure.

Besides the three lethal syndromes to be discussed,

two other events occur in total body irradiation. First is the *prodromal* radiation syndrome. The term *prodromal* means *running before*. It refers to the initial stage of a disease. The prodromal syndrome can occur with a dose as low as 50 cGy and occurs within a matter of minutes at high dose levels (in excess of 1000 cGy). This syndrome consists of nausea, vomiting, and diarrhea and is also called the NVD syndrome.

There may be a latent period following the prodromal syndrome. During this period the individual appears to be symptom-free; in reality, the last stage—death or recovery—is beginning. This period is a matter of hours at higher doses and weeks at lower doses. There are four basic stages: prodromal, latent, manifest, and recovery or death.

Hematopoietic Syndrome

At doses of radiation between 200 and 600 cGy, hematopoietic syndrome, also called the bone marrow syndrome, is induced. This syndrome is typified by failure of the bone marrow to produce sufficient cells to maintain survival much beyond approximately 30 to 60 days.

Gastrointestinal Syndrome

Between approximately 750 and 1500 cGy of radiation, gastrointestinal (GI) syndrome or death may be induced. This syndrome is characterized by nausea, vomiting, diarrhea, GI bleeding, and acute loss of electrolytes. Death occurs within 5 to 14 days. The mechanism of radiation injury depends both on the amount of damage to the preformed cellular elements and the profound suppression of cellular division in the progenitor cells of the gastrointestinal surfaces. Alimentary tract lining cell division is not restored in sufficient time to provide cellular recovery.

Central Nervous System Syndrome

At higher doses, symptoms may include hyperexcitability, lack of coordination, ataxia, respiratory distress, stupor, coma, vasculitis, meningitis, encephalitis, or brain edema. Symptoms result from breakdown of the integrity of the central nervous system. The symptom complex is referred to as the central nervous system (CNS) syndrome. This breakdown occurs in both the individual neurons and the supplying vasculature. Death is the inevitable outcome and occurs within one to three days.

Summary

At doses below 200 cGy, radiation induces a variety of sublethal and chronic alterations. These alterations may take the form of immunosuppression, genetic and

Stage 1	Stage 2	Stage 3	Stage 4
Prodromal ⟶	Latent ⟶	Manifest illness ⟶ Three possibilities:	Recovery or death*
		Hematologic syndrome	
		Gastrointestinal syndrome	
		CNS syndrome	

*Recovery is dose dependent and is seen only in the hematologic syndrome; this can take 3 weeks to 6 months, and many individuals will not survive.

FIGURE 18-9. Staging of acute radiation syndromes.

reproductive changes, and carcinogenesis. Thankfully, the bulk of this data has been collected within the confines of research laboratories rather than in general human populations. However, the atomic bombs used in World War II and radiation accidents such as that in Chernobyl have given us verification of these concepts for humans. Human data suggest that for doses in excess of 600 cGy, survival is virtually impossible, even with medical intervention. At doses between 200 and 600 cGy, survival is possible but requires intensive medical management. And finally, at doses of less than 200 cGy, survival is probable. These distinctions become more important if large populations have been irradiated and there is a scarcity of medical resources available—for example, following nuclear warfare. Since the probabilities in any radiation exposure suggest that sublethal changes are more likely to occur, large series of populations have been followed for the chronic changes following low doses of radiation. These data come not only from the survivors of Hiroshima, Nagasaki, and Chernobyl but also from patients treated with radiation for therapeutic purposes and radiation workers before the advent of strict regulatory standards.

IMMUNE SYSTEM

Cells making up the immune system are located throughout the body. Primary organs involved in immunocompetence are the bone marrow, spleen, thymus, lymph nodes, and Peyer's patches of the intestine. Organs involved in the immune system response are composed of connective tissue and vascular elements and a parenchyma. The parenchyma of the immune system is composed of lymphocytes. Lymphocytes are subdivided into two major categories, T and B lymphocytes. These two categories give rise to two distinct immune responses. T lymphocytes are thought to cause a cell-mediated response against foreign substances within the body. B lymphocytes produce an antibody response (humoral) to foreign substances. The reticuloendothelial cells provide important intermediary steps in degradation of foreign substances so that the immune system can respond to the individual components of these foreign structures.

The first point is that lymphocytes as a distinct cell population are highly sensitive to the lethal actions of ionizing radiations. Whole-body radiation exposures of 50 cGy have been found to decrease the lymphocyte count in circulating peripheral blood by 50% within 24 hours of exposure. Certain subpopulations of both T and B cells (pre-B and pre-T cells) may actually have an LD 50 of between 10 and 20 cGy. Total body exposures of 100 cGy, although sublethal, may induce a profound immunosuppression through the elimination of preformed lymphocytes. This exposure can also remove precursor cells that give rise to the immune responses. Immune suppression may last for variable periods of time. This depends on the total dose, the

number of preformed elements lethally injured, and the extent of damage to the precursor cells throughout the body. Established immune responses to previously recognized foreign substances are less sensitive to radiation than are newly developing immune responses.

REPRODUCTIVE SYSTEM

Radiation injury to the reproductive system is most likely to present a sublethal change to the individual affected. However, damage to the reproductive precursor cells, and the preformed elements may cause an increased number of chromosome mutations that may be either detrimental to the next generation or sufficient to impair fertility and subsequent fetal development. The specific processes involved in radiation injury of reproductive tissue is necessarily different in the male and female, since the nature of cell production is different. For the male, the development of mature sperm or spermatozoa is an ongoing process of cellular division, differentiation, and maturation. Adult female reproductive cellular injury is framed within the mutational effects of the radiation of immature oocytes that are arrested at the diplotene phase of the meiotic division cycle.

Male Reproductive System

This cellular renewal system is unique in comparison with other organs, since those cellular elements resulting from the division process are haploid (have only "N" quantity of the species chromosome number). The haploid quantity of chromosomes is of course required, because on fertilization, the female also contributes "N" quantity (i.e., any number or 1N male plus 1N female, equalling 2N or haploid number) of chromosomes, thereby restoring the diploid number of the species. Radiation injury of the male reproductive tissue takes two basic forms. First, low doses of radiation may impair cellular proliferation from types A and B spermatogonia stem cells, which in turn may decrease the number of mature spermatozoa that are formed.

Therefore, at some time after irradiation, a low sperm count may develop as a result of the previous injury and hypoplasia of the more immature precursor elements. The duration of this low sperm count is dose-dependent, and recovery requires survival and repopulation from surviving spermatogonia types A and B.

The second form of radiation injury to the male reproductive tissue is the induction of point mutations within mature spermatozoa. These mutations may be passed on to the next generation if the affected spermatozoa are used in fertilization of an ova. It is the combination of these two forms of radiation injury that leads to the suggestion that procreational attempts be delayed for approximately three to six months. This time delay will provide time for the existing spermatozoa that contain some point mutations to be absorbed within the normal cell turnover of the testes and will permit repopulation of the mature spermatozoa from surviving types A and B spermatogonia stem cells. This recommendation is not without controversy but should be considered. For the male, radiation doses as low as 3 cGy may cause detectable changes in spermatozoa count. Permanent sterility of the male is caused by the range of 600 to 1000 cGy.

Female Reproductive System

For the female, irradiation exposure of the reproductive tissues contained within the ovaries involves the irradiation of secondary oocytes and the polar bodies contained within the ovary. The actual number of oocytes are fixed before birth, and secondary oocytes are generated at each ovulation. Therefore, radiation exposure of the female reproductive tissue does not involve irradiation of an active cellular proliferation but does present the opportunity to induce sublethal mutations within the DNA. These sublethal mutations, although nonlethal to the irradiated individual, may pose the same genetic hazards to the next generation as previously discussed for the male. For the human female, a single dose of 50 cGy may induce temporary infertility.

However, a minimum dose of 400 cGy (or a fractionated dose of 1500 cGy over 15 days) produces permanent sterility in most women. Although it is sublethal in nature, it must be underscored that the principal radiation injury of reproductive tissue is the probability of mutational changes in the next generation. This probability is discussed more fully in the section concerning radiation effects on embryonic and fetal development.

CARCINOGENESIS

One of the principal long-term effects of radiation exposure is the increased risk of cancer and nonspecific life span shortening. It has been well documented throughout the years that exposure to radiation is associated with increased risks of various cancers. This was particularly true with diagnostic radiologists who practiced radiology during the first half of this century. During this time period, individuals who used radiation received 10 to 100 times more radiation per week than today's radiation worker. Throughout their working life, it has been estimated these individuals were exposed to hundreds of cGy.

Such high levels of radiation exposure occurred because of inadequate shielding of the radiation source, failure to appreciate the magnitude of the radiation exposure to the individual worker, and a lack of knowledge of radiation units. There was also a minimal understanding of the relationship between radiation and cancer and a severely restricted concept of cancer cells in general.

Although no single mechanism for carcinogenesis is presently universally accepted, two prominent hypotheses are currently in vogue. The first, genetic alteration, may involve the addition of new genetic material (such as viral genes) and the deletion of normal genes through various mutations and chromosome rearrangements. Once such a genetic alteration occurs, changes may develop in the growth-control mechanisms that favor accumulation of similarly altered cancer cells. This explanation may be helpful in understanding such cancers as retinoblastoma and renal and breast cancers in which specific chromosome alterations have been documented or specific *oncogenes* have been identified.

An alternative mechanism may be genetic activation. In this theory, cancer develops following the activation or repression of normal genes, rather than from a specific alteration of various DNA sequences. It may involve the activation of genes that previously were active only during embryonic life for noncancer cell populations. Specific examples may be the findings of cancer cell–related proteins. This theory also has the interesting implication that cancer may be a reversible process through genetic modulation (i.e., the reverse of genetic activation).

Although radiation may act through either of these mechanisms, it is likely that because of both single- and double-strand breaks of DNA following radiation exposure, genetic alterations can be more easily envisioned. Furthermore, it may also be possible that a combination of these mechanisms may be operative, each mechanism providing an increased probability that the cell will be converted into a cancer cell. These additional steps may be considered the result of cofactor, or co-*carcinogenic,* influences on the function of the cellular DNA.

Much information concerning radiation-induced cancer comes from extensive laboratory investigations. Such studies provide proper control groups and manipulation of important variables such as total dose, dose rate, sex of the individual, and age at the time of radiation exposure and other factors, such as dietary influences. Human data from epidemiological studies provide confirmation of the laboratory studies (Table 18–9). Human epidemiological studies have largely focused on early twentieth century radiologists, atomic bomb survivors, patients treated with x-rays along the spinal axis for an arthritic condition, children irradiated over the mediastinum in infancy for thymic enlargement, and groups of patients given repeated diagnostic radiation studies or irradiated for benign conditions.

An overview of the laboratory data suggests that the following generalizations can be made. First, rapidly renewing cell systems are more susceptible to carcinogenesis and have a shorter latent period for the development of radiation-induced cancers than slowing, renewing, or nondividing cell systems. Furthermore, comprehensive reviews of all radiation data periodically undertaken by the National Academy of Sciences

Table 18-9: STUDIES SHOWING EVIDENCE OF CARCINOGENESIS IN HUMANS

Group	Strong Association	Weak Association (Suggested)
Japanese A-bomb survivors	Leukemia, thyroid, breasts	Stomach, esophagus, bladder, salivary gland
Marshall Islanders		Thyroid
Radium-dial painters	Bone	Colon
Early radiologists	Leukemia, skin	Lymphoma, brain
Multiple chest fluoroscopies	Breasts	
Infants with enlarged thymus	Thyroid	Leukemia, skin, salivary gland
Thorotrast*	Leukemia, liver	Lungs, kidneys
In utero exposures	Leukemia	
Thyroid cancer patients ^{131}I therapy		Leukemia
Uranium miners	Lungs	

* Compound of thorium (a radioactive metal with a half-life of 10^{10} years) formerly used as contrast medium in radiology.

and reported in the Biological Effects of Ionizing Radiations (BEIR) have indicated that radiation induction of cancer occurs in organs that are normally at risk for cancer induction without a history of radiation exposures, such as female breasts, thyroid, lungs, bone marrow, and alimentary tract. However, notable exceptions have also been identified. Genital and urological cancers found in the male prostate and female uterus and cervix occur at fairly high rates without specific histories of radiation exposure. Analysis of various human groups given a wide range of radiation exposures for various purposes has indicated no increased incidents of cancer in these two sites as a result of the radiation exposure.

Classically, certain cancers have been considered highly sensitive to induction by radiation exposure. These are leukemia, skin cancers, thyroid, and breast cancer.

Leukemia

For the induction of leukemia, it has been determined that acute whole-body radiation doses are more leukemogenic than chronic or fractionated doses or the exposure of limited volumes of the body. The incidence of radiation-induced leukemia is somewhat proportional to the volume of the bone marrow exposed, and the incidence of all types of leukemia except chronic lymphocytic leukemia may be increased by exposure to ionizing radiations. Additionally, it is commonly accepted that radiation exposure of adults may produce an increased incidence of acute and chronic myelogenous leukemias, whereas children similarly exposed have a greater increase in the incidence of acute lymphoid and stem cell leukemias. The latency period for the induction of cancer appears to be five to seven years. The most controversial studies for radiation-induced leukemia relate to prenatal radiation exposures of 1 to 5 cGy delivered for diagnostic purposes. Skin cancers may also be radiation-induced; however, their latency period appears to be approximately 8 to 12 years and requires higher total doses of radiation.

Thyroid Cancer

Studies of thyroid cancers induced by radiation have largely come from the detailed follow-up of children subjected to external radiation therapy in the neck region to decrease the size of an enlarged thymus gland. These persons developed thyroid abnormalities approximately 10 to 20 years following exposure. The induced abnormalities include carcinomas, adenomas, and hyperplastic nodules. The other principal study group for thyroid cancers comes from the children on the Marshall Islands exposed to radioactive fallout following atmospheric testing of atomic weapons. In this group, children who were less than 10 years of age at the time of exposure, the incidence of thyroid nodules went from virtually zero to more than 80%, 8 to 16 years afterward. Less than 10% of those who were older than 10 years of age at the time of radiation exposure developed comparable lesions. This underscores the extremely important point that relative risks of cancer induction in various organs may change across the life span of an individual, although the same total doses and dose rates are employed.

Breast Cancer

The relationship between radiation exposure and the induction of breast cancer has also been intensely studied for generations. The highlights of these studies are

1. The induction of breast cancer occurs at cumulative doses of less than 100 cGy, and the incidence continues to increase through cumulated doses as high as 600 cGy.
2. Since the mode of radiation delivery was different for different groups studied, the effects of dose protraction and fractionation indicate that the radiation dose appears to be cumulative and that highly fractionated exposures were as effective at inducing breast cancer as unfractionated exposures. These points may become particularly important as we continually reassess the use of ioniz-

ing radiations for the early detection and diagnosis of breast cancer.

The overall assessment of the dose-response relationship for the induction of cancer suggests that carcinogenic changes do not occur within cells following a simple "one-hit" process that would provide a simple linear function with increasing radiation dose. Clearly, multiple data suggest that radiation may influence the process of carcinogenesis through a variety of aspects, depending on the particular conditions of the study.

FETAL IRRADIATION

The embryo and fetus pass through three basic stages of development (Fig. 18–10). The first is preimplantation, which in humans is the 10-day time period following conception. In this stage, the fertilized ovum is dividing, forming a ball of undifferentiated cells.

Stage two is organogenesis, in which the cells are implanted in the uterine wall. This stage occurs through the sixth week postconception. In this stage, cells begin differentiating into organs. For example, neuroblasts typically form on the 18th day of gestation and the eyes on the 20th day.

Stage three is the fetal or growth stage. This is the period following the sixth week postconception. It is, as the name implies, primarily a period of growth rather than new development. The main exception is the central nervous system (CNS), which is still highly undifferentiated in the fetus. Complete development of the CNS does not typically occur until the 12th year of life in humans.

The effects of radiation on the embryo and fetus are dependent on two factors: the stage of development and the radiation dose. The principal effects of radiation on an embryo or fetus are

- Embryonic, fetal, or neonatal death
- Malformations
- Retardation of growth
- Congenital defects
- Cancer induction.

For example, in the earliest stages of development, radiation exposure may destroy enough of the cells to terminate the pregnancy. However, since the cells are still undifferentiated (not specialized) at this point, if enough cells survive to continue to reproduce without chromosomal abnormalities, the only effect will be a delay in development. This is known as the all-or-none effect.

In middle stages of development, when organs and structures are not fully formed, radiation exposure may cause damage to a part or stunt its development. In later stages, when the fetus is growing, rather than developing, late effects of radiation are most common. Since the CNS remains highly undifferentiated, large doses of radiation (e.g., 25 cGy) can have a variety of effects on the CNS. Radiosensitivity begins to decrease at 20 weeks, but the fetus then becomes more susceptible to late and CNS effects.

Dekaban (1968) performed the most complete study of embryonic and fetal effects caused by large amounts of (therapeutic) radiation. His conclusions, based on a dose of 250 cGy or more, were

1. This dosage delivered before the second to third weeks of gestation will most likely result in prena-

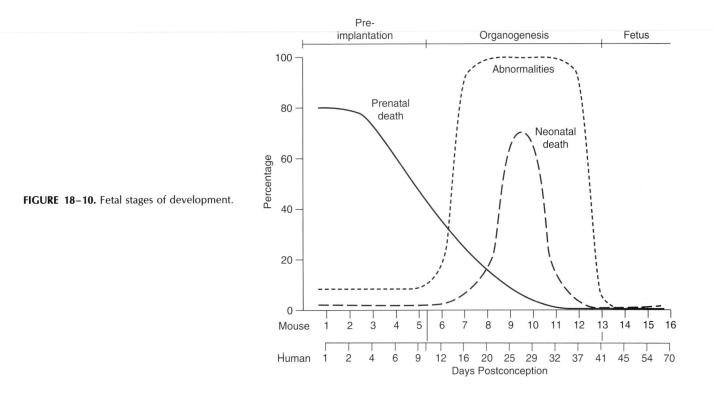

FIGURE 18–10. Fetal stages of development.

tal death, but few abnormalities will be seen in children carried to term.

2. Irradiation between the fourth and 11th weeks of gestation can result in severe abnormalities of multiple organs, especially the skeletal system and the CNS.

3. Mental retardation and microcephaly are frequent when the radiation is delivered from the 11th to 16th week of gestation.

4. Functional defects can result after the 20th week, although the fetus is in general less radiosensitive after that time.

Table 18–10 describes some anomalies related to human gestational days and radiation exposure. They are described in the following paragraphs.

Prenatal Death

Exposures of 5 to 15 cGy in the preimplantation stage can result in prenatal death, or death before birth. Ten cGy exposure in utero in the first two weeks can result in a spontaneous abortion. However, the natural occurrence of spontaneous abortion is 25% to 50%, and 10 cGy would raise this response by only 0.1%. Note that all these doses are to the embryo or fetus, not the external dose received by the mother.

In the preimplantation stage, there is typically an all-or-none response—either there is a radiation-induced spontaneous abortion or there are no effects. This type of all-or-none response usually requires high doses of radiation. At day one preimplantation, 200 cGy lead to death in 80% of humans; at day nine, this same dose leads to a 30% fatality rate. Embryonic resorption may occur, and the mother may never know she was pregnant.

Neonatal Death

Neonatal death is death at birth. It is considered a rare form of radiation response. According to mouse data, it appears to occur primarily from irradiation in the later stages of organogenesis and in the fetal stage, probably at high doses. In the fetal stage, the LD 50 approaches that of adults.

Congenital Malformation

Congenital abnormalities such as microcephaly (abnormally small head) or hydrocephaly (an expansion of the head because of an increased amount of fluid in the ventricles) can result from radiation exposure in the stage of organogenesis. This risk lessens somewhat in the fetal stage but remains high. It is not observed if irradiation occurs preimplantation. It has been said that 10-cGy exposure in this stage increases the number of abnormalities by 1%. A parallel can be drawn with exposure to rubella (German measles) and the drug thalidomide, which are thought to cause similar effects in the organogenesis stage.

In 1930 Murphy and Goldstein observed the children of women who had therapeutic radiation while pregnant. Twenty-eight of 75 children had abnormalities, primarily CNS and skeletal defects. A high percentage of microcephaly (16 of the 28) and hydrocephaly was observed.

Childhood Malignancy

In the fetal stage, few abnormalities are noted with radiation exposure. Instead, late effects of radiation such as cancer (especially leukemia) are more likely. However, it has also been stated that probably 50 cGy to the fetus are necessary to bring about an increase in late effects.

Diminished Growth and Development

Diminished growth and development are theoretically possible at all stages but primarily occur during the latter and possibly the very early stages of gestation. Hall (1988) states that growth retardation with irradiation will not be seen in the preimplantation stage, will be temporary in the organogenesis stage, and will be permanent if the fetus is irradiated during the fetal stage. During the later stages, growth retardation is thought to result from cell depletion with a consequent reduction in size. No congenital abnormalities are observed, but the individual has a somewhat reduced physical size. The children born at Hiroshima (after the bombing) were later noted to be about 7 lbs lighter, 1 inch shorter, and about 0.5 inch smaller in head circumference than nonirradiated controls.

Table 18–10: RADIATION DAMAGE IN TERMS OF GESTATIONAL DAYS

Anomaly	Gestational Days
Cataracts	0–6
Exencephaly (herniation of the brain)	0–37
Embryonic death	4–11
Anencephaly or microcephaly	9–90
Anophthalmia	16–32
Cleft palate	20–37
Skeletal disorders	25–85
Growth disorders	54+

Chapter Summary/ Important Concepts

Radiation biology is a combination of sciences, including biology, radiation physics, and epidemiology, that are used to describe the effects of radiation on living tissue. The cell is the basic unit of life, and is the basic unit of study in radiation biology. Damage to the cell may be sustained directly to the DNA or indirectly to the DNA through free radical information. High LET radiations are more likely to bring about direct damage to the DNA. The damage brought about by free radical formation can be altered by compounds that provide radiation protection, such as sulfhydryls, or by procedures that increase or mimic oxygen content, increasing radiosensitivity.

Three concepts allow the comparison of radiations and end points such as radiation damage. The first, linear energy transfer (LET), describes the amount of energy absorbed per unit path. The two categories of LET are low (examples: x-rays and gamma rays) and high (neutrons and alpha particles). Low LET radiations tend to travel far but produce fewer ionizations per unit distance travelled.

Relative biological effectiveness (RBE) compares a dose of test radiation needed to produce an effect with a standard radiation, usually 250-keV x-rays. This allows comparisons of radiation with different LETs. The oxygen enhancement ratio (OER) describes the increase in biological damage seen when oxygen concentration is increased.

Genetic effects include point mutations, gene mutations, and frameshift mutations, the gain or loss of one or more DNA bases. Muller's and the Russells' experiments indicated that mutations increase in quantity, but not quality, through radiation, most mutations caused by radiation are recessive, and a threshold is not observed. It appears that a dose-rate effect may occur in more complicated organisms. The doubling dose is the dose needed to double the amount of genetic mutations. The genetically significant dose, an average, is used to express the genetic effects to a population as a whole.

Cellular radiosensitivity has traditionally been defined in terms of the law of Bergonié and Tribondeau (1906) and by Ancel and Vitemberger's (1925) modification of that law. Bergonié and Tribondeau indicated that cells that are primitive, rapidly dividing, and have the potential to divide for extended periods are the most radiosensitive. Ancel and Vitemberger found that the stresses received before and after irradiation influence radiosensitivity and that the time to appearance of damage differs according to cell type.

Rubin and Casarett's (1968) classification of cells indicates that cells in a permanently nondividing state are the least sensitive to radiation—fixed postmitotic cells, which are highly differentiated, specialized, and do not divide.

The radiosensitivity of an organ depends on responses of individual components. This includes whether these components divide often or not and the composition of the parenchyma and stroma and surrounding vasculature.

Several time-related outcomes of radiation are possible. These are also dependent on dose. Following irradiation, mitotic activity ceases, leading to a parenchymal hypoplasia. This can lead to recovery or to other effects such as ulceration or necrosis or to late effects of radiation such as carcinogenesis.

Systemic or whole-body radiation effects include the prodromal syndrome, the central nervous system syndrome, the gastrointestinal syndrome, and the hematopoietic syndrome. These are seen at doses higher than are used in diagnostic imaging.

Lymphocytes are sensitive cells in terms of radiation response. A profound immunosuppression is possible with doses as low as 100 cGy.

In the male, doses as low as 3 cGy can cause a detectable decrease in sperm count, with permanent sterility occurring at 600 to 1000 cGy. In the female, temporary sterility can occur at 50 cGy, with a one-time dose of 400 cGy producing permanent sterility.

Carcinogenesis caused by radiation may occur as a result of genetic alteration or genetic activation. Radiocarcinogenesis has been shown in laboratory and epidemiological studies. Bone marrow (leukemia), skin (at high doses), the thyroid, and the breast are seen as highly radiosensitive in terms of carcinogenesis.

The fetus passes through three stages of development: preimplantation, organogenesis, and the fetal, or growth, stage. The effects of radiation on the fetus depend on two factors: the stage of development and the dose. Embryonic, fetal, or neonatal death; malformations; growth retardation; congenital defects; and cancer induction are all possible effects of radiation on the fetus.

Important Terminology

Carcinogenic. Producing carcinoma (cancer)

Centigray (cGy). A unit of absorbed radiation dose equal to one one-hundredth (0.01, or 1/100) of a gray; equivalent to one rad

Deoxyribonucleic Acid (DNA). A nucleic acid that constitutes the genetic material of all cellular organisms and the DNA viruses

Frameshift Mutation. A mutation resulting from an

addition or subtraction that is not an exact multiple of 3 base pairs in a DNA coding sequence. From the point of mutation onward, base triplets (codons) are read out of phase; the reading frame of the gene is changed, and a completely different set of amino acids is made into protein

Free Radical. An extremely reactive radical having a very short half-life (a nanosecond or less in an aqueous solution); it carries an unpaired electron

Genetically Significant Dose (GSD). An average calculated from actual gonadal doses received by the whole population, taking into account the expected contribution of individuals to exposed children; it is assumed that this dose, if received by every member of the population, would have the identical genetic effect of doses received by those individuals actually exposed to ionizing radiation

Gray (Gy). A unit of absorbed radiation dose equal to 100 rads; abbreviated Gy

Hypoplasia. Incomplete development or underdevelopment of an organ or tissue; it is less severe in degree than aplasia

In Vitro. Within a glass; observable in a test tube; in an artificial environment

In Vivo. Within the living body

Linear Energy Transfer (LET). The energy dissipation of ionizing radiation over a given linear distance; highly penetrating radiations, such as gamma rays, cause very few ionizations and thus have a relatively low LET; alpha particles have a relatively high LET

Linear Nonthreshold Dose Response. A graphic representation of the relationship between dose administered and biologic response, in which any dose of radiation can have some potential effect and there is a direct relationship between dose and response

Meiosis. A special method of cell division occurring in maturation of the sex cells, by means of which each daughter nucleus receives half the number of chromosomes characteristic of the somatic cells of the species

Mitosis. A method of cellular division, consisting of a complex of various processes, by means of which the two daughter nuclei normally receive identical complements of the number of chromosomes characteristic of the somatic cells of the species

Mutation. A change in form, quality, or some other characteristic; in genetics, permanent transmissible change in the genetic material, usually in a single gene; also, an individual exhibiting such a change

Necrosis. The sum of morphological changes indicative of cell death; it may affect groups of cells or part of a structure or an organ

Oncogene. A gene found in the chromosomes of tumor cells, activation of which is associated with the initial and continuing conversion of normal cells into cancer cells

Oxygen Enhancement Ratio (OER). A ratio measured by the comparison of the amount of cellular injury induced in the presence of oxygen versus that induced in the absence of oxygen; those radiations that require well-oxygenated conditions to exert their greatest effects are said to have a high OER

Parenchyma. "Anything poured in beside" the essential elements of an organ; used in anatomical nomenclature as a general term to designate the functional elements of an organ, as distinguished from its framework, or stroma

Point Mutation. A mutation resulting from a change in a single base pair in the DNA molecule, caused by the substitution of one nucleotide for another

Precursor. Something that precedes; in biological processes, a substance from which another, usually a more active or mature substance, is formed.

Prodromal. Running before; premonitory; indicating the onset of a disease or morbid state

Quality Factor. A multiplier that accounts for differences in biologic effects of different kinds of radiation

Radiosensitivity. Sensitivity of organs, cells, or tissues to ionizing radiation in terms of degree and quickness of response

Relative Biological Effectiveness (RBE). An expression of the effectiveness of other types of radiation in comparison with that of gamma or x-rays

Stroma. The supporting tissue or matrix of an organ as distinguished from its functional element, or parenchyma. The insoluble portion of the erythrocyte remaining after hemolysis, consisting of fragments of the cell membrane

Sulfhydryl. The univalent radical −SH

Telangiectasia. Permanent dilation of preexisting blood vessels, creating small, red focal lesions, usually visible in the skin or mucous membranes

Bibliography

Ancel, P.; Vitemberger, P. Sur la radiosensibilité cellulaire. CR Sociol Biol 92:517, 1925.

Arena, V. Ionizing Radiations and Life. St. Louis: CV Mosby, 1971.

Bacq, A.M.; Alexander, P. Fundamentals of Radiobiology, 2nd ed. New York: Pergamon Press, 1961.

Baker, M.; Dalrymple, G.V. Radiation and the fetus. In Hendee, W.R. Health Effects of Low-Level Radiation. Norwalk, CT: Appleton-Century-Crofts, 1984.

Bergonié, J.; Tribondeau, L. De quelques résultats de la radiothérapie et essai de fixation d'une technique rationnel. CR Acad Sci (Paris) 143:983, 1906.

Casarett, A.P. Radiation Biology. Englewood Cliffs, NJ: Prentice-Hall, 1968.

Dekaban, A.S. Abnormalities in children exposed to x-radiation during various stages of gestation; tentative time-table of radiation to the human fetus. J Nucl Med, Pt 1, 9:471, 1968.

Frankel, R. Radiation protection for radiologic technologists. New York: McGraw-Hill Book Co., 1975.

Hall, E.J. Radiobiology for the Radiologist, 3rd ed. Philadelphia: JB Lippincott, 1988.

Land, C.E. Estimating cancer risks from low doses of ionizing radiation. Science 209:1197–1203, 1981.

Lea, D.E. Actions of Radiation on Living Cells, 2nd ed. Cambridge, England: Cambridge University Press, 1956.

Moore, R. Ionizing radiations in chromosomes. J Coll Radiol Aust 9:272, 1965.

Muller, H.J. Artificial transmutation of the gene. Science 66:84, 1927.

Noz, M.E.; Maguire, G.Q. Radiation Protection in the Radiologic and Health Sciences, 2nd ed. Philadelphia: Lea & Febiger, 1985.

Puck, T.T.; Marcus, T.I. Action of x-rays on mammalian cells. J Exp Med 103:653, 1956.

Rubin, P.; Casarett, G.W. Clinical Radiation Pathology, Vols I and II. Philadelphia: WB Saunders, 1968.

Rugh, R. Ionizing radiations: Their possible relation to the etiology of some congenital anomalies in human disorders. Milit Med 124:401, 1959.

Russell, W.L. Genetic hazards of radiation. Proc Am Philos Soc 107:11, 1963.

Selman, J. Elements of Radiobiology. Springfield, IL: Charles C. Thomas, 1983.

Seltser, R.; Sartwell, P.E. Influence of occupational exposure to radiation on mortality of American radiologists and other medical specialists. Am J Epidemiol 81:2, 1965.

Travis, E.L. Primer of Medical Radiobiology, 2nd ed. Chicago: Year Book Medical Publishers, 1989.

Whalen, J.P.; Balter, S. Radiation Risks in Medical Imaging. Chicago: Year Book Medical Publishers, 1984.

⚡ Review Questions

1. A. Direct Damage   B. Indirect Damage
   Select the mechanism of energy transfer that is most closely associated with
   _____ Low LET radiations
   _____ Oxygen effect
   _____ Double-stranded DNA breaks
   _____ Free radical transformation
   _____ Irreparable radiation damage

2. True or False:
   _____ Any change in the linear sequence of DNA is a mutation
   _____ All mutations of DNA are detectable
   _____ All mutations of DNA are lethal
   _____ Single-strand breaks of DNA can be repaired without lethality

3. A profound immunosuppression can be seen with _____ centigrays (cGy)
   a. 50   c. 1000
   b. 100   d. 10,000

4. The most radiosensitive portions of the cell cycle are
   I. Mitosis.
   II. Mid-to-late S-phase.
   III. Transition from late G-1 into early S-phase.
   a. I and II only   c. II and III only
   b. I and III only   d. I, II, and III

5. Organ damage following radiation exposure
   a. can be predicted by the proportion of dividing compared with nondividing cells
   b. is independent of the proportion of cell division
   c. is seen sooner in organs composed of nondividing compared with dividing cells
   d. is easily detected immediately after radiation exposure

6. The law of Bergonié and Tribondeau states that
   1. stem cells are radiosensitive
   2. younger cells and tissues are more radiosensitive
   3. a high metabolic rate increases the radiosensitivity of cells
   a. 1 and 2 only   c. 2 and 3 only
   b. 1 and 3 only   d. 1, 2, and 3

7. Which of the following summarize the characteristics of radiation mutation?
   1. Radiation effects are specific.
   2. Most mutations are undesirable.
   3. Mutagenic effects are probably cumulative.
   a. 1 and 2 only   c. 2 and 3 only
   b. 1 and 3 only   d. 1, 2, and 3

8. In terms of cancer induction, which of the following are seen as especially radiosensitive?
   1. brain
   2. bone marrow
   3. thyroid

a. 1 and 2 only   c. 2 and 3 only
b. 1 and 3 only   d. 1, 2, and 3

9. Low LET radiations such as gamma and x-rays are also known as _____ radiation.
   a. sparsely ionizing   c. high RBE
   b. highly ionizing   d. particulate

10. Which of the following are considered relatively radiosensitive?
    1. Spermatogonia
    2. Erythrocytes
    3. Lymphocytes
    a. 1 and 2 only   c. 2 and 3 only
    b. 1 and 3 only   d. 1, 2, and 3.

11. Which of the following radiation effects are well understood?
    1. Cellular carcinogenesis
    2. Dosimetry
    3. Radiation production
    a. 1 and 2 only   c. 2 and 3 only
    b. 1 and 3 only   d. 1, 2, and 3

12. Which of the following were findings of Muller's experiments on fruit flies?
    1. There was an increase in the quality of mutations.
    2. Most mutations observed were recessive.
    3. No threshold was observed.
    a. 1 and 2 only   c. 2 and 3 only
    b. 1 and 3 only   d. 1, 2, and 3

13. The LD 50 of an embryo/fetus is similar to that of an adult
    a. in the preimplantation stage
    b. in organogenesis
    c. in the fetal stage
    d. not until birth

14. Ten cGy in utero exposure will raise the percentage of spontaneous abortions by _____%.
    a. 0.01   c. 1.0
    b. 0.1   d. 10

15. Growth disorders most likely occur following which conceptual days?
    a. 24   c. 44
    b. 34   d. 54

Exercises

1. Compare LET and RBE.
2. If 1 rad of 250-keV x-rays kills 50% of a cell colony and it takes 2 rads of a test radiation to produce the same effect, what is the RBE of the test radiation?
3. Describe the relative radiosensitivity of the hematologic system.
4. Why do we have a poor knowledge of some radiation effects?

5. What were the findings in the fruit fly (Muller's) experiments and the megamouse experiments? What was the main conflicting finding?

6. What factors must be calculated in the genetically significant dose?

7. What are the principal effects of radiation on an embryo or fetus?

8. What is the significance of CNS development in radiation effects in the fetus?

9. When will diminished growth and development most likely occur?

10. What is the difference between a point mutation and a frameshift mutation? What is their radiobiologic significance?

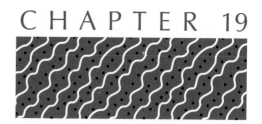

CHAPTER 19

Applying Radiation Biology to Clinical Practice

Steven B. Dowd, Ed.D., R.T.(R.)

Chapter Outline

Chapter Objectives

At the end of the chapter, you should be able to

- State potential radiation hazards.
- Describe the results of an epidemiological survey of radiologic technologists.
- Compare various types of risk expression.
- Draw various types of dose-response curves.
- Differentiate between linear, nonthreshold, and nonlinear threshold curves.
- Differentiate between stochastic and nonstochastic effects.
- Describe how early experiences with radiation led to radiation protection standards.
- Describe areas in which the theory of radiation biology has an effect on radiation protection practice, such as leukemia, fetal exposure, and mammography.

WHY STUDY RADIATION BIOLOGY?

Students sometimes ask why they need to study radiation biology, which to them at times appears to be an abstract science that has little to do with the clinical practice of radiography. Radiation biology is a science that is of more than mere academic interest to radiographers. Radiographers learn about radiation biology to be fully informed about the effects of ionizing radiation. This signifies true professionalism. Professionals are interested in all aspects of the science of their profession.

Sometimes patients still ask about the possibility of "x-ray burns," for example, which is a hold-over from the early days of radiology. It is certainly important that a radiographer know why this cannot occur at today's dose levels. Also, a radiation therapist should be able to describe the type of skin effects that can occur as a result of therapeutic radiation to patients.

Radiographers need to understand the potential risks of ionizing radiation. This necessitates a strong foundation in radiation biology. One of the roles of the radiographer is to minimize the risks of radiation to the patient and to him or herself while maximizing the benefits of diagnostic radiography. This is achieved through radiation protection, discussed in Chapter 21.

This chapter refines the theory of radiation biology introduced in the previous chapter while discussing specific risks of radiation. Chapter 18 presented the science of radiation biology. The focus of this chapter is to describe how this material has found use in the clinical setting by physicians, radiological physicists, radiological technologists, and others interested in improving the radiological health of the population. Even though we know that some uses of radiation hold little or no risk to the individual, we seek to understand potential risks and how to prevent them for professional practice. In some cases, all that radiation biology can provide us is a warning. This is sometimes strongly stated, sometimes not. It is the responsibility of each radiographer to evaluate these warnings and to translate them into radiation protection practice.

IDENTIFYING POTENTIAL RADIATION HAZARDS

This section briefly reviews the radiation hazards identified in the last chapter. These are divided into somatic effects (to the body); genetic effects to future generations; and fetal effects.

Somatic Effects

The somatic effects identified in the last chapter included, first, the very rare whole-body syndromes: hematopoietic syndrome, gastrointestinal syndrome, and central nervous system (CNS) syndrome. These are seen only at doses much higher than are used in diagnostic radiology. Next, effects to the immune system were described. However, the most important whole-body effect of interest to the radiographer working with diagnostic levels of radiation is carcinogenesis, especially leukemia, thyroid cancer, and breast cancer.

Genetic Effects

Genetic effects identified in the previous chapter included, first, two types of mutations—point mutations and frameshift mutations. Low LET radiations such as x-rays are more likely to be associated with sublethal, point mutations. Leukemia and other forms of neoplasm are possible effects, as are altered sex ratios, increased spontaneous abortions or stillbirths, increased infant mortality, increased congenital effects, and decreased life expectancy. Also, the dominant inheritable diseases of achondroplastic dwarfism, polydactyly, and Huntington's chorea can be caused by radiation exposure. The recessive inheritable diseases of cystic fibrosis, Tay-Sachs, hemophilia, and albinism are potential outcomes of radiation exposure.

Effects to the Fetus

Potential fetal effects of radiation include embryonic, fetal, or neonatal death; malformations; retardation of growth; congenital defects; and cancer induction. These are related to dose and the developmental stage of the embryo or fetus. In early stages of development, radiation will more than likely have an all-or-none effect that will terminate the pregnancy or simply delay development. In middle stages of development, radiation exposure is most likely to cause damage to a part or stunt its development. In later (growth) stages, late effects of radiation are most common.

An Epidemiological Study of Radiological Technologists

Population studies use an epidemiological approach. *Epidemiology* is the study of the distribution and determinants of disease in human populations. Epidemiology is an observational rather than an experimental science. This is an important distinction. That is, it collects information from a human population. Human populations do not separate themselves well into nicely discrete groups as is the case, for example, in experiments with laboratory animals. The basic question asked by any epidemiological study is whether those who have been exposed to an agent have a greater risk of developing a disease than those not exposed.

Epidemiological studies are used clinically to make value judgments about the use of radiation. As value judgments, rather than pure fact, there is some potential to make an incorrect decision.

One study, still in the preliminary stages, has explored the relationship between occupational exposure and risks such as cancer induction in radiological technologists. One hundred four thousand technologists participated in the study. These individuals were mostly female and white and had an average of 12 years work experience. Initial findings indicated a cancer incidence in 3.6% of respondents, with 1517 cases of skin cancer, 726 cases of cervical cancer, 665 cases of breast cancer, 242 cases of uterine cancer, 220 cases of thyroid cancer (9500 reported a "thyroid condition"), 76 reports of lung cancer, and 42 cases of leukemia.

Birthing experiences were similar in female technologists (9% observable defects) and spouses of male technologists (8%). A drawback of this study is that no comparison group was used to determine a "normal" incidence of effects. Also, data must be collected over time to show delayed effects.

Ninety-eight percent indicated wearing a monitor of some kind. Ninety-five percent wear lead aprons. Fluoroscopy or other procedures were not shown to increase mean scores of exposure. Ten percent indicated that their training had them take radiographs of other students. This should not occur today, for it would result in unnecessary radiation exposure. Average exposure in the 58% of technologists who could be traced through commercial dosimetry records was less than 1 rad. Finally, technologists were found to be more likely to use radiological services than the general public, increasing their overall dose.

This ongoing study should provide the profession with a better knowledge of the risks of low levels of radiation. A similar study of the effects of radiation on radiation workers has begun in Great Britain. As with most studies of radiation bioeffects that are conducted by looking back at groups of people instead of animals in a laboratory, the dosimetry problem has posed the largest threat to validity. That is, doses are not always known or comparable between types of radiation.

RISK VERSUS BENEFIT

Means of Expressing Risk

The idea behind comparing risk and benefit lies in the fact that, as human beings, we are willing to accept a risk as long as the potential benefit is greater. These kinds of comparisons are difficult to make, so we usually assign numbers to the risks. It would be better, of course, if we had one standard unit such as the roentgen to compare risk (the idea behind the BERT, described later), but this is only weakly possible.

We can say, for example, that the risk of 1 rad of radiation is equivalent to driving 220 miles on a freeway. That means that an equal number of people are thought to die from cancer due to radiation as those driving a distance of 220 miles on a freeway. Yet there are many confounding variables—the health status of the individual, the type of automobile driven, and so on—that weaken the validity of the comparison. With no other way to quantify risk, we are forced to use imperfect measures.

There are a variety of ways of expressing risk and benefit, and comparing the two. These are described in the following paragraphs.

Perceived Risk and Risk Comparisons

Two common means of expressing risk are by perceived risk and risk comparisons. Perceived risk asks individuals or groups of individuals to express their perception of risk. Perceived risk is an excellent teaching tool. For example, asking individuals first to rank, say, a list of five items in terms of potential risk allows them to express their opinion. Then the instructor or group facilitator provides the group with information that presents the actual risk of the item. This provides a basis for group discussion, disagreement, and critical thinking about items that did not agree with expert opinion.

In these and other cases, perceived risk is often used with risk comparisons. Risk comparisons make comparisons between two or more activities. For example, a chest x-ray can be compared with smoking a cigarette in terms of life span shortening. Table 19–1 lists some risk comparisons. One authority, Dr. John Cameron, has recommended the use of an actual unit called the BERT (background equivalent radiation time). This compares a chest x-ray, for example, with natural background radiation. A patient can be told that the chest x-ray received was worth 10 days of natural background radiation. This idea is somewhat sound, but falls short in that too many comparisons are made. First, as Cameron notes, "The values vary greatly from one medical center to another." Also, chest x-ray uses a different type of radiation, for the most part, than is seen in natural background radiation.

A League of Women Voters group rated nuclear power as the number one risk on a list of 30 potential risks (such as smoking, surgery, mountain climbing, pesticides), with diagnostic x-rays 23rd. College students ranked nuclear power first also, ranking x-rays 18th. Business and professional club members ranked nuclear power 9th and x-rays 24th. In terms of actual number of deaths, as risks x-ray is ranked 9th and nuclear power 20th. Each group overrated the potential danger of nuclear power and underrated the potential risk of diagnostic x-ray.

Cancer Risk

Based on population studies, we describe the risk of a group's developing cancer following irradiation three ways. *Absolute risk* is a common means of stating risk. It is expressed in terms of number of cases per 10^6 people per rad (centigray [cGy]) per year. Thus the value 4 cases per 10^6 people per rad per year would mean that if one million people were exposed to one rad, we would expect 4 more cases of the disease among those million people than would have normally been expected in the period of one year. This assumes a linear dose-response relationship.

Table 19–1: RISK COMPARISONS

Risk Cited and Outcome	Ionizing Radiation Risk and Outcome	Source
Smoking a cigarette (10 minutes life expectancy lost)	1 mr of radiation (1.5 minutes life expectancy lost)	(1)
Overweight by 20% (2.7 years of life expectancy lost)	1 rem occupational exposure (1 day life expectancy lost)	(1)
Home accidents (95 days life expectancy lost)	Medical x-rays (U.S. average) (6 days life expectancy lost)	(1)
Coal mining from age 20 (155 days life expectancy lost)	Radiation work at 5 rem/yr from age 20 (68 days life expectancy lost)	(2)
Construction employment from age 20 (94 days life expectancy lost)	Radiation work at 500 mrem/yr from age 20 (7 days life expectancy lost)	(2)

Source: Adapted from (1) Ruegesegger, D.R. Radiation exposure levels in an intensive care nursery. Pediatr Nurs 8:244–247, 1982; (2) Pizzarello, D.; Witcofski, R.L. Basic Radiation Biology, 2nd ed. Philadelphia: Lea & Febiger, 1975.
mrem = millirem (0.001 rem); mr = millirad (0.001 rad); rem = roentgen equivalents man (equivalent of 1 rad × relative biological effectiveness).

Excess risk describes risk in terms of the number of excess cases observed over what would be expected spontaneously (naturally) in a population. If 30 cases of a disease are observed in a population exposed to 400 rads and 17 were expected, then the excess risk is 13.

Relative risk is the term used when the dose to which a population has been exposed is not precisely known. The number of people in the exposed population is compared with those not exposed as a control group. A relative risk of 1 indicates no risk; relative risk rates tend to range from 1 to 10. It is expressed either as simply a number (e.g., 5) or as a ratio (e.g., 5:1).

Absolute risk and relative risk are the preferred models for expressing risk. Many texts list both values, because agreement does not exist as to which is the best means of expressing risk.

The Risk-Benefit Continuum

Radiation protection guidelines usually assume the lack of a *threshold* (a level below which no effects are seen). If no threshold is assumed, then any dose of radiation can have a potential effect. The concept of the lack of a threshold has led to risk-versus-benefit considerations for both patients and operators of radiological equipment. If a threshold is not assumed, then every use of radiation involves a small risk. However, the use of radiation in the healing arts results in such numerous benefits that if it is well used, the benefits of radiation greatly exceed the very small risk to the individual. Without ionizing radiation, the health of the population would decline, because we would lack the ability to diagnose disease and pinpoint trauma. A bell-shaped curve (Fig. 19–1) can be used to graphically represent this fact; the health of the population is shown to be low with non-use of ionizing radiation and high when radiation is well used but declines when radiation is overused.

A similar concept applied to the individual is the risk-benefit continuum (Fig. 19–2). This instrument assigns relative numbers at polar opposites to risks and benefits. Obviously, there is no need for an examination if it carries only a risk and no benefit. In this case, the patient should refuse the examination. However, when the risk is small and the potential benefit great, the patient should have the examination. Most radiological examinations carry a very small risk in relation to the potential benefit. The risk-benefit continuum is a useful tool for personal and classroom learning of risk versus benefit. For example, what personal, numerical value would the radiographer assign to a career in radiation work? How does that balance with the benefits to be received?

The goal of the risk-benefit continuum is not to show exactly the relationship between risk and benefit —that is not possible. The relationship between risk and benefit is a value decision that is only weakly quantified (i.e., expressed as some number). Thus the numbers are not really useful except to show the relative strength or weakness for the recommendation to conduct a specific radiological examination.

For example, a patient who will die without the use of radiation can be assigned a +3 in terms of risk. That is, if the patient does not have the examination, he or she will die. Thus any potential long-term effects such as cancer induction (5 to 20 years in the future) poses little threat to an individual who will die tomorrow if the examination is not undertaken. If the examination will, with an almost 100% degree of probability, find a curable cause of the disease, then that examination is assigned a +3 in terms of benefit. That total, +6, indicates that the examination should be done. However, even if the examination only has a weak chance of finding the cause (e.g., a +0.5; total of 3.5), the benefits still outweigh the risk.

As the numbers approach 0, the question of why an examination is performed must be asked. A classic example is the 98-year-old patient sent for a barium enema. Although the problem can be diagnosed, if no intercession is possible (that is, no surgery or other means is possible to cure the problem), then why subject the patient to the examination? This question is not easily answered, and certainly each physician has specific reasons for ordering a diagnostic examination that may not be apparent.

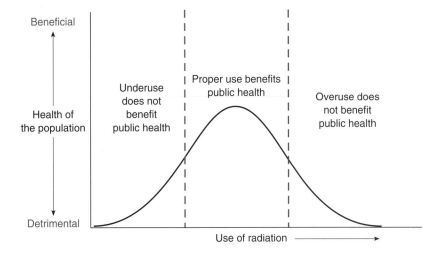

FIGURE 19–1. Bell-shaped curve showing the relationship between radiation exposure and health of a population. As radiation use increases the health of the population will rise up to a point, after which additional increases in radiation use drive down the health of the population.

```
        -3   -2   -1    0   +1   +2   +3
        ├────┼────┼────┼────┼────┼────┤
        100%                      0% risk
        risk

        -3   -2   -1    0   +1   +2   +3
        ├────┼────┼────┼────┼────┼────┤
        0%                        100%
        benefit                   benefit
```

Total

-6 Patient should not undergo examination

-3 Patient and physician may decide that patient should not undergo examination because of high risk-benefit ratio

0 Difficult decision for patient and physician; risk and benefit equal

+3 Good risk-benefit ratio; patient probably should undergo examination

+6 Patient should undergo examination

FIGURE 19-2. Risk-Benefit Continuum. (Dowd, Applied Radiology, Anderson Publishing Ltd., Vol. 13 #2, Port Washington, NY.)

Another example is the use of x-ray pelvimetry. Plain-film pelvimetry (an examination of the pelvic proportions by x-ray to determine whether a fetus can be delivered by the normal route) is an examination that students today are not likely to see in the clinical setting. The risks of the procedure are not great, but other examinations such as diagnostic medical ultrasound can provide the same or more information without ionizing radiation.

Remember that the continuum is just a learning tool, a way to help you think about the positive and negative uses of radiation. It definitely has its weaknesses and shortcomings and should be used for awareness, not as fact.

DOSE-RESPONSE CURVES

General Concepts of Dose-Response Curves

Dose-response curves plot effects observed in relationship to dose received. As dose increases, so will most effects. As with any other graphic representation of data, variables (numbers) are plotted along horizontal and vertical axes to show the relationship between the two quantities.

Dose-response curves vary in two basic ways (Fig. 19-3):

1. They are either linear, in which a proportional response is observed in relation to dose; or they are nonlinear, in which no proportional response is observed in relation to dose.
2. They are either threshold, which is a level below which no effects are observed; or they are *non-threshold*, in which even a small dose can theoretically cause an effect.

This chapter associates linear with threshold and one type of nonlinear *(sigmoid)* with nonthreshold in discussing three types of curves—linear, sigmoid, and linear-quadratic. There are more possible types, but this representation is to facilitate students' understanding of the relationship between dose and potential effects. Diagnostic radiology is primarily concerned with linear, nonthreshold dose–response relationships in terms of late effects.

Linear Dose-Response Curve

A *linear dose-response curve* (Fig. 19–3A) exhibits some effect, no matter how small the dose. Theoretically, even one photon could cause the effect to occur.

The observed effects, opposite to effects seen with a sigmoid curve, can be noticed even with no dosage, because there usually is a natural incidence of the effect. For example, leukemia is often seen as responding to the linear dose-response curve. It occurs naturally to a certain extent in the population; radiation serves to increase the incidence. This is also known as a *stochastic* effect, discussed in a subsequent section.

A direct proportion can be observed between dose and response for the linear (also called the linear nonthreshold) curve. Besides leukemia, breast cancer (at low doses), and genetic damage are assumed to follow this curve. It is because these three effects are assumed to follow this curve and because of its lack of a threshold, that we focus many of our radiation protection efforts on these effects. It is why we spend so

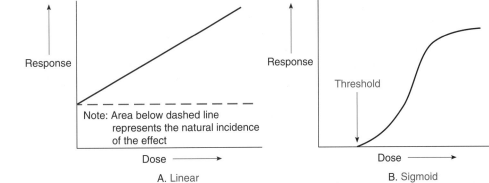

FIGURE 19-3. Types of dose-response curves. *A,* Linear dose-response curve, and *B,* Sigmoid dose-response curve

Response

Note: Area below dashed line represents the natural incidence of the effect

Dose ⟶

A. Linear

Response

Threshold

Dose ⟶

B. Sigmoid

much time studying the potential effects of mammography on breast cancer, even though the doses are low. For this reason, we focus strongly on having individuals wear lead aprons, because lead aprons cover most of the active bone marrow in the body.

Nonlinear Dose-Response Curves

Sigmoid Dose-Response Curve

The term *sigmoid* means S-shaped, a term probably familiar to radiography students from the sigmoid colon. This dose-response curve (Fig. 19-3B) applies primarily to high-dose effects, seen in radiotherapy. There is usually a threshold, a level (minimum dose) below which no observable effects occur. This minimum dose is different for different effects.

Since the curve is S-shaped, there is a nonlinear relationship between effect and dose, meaning that the frequency or intensity of an effect is not proportional to dose.

There is a partial recovery at low doses reflected in the tail of the curve. The curve eventually levels off and then turns downward at the highest doses as the affected animal or tissue dies before the effect can manifest (appear).

Linear-Quadratic Dose-Response Curves

The linear and quadratic curves do not hold true for all types of radiation responses. In 1980 the Committee on Biologic Effects of Ionizing Radiation (the BEIR Committee) proposed a model for certain types of responses. These responses include most cancers, also called solid tumors to differentiate them from leukemia. This curve is linear, or proportional, at the low-dose levels, becoming curvilinear at higher doses (Fig. 19-4). This curve has no threshold and is stochastic, since it is linear at the lowest levels.

A portion of the curve in which increases in dose show little or no increase in effects is called the toe. A segment of the top of the curve in which a plateauing or leveling off occurs, also showing little or no relationship between increases in dose and effect, is called the shoulder. Not all curves exhibit toes and shoulders, but they are a common part of nonlinear curves.

The danger in this model is that it can underestimate the low-dose effects of radiation, because the linear portion of the curve is somewhat "flattened." For this reason, some opt for the linear model, since it would err on the side of safety rather than being too liberal. Occupational recommendations for *maximum permissible doses* (MPDs), for example, assume that the linear curve holds for all effects, even though the effects of many cancers probably hold for the linear-quadratic curve.

Stochastic Effects

Stochastic effects are also called the statistical response. The probability of occurrence of effects increase in proportion to radiation dose of the entire population. It is assumed that stochastic effects do not exhibit a threshold. Stochastic effects are associated with both the linear and the linear-quadratic dose-response curves.

Thus a stochastic effect, especially at diagnostic levels in which doses are low, places the odds heavily in one's favor that no effect will occur. An unlucky, random few will experience an effect. Radiation risks from diagnostic imaging, with the exception of in utero exposure of a viable fetus, are considered to be stochastic. Heredity effects are considered to be stochastic as well as carcinogenic.

Nonstochastic Effects

Nonstochastic effects increase in severity with dose, and a threshold is assumed. This is also sometimes called the certainty effect. At high doses such as radiotherapy, it is assumed that certain effects such as skin erythema or cataracts will occur; thus the name certainty effect. This effect is associated with the sigmoid dose-response curve.

Cataract induction, nonmalignant damage to skin, hematologic deficiencies, and impairment of fertility are considered nonstochastic effects. The dose must be high enough to begin the effect, at which point the probability of an effect occurring is fairly certain. Some authorities indicate that a dose of 200 rad (cGy) is necessary to produce a nonstochastic effect; others indicate 100 rad (cGy).

APPLYING RADIATION BIOLOGY TO CLINICAL PRACTICE

Skin and Extremities

Because of radiation therapy and early uses of radiation, we have a good deal of information on skin

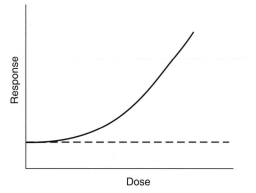

FIGURE 19-4. Linear-quadratic dose-response curves.

effects. Many of the early x-ray pioneers suffered x-ray burns to the skin. Patients also often suffered x-ray burns from exposures that used low-kV, unshielded tubes and several minutes of exposure time.

Radiodermatitis in the form of what were then called roentgen-ray burns was the cause of many lawsuits against untrained operators, including physicians. Thousands of dollars were awarded to individuals burned by x-rays. This led to certification of radiographers and the creation of physicians specializing in the use of x-rays for diagnosis and treatment.

Early Radiation Protection Guidelines

"Radiation biology" as practiced to bring about radiation protection practices in that day was self-experimental and experiential in nature. That is, individuals observed effects to themselves and to patients in order to determine, first, radiation effects and, second, the means to prevent these effects. For example, Henri Becquerel, the discoverer of radioactivity, noticed a skin burn on his chest two days after carrying a tube of radium in his pocket all day. One story associated with the incident is that a fellow researcher then offered to also carry a tube of radium in his pocket to see if the same effect would happen to him. Although the truth of this story cannot be verified, it is consistent with the approach taken to radiation effects in the early years of radiation exposure.

The first MPD has been called the erythema dose—the dose necessary to redden skin. Effects had to be readily observable before something was done about them. In some cases, nothing was done. For example, epilation (the loss of hair) caused by radiation was often not taken seriously, since the hair often grew back. It was thought to be a short-term effect that posed little danger to the individual.

Early techniques often used only a few (5 to 10) inches of focal-film distance with unshielded tubes and many minutes of exposure time. For example, the recommended x-ray technique in 1900 for the chest was 10 minutes and for the pelvis 20 minutes of exposure time.

The majority of effects on the extremities were noted in the hands of early radiologists, who often had multiple amputations of their fingers due to being unknowingly careless with fluoroscopy. Often operators had to put their hands in the beam to "prove" to the patient that the "x-ray light" did not hurt.

These operators contracted radiodermatitis, which often metastasized and resulted in death. M.K. Kassabian documented the deterioration of his hands because of radiodermatitis (these photographs are shown in Fig. 19–5). Dr. Kassabian died in 1910 from a metastatic malignancy of the axilla. However, before he died, he formulated a number of radiation protection measures based on his experiences, some of which are still used in modified form today. These include the use of lead protection, use of distance to minimize exposure, and having the operator go into an adjoining room.

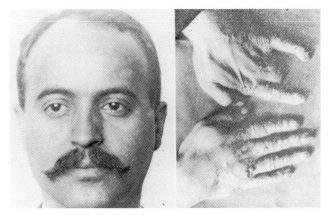

FIGURE 19–5. Radiodermatitis of M.K. Kassabian. (From Grigg, E.R.N. The Trail of the Invisible Light, 1965. Courtesy of Charles C Thomas, Publisher, Springfield, Illinois.)

Long-Term Effects

Chronic, long-term irradiation of the skin can result in nonmalignant changes. The early radiologists also developed hands and forearms that were "weathered," similar in appearance to individuals with many years of exposure to the sun. Sometimes the skin would become tight and brittle, leading to cracking and flaking.

Today's practice of diagnostic imaging and therapy does not lead to such changes. Currently, the group of individuals who must be most careful about the potential effects of radiation to the extremities are nuclear medicine technologists who hold syringes containing radioactive material during injection procedures.

Eyes

Radiation cataractogenesis is the formation of cataracts resulting from radiation exposure. Patients who received radiation therapy at high doses and cyclotron physicists have well-documented cases of cataractogenesis. This dose-response relationship is felt by most investigators to be a threshold, non-linear response. At 1000 rads (cGy) to the eye, 100% of those irradiated will develop cataracts. The threshold is believed to be about 200 cGy for a single dose, but this is not clear. For fractionated doses, it is thought to be as high as 1000 cGy.

Some technologists and physicians, especially those working in relatively high-dose areas such as angiography, wear protective lens shields. Although this may be unnecessary, each individual should practice personal radiation protection as he or she sees fit. For example, radiology residents can receive a high enough dose to the lens of the eye to warrant wearing protective lens shields. These individuals are not sufficiently experienced to keep doses to a bare minimum. There are also some high-dose examinations, such as conventional tomography of the head and neck, in which protective lens shields can be advocated for patient use.

Thyroid

The radiocarcinogenic thyroid dose is important for radiation protection purposes. Many individuals have opted for thyroid shields during fluoroscopy because of concern over the radiocarcinogenic dose. Radiation-induced thyroid tumors occur at a fourfold higher level in females than in males, a difference thought to be caused by the fluctuating hormonal status of women. This may make the need to wear thyroid shields more acute for women.

Leukemia

Ionizing radiation can cause leukemia and has been implicated in this disease more than in any other. As previously noted, leukemia, unlike many other cancers, apparently follows a linear, nonthreshold dose-response curve.

Leukemia has the shortest latent period of any malignant disease—5 to 7 years. The actual at-risk period is considered to be 20 years. Leukemia is considered to have an absolute risk, based on the A-bomb data of 1.5 cases per 10^6 people per rad per year. A study of ankylosing spondylitis patients treated with radiation therapy showed an absolute risk of 0.8 cases per 10^6 people per rad per year. The relative risk at 600 rads was 2.8 for the A-bomb survivors and 9.5 for a group of ankylosing spondylitis patients.

Genetic Effects

Gonadal shielding is provided, since genetic effects follow the linear curve—it can never be known if it was one stray photon that caused a genetic effect. For example, if we knew that genetic effects follow the sigmoid curve and thus do not exhibit any effects on future generations until a dose of possibly 5 rad, we could afford to be lax in gonadal protection. As it stands, we cannot be lax—to do so would jeopardize the future health of unborn children.

The potential genetic effects of radiation exposure, described in the previous chapter, are one of the strongest arguments for assuming the lack of a threshold and the resultant *ALARA* (as low as reasonably achievable) concept (to be described in greater detail in Chapter 20). ALARA means that each radiation exposure of the patient is to be scrutinized. A physician must have a valid reason for ordering the examination based on clinical need, not simply preventive malpractice. The radiographer must, in consultation with radiologists and radiological physicists, produce a film that provides a maximum amount of diagnostic information with as low a radiation exposure as possible.

One example of a sound practice of radiation protection that, unfortunately, has not found much favor is the use of personal records for diagnostic x-ray examinations. Such a record typically records the date, physician ordering the examination, location of facility, type of examination, and purpose of the examina-

tion (Fig. 19–6). Properly used, such records could eliminate potential repeats as well as limit the actual number of examinations. If a study is carefully reviewed before it is conducted, there is a greater chance that it will be conducted for a valid reason rather than performed at whim or to minimize patient or physician anxiety. The end result is less radiation dose to the patient.

Similarly, radiographers should view patient questions about equipment and certification status in a positive light. They should encourage patients to continue to ask such questions, regardless of where their examinations are performed. By making facilities and practitioners accountable to outside standards of quality, potential risk is minimized and potential benefit maximized.

If dose, especially gonadal dose, is maintained at low levels, the health of the population will benefit. Genetic effects are thought to hold to a linear nonthreshold dose-response relationship. Thus every exposure carries some risk. Fewer exposures mean less likelihood of genetic effects. The possibility of genetic effects from radiation could only be reduced to zero if no radiation exposure were used. However, this policy would decrease the health of the population in other ways. A balance (ALARA) must be achieved.

Fetal Exposure

In 1959 a scientist named Hammer-Jacobsen developed guidelines for therapeutic abortion after radiation exposure. Gaulden and Murphy refined these in 1980. They believed that before six weeks of development, 10 rad and above of exposure to the fetus was reason to suggest termination of a pregnancy. They noted that nothing should be done after six weeks in cases of low-dose exposures. They also stated that abortion should occur after high doses but did not specifically define high and low doses.

The "10 to 25" rule regarding radiation exposure and pregnancy has been developed by Bushong (1992), who developed this rule after he noted in a national women's magazine an article about a woman who had a two-view lumbar spine examination because of lower back pain. She later found that she was pregnant, and her physician informed her that he had consulted with a number of "experts" and recommended that she terminate the pregnancy because of the severe effects that could occur.

This examination probably resulted in a dose of about 100 millirad (mrad) to the fetus. The 10 to 25 rule uses both common sense and a knowledge of radiation biology. It states that

- Less than 10 rads should never be an indication to terminate a pregnancy
- Between 10 and 25 rads is a "gray area" in which the determination to terminate a pregnancy depends on the time of exposure
- Above 25 rads, termination of a pregnancy should be considered

PERSONAL MEDICAL EXPOSURE HISTORY

Name: _____

Address: _____   Birthdate: _____

Date	Physician	X-ray facility location	Examination	Purpose of examination	Technologist	Notes

FIGURE 19–6. An x-ray exposure record form.

Additionally, many experts think that the safest time to be irradiated in pregnancy is during the first two weeks—contrary to what many people believe. Because of the all-or-none effect (see earlier and Chapter 18) either a spontaneous abortion will occur or the child will be carried to term with no ill effects. Again, this is a value decision based on a knowledge of radiobiology—other individuals might consider the possibility of a spontaneous abortion unacceptable.

Mammography

Radiation can induce breast cancer. This has been and will continue to be important because of the possible development of breast cancer from diagnostic mammography. Some studies have indicated a relative risk for breast cancer as high as 10 to 1. The main data for the risk from mammography comes from the atomic bomb survivors of Hiroshima and Nagasaki. Why this group? Consider that mammography is a relatively new technology not widely used until the 1960s, when Wolfe refined and developed the carefulness of mammography as a tool to evaluate breast cancer. Mammography has gone through various in-carnations since that time using different film-screen types, tubes, and other changes.

Estimates based on atomic bomb survivors set the absolute risk at 1.5 cases per 10^6 persons per rad per year. In that same group, no increased risk was seen in the 40- to 49-year-old age group (Fig. 19–7). There were more young women in the first two groups. This would seem to indicate that breast irradiation in later years is safer. From this, it can be concluded that the benefit of mammography would appear to outweigh risk in women over age 40, although this cannot be conclusively determined from a few studies.

Risk-Benefit Considerations for Mammography

In 1976, Bailar suggested that the risk of radiation-induced breast cancer from mammography was greater than the benefit associated with the detection of breast cancer. His calculations showed that, with an average of 2 rad breast tissue dose per examination, in a group of one million women aged 35 to 49, 370 breast cancers could be induced. He also calculated 148 deaths from breast cancer in that group.

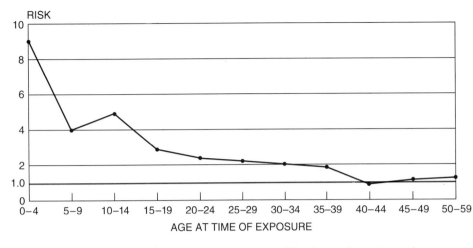

RISK

FIGURE 19–7. The relationship between age of exposure and breast cancer in Hiroshima survivors.

AGE AT TIME OF EXPOSURE

The red line, set at 1.0, is the natural incidence of the disease (breast cancer).

Also in 1976, however, what could be called the second generation of mammography screen-film was introduced. This film was 15 times faster than previous screen-film combinations. In 1978 a third generation of mammography film that reduced exposure by 50% was introduced. The American College of Radiology (ACR) recommends that the average dose in mammography be no more than 0.3 rad per view, and many facilities average 0.1 rad per view. With a four-view examination (two views of each breast), the average dose then ranges from 0.4 rad to 1.2 rad.

The guidelines from the American Cancer Society and the ACR for mammographic screening of asymptomatic women are

- A baseline mammogram between the ages of 35 and 40
- Mammograms at one- to two-year intervals from age 40 to 49
- Annual mammograms after age 50

These are not universally accepted, although they are based on reasonable assumptions of risk versus benefit. Some screening programs have found that younger patients could benefit from mammographic screening by detecting rarer but more aggressive malignancies sometimes found in younger ages. For example, women under the age of 40 account for 6.5% of breast cancers per year. A study conducted at Sloan-Kettering Memorial Hospital in New York found value for mammographic screening in women aged 35 to 39 years.

Other authors have suggested that mammograms are of no value for women under 50. These debates will continue as will efforts to minimize mammographic dose.

Patient dose can be minimized in mammography by observing a variety of factors, including using a high tube output and proper use of compression, grids, screen-film combinations, and developer time and temperature. Since mammography also allows for an expanded role of the radiographer in patient care and radiation protection, it is especially important that a mammographer understand the potential biological effects of radiation and how to reduce the dose.

Chapter Summary/ Important Concepts

Radiographers study radiation biology to learn about all types of radiation effects and how this translates into radiation protection practices and standards. Potential radiation hazards include somatic, genetic, and fetal effects.

One means of studying the effects of radiation on humans is through epidemiology, which looks back at effects that may have been caused by radiation. Often, control groups that have not been exposed to radiation are used to determine the effects of radiation.

Risk can be expressed in a variety of ways. This includes perceived risk, which simply asks an individual or group to express their perception of risk, and risk comparisons, which compare one risk to another. Population studies of radiocarcinogenesis use three basic measures: absolute risk, excess risk, and relative risk. The preferred models are absolute risk and relative risk. The risk-benefit continuum attempts to compare the opposites of risk and benefit to help in learning about risks and benefits of radiation. Like all models, it has a variety of imperfections.

Dose-response curves plot effects observed in relation to dose. A linear curve shows a proportional response in relation to dose; a non-linear curve does not. A curve with a threshold has a level below which no effects are observed; a nonthreshold curve does not. Radiation protection efforts are focused on three effects that are thought to follow a linear nonthreshold curve: leukemia, breast cancer, and thyroid cancer. Another type of curve developed to show responses for most solid tumors is the linear-quadratic curve.

Stochastic effects are random in nature and follow the linear and linear-quadratic dose-response curves. Nonstochastic effects are associated with a certainty of occurrence at a high dose.

Effects to the skin and extremities are rare to non-existent at today's dose levels. They are of interest because they helped to formulate early radiation protection standards. Nor should cataractogenesis occur at today's dose levels.

Thyroid effects are well documented through various populations. Since females have a potential lower threshold for the induction of thyroid tumors, they may be more prone to want to wear a thyroid shield. Certainly, all individuals exposed to radiation doses such as are seen in fluoroscopy should wear lead aprons to minimize the potential induction of leukemia.

Genetic effects are assumed to follow a linear, nonthreshold dose response curve. Since any dose of radiation can potentially cause an effect, and effects increase proportionally with dose, gonadal shielding should be provided whenever possible.

Although the fetus is sensitive to radiation, abortion is not an option simply because of radiation exposure. Most authorities set 10 rad as a guideline from which to begin considering abortion.

Mammography can induce breast cancer. However, most proof of radiation-induced breast cancer does not come from studies on mammography patients, it comes from other groups exposed to radiation. Currently, controversy exists as to the benefit of mammography in younger age groups.

Important Terminology

Absolute Risk. Expressed in terms of number of cases/10^6 people/rad (centigray)/year, assuming a linear dose-response relationship

ALARA. Acronym for "as low as reasonably achievable"; refers to the fact that all exposures should be kept as low as possible

Epidemiology. The study of the distribution and determinants of disease in human populations

Excess Risk. Risk in terms of the excess number of cases observed over what would be expected spontaneously (naturally) in a population

Linear Dose-Response Curve. A plotting of dose to response in which a proportional response is observed in relation to dose

Maximum Permissible Dose. Highest dose allowed by law or mandate to occupational workers and the general public

Nonlinear Dose-Response Curve. A plotting of dose to response in which no proportional response is observed in relation to dose

Nonstochastic. Describes an increase in severity with increased dose; a threshold is assumed; sometimes called the certainty effect

Nonthreshold. Refers to the fact that any dose of radiation can theoretically cause an effect

Radiodermatitis. Inflammation of skin caused by radiation

Relative Risk. Used when the dose to which a population has been exposed is not precisely known; the number of people in the exposed population is compared with a control group of those not exposed

Sigmoid. S-shaped; a type of nonlinear dose-response curve

Stochastic. Random in nature; also called the statistical response, indicating that the probability of occurrence of effects increases in proportion to radiation dose of the entire population

Threshold. A level below which no effects are observed on a dose-response curve

Bibliography

Bacq, A.M.; Alexander, P. Fundamentals of Radiobiology, 2nd ed. New York: Pergamon Press, 1961.

Baker M.; Dalrymple, G.V. Radiation and the fetus. In Hendee, W.R., Health Effects of Low-Level Radiation. Norwalk, CT: Appleton-Century-Crofts, 1984.

Bushong, S.C. Quality assurance in mammography. Paper presented at the Annual Meeting of the Alabama State Society of Radiologic Technologists, 1992.

Cameron, J. Are we exaggerating fear? Radio Technol 62:336, 1991.

Casarett, A.P. Radiation Biology. Englewood Cliffs, NJ: Prentice-Hall, 1968.

Dowd, S.B. A continuum for evaluating risks and benefits of ionizing radiation. Appl Radiol 13:81–82, 1984.

Dowd, S.B. The basics of radiation protection for hospital workers. Hosp Top 69:31, 1991.

Fischoff, B. et al How safe is safe enough? A psychometric study of attitudes toward technological risks and benefits. Pol Sci 9:127, 1978.

Gaulden, M.E.; and Murray, R.C. Medical radiation and possible adverse effects on the human embryo. In Meyn, R.E.; Withers, R., eds. Radiation Biology in Cancer Research. New York: Raven Press, 1980.

Hall, E.J. Radiobiology for the Radiologist, 3rd ed. Philadelphia: J.B. Lippincott, 1988.

Hammer-Jacobsen, E. Therapeutic abortion on account of x-ray examination during pregnancy. Dan Med Bull 6:113, 1959.

Land, C.E. Estimating cancer risks from low doses of ionizing radiation. Science 209:1197, 1981.

Merriam, G.R.; Focht, E.F. Clinical study of radiation cataracts and the relation to dose. AJR 77:759, 1957.

Noz, M.E.; Maguire, G.Q. Radiation Protection in the Radiologic and Health Sciences, 2nd ed. Philadelphia: Lea & Febiger, 1985.

Palmer, L. Exposed (Synopsis of a presentation by S.C. Bushong). RT Image June 22, 1992, p. 32.

Payne, J.T.; Loken, M.K. A survey of the risks and benefits of ionizing radiation. CRC Crit Rev Clin Radiol Nucl Med 6:425, 1975.

Pizzarello, D.; Witcofski, R.L. Basic Radiation Biology, 2nd ed. Philadelphia: Lea & Febiger, 1975.

Ruegesegger, D.R. Radiation exposure levels in an intensive care nursery. Pediatr Nurs 8:244–247, 1982.

Selman, J. Elements of Radiobiology. Springfield, IL: Charles C Thomas, 1983.

Travis, E.L. Primer of Medical Radiobiology, 2nd ed. Chicago: Year Book Medical Publishers, 1989.

Whalen, J.P.; Balter, S. Radiation risks in medical imaging. Chicago: Year Book Medical Publishers, 1984.

▰▰ Review Questions

1. The study of the distribution and determinants of disease in a population is known as
   - a. epidemiology
   - b. pathology
   - c. experimentation
   - d. philosophy

2. The number of cases per 10^6 people per rad per year is a means of expressing _____ risk.
   - a. absolute
   - b. excess
   - c. beneficial
   - d. relative

3. A dose-response curve that assumes that any amount of radiation could have an effect and shows a proportional response to dose is a _____ curve.
   - a. linear threshold
   - b. linear nonthreshold
   - c. nonlinear threshold
   - d. nonlinear nonthreshold

4. If an effect occurs naturally in a population, and radiation increases the incidence, it is a _____ effect.
   - a. stochastic
   - b. nonstochastic

5. The 1980 BEIR Committee proposed a model for solid tumors. This is the _____ curve.
   - a. linear threshold
   - b. sigmoid nonthreshold
   - c. sigmoid plateau
   - d. linear-quadratic

6. An effect that is certain to occur with a specific dose is known as a _____ effect.
   - a. stochastic
   - b. nonstochastic

7. The nonfractionated dose at which 100% of the population will develop cataracts is _____ centigray.
   - a. 200
   - b. 400
   - c. 800
   - d. 1000

8. Many individuals, because of the all-or-none effect, consider which of the following time periods as the safest for occupational exposure of a pregnant worker?
   - a. first two weeks
   - b. second two weeks
   - c. first two months
   - d. last two months

9. The fact that *any* exposure to radiation can cause a potential effect is seen in which of the following?
   - I. Threshold
   - II. ALARA
   - III. Linear-quadratic curve
   - a. I and II only
   - b. I and III only
   - c. II and III only
   - d. I, II, and III

10. Which form of risk is commonly used for radiocarcinogenesis when the dose to which a population has been exposed is not known?
    - a. absolute risk
    - b. excess risk
    - c. relative risk
    - d. comparative

Exercises

1. What is the primary difference between linear nonthreshold and nonlinear threshold curves? What is the significance of each of these models?
2. Compare stochastic effects with nonstochastic effects.
3. Describe how radiation protection principles based on radiobiology were first formulated.
4. What is the "10 to 25" rule?
5. What studies have been used to determine the risk of mammography? What are some of the limitations of these studies?
6. Based on the risk-benefit continuum, determine the safety of radiography as a profession.
7. Why cannot the epidemiological study of radiological technologists described in this chapter be used to determine the cancer incidence of radiological technologists?

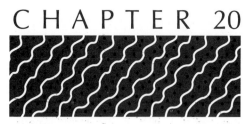

CHAPTER 20

Radiological Health Physics

Michael A. Thompson, M.S.

Chapter Outline

Chapter Objectives

On completion of this chapter, you should be able to

- Indicate the national and international advisory bodies who make recommendations regarding radiation protection standards.
- Indicate how radiation protection regulations come into existence and the agencies that enforce them.
- Explain the difference between exposure, absorbed dose, and dose equivalent, indicating units in which each is measured.
- Calculate absorbed dose and dose equivalent from an exposure measurement and other pertinent information.
- Explain what is meant by the ALARA concept and its role in a radiation protection program.
- Indicate common types of personnel dosimetry, how they measure occupational exposure, and their relative advantages and disadvantages.
- List specific actions that must be taken to assure that personnel dosimetry devices provide accurate estimates of occupational exposure.
- Indicate how personnel dosimetry readings are used to indicate compliance with radiation protection standards regarding occupational exposure.
- Explain how time, distance, and appropriate shielding can be used to reduce occupational exposure from any radiation source.
- Perform simple calculations regarding the use of distance and shielding in the reduction of radiation exposure.
- Describe the importance of using proper handling and storage techniques for lead aprons and lead gloves.
- Identify commonly found radiation warning signs as to the type and level of hazard associated with each.
- Indicate the difference between a primary and secondary barrier as used in a radiographic imaging room.
- Indicate the importance of radiation protection standards to the pregnant technologist and measures that can be taken to assure her safety.

THE NEED FOR RADIATION PROTECTION STANDARDS

Perhaps no other discovery in the history of science has had the impact on medicine and society as has the discovery of x-rays by Wilhelm Röntgen in November of 1895. Röntgen's work eventually culminated in his demonstration of the ability of the newly discovered "x-rays" to produce anatomical images unlike any seen before. The excitement created by this major discovery produced a rush to use this newly discovered phenomenon in both medical diagnosis and therapy. In contrast to the numerous tests today that must be conducted prior to using any new mode of treatment on humans, the first medical x-ray made in the United States (U.S.) was produced at Dartmouth College in February, 1896, just three months after Röntgen's initial discovery. Within weeks another radiograph was used to aid a surgeon in the removal of a bullet from a patient's leg. These early radiographs required exposure times of approximately 20 minutes to one hour to obtain the desired images, compared with today's exposure times of a second or less. Today's shorter exposure times greatly reduce radiation dose to the patient.

Therapeutic use of x-rays possibly began even earlier than their diagnostic use. Physicians at Hahnemann Medical College of Chicago had suggested the use of x-rays to destroy pathological conditions such as cancer and lupus. As early as January, 1896, a case of lupus and breast cancer were treated unsuccessfully with x-rays at a time when there were more unknowns than knowns about this new form of energy.

Capitalizing on the tremendous interest and the potentially wide range of applications, commercial production of x-ray tubes within the United States began in 1897. Initially, it was the joint opinion of the medical and scientific communities that there were no adverse health effects associated with x-ray exposure. As a result, x-ray tubes were made available to large numbers of individuals who knew little of the associated dangers.

As early as March 1896, Thomas Edison reported eye irritation as a result of his work with x-rays and indicated that precautions should be taken with their use. Although Edison abandoned his work with x-rays, it was too late to prevent the overexposure of his assistant, Clarence M. Dally, who died in 1904 as a result of x-ray–induced dermatitis.

Another important event occurred in March 1896 that played a major role in the development of radiation protection standards. This was the discovery of radioactivity by Henri Becquerel. Becquerel's discovery was almost eclipsed by the widespread interest and publicity accorded to Röntgen's discovery of x-rays. Becquerel's discovery did capture the interest of Pierre and Marie Curie who later successfully chemically isolated two new radioactive elements, radium and polonium. By the end of 1904, some 20 radionuclides had been isolated, and fundamental laws of radioactive decay had been formulated.

The amazing properties of x-rays and the closely associated properties of radioactive materials quickly captured public attention and fascination. This fascination resulted in exaggerated claims of curative powers, unsupervised applications, and unrestricted use. Lack of control of radiation sources often led to tragic consequences.

Many saw x-ray units as new sources of public amusement. Soon after Röntgen's discovery, thousands viewed their own bones, using a fluoroscopic device developed by Thomas Edison, at the New York Electrical Exposition held in early 1896. For years thereafter, mystic and curative powers were attributed to the new radiations. Claims were made that x-ray "baths" could be used to cure diseases such as tuberculosis,

cancer, and even criminal behavior. Another popular use of x-rays was as a depilatory. This application produced numerous cases of young women with faces showing the disfigurement produced by these x-ray treatments. Even with this evidence of the potentially biologically damaging effects of radiation overexposure, the practice continued well into the 1930s. Fluoroscopic devices remained in shoe stores to allow children and adults to view their toes inside a new pair of shoes through the 1950s.

Mystical powers were also ascribed to the newly discovered, highly radioactive element radium. Although not condoned by the medical community at the time, many false claims were made regarding the beneficial health effects of drinking and bathing in radioactive waters. These radioactive waters were sold to the general public during the early 1900s. The obvious hazard associated with these "medications" was the radiation dose that would result from ingestion of the radiation-producing substances. In 1932 attention was focused on the hazards of radium ingestion with the death of a wealthy young businessman who had consumed several bottles of radium-containing medications each day for several years. His death, along with the increased incidence of cancer in the radium dial–painting industry in the 1920s, emphasized the need for radiation protection standards to protect public health.

The late 1890s and early 1900s saw a significant rise in the recognition of the hazards associated with radiation exposure. John Dennis, a well-versed reporter, wrote a series of articles describing the widespread and uncontrolled use of x-rays and presented his findings at the meeting of the Seventh District Dental Society of the State of New York in April 1899. Dennis was perhaps the first to recommend state licensing in an effort to limit x-ray usage to qualified users alone. He also strongly suggested that causing injury to an individual with a radiation source or a radiation-producing device should be considered a criminal act. Professional societies such as the American Roentgen Ray Society and the British Röntgen Society, whose members included physicians, engineers, and other scientists, called for the adoption of stringent rules to protect both patients and x-ray personnel. In 1922 it was suggested that radiation workers routinely carry an unexposed dental x-ray film in their breast pocket as a means of estimating skin dose to the worker. These films were to be processed at two-week intervals and the degree of darkening was to be used to estimate the skin dose. Today, this method has been perfected by the addition of filters to better estimate the energy of the radiation to which the wearer has been exposed. This is discussed in more detail later in this chapter.

In 1928 the United States decided to centralize its radiation protection efforts through the National Bureau of Standards (NBS). In early 1929 a committee of eight individuals, representing radiological professional societies, the American Medical Association (AMA), x-ray equipment manufacturers, and the NBS, was formed to produce radiation protection guidelines. From this committee grew the *National Council on Radiation Protection and Measurements (NCRP)*. On its formation, the NCRP became a more encompassing body with a wider range of radiation protection interests. To this day, the NCRP is very active in the production and distribution of technical guides to assist the clinician and scientist in matters of radiation protection. As described in the next section, the NCRP plays an important role in the regulations to which all users of radiation must conform.

ADVISORY AND REGULATORY AGENCIES

The state and federal regulations under which all users of radiation work typically originated as a recommended radiation protection standard. A radiation protection standard refers to a recommended practice or limit to minimize any potential harmful effects of radiation exposure to workers and members of the general public. Although many groups, both official and unofficial, become involved in the proposal of specific standards, two organizations deserve special attention: *International Commission on Radiological Protection (ICRP)* and the previously mentioned National Council on Radiation Protection and Measurements (NCRP).

Established in 1928, the ICRP assumes the fundamental responsibility of providing general guidance in radiation protection matters. Although originally concerned primarily with radiation protection in medical radiology, its scope expanded with the widespread use of radiation both in and outside the field of medicine. The commission is composed of international scientists recognized for their expertise in specific areas of radiation protection. This organization issues its recommendations in the form of reports published in the appropriate professional journals. It is the policy of the ICRP to make recommendations only and to leave the responsibility of developing and enforcing specific regulations to the individual nations.

In the U.S., the NCRP reviews the recommendations of the ICRP and then makes its own suggestions as to how the information should best be incorporated into the nation's radiation protection standards. Like the ICRP, the NCRP consists of radiation protection technical experts and scientists in closely related disciplines. The NCRP consists of a Main Committee and some twenty subcommittees. Each of the individual subcommittees is responsible for issuing recommendations in its own area of expertise. The approved recommendations are published as *NCRP Reports* and are available for purchase by interested groups. Although the NCRP is not an official government agency, its recommendations are commonly adopted by federal and state agencies that regulate radiation sources and their use.

Other professional groups that have played an important role in the formulation of radiation protection standards include

- Advisory Committee on the Biological Effects of Ionizing Radiation (BEIR) of the National Academy of Sciences–National Research Council
- International Atomic Energy Agency (IAEA)
- United Nations Scientific Committee on the Effects of Atomic Radiation (UNSCEAR)
- Health Physics Society

United States Regulatory Agencies

Before about 1950, the United States had no formal regulatory codes regarding radiation protection practices. Court cases involving alleged misuse of radiation sources and subsequent evaluation of the extent of damages were often settled by referring to an appropriate *NCRP Report*. This left many questions open to interpretation by individuals who had no experience in the area of radiation protection. One of the first governmental attempts to protect public health was made by the United States Food and Drug Administration (FDA) when it required hazard warning labels to be attached to certain x-ray–producing devices.

Great advances were made in the practical aspects of radiation protection during the concluding years of World War II (1941 to 1945). Many of the advancements occurred as a result of the Manhattan Project, the project to develop the atomic bomb. Radiation protection standards had to be developed to protect the workers on this important task.

Recognizing the rapid growth and development of both medical and nonmedical applications utilizing radiation sources, legislation was passed in 1946 that established the Atomic Energy Commission (AEC). This congressional act did not however give the AEC the authority to establish regulations for the control of radiation sources. Consequently, it took no regulatory action for the next seven years. Finally, the Atomic Energy Act of 1954 better defined the role of the AEC and gave the AEC control over specific categories of radioactive materials and their use. The AEC did not have jurisdiction over x-ray machines.

The AEC was abolished in 1974, and its regulatory responsibilities were turned over to the newly created Nuclear Regulatory Commission (NRC). Like the old AEC, the NRC does not regulate or inspect x-ray facilities but has jurisdiction over uses of radioactive materials such as those employed in nuclear medicine, radiation therapy, industrial radiography, and so forth. Many of its regulations regarding *occupational radiation exposure* have however been adopted by many state and county regulatory agencies in their efforts to provide radiation protection standards for diagnostic radiology. It should be noted that at the present time there is no federal agency comparable to the NRC that is involved in the regulation of radiation machine users.

Specific federal regulations regarding occupational radiation exposure are found in Title 10 of the *Code of Federal Regulations,* Part 20, abbreviated as 10CFR20 (Note: Title 10 is designated Energy). Specific federal regulations as they pertain to the x-ray equipment manufacturer, are found in Title 21 of the Code of Federal Regulations, Part 1020, abbreviated 21CFR1020 (Title 21 is named Food and Drugs; recall that it was the FDA that first required warnings on x-ray units). Copies of these regulations are available from one of the following sources:

- Your institution's *radiation safety officer (RSO)*
- Your state regulatory agency
- Your county regulatory agency
- The United States Government Printing Office (USGPO) in Washington, D.C., or one of its local bookstores

In the remainder of this chapter, we discuss the general philosophy of radiation protection, some of the more important regulations as they pertain to the radiographer and the techniques used to monitor occupational radiation exposure to assure the safe use of x-rays in the workplace.

UNITS OF RADIATION PROTECTION

Exposure: Roentgens and Coulombs/kg

In order to explain regulatory dose limits, the units in which these measurements are made and their meanings must first be considered. When ionizing radiation such as x-rays pass through air, *ion pairs* are formed. Recall that an ion pair consists of an electron and the atom from which the electron was removed. Each component of the ion pair carries a charge. The ejected electron carries a charge of -1.6×10^{-19} coulomb (C) while what remains of the atom carries a charge of $+1.6 \times 10^{-19}$ C (i.e., a charge corresponding to a neutral atom from which a single electron has been removed). Thus the amount of charge produced in a known volume of air can be used as a measure of the amount of radiation to which the volume of air has been exposed.

The unit of *radiation exposure* most commonly used is the *roentgen (R)* and is defined as that quantity of x- or gamma (γ) radiation that produces a charge (of either sign) of 2.58×10^{-4} C per kilogram of air. That is,

$$1 \text{ roentgen (R)} = 2.58 \times 10^{-4} \text{ C/kg air}$$

It is important to recognize that this unit is defined only for x- or γ-rays having energies of less than 3 MeV, which certainly includes those energies commonly used in medical diagnosis. In the SI system of units, radiation exposure is measured in units of coulombs/kg. At the current time, this SI quantity has no special name. In making conversions from the roentgen to the SI unit, the following conversion factor should be used:

$$\boxed{1 \text{ C/kg} \cong 3876 \text{ R}}$$

))))) EXAMPLE

The NCRP has recommended that x-ray technologists should not receive an annual occupational exposure exceeding 5R. Members of the general public should not exceed an annual exposure of 100 mR. Express these exposures in SI units.

For the x-ray technologist, 5R corresponds to

$$5R \times \frac{1 \text{ C/kg}}{3876 \text{ R}} = 1.29 \times 10^{-3} \frac{\text{C}}{\text{kg}} = 1.29 \frac{\text{mC}}{\text{kg}}$$

For members of the general public, 100 mR corresponds to

$$(100 \times 10^{-3}) \times \frac{1 \text{ C/kg}}{3876 \text{ R}} \cong 25.8 \times 10^{-6} \frac{\text{C}}{\text{kg}} = 25.8 \frac{\mu\text{C}}{\text{kg}}$$

Exposure (R or mR) or exposure rate (R/hr or mR/hr) readings are the first actual measurements that are commonly made. These measurements are typically made with an ionization chamber. After taking this measurement, absorbed dose can then be determined.

Radiation Absorbed Dose: Rads and Grays

When an individual is exposed to ionizing radiation, the potential for biological effects is dependent on the amount of energy absorbed by the tissues. The amount of energy absorbed depends on

- Type of radiation
- Energy of the incident radiation
- Type of material and its energy absorption characteristics

The CGS unit of absorbed dose is the *rad* (an acronym for radiation absorbed dose), defined as the quantity of radiation needed to deposit 100 ergs of energy per gram of irradiated absorber. That is,

$$1 \text{ rad} = 100 \text{ ergs/gm of absorber}$$

or since the joule (J), the SI unit of energy, is equivalent to 10^7 ergs,

$$1 \text{ rad} = \frac{100 \text{ ergs}}{\text{gm}} \times \frac{1 \text{ J}}{10^7 \text{ ergs}} \times \frac{10^3 \text{ gm}}{1 \text{ kg}} = 10^{-2} \frac{\text{J}}{\text{kg}}$$

The SI equivalent of the rad is the *gray (Gy)* defined as

$$1 \text{ gray (Gy)} = 1 \text{ J/kg of absorber}$$

or since $1 \text{ rad} = 10^{-2} \text{ J/kg}$,

$$\boxed{1 \text{ Gy} = 100 \text{ rads}}$$

or

$$\boxed{1 \text{ rad} = 1 \text{ centigray (cGy)}}$$

As previously mentioned, when one is exposed to ionizing radiation such as x- or γ-rays, the fraction of the energy absorbed depends on both the energy of the radiation and the characteristics of the absorbing medium. If the exposure level in roentgens is known at a specific location, the absorbed dose in rads can be estimated using the f-factor. F-factor values, as indicated in Table 20–1, allow the conversion of roentgens to rads as follows:

$$\text{Absorbed dose (rads)} = (\text{f-factor}) \times (\text{exposure in roentgens})$$

Similarly, absorbed dose in SI units can be estimated using the f-factor (SI), also indicated in Table 20–1, in order to convert coulombs/kg to grays. That is

$$\text{Absorbed dose (Gy)} = [\text{f-factor(SI)}] \times (\text{exposure in coulombs/kg})$$

))))) EXAMPLE

Determine the absorbed dose in rads which results from an exposure of 10R to soft tissue. Assume the exposure results from 50 keV x-rays and that the radiation absorption characteristics of soft tissue are similar to those of water.

From Table 20–1, the f-factor for 50 keV photons in water is 0.90. Therefore,

$$\text{Absorbed dose} = (0.90) \times (10 \text{ R})$$
$$= 9 \text{ rads}$$

))))) EXAMPLE

Determine the absorbed dose in grays which results from an exposure of 2.58×10^{-3} C/kg to muscle. Assume the exposure results from 80 keV x-rays.

From Table 20–1, the f-factor (SI) for 80 keV photons in muscle is 36.8. Therefore,

$$\text{Absorbed dose} = (36.8) \times (2.58 \times 10^{-3} \text{ C/kg})$$
$$\cong 9.5 \times 10^{-2} \text{ Gy or } 9.5 \text{ cGy}$$

Dose Equivalent: Rems and Sieverts

Once the fraction of energy to which one has been exposed has been determined, the fact that all types of radiation are not equally biologically hazardous must be taken into consideration. To account for these differences, the concept of *dose equivalent* was formulated. Dose equivalent is defined as follows:

$$\boxed{\text{Dose equivalent} = \text{absorbed dose} \times \text{quality factor}}$$

The *quality factor* (typically designated by Q or QF) is used to evaluate the relative hazard associated with different types of radiation. Its numerical value, as determined by advisory bodies such as the ICRP and the NCRP, is based on recognition that the ability of different types of radiation to produce specific chemical or biological effects depends to a large extent on how the energy is distributed, such as that described by the *linear energy transfer (LET)*. Typically, as the LET and associated specific ionization (SI) increase, so does the assigned value of the quality factor. Quality factors recommended by the NCRP are listed in Table 20–2. The use of the quality factor in the calculation of dose equivalents is illustrated in the following examples.

))))) EXAMPLE

An individual receives an absorbed dose of 10 rads as a result of exposure to thermal neutrons. Determine the dose equivalent.

$$\text{Dose equivalent} = (Q) \times (\text{absorbed dose})$$
$$= (5)(10 \text{ rads})$$
$$= 50 \text{ rem}$$

))))) EXAMPLE

An x-ray technologist receives an absorbed dose of 0.25 Gy to the hands while working in the emergency room. Determine the dose equivalent.

Table 20–1: f-FACTORS FOR SELECTED PHOTON ENERGIES IN VARIOUS ABSORBING MEDIA

Photon Energy (keV)	Water		Compact Bone		Muscle (Striated)	
	f-Factor	f-Factor (SI)	f-Factor	f-Factor (SI)	f-Factor	f-Factor (SI)
10	0.90	35.2	3.6	141	0.92	35.8
20	0.87	33.9	4.2	163	0.91	35.3
30	0.88	34.1	4.2	164.7	0.90	35.2
40	0.88	34.3	4.0	154.1	0.91	35.5
50	0.90	34.9	3.5	134.2	0.92	35.9
60	0.91	35.5	2.8	110.8	0.94	36.4
80	0.94	36.5	1.9	74.8	0.94	36.8
100	0.95	37.0	1.4	56	0.95	37.0
150	0.96	37.5	1.1	41.3	0.96	37.2

Absorbed dose (rads) = (f-factor) (exposure in roentgens); absorbed dose (grays) = (f-factor [SI]) (exposure in coulombs/kg).

Table 20–2: RECOMMENDED QUALITY FACTORS FOR DIFFERENT TYPES OF RADIATION

Type of Radiation	Quality Factor (Q)
X-rays, γ-rays, and β-particles	1
Thermal neutrons (E $\simeq$ 0.025 eV)	5
Neutrons (other than thermal) of unknown energy	20
Protons (low energy—e.g., those generated in tissue by fast neutrons)	20
α-Particles and multiple charged particles of unknown energy	20

Source: Recommendations on Limits for Exposure to Ionizing Radiation (NCRP Report No. 91). Bethesda, MD: National Council on Radiation Protection and Measurements, 1987.

$$\text{Dose equivalent} = (Q) \times (\text{absorbed dose})$$
$$= (1) \times (0.25 \text{ Gy})$$
$$= 0.25 \text{ sievert}$$

Note. From Table 20–2, the quality factor is 1 for x-rays.

The previously derived relationship between rads and grays is also valid between units of dose equivalent. That is,

$$1 \text{ sievert (Sv)} = 100 \text{ rem}$$

or

$$1 \text{ rem} = 1 \text{ centisievert (cSv)}$$

RADIATION PROTECTION PHILOSOPHY

It is the basic goal of radiation protection to minimize the potential for biological harm to individuals exposed to radiation and to their offspring. Radiation protection standards that can be considered reasonable and acceptable in relation to the benefits from activities involving radiation exposure are then established.

Radiation exposure limits to individuals, excluding medically prescribed radiation, are established to minimize the potential for two specific types of biological effects from radiation exposure:

- Prompt effects—those types of biological effects that tend to occur soon after exposure to high doses of radiation (e.g., blood changes, decrease in sperm count, lens opacification); the severity of the effect tends to increase with increasing dose; also referred to as *nonstochastic effects*)
- Delayed effects—those types of biological effects the probability of whose occurrence increases with increasing absorbed dose; but the severity of the effect is independent of dose magnitude (e.g., induction of

cancer and genetic effects); also called *stochastic effects.*

Individual dose-equivalent limits are established for those persons exposed both occupationally and nonoccupationally. These limits are established with the assumption that the risk to a person's health increases with dose. It also assumes that there is no level of radiation exposure without risk. This is only a cautious assumption made for radiation protection purposes.

In 1987 the NCRP issued new recommendations for individual dose-equivalent limits in its NCRP Report No. 91, titled *Recommendations on Limits for Exposure to Ionizing Radiation.* These recommendations are based on the most up-to-date scientific information regarding radiation exposure and its associated risks. As a result of these recommendations, the United States Nuclear Regulatory Commission has revised its regulations regarding individual dose-equivalent limits for the first time in some 30 years. These new regulations go into effect in January 1994 and will affect all users of radiation. Selected dose-equivalent limits are indicated in Table 20–3. Some limits have been raised, whereas others have been lowered. These modifications reflect scientific findings regarding the relative radiosensitivity of various parts of the body and the relative risks associated with radiation exposure. Occupational exposure is monitored by the use of *film badges* (to measure whole-body exposure) and *finger ring thermoluminescent dosimeters* (to measure exposure to the hands) which are worn by the technologist during working hours. These devices are monitored on a monthly basis, and *dosimetry reports* are returned to the department, indicating the employee's radiation dose equivalent for each specific month. These reports are typically reviewed each month by the facility's radiation safety officer (RSO) before posting in the department. It is the RSO's responsibility to assure safe working conditions and that no individual exceeds occupational exposure limits. This person must also ensure that members of the general public are also adequately protected against radiation exposure while in the medical facility.

As early as 1966 but with clearer definition in 1977, the ICRP introduced the concept that all radiation exposure (except that medically prescribed) should be maintained as low as reasonably achievable, known by the acronym *ALARA.* The ALARA concept was based on three basic ideas:

- No practice involving radiation exposure shall be adopted unless its introduction produces a net positive benefit
- All radiation exposures should be kept as low as reasonably achievable, economic and social factors being taken into account
- The dose equivalent to individuals shall not exceed recommended dose limits for the appropriate circumstances

As this concept was incorporated into radiation protection philosophy, there was some difficulty in its implementation; without specific numerical guidelines, it

Table 20–3: COMPARISON OF SELECTED INDIVIDUAL DOSE-EQUIVALENT LIMITS BEFORE AND AFTER JANUARY, 1994.

	Before January 1994	After January 1994
Occupational Exposures (Annual)		
Effective dose-equivalent limit (stochastic effects): whole body (external and internal)	5 rem (50 mSv)	5 rem (50 mSv)
Dose-equivalent limits for tissues and organs (nonstochastic effects):		
lens of the eye	5 rem (50 mSv)	15 rem (150 mSv)
hands	75 rem	50 rem (500 mSv)
forearms	30 rem	50 rem (500 mSv)
skin	15 rem	50 rem (500 mSv)
gonads	5 rem (50 mSv)	50 rem (500 mSv)
red bone marrow	5 rem (50 mSv)	50 rem (500 mSv)
Long-term accumulation dose guidance: cumulative exposure not to exceed	5 rem (Age − 18) 50 mSv (Age − 18)	Discontinued 1 rem × age (yrs) (10 mSv × age [yrs])
Exposures to Members of the General Public (Annual)		
Effective dose-equivalent limit, continuous or frequent exposure	0.5 rem (5 mSv)	0.1 rem (1 mSv)
Effective dose-equivalent, infrequent	—	0.5 rem (5 mSv)
Dose to Embryo-Fetus		
Total dose equivalent	0.5 rem (5 mSv) in gestation period	0.5 rem (5 mSv)
Dose-equivalent limit per month	Not specified	0.05 rem (0.5 mSv)

Source: Recommendations on Limits for Exposure to Ionizing Radiation (NCRP Report No. 91). Bethesda, MD: National Council on Radiation Protection and Measurements, 1987.

was difficult to determine just when the ALARA concept had been achieved. Past regulations involving the safe use of radiation indicated that users were to comply with exposure limits and make every effort to make all exposures as low as reasonably achievable. The most recent regulation revision incorporates the ALARA concept more strongly. It states that the user of radiation shall use, to the extent practical, procedures and engineering controls based on sound radiation protection principles to achieve both occupational doses and doses to the general public that are as low as reasonably achievable. The ALARA concept is thus becoming an integral part of radiation protection practice.

PERSONNEL DOSIMETRY

Dosimetry refers to the measurement of radiation dose to an individual. External radiation dose (i.e., radiation dose delivered to an individual by radiation sources outside the body) is measured using a *personnel dosimeter*. Perhaps the most commonly used personnel dosimeters found in medical facilities are the film badge, the *thermoluminescent dosimeter* and the *pocket dosimeter*.

Film Badges

The film badge is the primary dosimeter provided to technologists to measure occupational radiation exposure. Its use is based on the fact that the more radia-

tion to which the badge is exposed, the darker the film when it is processed. If the film badge, shown in Figure 20–1, is worn in an appropriate location during working hours, it will then provide an accurate estimate of the occupational radiation exposure to the individual during the time period that the badge was worn. After processing, the degree of darkening of the individual's badge is compared to other similar films exposed to known amounts of radiation. These comparisons are used to estimate the radiation dose to the individual.

Film badges typically consist of a piece of film sealed in a light-tight packet. The film packet, which is replaced each month, fits inside a plastic holder which can be clipped to the individual's clothing. Various types of filters (e.g., lead, copper, aluminum) can be positioned inside the holder as shown in Figure 20–2 to shield certain sections of the film. Any darkening of the film in these areas can then be used to determine the energy of the radiation to which the individual has been exposed. This type of information can be used to evaluate the radiation dose as shallow (nonpenetrating) or deep (penetrating).

In order for the film badge to provide an accurate estimate of an individual's whole-body occupational dose, film badges should

- Be worn at the collar level; if a lead apron is worn, the film badge should be worn at collar level outside the lead apron
- Never be worn during medical or dental radiographic procedures when you are the patient
- Never be stored near radiation sources
- Never be stored near heat sources or areas of high humidity

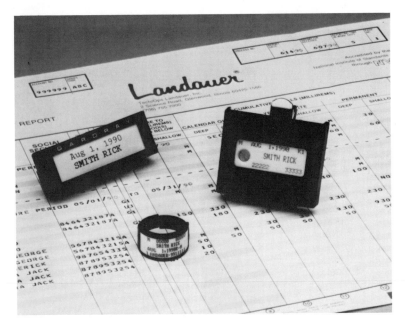

FIGURE 20–1. Personnel dosimetry devices: Two types of film badges and a thermoluminescent dosimeter (TLD) finger ring. (Courtesy of Landauer, Inc., Glenwood, IL.)

- Be worn only for the assigned time period
- Be worn only by the individual to whom the badge has been assigned

Relative advantages and disadvantages associated with film badges are summarized in Table 20–4.

Thermoluminescent Dosimeters

Thermoluminescent dosimeters (known also as TLDs) are commonly used as finger rings in order to measure occupational exposure to the hands. This is an important measurement for the radiation therapy and nuclear medicine technologist, since a greater part of their occupational exposure can occur to the hands. For the x-ray technologist, hand exposures can occur on those rare (it is hoped) occasions when a patient must be held during a radiographic procedure. Rather than a piece of film, the TLD contains crystals of lithium fluoride (LiF) or calcium fluoride (CaF_2). When the crystals are exposed to ionizing radiation, energy is stored within the crystal. This energy is trapped within the crystal until it is heated above approximately 190°C. As the crystal is heated (a process known as annealing), it releases the trapped energy in the form of light. The intensity of the emitted light is directly proportional to the radiation dose.

TLDs have several advantages over film badges including the following:

- TLDs tend to be accurate over a wide range of absorbed doses
- TLDs can be reused after each annealing process

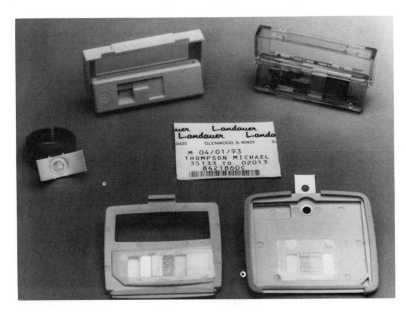

FIGURE 20–2. Film badge holders showing filters within the holder frame. Also shown is a thermoluminescent dosimeter (TLD) ring badge with the crystal exposed.

Table 20–4: CHARACTERISTICS OF SEVERAL TYPES OF DOSIMETRY DEVICES COMMONLY USED FOR MEASURING OCCUPATIONAL EXPOSURE

Characteristics	Film Badges	Thermoluminescent Dosimeters (TLDs)	Pocket Dosimeters (Direct-Reading)
Principle of operation	Magnitude of exposure based on degree of darkening of photographic film	LiF or CaF_2 crystal; amount of light emitted from crystal when heated is representative of exposure	Based on the principle of the electroscope; as air within the chamber is ionized, charge is neutralized in proportion to dose received
Types of radiation detected	X-rays, γ-rays, higher energy β-particles	X-rays, γ-rays, higher energy β-particles	X-rays and γ-rays
Time period typically worn	One month	One month or longer	Minutes to hours
Adversely affected by	Light leaks, heat, high humidity	Extreme heat	Mechanical jarring and high humidity
Reusable?	No	Yes	Yes
Method of recording exposure	Processed film provides a hard copy of the exposure	No hard copy; requires manual or computer recording of the exposure	No hard copy; requires manual recording of the exposure
Energy discrimination capabilities?	Yes	No	No
Advantages	1. Processed film provides a permanent record of the exposure 2. Use of filters allows energy discrimination	1. LiF approximately tissue equivalent 2. Accurate over a wide range of exposures 3. Not affected by normal heat or humidity 4. Can be reused after annealing	1. Provides a direct, immediate measurement of exposure 2. Can be reused after charging
Disadvantages	1. Film can give false readings if exposed to light, heat or humidity 2. Must wait for film to be processed to obtain readings	1. Must wait for badges to be processed to obtain readings 2. Tend to be more expensive than film badges	1. Can give high readings if dropped or used in high humidity 2. Exposures must be manually read and recorded 3. Must be recharged prior to each use

CaF_2 = calcium fluoride; LiF = lithium fluoride.

- LiF is nearly tissue equivalent
- TLDs are relatively insensitive to environmental changes

Unlike film badges, however, TLDs do not provide a permanent record once the crystals have been annealed. A summary of advantages and disadvantages is indicated in Table 20–4.

Pocket Dosimeters

Although it is not a commonly used method of personnel dosimetry within a medical facility, the pocket dosimeter warrants discussion because of its use during emergency situations. The direct-reading pocket dosimeter operates on the principle of the simple electroscope (see Chapter 4). This simple dose-measuring device is mounted in a pen-type holder, as shown in Figure 20–3, which can be readily clipped on an individual's clothing. Within the dosimeter housing is a thin quartz fiber. The fiber is electrostatically repelled from a central electrode when the unit is charged with a charging base. The charge is adjusted until the quartz fiber is moved across a visible scale to the zero position. As x- or gamma-radiation enters and ionizes the air, charges on the fiber and electrode are neutralized. This allows the fiber to move across a calibrated scale, indicating exposure dose. Unlike the film badges or TLDs, pocket dosimeters can be read directly by viewing the scale through the eyepiece of the dosimeter. It provides a measurement of cumulative dose and can be reused after charging. This makes it especially useful in emergency situations in which exposure limits for personnel may be reached in a short time.

However, these devices are not without their own problems. Pocket dosimeters

- Require accurate record-keeping of doses to individuals to whom the dosimeters have been assigned
- May provide erroneously high readings if dropped or used in areas of high humidity
- Require a properly operating charging base to charge dosimeters before each use

Relative advantages and disadvantages of this type dosimeter are compared with other types of dosimeters in Table 20–4.

Proper Care of Personnel Dosimeters

Regardless of the type of personnel dosimetry device assigned, it is the wearer's responsibility to assure that it is cared for properly. In order for the device to give an accurate estimate of the wearer's occupational exposure, the following precautions must be observed:

- Dosimetry devices must be worn only by the persons to whom they are assigned and for the period designated
- Film badges should be worn at collar level or if a lead apron is worn, at collar level outside the lead apron

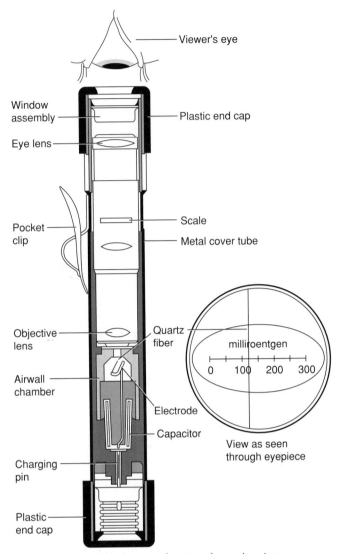

FIGURE 20–3. Schematic drawing of a pocket dosimeter.

- Dosimetry devices should not be worn when having personal medical or dental x-ray procedures, since this is not occupational exposure
- When not in use, dosimetry devices should be stored in a location away from heat, humidity, and sources of stray radiation
- If the badge or other dosimetry device is lost or anything happens to it that could lead to a false reading, your RSO, your supervisor, or both should be notified

Great care should always be taken with any personnel dosimetry device, since this provides the wearer's radiation exposure history and is the only way to assure that the wearer does not exceed maximum occupational exposure limits.

The Dosimetry Report

Film badges and TLDs are collected at the end of the wearing period for processing. Typically, devices

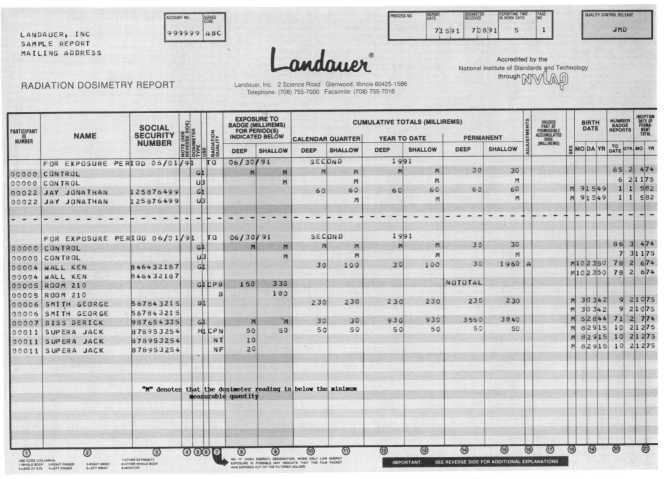

FIGURE 20–4. A typical dosimetry report. (Courtesy of Landauer, Inc., Glenwood, IL.)

are collected at the end of each month and are replaced with new badges. The old badges are shipped to the respective film badge company, where the badges are processed and exposures are determined. Films from badges are carefully compared to similar films exposed to known levels of radiation. The degree of film darkening under the various filters gives an indication of the energy and penetrating power of the radiation to which the wearer has been exposed. From this information, deep (penetrating) and shallow (nonpenetrating) doses to the individual wearer can be determined.

Within several weeks after badges have been collected for processing, a dosimetry report like that shown in Figure 20–4 is sent to your department. These reports are required to be posted where workers can review their occupational exposures. In this report, which all radiation workers are encouraged to review on a periodic basis, one typically finds the following:

- Exposure period, indicating the period of time during which the radiation dose was received
- Name and social security number are used to identify the individual who received the dose
- Dosimeter type, indicating whether the radiation dose was measured on a standard whole-body badge, a ring badge, a TLD, and so forth; abbreviations used vary from one company to another

- Exposure for the period indicated states the dose equivalent (in millirems) to the individual for the time period under consideration
- Cumulative totals, or cumulative dose equivalents (in millirems) for the calendar quarter, for the year to date, and the total dose equivalent for the person since the beginning of his or her occupational exposure

The information contained in these reports should be transferred whenever you change employment site so that your occupational exposure records are always up to date. This is usually accomplished simply by making a request in writing to the facility's radiation safety officer or the film badge company. The dosimetry report is a permanent record that should be kept on file indefinitely.

REDUCING OCCUPATIONAL RADIATION EXPOSURE: TIME, DISTANCE, AND SHIELDING

As an employee who works with radiation within a medical facility, the radiological technologist must be aware that x-ray machines are not the only sources of radiation within such a facility. Situations may arise in which the technologist must be knowledgeable and take quick action involving other sources of radiation in order to minimize exposure to employees, patients, and the public.

Radiation sources within a medical facility generally fall into three categories:

- Radiation-producing machines
- Sealed sources
- Unsealed sources

Radiation-producing machines include x-ray machines and linear accelerators used in radiation therapy. Linear accelerators are devices used to produce high-energy electrons or high-energy x-rays in the treatment of cancer. Radiation-producing machines do not produce radiation unless they are activated.

Sealed sources refers to radiation sources contained in plastic rods or disks or metal capsules. Such sealed sources are found in both nuclear medicine departments, where they are used for calibration and equipment checks, and in radiation therapy departments, where they are used in cancer *(brachytherapy)* treatment procedures. The radiation emitted from the sealed sources used in nuclear medicine is of relatively low intensity compared with that used in radiation therapy. Brachytherapy sources commonly contain the radioactive material cesium (^{137}Cs), which emits 662-keV gamma photons. These sources emit high intensities of penetrating radiation and must be appropriately shielded to avoid high radiation exposure. Sealed sources can thus produce high radiation intensities but do not produce contamination problems.

Unsealed sources are most commonly found in nuclear medicine departments and, on occasion, in radiation therapy departments. These are radioactive materials that may be in any physical form—solid, liquid, gas, powder, and so forth. They may pose both an exposure problem and possible contamination problems. Contamination implies the spread of radioactive materials to places where it should not be—for example, floors, countertops, skin, clothing.

Regardless of the type of radiation source, there are always three basic ways to reduce radiation exposure to yourself and others in the area:

Time

Reduce the time spent in the area of the radiation source. Although this is not a primary method of reducing radiation exposure for the radiographer (since x-ray units produce radiation only when energized), it is an important method of protection when a source continuously emits radiation. This is the case with sources containing radioactive materials such as those used in nuclear medicine and radiation therapy. One can thus reduce exposure to such sources by simply reducing the time spent near such sources. This concept is applicable in fluoroscopic examinations in which an x-ray tube may be on for minutes at a time. Fluoroscopic equipment is required to be equipped with a 5-minute timer, which produces an audible sig-

nal at the completion of each 5-minute period that the tube is on. The sound makes the radiologist aware of the time that has passed. The required timer is an effort to reduce exposure time to both the patient and attending personnel.

Distance

One of the simplest methods to reduce radiation exposure is to move away from the radiation source. In earlier discussions on the various types of particulate radiation (i.e., alpha and beta particles), it was shown that charged particle radiation tends to have limited ranges in air, as shown in Table 20–5. For those radiation sources that emit only alpha or negative beta radiation, distance alone may be sufficient to minimize exposure. For positron emitters one must be concerned about the penetrating 511-keV annihilation photons. In this case and for other sources that continuously emit x- or gamma rays, increasing the distance from the source greatly reduces radiation exposure.

Always recall that for a point source of radiation (i.e., radiation that is emitted isotopically or equally in all directions from a source), the inverse square law discussed in earlier chapters and given as

$$I_1 d_1^2 = I_2 d_2^2$$

can be used to determine variations in radiation intensity as distances are varied.

Appropriate Shielding

When it is available and practical, appropriate shielding can also be used to reduce radiation exposure. The use of shielding effectively allows technologists to work closer to the radiation source while reducing their exposure. The technologist employs both distance and shielding when the radiograph is made in that the control console is located a distance away from the x-ray unit and is positioned behind a lead (Pb) shield.

In the event that a patient must be held (e.g., a trauma case in the emergency room) during a radiographic procedure, a family member rather than the technologist should be asked to hold. If a family member is not available, the technologist holding should wear a lead apron, as shown in Figure 20–5, and lead gloves.

Lead aprons, depending on their thickness, typically range from 2 to 4 HVLs for diagnostic energy x-rays. Recall from Chapter 9 that the intensity of the radiation transmitted through an absorber can be described by

$$I = I_0 e^{-\mu_l x}$$

or

$$I = I_0 (0.5)^N$$

where N in the latter equation represents the thickness of the absorber in HVLs.

Table 20–5: BASIC CHARACTERISTICS OF THE MOST COMMON TYPES OF RADIATION

Radiation	Symbol	Classification	Charge ($\times 1.6 \times 10^{-19}$ C)	Method of Interaction in Matter	Range in Air	Methods of Shielding	Emitted From	Hospital Departments Using this Type of Radiation	Medical Uses
Alpha	α	Particulate (particle)	+2	Electrical	~1 cm/MeV (≈0.5 in/MeV)	Use distance—move away from source; low Z shielding such as paper, cardboard, plastic, etc.	Radioactive materials	None	None (due to its low penetrating power)
Beta (negatron)	$\beta-$	Particulate (particle)	−1	Electrical	~3.7 m/MeV (~12 ft/MeV)	Use distance—move away from the source; low Z shielding such as cardboard or plexiglas; do not use Pb since bremsstrahlung can be produced	Radioactive materials	Nuclear medicine, radiation therapy (limited use)	Cancer therapy and hyperthyroid conditions
Beta (positron)	$\beta+$	Particulate (particle)	+1	Electrical; annihilation events	Millimeters	Use sufficiently thick pieces of Pb to shield against the 511-keV photons produced in positron annihilation events	Radioactive materials	Nuclear medicine (limited use)	Positron-computed tomography (PET)
X-rays or gamma rays	x or γ	Photon	0	Direct interactions with atoms, nuclei, shell electrons	Meters (depending on energy of photon)	Use sufficiently thick pieces of Pb or other high-Z absorbers	Radioactive materials or radiation-producing machines	Radiology, nuclear medicine, and radiation therapy	Medical x-rays, nuclear medicine, imaging, and cancer therapy

Pb = lead.

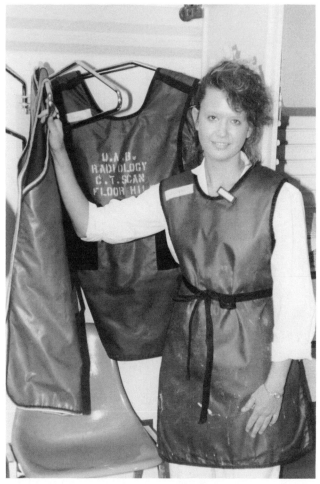

FIGURE 20–5. Lead aprons should be handled carefully and stored on special holding racks when not in use. Film badges should be worn at collar level outside the lead apron.

PROPER CARE OF LEAD APRONS AND LEAD GLOVES

Lead aprons and lead gloves are commonly found in almost every radiology department. These protective articles are worn by persons who perform fluoroscopic, portable radiographic, and special procedures and by those who on occasion may have to hold a patient. If the aprons and gloves are to provide the protection for which they were intended, these articles must be handled carefully. Aprons are typically manufactured with lead-equivalent thicknesses of 0.25 mm and 0.5 mm. Such aprons weigh between 3 and 15 lbs (~1.4 to 6.8 kg) and can reduce radiation exposure by 75% or more.

However, lead is a soft metal that is easily bent and folded when it is in the form of thin sheets. If the aprons or gloves are continuously folded or piled in a storage area when not in use, they can develop cracks and holes. For this reason, these protective articles should always be stored on racks designed for that purpose. In addition, gloves and aprons should be fluoroscoped or radiographed (at a high-kVp technique) at least on an annual basis to check for cracks or holes. If cracks are found in aprons or gloves, their

It is also important to note that there are cases in which the use of shielding is not recommended. Such instances include the following:

- When the use of shielding interferes with proper patient care
- When only inappropriate shielding is available (e.g., thin lead shielding is available to shield against high-energy photon radiation). In such cases, it may be better to use no shielding rather than produce lower energy scatter radiation that would have a greater chance of being absorbed within the body

In each of these situations, if shielding is either inappropriate or unavailable, time and distance should be used to advantage to minimize one's own occupational exposure and to reduce radiation exposure to patients and other nonoccupationally exposed persons.

The radiological technologist can always use any of these methods to reduce radiation exposure and in doing so, can implement the ALARA concept. These techniques for reducing radiation exposure can be applied to any radiation source in a medical facility.

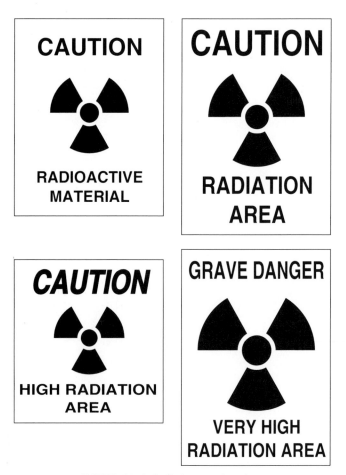

FIGURE 20–6. Radiation warning signs.

use should be discontinued and the articles should be replaced.

POSTING REQUIREMENTS

State and federal regulating agencies define a *restricted area* as an area to which access is limited for the purpose of protecting individuals against undue risk from radiation exposure. Within a medical facility, restricted areas include rooms in which radiographic procedures are performed, nuclear medicine departments, and rooms in which radioactive materials are used or stored. *Unrestricted areas* are those areas to which access is not limited because of the presence of radiation or radiation sources. Unrestricted areas commonly include hallways, stairwells, patient waiting areas, and the like. Radiation exposure rates should not exceed 2 mR/hr (0.02 mSv/hr) in unrestricted areas.

Regulations require that restricted areas be properly posted with signs and labels to warn individuals entering such areas of the potential for radiation exposure or the possibility of radioactive contamination or both. The radiation symbol, a magenta or black tri-blade on a yellow background, is the internationally recognized symbol of radiation. Signs indicating various levels of radiation hazard may be found in a medical facility,

and it is important that all users of radiation recognize and heed these warnings. The requirements for each type of sign shown in Figure 20–6 are given below:

- Caution—Radioactive Materials. Required to be posted at the entrance to rooms where radioactive materials are used, stored, or both; indicates the presence of radioactive materials and the possibility of radioactive contamination.
- Caution—Radiation Area. Required to be posted at the entrance to rooms in which radiation levels could result in a person's receiving a dose equivalent in excess of 5 mrem (0.05 mSv) in one hour at 30 cm from the source or any surface that the radiation penetrates.
- Caution—High-Radiation Area. Required to be posted at the entrance to rooms in which radiation levels can result in a dose equivalent in excess of 100 mrem (1 mSv) in one hour at 30 cm from the source or any surface that the radiation penetrates.
- Grave Danger—Very High Radiation Area. Required to be posted at the entrance to rooms in which radiation levels could result in an absorbed dose of 500 rads (5 grays) in one hour measured at a distance of 1 m from the radiation source or from any surface that the radiation penetrates.

Other important types of labels are those required by the United States Department of Transportation (DOT) to be posted on shipping boxes containing radiation sources (Fig. 20–7). DOT labels are used to

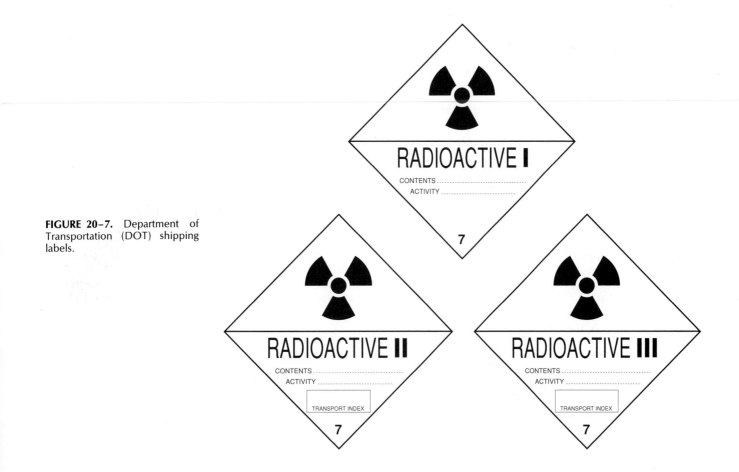

FIGURE 20–7. Department of Transportation (DOT) shipping labels.

Table 20–6: U.S. DEPARTMENT OF TRANSPORTATION (DOT) EXPOSURE RATE LIMITS FOR DOT CLASSES I, II, AND III PACKAGES

DOT Class	Exposure Rate at Contact Cannot Exceed	Exposure Rate at 3 Ft From Surface of Package Cannot Exceed
Class I (white label)	0.5 mR/hr	No detectable radiation (NDR)
Class II (yellow label)	50 mR/hr	1 mR/hr
Class III (yellow label)	200 mR/hr	10 mR/hr

indicate exposure rates at the surface of the shipping container and at a distance of 3 ft (~1 m). The exposure rate limits for each label are shown in Table 20–6. These labels are useful in recognizing potential exposure rates from shipping boxes containing radioactive materials used in medicine. Boxes should never be discarded after the sources have been removed without removing or defacing these labels. If such containers are ever found in an unsecured area, security personnel should be notified immediately and the containers secured until the RSO can arrive and assess the situation.

OTHER PROTECTIVE BARRIERS AGAINST MEDICAL GAMMA AND X-RAY SOURCES

In a previous section, the use of lead aprons and gloves by technologists to reduce their radiation exposure during certain radiographic and fluoroscopic procedures was discussed. In most cases, in standard radiographic procedures the technologist makes the exposure while standing behind a lead shield. The patient can be viewed through a window of leaded glass. This is called a *fixed protective barrier.*

The establishment of effective dose equivalents for both occupationally and nonoccupationally exposed individuals allows the determination of proper wall or shielding thicknesses or both needed to reduce exposure rates to acceptable limits. This allows rooms and hallways adjacent to the x-ray units and other medical radiation sources to be used for other purposes. The adjacent areas can then be designated as either controlled areas (i.e., occupied solely by occupationally exposed individuals) or noncontrolled areas (i.e., occupied by nonoccupationally exposed individuals who are not under the control of the RSO).

In a room where an x-ray unit is housed, the walls, ceiling, and floors serve as protective barriers. In shielded rooms, a *primary barrier* is one that is con-

structed to attenuate radiation from the primary beam. These are commonly ceilings, floors, or specific walls in an imaging room toward which the primary beam may at some time be directed during a radiographic study. Such barriers (Fig. 20–8) are required to provide more substantial shielding since the highest energy radiation in the primary beam is typically directed toward these barriers. This is in contrast to *secondary barriers,* which provide shielding against scatter and leakage radiation. In an imaging room, secondary barriers include the stationary, fixed barrier behind which the technologist stands while making an exposure and those walls toward which the primary beam is never directed.

In the determination of thickness requirements for specific barriers, several important factors must be taken into consideration. These factors include the following:

- The average mA and length of time the tube is in actual operation per week, described as the workload
- The distance between the x-ray unit and the location of interest as a result of the inverse square law with distance
- The intensity of radiation output from the x-ray unit
- The fraction of the operating time that the location of interest is actually occupied by personnel or members of the public; this is called the occupancy factor
- The fraction of the operating time that the x-ray beam is directed toward the location of interest; this is referred to as the use factor

Each of these factors enters into calculations performed by the medical facility's RSO or medical physicist in the determination of proper barrier thicknesses.

Other types of protective barriers used in medical facilities to reduce radiation exposure include the following:

- Lead "pigs," or containers, used to shield radioactive materials used in nuclear medicine and radiation therapy
- Syringe shields made from lead, tungsten, depleted uranium, or leaded glass used to protect the hands of nuclear medicine technologists when injecting radiopharmaceuticals
- Bedside shields used to reduce radiation exposure to nursing staff as a result of radiation emitted from brachytherapy (radiation therapy) implants
- Lead barrier shields (L-blocks) used in radiation therapy and nuclear medicine departments to protect technologists when drawing up doses and working with brachytherapy sources

It is important in implementing an effective ALARA program that the technologist utilize protective barriers such as those discussed in this chapter as a means of reducing radiation exposure. The wise use of shielding, time, and distance can make significant contributions to reducing one's occupational radiation exposure.

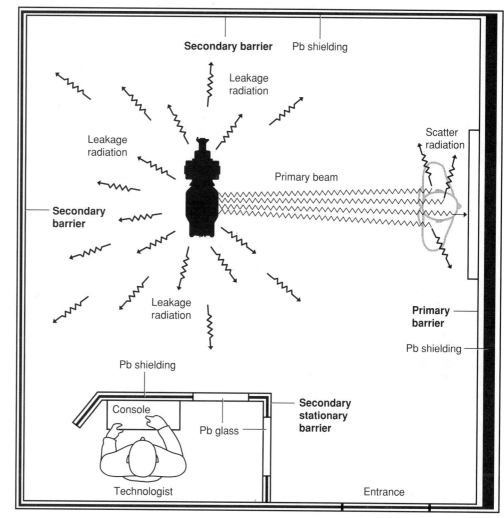

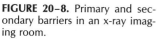

FIGURE 20–8. Primary and secondary barriers in an x-ray imaging room.

PREGNANCY AND RADIATION PROTECTION POLICY

Recognizing the effect of ionizing radiation on rapidly dividing cells and the litigation that can arise when individuals work in unsafe conditions, agencies that regulate the safe use of ionizing radiation have tried to generate regulations to safeguard the developing fetus without denying the pregnant technologist her means of a livelihood. Such regulations also seek fairness to employers in their desire to operate an efficient radiology, nuclear medicine, or radiation therapy department.

Regulations make reference to the relatively new term *a declared pregnant woman.* Regulations now (after January 1994) require that the pregnant, occupationally exposed worker notify her employer, voluntarily and in writing, of her pregnancy and the estimated date of conception. Such voluntary, formal notification is necessary in order that the employer has the pertinent information needed to limit the radiation dose to the developing fetus. Regulations state that during the entire pregnancy, the occupational dose to the embryo and fetus cannot exceed 0.5 rem (0.5 mSv per month). In the event that the pregnant worker does not make formal notification of the pregnancy until the allowable 500 mrem has been exceeded, the employer is required to limit exposure during the remainder of the pregnancy to less than 50 mrem (0.5 mSv).

On formal notification of the pregnancy, the supervisor should review with the technologist her radiation exposure history within the department. The supervisor may recommend the wearing of a lead apron, possibly a temporary change of duties within the department, and that the technologist be double-badged. The technologist may be asked to wear a film badge at collar level and a film badge at waist level under the lead apron as a way of monitoring fetal exposure during the pregnancy. The technologist may also be asked to sign a statement indicating that she received counseling and was advised of any necessary precautions required during the course of the pregnancy. Policy varies from institution to institution. It is the responsibility of both the employer and employee to work together during the pregnancy to assure continued implementation of the ALARA principle. Every technologist of child-bearing age who works with ionizing radiation in any form should become familiar with her individual department's pregnancy policy.

Chapter Summary/ Important Concepts

Early recognition of the hazards associated with uncontrolled use of radiation established the need for radiation protection standards. Radiation protection standards are under continuous review and are revised as scientific investigation and evidence warrant. At the international level, the International Commission on Radiological Protection (ICRP) makes recommendations on radiation protection standards. In the United States, these are reviewed by the National Council on Radiation Protection and Measurements (NCRP), which makes its recommendations. These recommendations are reviewed by various regulating agencies, such as the United States Nuclear Regulatory Commission (NRC), state health departments, and so forth, and are then incorporated into state and federal regulations.

When radiation measurements are made, three quantities are of specific interest:
Exposure: measured in units of roentgens (R) or coulombs (C)/kg
Absorbed dose: measured in units of rads or grays (Gy)
Dose equivalent: measured in units of rems or sieverts (Sv)

Once an exposure reading is determined, determination of absorbed dose and dose equivalent are made by using the following:

Absorbed dose = (exposure) × (appropriate f-factor)

and

Dose equivalent = absorbed dose × appropriate quality factor

Radiation protection standards for occupational radiation exposure are established to minimize the potential for both prompt (nonstochastic) effects and delayed (stochastic) effects. The general philosophy of radiation protection is that occupational radiation exposure should be kept as low as reasonably achievable, which is known as the ALARA concept. Regardless of the type of radiation sources encountered, occupational exposure can be reduced by the effective use of time, distance, and appropriate shielding.

The measurement of radiation dose to an individual is known as dosimetry. The measurement of occupational radiation exposure is accomplished with the use of personnel dosimeters such as film badges, TLDs, and, when immediate measurements are needed, pocket dosimeters. Personnel dosimeters should be cared for properly so that they will provide an accurate assessment of occupational radiation exposure as recorded on the monthly dosimetry report.

Regulations provide a set of effective dose equivalent limits (i.e., maximum allowable occupational exposure limits) that apply to all radiation workers. All technologists who employ radiation (e.g., x-ray technologists, nuclear medicine technologists, radiation therapy technologists) should utilize time, distance, and appropriate shielding in the performance of their work to minimize their occupational exposure.

Certain areas within the medical facility are considered restricted areas for radiation protection purposes. Within such areas a variety of radiation warning signs are used to indicate specific radiation hazards. Each type of warning label is used for a specific set of conditions. The level of radiation hazard must always be evaluated before radiation warning labels are posted.

A variety of barriers are used in the medical facility to reduce radiation exposure to individuals. Barriers that are constructed to attenuate radiation from the primary beam of an x-ray unit are called primary barriers. Those constructed to attenuate scatter and leakage radiation are referred to as secondary barriers. Other specific types of barriers are used in radiation therapy and nuclear medicine departments.

Radiation exposure is of special concern to the pregnant technologist. The technologist and her supervisor, after the formal notification of pregnancy, must work together to ensure that the radiation dose to the fetus remains below allowable limits. With proper precautions, this can easily be accomplished, usually without major changes in work schedule.

Important Terminology

ALARA. Philosophy of radiation protection asserting that occupational radiation exposure should be kept "as low as reasonably achievable"

Brachytherapy. A form of radiation therapy in which radioactive implants in the form of sealed sources are placed short distances from lesions or tumors for specified periods of time; high radiation exposure rates are typically associated with this type therapy, but there is minimal chance of radioactive contamination

Code of Federal Regulations (CFR). Documents that contain all federal regulations; regulations regarding occupational radiation exposure are found in Title 10 (i.e., 10CFR)

Dose Equivalent. The product of absorbed dose times an appropriate quality factor; measured in units of rem or sieverts (Sv); used for radiation protection purposes

Dosimetry. The measurement of radiation dose to an individual

Dosimetry Report. The printed report indicating the occupational radiation exposure of a person or group of persons incurred during a specified time period as measured on a personnel dosimeter

Film Badge. A method of personnel dosimetry used to provide a measure of a person's occupational radiation exposure by comparing the degree of darkening of a piece of radiographic film worn by the individual with similar films exposed to known quantities of radiation; typically worn for periods of one month

Finger Ring Dosimeter. A personnel dosimeter used to measure occupational radiation exposure to the hands

Fixed Protective Barrier. A nonmovable device used to provide protective shielding against radiation exposure

Gray (Gy). SI unit of absorbed dose equivalent to one joule of energy absorbed per kilogram of absorber; also equivalent to 100 rads

International Commission on Radiological Protection (ICRP). The primary organization for setting radiation protection standards at the international level; it is the recommendations of this body that are reviewed by the NCRP and become the basis for new regulations in the United States

Ion Pairs. Charge pairs produced when electrons are removed from neutral atoms as a result of interaction with ionizing radiation

Linear Energy Transfer (LET). The quantity of energy lost per unit distance travelled as radiation passes through matter

National Council on Radiation Protection and Measurements (NCRP). The nongovernmental body in the United States that reviews recommendations of the ICRP and makes its own recommendations to regulating agencies regarding radiation protection standards

NCRP Reports. Recommendations of the NCRP regarding specific issues in radiation protection

Nonstochastic Effects. Observable effects of radiation that occur to all or nearly all individuals receiving a specific dose; such effects are dose-dependent and have a threshold dose below which the effect is not observed; typically associated with high doses (e.g., erythema, epilation, sterility, death)

Occupational Radiation Exposure. Radiation exposure received in the course of one's employment

Personnel Dosimeter. Any device (e.g., film badge, TLD, pocket dosimeter) worn by a person in the performance of his or her work to measure occupational radiation exposure

Pocket Dosimeter. A personnel dosimetry device that can typically be read directly to obtain an immediate estimate of one's radiation exposure

Primary Barrier. Protective shielding constructed to attenuate the primary beam from a radiation source

Quality Factor (Q or QF). A dimensionless quantity used to convert absorbed dose to dose equivalent; created specifically for radiation protection work to reflect the potential biological impact of various types of radiation

rad. Radiation absorbed dose; centimeter-gram-second (CGS) unit of absorbed dose equivalent to 100 ergs of energy absorbed per gram of absorber

Radiation Exposure. A measure of the energy carried by ionizing radiation incident on an individual or other type absorbing medium

Radiation-Producing Machine. Any type device whose operation results in the production of ionizing radiation (e.g., x-ray unit or accelerator)

Radiation Safety Officer (RSO). The individual in a department or institution who supervises and enforces the facility's radiation protection program

Restricted Area. Location within a facility to which access is restricted for the purpose of protecting persons against undue risks from exposure to radiation or radioactive materials (e.g., nuclear medicine department, x-ray examination room, room in which a CT unit is used)

Roentgen (R). Unit of radiation exposure; defined as the quantity of x- or gamma radiation that would produce a charge (of either sign) of 2.58×10^{-4} C/kg of air

Sealed Source. A radioactive source sealed within a plastic or metal casing; may produce high radiation exposure but minimal, if any, contamination

Secondary Barrier. A barrier constructed to provide protective shielding against scatter or leakage radiation

Stochastic Effect. An effect for which the probability of occurrence, rather than the magnitude or severity of the effect, is proportional to the dose received (e.g., cancer induction and genetic effects)

Thermoluminescent Dosimeter (TLD). A personnel dosimetry device commonly containing a lithium fluoride or calcium fluoride crystal that stores incident radiation energy and re-emits it as light when the crystal is heated; the intensity of the emitted light is proportional to the radiation dose received

Unrestricted Area. Site within a department or facility to which access is not restricted for radiation protection purposes (e.g., most hallways, stairwells, patient waiting areas)

Unsealed Source. Generally refers to radioactive materials (solids, liquids, or gases) not encased in plastic or metal casings; an unsealed source may produce not only high radiation exposure but may also carry the potential for radioactive contamination

Bibliography

Brodsky, A. CRC Handbook of Radiation Measurement and Protection, Vol 1. Boca Raton, FL: CRC Press, 1978.

Bushong, S.C. Radiologic Science for Technologists: Physics, Biology, and Protection, 5th ed. St. Louis: C.V. Mosby, 1993.

Cember, H. Introduction to Health Physics, 2nd ed. New York: Pergamon Press, 1983.

Hendee, W.R.; Ritenour, R. Medical Imaging Physics, 3rd ed. St. Louis: Mosby–Year Book, 1992.

Kathren, R.L. Radiation Protection: Medical Physics Handbook 16. Boston: Adam Hilger, 1985.

Noz, M.E.; Maguire, G.Q., Jr. Radiation Protection in the Radiologic and Health Sciences, Philadelphia: Lea & Febiger, 1979.

Recommendations on Limits for Exposure to Ionizing Radiation (NCRP Report No. 91). The National Council on Radiation Protection and Measurements, Bethesda, MD: NCRP Publications, 1987.

Shapiro, J. Radiation Protection: A Guide for Scientists and Physicians, 3rd ed. Cambridge, MA: Harvard University Press, 1990.

Statkiewicz, M.A.; Ritenour, E.R. Radiation Protection for Student Radiographers. Denver: Multi-Media Publishing, 1983.

Review Questions

1. Regarding radiation protection standards, indicate
   a. the primary international body that makes recommendations in radiation protection matters
   b. for the U.S., the primary national body that makes recommendations about radiation protection matters
   c. two agencies in the U.S. that regulate the safe use of radiation and radiation sources
2. Explain briefly how absorbed dose and dose equivalent are determined from an exposure reading.
3. A technologist receives an exposure of 60 R to the hands as a result of an accident involving a radiation source that produces a monoenergetic beam of 100-keV photons.
   a. Use Table 20–1 to determine the absorbed dose. Assume soft tissue to be equivalent to water in its radiation absorption characteristics.
   b. Use Table 20–2 to determine the dose equivalent.
   c. If this accident occurred on February 15, 1994, does this dose exceed the maximum allowable dose? (See Table 20–3)
4. A radiation worker receives an exposure of 9×10^{-4} C/kg to the whole body as a result of an accidental exposure from a gamma source.
   a. Use Table 20–1 to determine the absorbed dose in grays. Assume soft tissue to be equivalent to water in its radiation absorption characteristics.
   b. Use Table 20–2 to determine the dose equivalent in sieverts (Sv).
   c. If this exposure occurred February 20, 1994, does this dose exceed the maximum allowable dose?
5. Make the following conversions:
   a. 100 mSv to rem
   b. 2 mrem to mSv
   c. 10 cGy to rads
   d. 400 mrem to mSv
   e. 600 R to C/kg
6. Briefly explain what is meant by the ALARA concept.
7. Briefly indicate how occupational radiation exposure is most commonly measured.
8. How do radiological technologists determine their occupational radiation exposure for a particular month?
9. Briefly describe three common types of personnel dosimetry and how they are used to estimate occupational radiation exposure.
10. Should personnel dosimeters be worn when technologists themselves undergo medical or dental x-ray procedures? Why or why not?
11. Indicate advantages and disadvantages of film badges, TLDs, and pocket dosimeters.
12. For whole-body radiation exposure, what should be the *monthly* maximum occupational level?
13. Indicate three ways a technologist can reduce radiation exposure from any source of radiation.
14. Indicate the proper sign or label that should be posted for each of the following:
    a. a room which houses cobalt-60 (^{60}Co) teletherapy sources; exposure rates in the room are as high as 700 R/hr when in use.
    b. a room used to store nuclear medicine radiopharmaceuticals; exposure rates in the room measure 5.8 mR/hr.
    c. a laboratory which used unsealed radiation sources; exposure levels in the room never exceed 0.5 mR/hr.
    d. a shipping container containing a radioactive source; exposure rates at the surface of the container read 0.9 mR/hr and NDR at 3 feet.
    e. a shipping container containing a radioactive source; exposure rates at the surface of the container read 25 mR/hr and 1.5 mR/hr at 3 feet.
    f. a room which houses an x-ray unit; exposure rates in the room may reach 20 mR/hr during operation
15. a. Describe what is meant by a primary and a secondary barrier.
    b. How does one distinguish between the two when designating these within an imaging room?
    c. How does the effective thickness of a primary barrier differ from that of a secondary barrier?
16. List measures that can be taken to ensure that a declared pregnant technologist minimizes fetal radiation exposure while still performing her duties within the radiology department.

Exercises

1. A radiation source produces an exposure rate of 50 mR/hour at a distance of 3 m from the source. At what distance will the exposure rate drop to 2 mR/hour?
2. The exposure rate from a brachytherapy patient (i.e., a patient having radioactive implants) is measured at 20 mR/hour at a point where a nurse would stand when working with the patient. How long could a nurse stand at that location before receiving a dose equivalent of 50 mrem. (Assume the radiation implants are ^{137}Cs, which emits 662-keV photons.)
3. Determine the dose equivalents for each of the following:
   a. 10 rads resulting from alpha radiation
   b. 3 rads resulting from thermal neutrons
   c. 5 cGy resulting from beta radiation
   d. 15 R exposure resulting from gamma radiation (assume f-factor ≈ 1)
   e. 3.5 R exposure resulting from x-rays (assume f-factor ≈ 1)
4. If the HVL of a 100-kVp x-ray beam in Pb is 0.24 mm and in concrete is 1.5 mm, determine

a. the exposure rate transmitted through a lead sheet 1 mm thick if the initial exposure rate (with no shielding) is 120 mR/hour.

b. the thickness of concrete needed to reduce the exposure rate from this unit from 120 mR/hour to 2 mR/hour.

c. the number of HVLs needed to reduce the initial intensity to 1% of its initial value.

5. If the HVL of an 80-kVp x-ray beam in lead is 0.19 mm, what percent of its initial intensity if transmitted by a lead apron 0.25 mm thick? 0.5 mm thick? 1.0 mm thick?

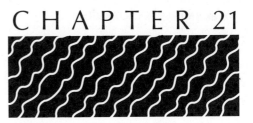

C H A P T E R 21

Radiation Protection

*Steven B. Dowd, Ed.D.,
R.T.(R.)*

Chapter Outline

Chapter Objectives

On completion of this chapter, you should be able to

- Describe how time, distance, and shielding can be used for radiation protection of the operator and patient.
- State the relative hazard to the fetus from radiation exposure, and describe means to minimize that exposure.
- State the first rule of mobile radiography.
- Explain how proper technique selection can be used in radiation protection.
- Describe the effect of filtration on the beam and patient dose.
- State a use for a compensating filter.
- Describe the effect a grid has on radiation dose.
- List examinations in which opposite projections (e.g., PA and AP) can be used to minimize patient dose.
- Describe the effect of film-screen combination on patient dose.
- List means of collimation and their effect on patient dose.
- Describe the appropriate use of gonadal shielding and types of shields.
- Describe the value of (a) immobilization and (b) patient instructions in minimizing patient dose.
- Explain how minimizing repeats will decrease patient dose.
- State the need for certification and education in reducing patient dose.
- Describe means of protecting the pregnant or potentially pregnant patient.

THE BASIS OF RADIATION PROTECTION

All human activities have both risks and benefits. We freely decide to engage in activities such as airline travel, because we perceive the benefit of such an activity to outweigh the potential risk. Although there is more potential risk associated with air than rail travel, most people would choose the quicker route. Similarly, the amount of information provided by a diagnostic radiograph ordered by a physician having reason to suspect a disease process far outweighs the potential risk. Radiation protection is an art based on sound scientific principles. Radiation protection seeks to limit the exposure of patients to a level that is as low as reasonably achievable (the *ALARA* concept) while providing a maximum amount of diagnostic information. Many of the techniques used to limit patient dose also reduce operator exposure.

Many of the items described here—for example, three-phase generators, fluoroscopy, half-value layer (HVL)—have been discussed in greater detail, although not always in relation to radiation protection, in other chapters of this text. If it remains unclear how radiation protection can be practiced using these items, the student may wish to review those individual chapters.

PROTECTING THE RADIOGRAPHER

Although the patient should be the only individual exposed to the primary beam, personnel may be exposed to secondary or leakage radiation from the tube. Examinations with the possibility of greater exposure to the worker include interventional procedures, fluoroscopy, and mobile radiography.

Radiographers should not routinely hold patients unable to cooperate during a procedure. Some regulatory agencies require workers to document any holding of patients during procedures. If immobilization devices are unavailable or cannot be used, assistance should be secured from nonradiation workers, preferably a family member or friend. No one should ever routinely hold patients. Any individual holding a patient should remain at right angles to the primary beam. Most scatter radiation is backscatter as illustrated in Figure 21–1. Persons holding patients should also wear a lead apron and if possible, lead gloves (see the section on immobilization for additional guidelines on using human immobilizers).

The three cardinal, or most important, principles of radiation protection are time, distance, and shielding. These are discussed in greater detail in the following paragraphs.

Time

The radiographer must reduce the amount of time spent in the area of the radiation source. *Time* and radiation exposure are directly proportional; that is, if the amount of time spent in the area of the source doubles, the radiation exposure to the individual also doubles. Exposure is a function of time and is directly proportional to it. The less time spent near the source of radiation the less exposure is received.

Distance

Distance is the most effective means of reducing radiation exposure. At a distance of 1 m from the scattering object (the patient), the intensity of scatter radiation in fluoroscopy decreases to 0.1% (one thousandth) of the intensity measured at the scattering object.

The inverse square law, which states that radiation intensity varies as the inverse of the square of the distance, holds true for the primary beam, which is considered a point source of radiation and after about 1 m for scatter radiation. Thus an intensity of 100 mrad (1 mGy) at 20 inches diminishes to 25 mrad (0.25 mGy) at 40 inches. This does not hold true for scatter radiation because the patient is an extended source of radiation. How scatter radiation behaves depends roughly on the area of the scattering medium (in this case, the patient). However, the basic concept is the same: remain as far from the source (patient) as possible. For this reason, the cord on fixed radiographic equipment is short to keep the operator behind the control booth.

Shielding

Shielding consists of either fixed structural barriers (made of lead, concrete, or both) or nonfixed devices such as mobile shields, lead aprons, gloves, and the like. Lead is the material preferred for shielding. Its high atomic number (82) is a major factor in low-energy x-ray absorption interactions. Lead aprons, for example, should consist of a minimum of 0.25 mm lead equivalent (Pb eq). Most facilities use lead aprons consisting of 0.5 mm Pb eq; aprons of 1.0 mm Pb eq are also available.

Shielding is measured in terms of *half-value layers (HVLs)* and *tenth-value layers (TVLs)*. These terms refer to the thicknesses of lead that will transmit 50% and 10%, respectively, of the incident x-radiation. For lead aprons to be effective, the lead must not be cracked; thus aprons should not be handled carelessly or folded.

Fixed barriers are classified as either primary or secondary barriers. A primary barrier can be struck by the primary beam and must cover the wall from the floor to a height of at least seven feet. The primary beam

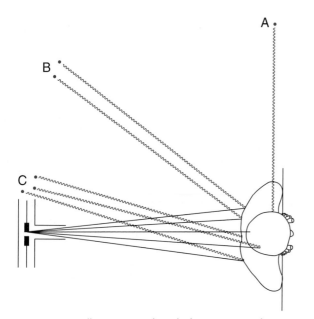

FIGURE 21–1. *A* illustrates a relatively low amount of scatter at 90°. *B* and *C* show the amounts of scatter behind the patient.

should not be directed toward secondary barriers, which can only provide protection against secondary radiation. The control booth is usually considered a secondary barrier; the ceiling always is a secondary barrier in a radiology room. This is not true, for example, during mobile radiography in the emergency room.

When a control booth is considered a secondary barrier, x-rays will have scattered at least twice before entering. This reduces the intensity of the beam to one millionth (one one-thousandth × one one-thousandth; see earlier) of the original value.

The Pregnant Radiographer

The working habits of pregnant radiographers should be based on previous radiation exposure history and the current work setting. It is usually best to rotate the radiographer out of areas such as fluoroscopy and mobile radiography because of the potential for greater exposure in those areas. An additional monitor can also be provided to be worn at waist level under the lead apron to determine fetal dose. Pregnant radiographers should never hold patients, although this is a decision to be made by the worker.

Rotation changes are best made in conjunction with the radiographer, the radiographer's personal physician, and the radiation safety officer, although the final decision rests with the radiographer. The most important factor is the relationship between the employer and employee. The employer is responsible for providing a safe work setting; however, the employee must also observe rules of safe practice.

In no case can a radiographer be fired simply because she is pregnant. The National Council on Radiation Protection and Measurement (NCRP) has recommended a dose limit to the fetus of 0.5 rem, or 5 millisieverts (mSv), based on the view of the embryo and fetus as an "involuntary visitor" brought into a radiation area as a result of the mother's occupational exposure. NCRP Report No. 91 (1987) states that the dose should not exceed 0.5 mSv (50 mrem) in any month; not more than 5 mSv (0.5 rem) during gestation. These limits are subject to change as the results of scientific studies are analyzed and incorporated into existing regulations.

It is important to realize that there is no such thing as a "radio-unique" effect; that is, a variety of other factors such as air pollution, food additives, tobacco, and stress can all lead to the same effect to the fetus as radiation exposure. It is as difficult to mandate a "safe" dose for the fetus as for the adult, even though we know that developing cells are more sensitive to radiation. The National Academy of Science has stated that it is uncertain that a dose of less than one rad would have any effect at all on the fetus.

Even at 5 rads, there is only a small risk of congenital anomalies and malformations. The risk of carcinogenesis is much lower than other risks associated with pregnancy.

Radiation Protection During Mobile Radiography

This section describes mobile or portable radiography—the use of units brought to patients' rooms as opposed to other forms of radiography on wheels (e.g., mobile mammography units contained within vans that travel from site to site). The intensity of radiation 1 m from the patient in portable radiography is so small that a radiation worker standing at this distance in one study would have to have been exposed to approximately 2000 films a month to reach the dosage allowed the general public. Scatter from the patient is the main source of exposure to the operator and others present. This is normally very small. If the exposure for a portable chest is 40 mR, then at 1 m scatter would equal 0.04 mR. At 2 m, according to the inverse square law, exposure would be reduced to 0.01 mR. However, mobile radiography still constitutes a potential radiation hazard for patient rooms and surgical suites, which unlike the radiology department are not usually designed for radiation protection. These rooms are not shielded and do not have *lead aprons* or other means of protection available unless brought by the radiographer.

The first rule of mobile radiography is the same as the first rule of regular radiography—secure the cooperation of and establish communication with the patient. On arrival at the patient's room, the mobile unit should be left in the hall, and the radiographer should assess the patient's condition and ability to cooperate and should attempt to establish rapport. Before making the required radiographs, all nonessential persons should be asked to leave the area. Individuals remaining, including the patient, should be shielded. Be certain to tell those persons previously asked to leave when the radiographic procedure is finished.

Distance, as always, is the most effective means of protection in mobile radiography. When performing mobile radiography, the radiographer is expected to stand 6 ft from the source, using a cord long enough to allow this distance. Exposure time can also be reduced, with a corresponding decrease in operator and patient exposure, by using the fastest screen-film combination possible.

Health educators talk about "teachable moments," or situations in which individuals can be taught good health practices. Here mobile examinations can be used to show that a radiographer is a professional concerned with the radiological health not only of the patient but also of family members, nurses, and physicians. Sometimes family members ask to stay, for example, possibly with an apron (many people feel that lead aprons provide some sort of absolute protection against radiation). Explain to them the greater value of distance in radiation protection.

For professional workers such as nurses, the "teachable moment" more often consists of letting these individuals know that the radiographer practices sound radiation protection principles by reassuring them that you will not make an exposure while they are present. This establishes the radiographer as a professional.

Radiation Protection During Fluoroscopy and Angiography

Fluoroscopy is a dynamic imaging technique (see Chapter 15) that allows the viewing of motion and location in real time. In addition to fluoroscopy in the radiology department, mobile fluoroscopy is often performed in the operating room for surgical procedures such as fixation of long-bone fractures and hip pinnings. Means to reduce patient dose in fluoroscopy include

- Exposure rate at tabletop cannot exceed 10 R/min and should not exceed 5 R/min
- Using a minimum focal distance of at least 30 cm (12 inches) for mobile units and 38 cm (15 inches) for fixed units
- Collimating the beam to expose only the clinical area of interest
- Optimizing technical factors; using appropriate mA and kVp
- Providing sufficient beam filtration to meet regulatory requirements

Fluoroscopic units are equipped with five-minute reset timers to remind the operator that a certain recommended time limit has elapsed for *beam-on time*. This does not mean that it is illegal to exceed five minutes of fluoroscopic time. The timer is designed to serve only as a reminder that this block of time has been exceeded. Also, fluoroscopic foot switches are designed to terminate the exposure once the foot is released from the switch. This is referred to as a *deadman switch.*

In fluoroscopy, scatter at 90° and just to the front of the patient is greatest; the patient's body filters some of the radiation. Scatter production in fluoroscopy is illustrated in Figure 21–2. Also, the preponderance of dose to the radiographer from the patient is at the level of the operator's gonads. The best means of radiation protection for the radiographer during fluoroscopy is to stand behind the radiologist. However, the motion of the radiologist is not always predictable, so that distance should also be used to ensure lower doses. This is in addition to a lead apron and the lead gloves that should be worn if the hands will be placed in the primary beam. Only those persons required for the examination should be in the room, and they should wear lead aprons.

Wearing a lead apron is important, because with an apron of normal length, approximately 80% of the active bone marrow in the body is covered. "Wraparound" aprons are essential for radiographers who may have to move around the room during fluoroscopy. This reduces the possible *oncogenic* effect of radiation on bone marrow (i.e., the development of leukemia).

Many states have restrictions on the use of fluoroscopy. Certain states allow radiographers to become certified in the limited use of fluoroscopy. However, some states do not allow anyone not licensed to practice medicine to operate fluoroscopic equipment, except for static functions (e.g., spot-filming) when performed under the direct supervision of a radiologist who is physically present.

Angiographic studies are modified fluoroscopic studies. In such studies, catheters are placed in the patient and monitored under fluoroscopic control. As a result, patient doses tend to be high because of the long fluoroscopic times required for catheter insertion and the many images needed to record anatomical structures.

Cardiac cineangiography is one example of a high-dose study. Typically, 13 minutes of fluoroscopy and 110 seconds of cinefluorography are used, although this of course varies with the physician. The entrance skin dose for cinefluorography is usually 2 mR per frame. If 60 frames are used per second, this translates into about 7.2 R/min or about 13.2 R total, assuming 110 seconds of cinefluorography. With tabletop doses ranging from approximately 1 to 3 R/min for most fluoroscopic equipment (with a maximum of 10 R/min), patient dose could easily range from 26 to 52 R per examination. For this reason, speed and efficiency are imperative in cardiac cinefluorography.

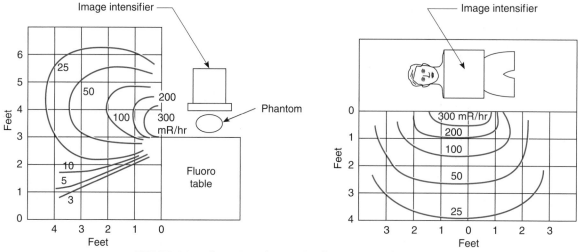

FIGURE 21–2. Illustration of scatter (isodose curve) in fluoroscopy.

PATIENT PROTECTION

A variety of basic principles, many of which are under the control of the radiographer, can be used to minimize patient exposure while retaining a diagnostic image. These are described in the following paragraphs.

Technique Selection

Tube current (milliamperage, or mA), time (s), and kilovoltage (kVp) should be selected in unison to produce an image that is diagnostically acceptable to the physician while maintaining good radiation protection practices. High kVp is preferred, yet it should not be so high as to degrade image quality through the production of excess scatter radiation and excessively long-scale contrast. Most examinations have an optimum kVp setting beyond which the contrast scale is degraded. *Fixed–kVp technique systems* allow a lower average mAs, since kVp values are generally higher than those used in *variable–kVp technique systems.*

For example, equivalent density is achieved by using a fixed-kVp technique of 20 mAs and 80 kVp, whereas a variable technique chart might require 40 mAs and 68 kVp. Using the fixed-kVp technique can reduce patient dose by about 56 mR.

The relationship between mAs, density, and intensity is direct; as mAs is doubled, density and intensity also double. The relationship between kVp and intensity is more complex:

$$\left(\frac{kVp_1}{kVp_2}\right)^2 = \frac{I_1}{I_2}$$

)))))) EXAMPLE

To illustrate the use of these relationships, consider the previously mentioned example. If a variable technique of 40 mAs and 68 kVp provides an intensity of 180 mR, the intensity of the second technique can be calculated as follows:

Step 1: mAs is being halved; therefore, the intensity due to mAs decreases to one half of the original value.

$$\frac{mAs_1}{mAs_2} = \frac{I_1}{I_2}$$

$$\frac{40}{20} = \frac{180}{x}$$

$$x = 90 \text{ mR}$$

Step 2: kVp is being increased; thus intensity now increases as follows:

$$\left(\frac{kVp_1}{kVp_2}\right)^2 = \frac{I_1}{I_2}$$

$$\left(\frac{68}{80}\right)^2 = \frac{90}{x}$$

x = 124.6 mR, a total
decrease of about 56 mR

When manually selecting techniques, the time of exposure should be minimized to keep the degrading effects of motion as low as possible. Tube current (mA) can be increased to compensate in direct proportion. A technique of 200 mA and 0.1 seconds (20 mAs) is equivalent to 400 mA and .05 seconds. Both will provide equivalent density.

When phototiming (i.e., using automatic exposure control devices), it is important to use a balance between mA and time that cannot potentially overexpose the patient. For example, it is unwise to choose 400 mA and 1 second *back-up time* for a phototimed abdominal film, for if a malfunction occurs, the patient would receive the full 400 mAs. Assuming that about 40 mAs is necessary, it would be wiser to select 200 mA and 1 second to minimize the possibility of grossly overexposing the patient. Some authorities recommend using only 1.5 times the expected mAs.

Another potential disadvantage of phototiming is that it is not always as precisely reproducible as manual timing. If positioning is not duplicated exactly for the repeat exposure, and the technical setting has been changed (e.g., density setting changed to $1\frac{1}{4}$), that film may be unacceptable because the amount of tissue over the photocell has changed as illustrated in Figure 21–3.

Filtration

A filter is a device placed at the *x-ray port* to absorb low–energy x-ray photons (Fig. 21–4) that do not contribute to the diagnostic value of the image but contribute radiation dose to the patient. Removing these low-energy photons decreases the overall patient dose. As filtration is added to a tube, the patient dose decreases, given equivalent techniques. *Total filtration*

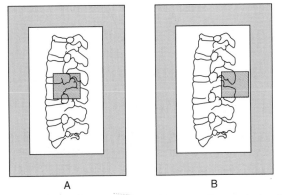

FIGURE 21–3. *A,* The part is correctly centered over photocell. *B,* This part is incorrectly centered over photocell, which will lead to excessive radiation exposure.

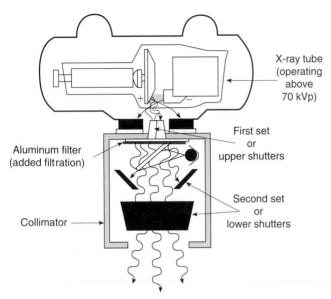

FIGURE 21–4. Filtration in the x-ray tube.

is a sum of that filtration added to the tube (placed at the x-ray port) and the inherent filtration of the tube itself. Regulations require that equipment operating above 70 kVp must have a 2.5-mm aluminum equivalent (Al eq) total filtration. Aluminum is a preferred absorber for filtration because of its low atomic number (13). As a result, it absorbs low-energy but not high-energy photons.

If increases in filtration of the beam are compensated for by an advance in mAs, then patient dose increases if the added filtration is 1.0 mm Al eq or less. Instead, kVp should be increased to maintain image density, which will lower patient dose. This will also lower contrast, reducing image quality. There is a practical limit to this concept.

Compensating filters are used to compensate for variations in patient density. For example, wedge filters (Fig. 21–5) are employed in foot radiography with the thick portion of the wedge over the toes and the thin portion toward the heel to provide for even density on the film. Other means of compensating filtration include the use of special cassettes with two types of intensifying screens, or the addition of a piece of paper to a screen to limit the amount of light produced in one section. Correct use of compensating filters can cut the patient's exposure in half by eliminating the need for two films.

Grids

Grids are placed between the patient and image receptor to absorb scatter radiation (Fig. 21–6). They are usually employed when the thickness of the part of the body under examination exceeds 10 to 13 cm (depending on the preferences of the radiologist). Using a grid requires an increase in technical factors; it is not a device to minimize radiation exposure. It does im-

prove image quality by removing unwanted scatter radiation. A Bucky (moving) grid absorbs about 10% more radiation than the equivalent stationary grid.

If various grid ratios are available, it is the responsibility of the radiographer to choose the lowest possible grid ratio that will reduce scatter yet not require overly high technical factors. One example of how grid choice can lead to radiation protection of the patient is to use an 8:1 grid instead of a 12:1 grid for a child. A child, because of size, may not need as high a grid. In this example, mAs can be reduced by 20% with an equivalent density.

Employment of an air-gap technique instead of a grid also provides a slightly lower patient dose than the grid technique. The air-gap technique uses an increased object-to-film distance to remove scatter from the film (Fig. 21–7).

Position and Projection

Certain projections are superior in terms of radiation protection. An approximate reduction of 95% in radiation exposure to the lens of the eye (important for potentially preventing cataracts) is possible by using the posteroanterior (PA) projection of the cranium instead of the anteroposterior (AP). In a female patient undergoing an intravenous pyelogram (IVP) or a cystogram, the contrast-filled bladder serves as a gonadal shield in the AP projection, whereas it does not do so in the PA projection. Using the PA rather than the AP projection for juvenile scoliosis examinations reduces

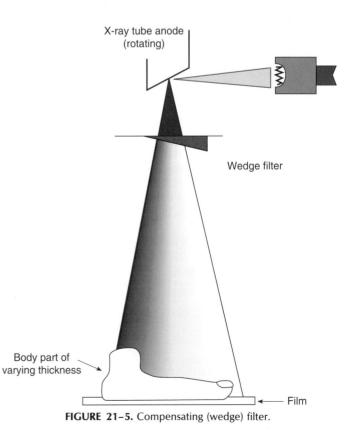

FIGURE 21–5. Compensating (wedge) filter.

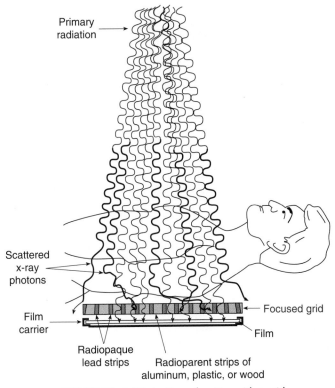

FIGURE 21–6. Elimination of scatter with a grid.

Primary radiation

Scattered x-ray photons

Film carrier

Radiopaque lead strips

Radioparent strips of aluminum, plastic, or wood

Focused grid

Film

exposure to the breasts to approximately 1% of the original value.

A use of positioning to minimize radiation exposure is the centering on T-6 rather than T-4 in a PA chest radiograph exposed with an automatic exposure control. Because of the position of the photocell in relation to anatomical parts, this position provides a radiograph with a longer scale of contrast, less patient dose, and better visualization of cardiac outlines and fluid levels. If the positions and projections used in the institution employing the radiographer do not make good use of radiation protection practices, it is the responsibility of the radiographer to tactfully lobby for their use.

Image Receptors

As the speed of an image receptor increases, the amount of radiation needed to expose the film decreases. On a negative note, as the speed of the film-screen system becomes greater, diagnostic quality is reduced. The highest possible film-screen combination still able to achieve the needed diagnostic quality should be selected to minimize risk (radiation exposure) and maximize benefit (the quality of the examination).

As an example, changing from a 200- to a 400-speed system can reduce radiation in terms of entrance skin exposures by 20% to 50%, according to the text *Average Patient Exposure Guides: 1988*. On an AP abdominal film, for example, entrance skin exposure can be

reduced by 50% with this change. After selection of the appropriate kilovoltage, the most effective technique for reducing patient dose is the use of faster film-screen combinations. Figure 21–8 illustrates the use of a 400- and 600-speed film-screen system on a phantom abdomen. Forty mAs was used for the 400-, 25 mAs for the 600-speed, with an equivalent density. Assuming 300 mR skin entrance exposure on the 400-speed film, the 600-speed film should show a skin entrance exposure of 200 mR, a decrease of 50%.

Beam Limitation (Collimation)

Most modern x-ray units are equipped with *positive beam limitation (PBL),* which automatically collimates, or limits, the beam to the size of the film when using the Bucky grid. Most of this equipment also allows the radiographer to further minimize the beam size. Proper collimation reduces patient exposure and improves image quality. Differences in scatter caused by beam size are illustrated in Figure 21–9. Other means of collimation include cones and cylinders (Fig. 21–10), which are attached to the tube housing to further limit beam size; aperture diaphragms, which are used for machines lacking collimators; and lead blockers, which are placed in the beam to absorb scatter radiation.

The radiographer should always seek to limit the beam size to the area of clinical interest. Regulations

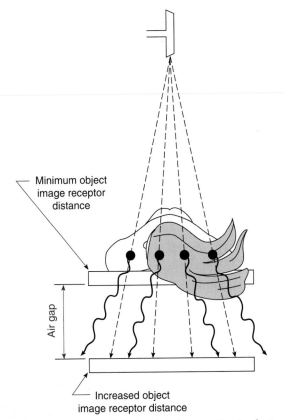

Minimum object image receptor distance

Air gap

Increased object image receptor distance

FIGURE 21–7. Air-gap technique. Note how scatter is eliminated through the use of a greater object-film distance.

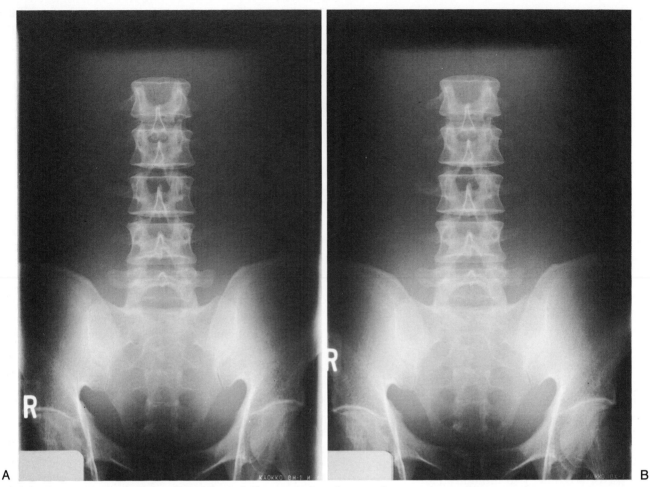

FIGURE 21-8. Two anteroposterior (AP) abdominal films, equivalent density. Film in *A* demonstrates use of a 400-speed film/screen system. Film in *B* used a 600-speed system.

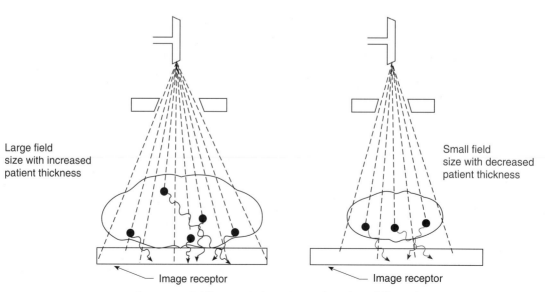

FIGURE 21-9. Illustration of differences in intensity resulting from different beam sizes.

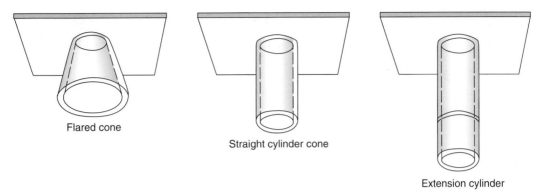

FIGURE 21-10. Cone and cylinders.

require collimation to be accurate to within 2% of the focal film distance. Proper collimation contributes to image quality and radiation protection of both patient and operator by reducing the amount of scatter radiation.

Shielding

One of the most important means of minimizing the potential effects of radiation exposure on future generations is shielding of the ovaries and testes (gonads). This is important for all individuals of reproductive age and younger. Some facilities recommend that all males and all females younger than age 65 be shielded. A variety of examinations are associated with high gonadal doses, including barium enema, hip, femur, lumbar spine, sacrum, coccyx, and urography. It is therefore important that appropriate patient shielding be used especially in such examinations.

Some facilities routinely use gonadal shielding unless it interferes with the diagnostic quality of the beam. The shielding can be used to minimize patient anxiety associated with radiation exposure. Often, gonadal shielding is an excellent public relations tool even when exposure to the gonads is minimal. As a rule, gonadal shielding should be used when the gonads are within 5 cm (~2 in) of the primary beam, unless this would compromise diagnostic quality of the film.

There are three basic types of gonadal shields. Flat contact shields are usually made of lead-impregnated vinyl and are placed directly over the patient's gonads.

Shaped contact shields are used for male gonadal shielding (Fig. 21-11). They are cup-shaped to provide for maximum protection in a variety of settings. Shadow shields cast a "shadow" in the beam and are mounted at the tube or on the tube housing and support structures (Fig. 21-12).

Shadow shields have some definite advantages over the other types. They are relatively easy to use, even when the patient is uncooperative. Also, they do not require the radiographer to touch a patient on or near a "private" area, preserving the patient's modesty. Finally, they are ideal for use during sterile procedures, since the radiographer does not have to insert the shield into a sterile field. Their main disadvantage is that they cannot be used during fluoroscopy; since the tube is under the table, positioning of a shadow shield would be essentially impossible.

Male gonadal shielding should be used in examinations of the pelvis, hip (except obliques), and upper femur, unless it interferes with the examination. Male gonadal shielding is not usually used on retrograde urethrograms, voiding cystourethrograms, and visualization of the rectum. It is more difficult to provide gonadal shielding to female patients because of the internal nature of the female gonads.

Other types of shielding include contact lens shields for the lens of the eye and breast shields for juvenile scoliosis examinations. Shielding can be used in conjunction with other methods to further minimize exposure; for example, a combination of fast rare earth screens, compensating filters, and breast shields will lower patient dose during juvenile scoliosis radiography.

FIGURE 21-11. Flat (A) and shaped (B) contact shields.

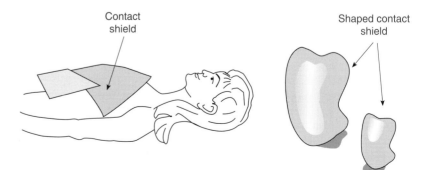

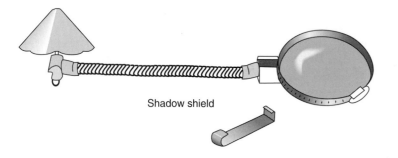

FIGURE 21–12. A shadow shield.

Shadow shield

Immobilization

Immobilization is sometimes needed to prevent the image-degrading effects of *voluntary motion.* Another type of motion, *involuntary* (physiologic) *motion* of organs is best handled by shortening the time of exposure.

Far superior to immobilization is the use of effective communication (described in the next section) and positioning aids such as sandbags, angle sponges, foam pads, and the radiographer's standby tape.

However, the patient unable to cooperate must be immobilized. Patient ability to cooperate must be ascertained by the radiographer, who will then decide on appropriate means of immobilization. An adult may be unable to hold the forearm still and may need sandbags applied to each end of the arm to prevent image-degrading motion. Obviously, a six-month-old infant will be unable to cooperate and may need immobilization in the form of a Pigg-O-Stat (Fig. 21–13) for a PA and lateral chest x-ray.

Using people as immobilizers is the last resort. Radiographers are the last choice for holding patients and no one should be responsible for routinely holding patients. Relatives, especially males, are the first choice for holding patients. After that, nonradiology hospital personnel are the next choice over "other" radiology personnel such as patient transporters.

Human immobilizers must be provided with shielding—minimally, lead aprons and gloves. They should also wear a monitoring device. The International Committee for Radiologic Protection (ICRP) also recommends that the individual holding a patient be older than the "normal" reproductive age. The ideal device for assistants who do not normally wear a badge would be a pocket dosimeter. If this is not available, then the procedure and the specific exposures they hold for should be documented. Also, time should be taken to explain some of the basic principles of personnel protection to the individual holding the patient. This display of professional concern will be appreciated, and will be helpful if problems arise in the future.

One positive aspect of immobilization is the use of *compression bands* in abdominal radiography. Their employment results in less tissue density and less scatter radiation, which minimizes patient dose and gives a more appropriate scale of contrast.

Patient Instructions

It is extremely important that the patient who is able to cooperate be allowed to do so. Experienced radiographers know the value of securing patient cooperation and the extent to which this minimizes repeat examinations. Taking a few extra seconds to secure patient

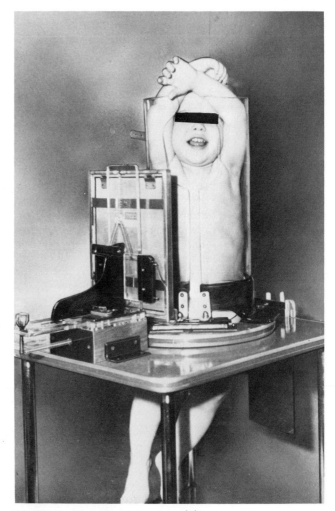

FIGURE 21–13. A Pigg-O-Stat immobilizer.

cooperation and consent and instill a sense of trust in the radiographer can easily save time on repeat films. In fact, securing cooperation and communicating with the patient should be the first rule of radiography.

Radiographers need to adopt a professional approach to patient instruction, which involves a combination of visible technical competence, showing a caring and consumer-oriented attitude, and effective communication skills. The following activities can establish a communication process and facilitate patient cooperation:

- Use appropriate vocabulary. Some patients may not understand more complicated terms. On the other hand, "talking down" to some patients minimizes cooperation.
- Organize your thoughts. The radiographer should have a pre-planned routine that can be altered as needed. Never ramble, or appear to be unprepared for the patient.
- Use appropriate voice tone and volume. Experienced radiographers know that some elderly patients become uncooperative when spoken to in a loud voice as they resent the assumption that they are deaf. Other patients may resent a healthcare worker they find too "enthusiastic" and thus by assumption, unprofessional.
- Effective listening. Always listen first. Moving through an examination without listening can cause resentment and a loss of cooperation.

Patients have the right to refuse examinations (with certain exceptions, such as minors), but the radiographer cannot advocate refusal to the patient. The radiographer may

- Question the validity of the request for the examination with the appropriate personnel involved in the care of the patient. In many cases, this is in the patient's best interest. For example, the patient may have pain in the right wrist but a radiographic examination of the left wrist was ordered. In this case, the referring physician, the radiologist, or the nurse in charge of the patient may be questioned as to the validity of the request.
- Provide the patient with information indicating that the benefits of diagnostic examinations tend to outweigh the risks (for example, the information relative to patient doses given in this and earlier chapters). Don't overdo it, however; just give information that is relevant and understandable to the patient.

Repeat Exposures

An "average" repeat rate for radiographs ranges from about 4% to 15%, although authorities cite a variety of rates. A variety of factors influences repeat rate, including the experience level of the radiographer and the radiologist's opinion of image quality. The purpose of a departmental quality assurance program is to reduce repeats and improve image quality. Abdominal and thoracic-lumbar spine radiographs are the sources of the most repeats.

A very low repeat rate may indicate that poor quality films are being passed. Repeat exposures because of improper film processing, poor positioning, improper exposure factors, and poor patient instruction are under the control of the radiographer. In line with a risk versus benefit consideration, radiographs should be repeated only when the quality of the film is unacceptable. For example, although not marking or improper marking of films is contrary to professional practice, it is not grounds for a repeat exposure of the patient.

Film critique is one method to determine the acceptability of a film and reduce patient dose. Simply tracking repeat films to determine the cause is a good quality assurance measure. This information can be used to educate staff and to improve the quality of films. Although the radiographer never attempts to diagnose, in order to produce the best possible image for the radiologist, the radiographer must understand the needs of the radiologist in order to produce what he or she considers to be a diagnostic image.

Film critique for the radiographer involves the use of critical thinking skills. A technologist performing radiography must be attuned to a variety of image factors. For example, are changes seen in the regular 6 AM portable chest x-ray on a patient in the intensive care unit caused by pathology, patient improvement, or improper technique? In trauma radiography, Drafke (1990) has applied educational principles of critical thinking and problem solving to film evaluation:

1. Define the problem. What are the constraints or limitations? Why did the usual solution (method) not work?
2. List alternatives. List all the possibilities without judging them. List the opposite for each—many problems that cannot be solved in one way can be solved by turning them 180 degrees.
3. Evaluate each. Look for things that would make a solution work or would prevent a solution from working.
4. Select the best solution and try it.
5. Critique the results. If it worked, make a note of it. If it did not work, find out why, re-evaluate the method for the remaining alternatives, and try again.

Proper use of film critique is one important means by which the radiographer can assure diagnostic quality and patient radiation safety. Repeat films should always be documented. A radiographer with an understanding of why films need to be repeated and with the knowledge to correct the factors that lead to substandard films provides the best possible films at the lowest possible patient dose.

Equipment

A radiographer should report all equipment problems as soon as possible. He or she may also be involved in quality assurance checks of equipment. For many procedures, a radiation physicist should assess the radiation safety characteristics of the machine. One study (Brown and Greenberg, 1981) found that in a one-year period, the output of about one third of the fluoroscopic machines studied varied by as much as 100%. It is to be hoped that with state inspections of radiology equipment, this is no longer true.

Many states have a variety of equipment regulations and recommendations for safe practice. These recommendations and regulations encourage an understanding of equipment that promotes safe daily practice and gives an ability to handle emergencies that may arise. For example, all operators of equipment must be aware of the following operational controls and emergency procedures:

- Emergency off-switch and electrical power switch
- Source-to-image distance indicator and beam limitation devices
- Proper operation of the beam-on indicator
- The manufacturer's recommended operation procedures

Processor maintenance and proper darkroom procedures also help to keep patient doses low. These measures include the proper balance of time, temperature, and replenishment of processor chemicals. Although it is not usually possible to increase these factors to minimize patient dose, maintaining a balance of time, temperature, and replenishment keeps patient dose low by maintaining imaging standards, thus reducing the need for repeat films. Also, the darkroom must be kept light tight, and safelight illumination must be enough for viewing but not enough to fog the film.

Some authorities claim that using three-phase equipment because it allows for production of photons of higher average energy results in greater radiation protection of the patient. That is, with the average photon energy being higher for a given kVp, mAs can be reduced to one half the original value from a single-phase to a three-phase generator.

Patient Doses

Radiographers should be familiar with estimated doses of representative examinations. Because the radiographer is able to control factors that lead to this dosage and patients may be interested in their exposure, this information is valuable to the professional.

Patients vary greatly in the amount of information they want to know about their examination. Often, the "trigger" for wanting more information is a recent television program or magazine article on the hazards of radiation. Sometimes college students have recently covered the topic of radiation exposure in a course and want to know more from curiosity, not from resistance to an examination. Never confuse curiosity with refusal of an examination. A radiographer's not knowing the information or appearing incompetent may make the patient have second thoughts about the examination, however.

Table 21-1: REPRESENTATIVE EXPOSURES FOR RADIOLOGICAL EXAMINATIONS

Examination	Skin Dose	Gonadal Dose Male	Female
PA chest	10–20 mrad	1 mrad	<0.5 mrad
	0.1–0.2 mGy	.01 mGy	<.005 mGy
AP abdomen	250–500 mrad	100 mrad	225 mrad
	2.5–5.0 mGy	1 mGy	2.25 mGy
Lateral skull	100–200 mrad	<0.5 mrad	
	1–2 mGy	<.005 mGy	
Extremity	50–200 mrad	15 mrad	<0.5 mrad
	0.5–2.0 mGy	.15 mGy	<.005 mGy
		(lower extremity)	
		<0.5 mrad	
		<.005 mGy	
		(upper extremity)	

Source: Bushong, S.C. Radiation protection. In Ballinger, P.W., ed. Atlas of Radiographic Positions and Radiologic Procedures, 5th ed. St. Louis: C.V. Mosby, 1982.
These values vary, depending on a variety of items, including screen-film combination, patient factors, technical factors, and the like.
mGy = milligray; mrad = millirad.

A variety of means exist to inform patients about the doses they receive. In some departments, this information is released only by the radiologist or physicist. In any case, the radiographer should know what type of information about dose is to be provided to patients, who provides it; also, the technologist should know representative dose values for professional use. Some of these values are listed in Table 21-1.

Certification and Education

As professionals, radiographers should engage in performing only procedures for which they have received education, training, and certification. Various reports have shown the value of education in radiation protection to the patient. For example, it has been found that those who engaged in continuing education were more likely to provide radiation protection to patients.

Another study, by Williamson and Le Heron, found that limited radiography in small-practice settings, performed primarily by nurses, led to a 55% rejection rate by radiologists. Although only 18% of these radiographs were "completely undiagnostic," it seems reasonable that patients should be provided only with films that are completely diagnostic. The nonradiological personnel had rates for unacceptable films that are much higher than are seen with even the most inexperienced radiographers.

The purpose of state licensing of radiographers and voluntary certification by the American Registry of Radiologic Technologists (ARRT) is to ensure that patients are provided with competent practitioners able to protect the patient from excessive radiation. The overall effect is to decrease risks to the health of the population.

It seems reasonable that the best angiographers (special procedures technologists), for example, are those who undertake additional training and experience in this area and attempt to be certified as advanced practitioners in this field through the ARRT examination in cardiovascular and interventional technology (CVIT). In the long run, it is the patient who benefits most from this process.

The Pregnant and Potentially Pregnant Patient

As noted earlier, at low doses (below 1 rad or rem), the risk to the fetus is considered minimal to nonexistent. For patients who may receive more than one rad the risk is greater. Still, the risk of 5 rads is negligible when compared with other risks of pregnancy, with the risk of malformation increasing significantly above 15 rads. Radiation exposure is rarely cause for terminating a pregnancy. These cases require a variety of considerations. The most vulnerable time for the fetus is from the 10th day to the 10th week postconception. Some women might consider abortion with a fetal exposure of 25 rads four weeks after conception. Others would never consider such an option. Certainly, a dose of 5 rads in the 20th week would rarely suggest termination of a pregnancy. Baker and Dalrymple (1984) believe that three pieces of information must be gathered before a decision to terminate a pregnancy can be made:

1. The exact gestational time of radiation exposure must be known.
2. A reasonably accurate estimate of fetal dose is needed.
3. A variety of patient factors such as age, general health, and attitude toward pregnancy and abortion must be assessed.

The ten-day rule seeks to eliminate potential radiation exposure to the embryo by postponing elective abdominal x-rays of fertile women until the ten-day period following the onset of menstruation. This rule, however, has not found much favor recently. Instead, the potential pregnancy status of female patients is determined with steps taken to minimize fetal and embryonic exposure. Often, a radiation physicist calculates the actual fetal dose when procedures are deemed absolutely necessary.

The radiographer is often responsible for ascertaining that a pregnancy test has been performed on female patients, questioning patients relative to their pregnancy status, or both. This is the most effective means of avoiding fetal exposure. It is the radiographer's responsibility to do so professionally and to reassure the patient that appropriate safety measures are taken regardless of pregnancy status. The radiographer should be extremely cautious about providing information, and patients wanting specific information should be referred to the institution's radiation safety officer. This is a delicate area, and the potential stress associated with radiation exposure can easily lead to misunderstandings.

Chapter Summary/ Important Concepts

All human activities carry both risk and benefit. The amount of information provided by a diagnostic radiograph may be required by a physician having reason to suspect a disease process that outweighs the potential risk.

The three cardinal, or most important, principles of radiation protection are time, distance, and shielding. Time and radiation exposure are directly proportional. Distance is the most effective means of reducing radiation exposure. Shielding consists of either fixed structural barriers (made of lead and/or concrete) or devices such as mobile shields and lead aprons, lead gloves, and thyroid shields.

Employment of a radiographer cannot be terminated because of pregnancy. Rotation changes are best made in conjunction with the radiographer, the radiographer's personal physician, and the radiation safety officer. Although the employer must provide a safe working environment, the employee must also practice sound radiation safety procedures. It is recommended that the fetus receive no more than 50 mrem/month and no more than 0.5 rem (5 mSv) during the gestational period.

Mobile radiography constitutes a potential radiation hazard, since patient rooms and surgical suites are not usually designed for radiation protection. The first rule of mobile radiography is to establish communication with the patient, if possible. Special attention must be paid to persons such as visitors, nurses, and doctors, who must often be instructed in proper radiation protection practices.

Thirteen factors that the radiographer can use to limit patient dose have been described in this chapter. The application of these scientific principles is part of the professional practice of the radiographer.

Technique selection is the primary means by which the radiographer can minimize patient dose; mAs and kVp must be selected in unison to produce an acceptable image while protecting the patient. Phototiming must be selected with care because of the possibility of grossly overexposing the patient with excess mAs and the lack of precisely reproducible exposures.

Filtration absorbs low-energy (low-kV) radiation that does not contribute to the image. When filtration is increased, kVp should also be enhanced to maintain film density. Compensating filters are a type used to adjust for variations in patient density.

Grids absorb scatter and require an increase in technical factors. The radiographer must choose the grid that does not require overly high technical factors and provides the desired scale of contrast.

Flexibility in the use of alternative positions and projections can decrease exposure to sensitive organs such as gonads, eyes, and juvenile breasts to less than 1% of original value.

Using a higher-speed film-screen system can reduce patient exposure. The loss in image quality with faster speeds must be balanced with the decrease in patient dose in accordance with risk versus benefit.

A radiographer must seek to secure patient cooperation by exhibiting professional competence and a caring, consumer-oriented attitude in conjunction with effective communication skills. The first rule of radiography should be to establish communication with the patient. If this does not produce the desired result, immobilization may be necessary as a last resort. Immobilization devices should always be used rather than personnel to hold patients.

A radiographer must strive for a repeat rate in accordance with department and professional standards. He or she is a professional who uses scientific knowledge of image factors with critical thinking skills (film critique) to produce a diagnostic image that provides the least exposure to the patient. Equipment problems must be reported to appropriate personnel as soon as possible.

Familiarity with estimated radiation doses of examinations further establishes the radiographer as a knowledgeable professional. This professional should also engage only in examinations for which he or she is educated, licensed, and competent as determined by outside authorities.

The most vulnerable time for the fetus is from the tenth day to the tenth week postconception. Above 15 rads, the risk of potential malformations increases significantly. The radiographer does not advocate specific actions for the patient but reassures the patient and refers her to the radiation safety officer if she wishes additional information.

Important Terminology

ALARA. As low as reasonably achievable; a philosophy of radiation protection that seeks to keep doses to the lowest possible level

Back-up Timer. Used with phototimers (automatic exposure controls) to ensure that an exposure will be of at least a minimum amount

Beam-on Time. The amount of time the beam is actually energized or producing radiation; see also *time*

Compensating Filters. Devices used to provide a more homogeneous thickness

Compression Band. A device that compresses the size of a part; often used with intravenous pyelograms to retain contrast in the kidneys

Dead-Man Switch. A switch that terminates exposure when pressure is no longer applied (thus "dead man")

Distance. There is an inverse relationship between distance and radiation exposure for point sources of radiation

Fixed Barriers. Barriers such as lead, concrete, or both that remain in place

Fixed-kVp Technique System. A system of exposure that relies on using one kilovoltage for each body part; mAs is varied in response to increases or decreases in size of the part

Half-Value Layer (HVL). The amount of shielding that reduces the intensity of radiation to one half its original value

Involuntary Motion. Motion that cannot be controlled such as that of the heart or intestines

Lead Apron. A cover containing a certain thickness of powdered lead in rubber designed to reduce radiation exposure

Mobile Shield. A device that is movable and usable in various settings as opposed to fixed barriers such as lead in a wall

Oncogenic. Pertaining to the production of cancer

Positive Beam Limitation (PBL). Also called automatic collimation; a device that limits the size of the beam to the size of the cassette inserted in the Bucky

Shielding. Materials used to absorb radiation

Tenth-Value Layer (TVL). The amount of shielding that will reduce an original intensity of radiation to one tenth of the original value

Time. There is a direct relationship between radiation exposure and the time of exposure

Total Filtration. The sum of inherent (with the tube) and added filtration; the total filtration needed depends on the maximum kVp available

Variable–kVp Technique System. A system of exposure that relies on using one mAs for each part; kVp is varied by two kVp for each centimeter in response to increases or decreases in size of the part.

Voluntary Motion. Motion that is under the control of the patient

X-ray Port. The area at the collimator from which x-rays emanate

Bibliography

Baker, M.; Dalrymple, G.V. Radiation and the fetus. In Hendee, W.R. Health Effects of Low-Level Radiation. Norwalk, CT: Appleton-Century-Crofts, 1984.

Barnett, M.; Eccleston, R. Radiation Protection During Medical X-ray Examinations. Rockville, MD: U.S. Department of Health, Education, and Welfare, 1976.

Brown, M.R.; Greenberg, L.H. Fluoroscopic Measurement in Saskatchewan. J Can Assoc Radiol 32:118, 1981.

Bushong, S.C. Policies for managing the pregnant employee. Radiology Management 6:2, 1984.

Bushong, S.C. Radiation protection. In Ballinger, P.W., ed. Merrill's Atlas of Radiographic Positions and Radiologic Procedures, 5th ed. St. Louis: C.V. Mosby, 1982.

Bushong, S.C. Radiologic Science for Technologists, 4th ed. St. Louis: C.V. Mosby, 1988.

Butler, P.F.; Thomas, A.W.; Thompson, W.E.; et al. Simple methods to reduce patient exposure during scoliosis radiography. Radiol Technol 57:411, 1986.

Caprio, M.L. The pregnant x-ray tech—providing adequate radiation protection for the fetus. Radiol Technol 52:161, 1980.

Carlton, R.R.; McKenna-Adler, A. Principles of Radiographic Imaging. Albany, NY: Delmar Publishers, 1992.

Carroll, Q.B. Fuchs's Principles of Radiographic Exposure, Processing, and Quality Control, 3rd ed. Springfield, IL: Charles C Thomas, Publishers, 1985.

Conference of Radiation Control Program Directors, Inc.: Average patient exposure guides, 1988. Frankfort, KY: CRCPD Publication, 1988, p 88.

Cusworth, R.J. Quality Assurance in Diagnostic Radiology: An Eight-Step Methodology. Denver: Multi-Media Publishing, 1983.

DeVos, D. Basic Principles of Radiographic Exposure. Philadelphia: Lea & Febiger, 1990.

Donohue, D.P. An Analysis of Radiographic Quality. Baltimore: University Park Press, 1980.

Drafke, M.W. Trauma and Mobile Radiography. Philadelphia: F.A. Davis, 1990.

Frank, E.; Stears, J.; Gray, J.; et al. Use of the PA projection: a method of reducing x-ray exposure to specific radiosensitive organs. Radiol Technol 54:343, 1983.

Frankel, R. Radiation Protection for Radiologic Technologists. New York: McGraw-Hill, 1975.

Hale, J.; Thomas, J.W. Radiation risks for patients having x-rays. Nurse Pract 10:16, 1985.

Holmes, P. Off-beam. Nurs Times, 87:20, 1991.

Land, C.E. Estimating cancer risks from low doses of ionizing radiation. Science 209:1197, 1981.

Martigoni, K.; Nitschke, J. A new radiation protection dose limit for occupationally exposed personnel in the Federal Republic of Germany. Radiologe 31:235, 1991.

McLemore, J. Quality Assurance in Diagnostic Radiology. Chicago: Year Book Medical Publishers, 1981.

Mole, R.H. The ten-day rule: a misnomer. Radiography 50:229, 1984.

NCRP Report No. 54. Medical Exposure of Pregnant and Potentially Pregnant Women. Bethesda, MD: NCRP Publications, 1977.

NCRP Report No. 91. Recommendations on Limits for Exposure to Ionizing Radiation. Bethesda, MD: NCRP Publications, 1987.

NCRP Report No. 102. Medical X-ray, Electron Beam and Gamma-Ray Protection for Energies up to 50 MeV (Equipment Design, Performance, and Use). Bethesda, MD: NCRP Publications, 1989.

Noz, M.E.; Maguire, G.Q. Radiation Protection in the Radiologic and Health Sciences, 2nd ed. Philadelphia: Lea & Febiger, 1985.

Payne, J.T.; Loken, M.K. A survey of the risks and benefits of ionizing radiation. Proposed rules, specific area: gonad shielding, guidelines for use on patients during medical diagnostic x-ray procedures. CRC Crit Rev Clin Radiol Nucl Med 1975.

Federal Register, 40:42749, September 16, 1975.

Riley, S.A. Radiation exposure from fluoroscopy during orthopedic surgical procedures. Clin Orthop 248:257, 1989.

Rossi, R.P. Radiation protection. In Carlton, R.R.; Adler, A. Principles of Radiographic Imaging: An Art and a Science. Albany, NY: Delmar Publishers, 1992.

Ruegesegger, D.R. Radiation exposure levels in an intensive care nursery. Pediatr Nurs 8:244, 1982.

Selman, J. Elements of Radiobiology. Springfield, IL: Charles C Thomas, Publishers, 1983.

Statkiewicz, M.A.; Ritenour, E.R. Radiation Protection for Student Radiographers. Denver: Multi-Media Publishing, 1983.

Tilson, E.R. Educational and experiential effects on radiographers' radiation safety behavior. Radiol Technol 53:321, 1982.

Whalen, J.P.; Balter, S. Radiation Risks in Medical Imaging. Chicago: Year Book Medical Publishers, 1984.

Williamson, B.D.P.; Le Heron, J.C. Radiographic quality and radiation protection in general medical practice and small hospitals. New Zealand Med J, 102:104, 1989.

Woodruff, K. Here's a way to make filters. ADV Radiol Sci Professionals, 4:23, 1991.

Review Questions

1. In general, patient dose may be reduced (while maintaining radiographic density) through the use of _____ techniques.
   - a. high kVp, low mAs
   - b. high kVp, high mAs
   - c. low kVp, low mAs
   - d. low kVp, high mAs

2. The greatest radiation exposure, given otherwise identical technical factors, would result from which of the following primary beam sizes?
   - a. 4 inches × 4 inches
   - b. 5 inches × 5 inches
   - c. 8 inches × 10 inches
   - d. 10 inches × 12 inches

3. Which of the following structures would receive the *least* exposure from an AP abdomen?
   - a. stomach
   - b. small bowel
   - c. liver
   - d. kidney

4. The basic types of gonadal shields are I. flat contact II. shaped contact III. shadow
   - a. I and II only
   - b. I and III only
   - c. II and III only
   - d. I, II, and III

5. If 1 mm of aluminum filtration is added to a tube housing and mAs is added to compensate for that added filtration, then patient radiation exposure will increase
   - a. true
   - b. false

6. Above _____ rad, the risk of potential malformations increases significantly, which might indicate therapeutic abortion for some patients.
   - a. 5
   - b. 10
   - c. 15
   - d. 20

7. Voluntary motion is best controlled by limiting exposure time.
   - a. true
   - b. false

8. Which of the following is not a radiation protection measure?
   - a. high-speed screens
   - b. shielding
   - c. grids
   - d. high-kVp techniques

9. An expected patient dose for a PA chest might be:
   - a. 10 mrad
   - b. 100 mrad
   - c. 1000 mrad
   - d. 10 rad

10. Radiation is assumed to have scattered twice before entering the control booth. This reduces the beam to less than _____ of its original value.
    - a. one hundredth
    - b. one thousandth
    - c. one millionth
    - d. one billionth

Exercises

1. Calculate the reduction in dose from switching from a technique of 10 mAs and 70 kVp to 5 mAs and 80 kVp. The original dose was 55 mR.

2. If the original exposure was 20 mrad at 1 m, what would be the more effective change: (a) adding a half-value layer apron or (b) stepping back to 2 m?

3. Based on the information in this chapter, ask for the pregnancy policy from a local healthcare institution. Does it seem to be appropriate? What changes could be made to make it a better policy?

4. What are the two most effective factors for reducing patient dose? List examples of how these could be used in actual clinical practice.

5. What is the ultimate goal of state licensing and voluntary certification?

6. Why is establishing communication important in radiation protection?

7. What factors influence the repeat rate?

8. Who can refuse a radiograph? How can the radiographer best indicate to the patient the need for an examination?

9. What is the value of using "teachable moments" in mobile radiography? Why is it especially important in this setting?

10. How can the potential disadvantages of phototiming (in relationship to radiation exposure) be minimized?

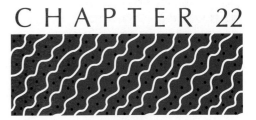

CHAPTER 22

Other Imaging Modalities

Michael A. Thompson, M.S.

Chapter Outline

Chapter Objectives

On completion of this chapter, you should be able to

- Describe the basic components and method of operation of a CT unit.
- Describe how CT images are generated.
- Indicate the most common body plane imaged with CT.
- Specify the difference in the method by which CT images are generated compared with conventional radiography.
- Indicate how nuclear medicine images are produced and what these images represent.
- Describe the operation of a scintillation camera.
- Describe the differences and similarities that exist between radiography and nuclear medicine in regard to radiation protection considerations.
- Indicate the basic components of an MRI unit.
- Describe the differences between images produced by magnetic resonance and those generated by conventional radiography.
- Describe how sound waves are used to generate images.
- Indicate strengths and weaknesses of ultrasound compared with conventional radiography.
- Explain what is represented by a thermographic image.

COMPUTED TOMOGRAPHY

*C*omputed tomography (CT) represents a blend of conventional x-ray units, x-ray detectors, and the digital computer. In many cases, lesions or pathological structures may be missed when conventional two-dimensional radiographic images are used to view three-dimensional structures such as the human body. Thus tomographic imaging methods are used in an attempt to isolate individual planes and produce thin-slice images of the body.

It is important to realize several major differences between CT and conventional radiography:

- Conventional radiography produces images on radiographic film by the direct action of transmitted x-rays on the photographic emulsion; CT produces its images using mathematical techniques performed by a computer
- Conventional, linear tomographic techniques create thin, body section images by "blurring" information from regions outside the area of interest; CT images are mathematically constructed with the aid of the computer so that information from unwanted areas is totally eliminated
- Radiographers must use their technical knowledge of kVp, mA, and exposure time to determine the best combination that will produce the best image contrast; once the image

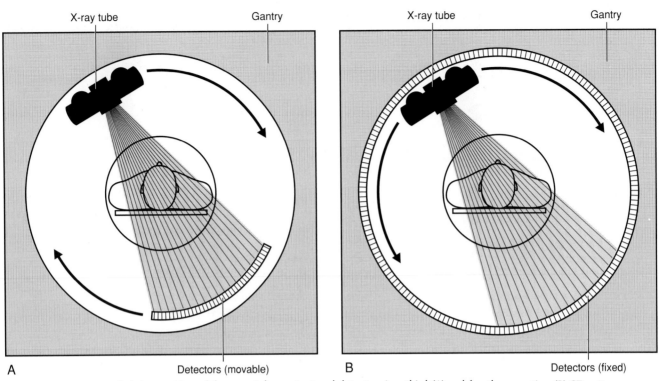

X-ray tube   Gantry

A   Detectors (movable)

X-ray tube   Gantry

B   Detectors (fixed)

FIGURE 22–1. Relative position of the x-ray tube, patient and detectors in a third (A) and fourth generation (B) CT unit.

information has been collected, CT image contrast can be manipulated electronically without additional radiation exposure to the patient

Principles of Computed Tomographic Image Production

Computed tomographic (CT) image information collection begins when a thin, fan-shaped x-ray beam is passed through the edge of the selected body slice. The radiation transmitted through this slice is collected by an array of radiation detectors. The information collected at this position of the tube and detectors does not produce a complete image of the slice rather only a "profile" of the slice from that specific angle. In order to obtain sufficient information to produce the final complete image, the x-ray tube is rotated around the patient, as illustrated in Figure 22–1, and data profiles are collected from many angles. Several hundred views are commonly taken, and the information obtained is stored in computed memory. All these individual views are typically collected in a matter of seconds.

Once the data from the different views have been collected, the process of image reconstruction begins. Image reconstruction is performed with a digital computer. The computer takes the information acquired from the different views and converts this into a numerical representation known as *digital image*. The image generated is composed of a number of individual picture elements known as *pixels*. Each pixel is assigned a specific numerical value, known as the CT

number, which is related to the tissue density in its corresponding volume element, or *voxel*. This concept is illustrated in Figure 22–2.

The digital image generated can then be displayed on a cathode ray tube (CRT) screen, where it can be viewed by the imaging technologist. Image brightness

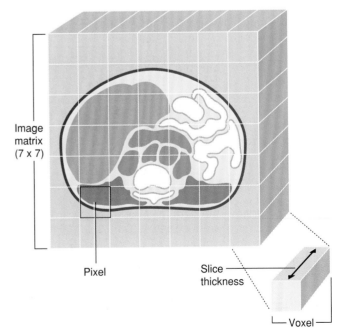

Image matrix (7 x 7)

Pixel

Slice thickness

Voxel

FIGURE 22–2. Elements of a digital image. For a CT image, the shade of gray assigned to a particular pixel depends on the CT number assigned to that pixel and the gray scale used.

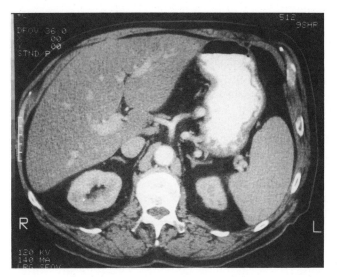

FIGURE 22–3. A CT image of the abdomen.

and contrast can be electronically manipulated by adjusting the gray scale to the range of CT numbers. On attaining appropriate image brightness and contrast, hard copies of the images can then be produced on radiographic film. Because of the manner in which CT images are acquired, CT images are commonly restricted to transverse cross-sectional slices (Fig. 22–3). Today, other imaging planes can be obtained by computer manipulation of the acquired data to produce other body planes and even three-dimensional images of body structures.

Computed Tomographic Imaging Equipment

A typical CT imaging system consists of an x-ray tube mounted on a circular gantry assembly, which allows the tube to rotate around the patient's body. Also mounted within the gantry are detectors that measure the x-ray transmission through the patient's body at the various angles. Since the introduction in 1971 of the CT unit as a feasible method of producing tomographic images, the basic CT unit design has changed several times. Third-generation scanners utilize a rotating detector configuration, whereas those of the fourth generation employ a ring of detector elements that totally encircle the patient's body. In this latter arrangement, only segments of the detector array are in use at any one time as the x-ray tube rotates. Although each CT unit design is different, one is not necessarily better than the other in terms of the quality of images produced.

X-ray tubes used in CT units are of rotating anode design. These tubes are also required to have large heat-loading capabilities and the ability to dissipate heat quickly. Tubes having anode heat capabilities as high as several million heat units are not unusual.

The detectors in fourth generation scanners are scintillation detectors. Recall from previous chapters that this type of detector employs a crystal such as cadmium tungstate or cesium iodide, which produces flashes of light (or scintillations) when x-rays are absorbed. Photomultiplier tubes (PMTs) have in most cases been replaced in CT units by the smaller, less expensive photodiode. These are highly efficient photon detectors.

Another type of detector used in a large number of third-generation scanners is the xenon gas detector. These detectors utilize the ionization of the gas by the incident radiation as a way of producing an electrical signal. Such gaseous detectors are operated at relatively low voltages, so that the magnitude of the current produced is proportional to the intensity of the x-rays incident on the detector. Although these are not as efficient as scintillation detectors, the choice of detector usually lies with the manufacturer. It is generally considered that the type of detector has little or no effect on the quality of the CT image.

Collimation of the x-ray beam occurs at two specific locations. The first point of collimation occurs near the x-ray tube and the second at the detector. It is at the second point that scatter radiation is controlled. Collimation also controls slice thickness. Most scanners allow variation of slice thickness to selected values such as 1, 2, 5, or 10 mm.

The other major component of the CT unit is the digital computer. Once the scan sequence has been initiated by the technologist, the imaging continues under computer control. The computer coordinates the full sequence of events required for data collection, image reconstruction, data storage, and data retrieval. The technologist can also manipulate the data once it is collected in order to vary brightness, contrast, magnification, and rotation of the image.

NUCLEAR MEDICINE

Like radiology, nuclear medicine also uses ionizing radiation to obtain medical images. Unlike radiology, nuclear medicine utilizes gamma radiation from radioactive materials, primarily from a radioisotope of the element technetium known as *technetium-99m (^{99m}Tc)*. This particular radionuclide emits a 140-keV gamma photon used in the imaging process. This is comparable in energy to x-ray photons used in diagnostic radiography. Radiography has the capability of changing x-ray energies by varying kVp. In nuclear medicine, to change the energy of the radiation used, one must change the radionuclide.

Nuclear Imaging Principles

Nuclear medicine procedures perform what is referred to as physiological imaging. This indicates that the clinical studies are designed to tell the physician whether a specific organ (e.g., lungs, heart, liver) is functioning properly.

Imaging is performed by injecting the patient with an appropriate *radiopharmaceutical*. The radiopharmaceutical is a drug or compound that has been "labeled" or "tagged" with a radioactive atom such as ^{99m}Tc. When injected into the bloodstream, the body responds to the chemical composition of the pharmaceutical, not the fact that it is radioactive. For example, a pharmaceutical that behaves chemically like calcium is incorporated into bone. If the compound is radioactive and emits radiation, a "bone image" can be obtained with appropriate radiation detectors. A list of commonly used radiopharmaceuticals and clinical information regarding each is shown in Table 22–1. The table contains only a partial list of the radiopharmaceuticals used in nuclear imaging procedures. The list of radiopharmaceuticals continues to change as new and better imaging agents are produced.

Once a patient has been referred for a nuclear study by his or her physician, the specific radiopharmaceutical is prepared by either a technologist within the nuclear medicine department or a nuclear pharmacy. The patient is positioned on the imaging table, and the technologist injects the radiopharmaceutical into the patient's bloodstream. The imaging process begins.

Imaging Equipment

Unlike radiography, nuclear imaging equipment does not produce radiation. Instead, the patient is the radiation source and the nuclear "cameras" used are large, sensitive radiation detectors. A nuclear camera is shown in Figure 22–4. Gamma photons emitted from the patient's body first encounter a lead collimator mounted on the face of the camera. The collimator typically is a thickness of lead into which holes of equal size and equal spacing have been drilled. These devices act in the same way as grids in radiography and are used to reduce the amount of scatter included in the final image. Only gamma photons that travel along certain directions enter the detector, whereas others are absorbed in the lead of the collimator.

Photons that enter the detector next strike a large sodium iodide (NaI) crystal, which gives off tiny flashes of light (known as scintillations) when the energy of the incident photons is absorbed by the crystal. Nuclear imaging cameras are also known as *scintillation cameras* for this reason. These faint flashes are detected by sensitive photomultiplier tubes (PMTs) located behind the crystal face. Most modern scintillation cameras employ any number from 37 to 91 PMTs, depending on the size of the camera. The PMTs convert the scintillations into electrical pulses. These electrical pulses are then electronically sorted and are used to generate a visible light image. The image appearing on a CRT screen represents the distribution of the radiopharmaceutical within the patient's body. This visible light image then exposes a piece of radiographic film. The film is processed in an automatic film processor, and a "hard copy" of the patient's study is obtained. A typical nuclear medicine study is shown in Figure 22–5. Because of the manner in which the image is transferred to the film, unlike radiography in which images are light on a dark background, nuclear images are dark on a light background.

Many commonly performed nuclear studies trace the movement of specific radiopharmaceuticals through organs such as the kidneys, heart, and lungs. In many such cases in which the movement of the radiopharmaceutical occurs extremely rapidly, the imaging process is computer-controlled. This method allows imaging to occur at a much faster rate, and the

Table 22–1: RADIOPHARMACEUTICALS COMMONLY USED IN NUCLEAR MEDICINE

Pharmaceutical	Radionuclide Tag	Principal Photon Energy	Physical Half-Life	Clinical Use
Diagnostic Applications				
Thallous chloride	^{201}Tl	68–80 keV	73.1 hr	To evaluate myocardial perfusion and ischemia
Sestamibi	^{99m}Tc	140 keV	6 hr	
Pyrophosphate	^{99m}Tc	140 keV	6 hr	To evaluate acute myocardial infarction
DTPA	^{99m}Tc	140 keV	6 hr	Brain imaging
Gluceptate	^{99m}Tc	140 keV	6 hr	
Sodium iodide	^{123}I	159 keV	13 hr	Thyroid imaging
Sodium pertechnetate	^{99m}Tc	140 keV	6 hr	
Sulfur colloid	^{99m}Tc	140 keV	6 hr	Liver/spleen imaging
Mertiatide (MAG$_3$)	^{99m}Tc	140 keV	6 hr	Renal imaging
Succimer (DMSA)	^{99m}Tc	140 keV	6 hr	
MAA particles	^{99m}Tc	140 keV	6 hr	Lung perfusion studies
Xenon gas	^{133}Xe	80 keV	5.3 days	Lung ventilation studies
MDP	^{99m}Tc	140 keV	6 hr	Bone imaging studies
Oxidronate	^{99m}Tc	140 keV	6 hr	
Therapeutic Applications				
Sodium iodide	^{131}I	364 keV	8 days	Treatment of hyperthyroidism and thyroid cancer
Chromic phosphate	^{32}P	1.71 MeV (β^-)	14 days	Treatment of peritoneal and pleural effusions
Sodium phosphate	^{32}P	1.71 MeV (β^-)	14 days	Treatment of certain leukemias and bone metastases

keV = kiloelectron volts; MAA = macroaggregated albumin; MDP = methylene diphosphate.

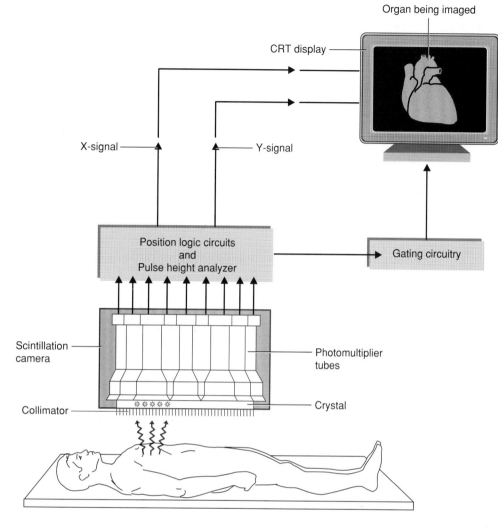

FIGURE 22-4. A scintillation camera used in nuclear medicine procedures in a sensitive radiation detector.

images acquired are much more representative of the true flow rates and clearance times (i.e., the time required for a radiopharmaceutical to be cleared from an organ). Computers play a major role in many standard studies, not only in the acquisition of data but in the processing and analysis of the images obtained.

Two additional nuclear imaging techniques that employ the computer in the generation of images are *SPECT* and *PET.* SPECT (single photon emission computed tomography) is the nuclear medicine version of CT (i.e., x-ray computed tomography). It uses a scintillation camera capable of rotating about the body. As in standard nuclear medicine procedures, the patient is injected with an appropriate radiopharmaceutical, depending on which organ is being imaged. SPECT allows functional imaging of an organ one thin slice at a time. Slice imaging (i.e., *tomography*) possibly allows the physician to see lesions and defects that might otherwise have been missed when viewing a single image of the entire organ.

PET (positron emission tomography) is currently performed only in specific cities in the United States. It is a highly specialized nuclear imaging procedure

that utilizes positron (β^+)-emitting radiopharmaceuticals. Because of the short physical half-lives (Table 22-2) and the special techniques required for radiopharmaceutical preparation, most PET centers have been located near the production sites of the radiopharmaceuticals. Another factor which has limited the use of PET is that the scintillation cameras employed are very different from standard nuclear medicine cameras. Recall that when a positron is emitted, annihilation radiation soon results when the positron encounters an electron. It is the two 511-keV photons, emitted in opposite directions, that are detected and used in image formation. Greater radiation protection precautions must be taken by imaging personnel because of the 511-keV photon radiation produced.

Recent developments in availability of positron-emitting radiopharmaceuticals will allow more facilities to employ PET techniques if they wish to do so. The advantages of PET lie in the fact that the radionuclides used (e.g., oxygen, nitrogen, carbon) are natural components of the body. PET holds great promise in early detection of coronary artery disease (CAD), brain metabolism studies, and studies in neurological disorders.

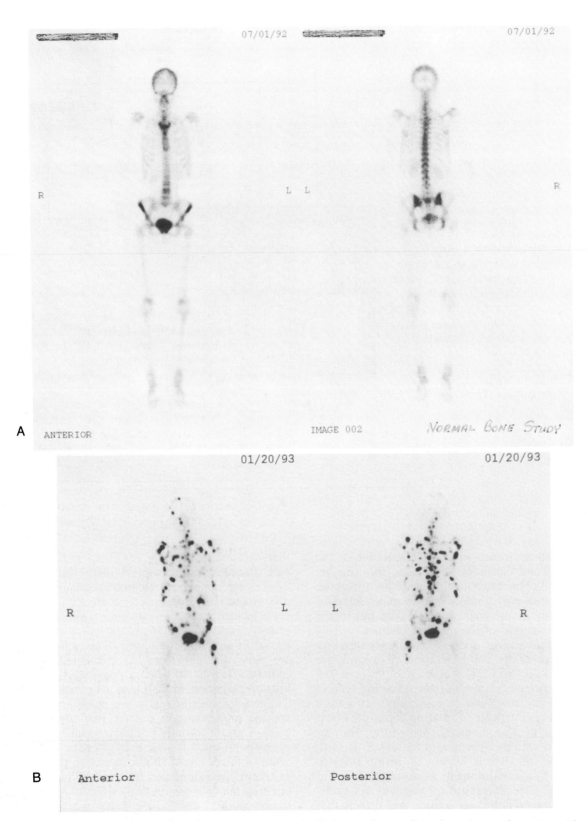

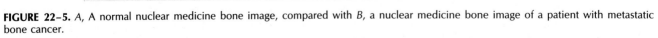

FIGURE 22–5. *A*, A normal nuclear medicine bone image, compared with *B*, a nuclear medicine bone image of a patient with metastatic bone cancer.

Table 22-2: RADIOPHARMACEUTICALS COMMONLY USED WITH PET IMAGING SYSTEMS

Pharmaceutical	Radionuclide Tag (β^+)	Physical Half-Life	Clinical Use
Deoxy-D-glucose	^{18}F	110.0 min ⎫	Brain metabolism studies
	^{11}C	20.3 min ⎭	
Ammonia	^{13}N	10.0 min	Perfusion studies
Thymidine	^{11}C	20.3 min	DNA synthesis studies
Carbon dioxide	^{15}O	2.0 min	Oxygen utilization studies
Oxygen gas	^{15}O	2.0 min	Oxygen utilization studies

C = carbon; DNA = deoxyribonucleic acid; F = fluorine; N = nitrogen; O = oxygen.

Radiation Protection in Nuclear Medicine

Radioactive materials come in all physical forms—solids, liquids, and gases. Those used in nuclear medicine are primarily in liquid form, but gases are used for ventilation studies. Thus in addition to using time, distance, and shielding to reduce radiation exposure, nuclear medicine personnel must always be aware of potential *contamination*—the unacceptable spread of radioactive material to such areas as countertops, floors, personnel, imaging tables, and the like. Daily checks are made to minimize the possibility of radioactive contamination. This is not a life-threatening problem, but contamination potentially may lead to misdiagnosis of a patient. It therefore is imperative that potential contamination problems be controlled.

For nuclear medicine personnel the greatest radiation dose occurs to the hands as a result of preparing and injecting radiopharmaceuticals. To minimize hand exposure, syringes can be inserted into syringe shields made of lead, tungsten, or depleted uranium. The highest whole body doses are usually received by technologists who prepare the radiopharmaceuticals. However, with the advent of nuclear pharmacies in almost every major city, this exposure to the technologist has been greatly reduced.

MAGNETIC RESONANCE IMAGING

Magnetic resonance imaging (MRI) is the newest of the medical imaging modalities even though it has been in use in the United States for a number of years. MRI is based on the principles of the phenomenon known as nuclear magnetic resonance (NMR), which was first described by physicists Felix Bloch at Stanford University and Edward Purcell at Harvard. Although originally used as an analytical tool on test tube samples in physics and chemistry, the principles were later extended to medical imaging as the technology of designing large-bore magnets developed. The imaging modality utilizes strong magnetic fields, radiofrequency (RF) radiation, and computers to generate some of the most diagnostically useful images ever produced in medicine—images like those shown in Figure 22-6.

MRI does not employ ionizing radiation, but it does use nonionizing radiofrequency radiation like FM radiowaves. As discussed in the next section, bone poses a problem for ultrasound. This is not the case for proton MRI images, in which bone is invisible. Additional advantages of MRI include the following:

● Images in almost any plane of the body (i.e., transverse, sagittal, coronal, and angular cuts) can be produced with MRI

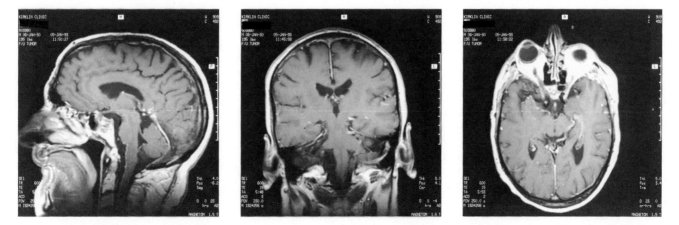

FIGURE 22-6. Magnetic resonance (MRI) images of the head in the sagittal (*left*), coronal (*middle*), and transverse (*right*) planes. MRI can provide images in almost any body plane.

- Chemical changes that occur within body tissues as a precursor to certain disease states can potentially be visualized with MRI
- Risks associated with exposure to ionizing radiation are not present with MRI

However, the technology of MRI does have certain limitations:

- Some patients are eliminated as candidates for MRI studies—those who are claustrophobic or who have cardiac pacemakers, aneurysm clips, or a metal prosthesis
- MRI units must be located in areas with minimal radiofrequency interference or RF shielding must be used
- MRI units must be located away from instruments affected by strong magnetic fields (e.g., CRTs, computers, magnetic tapes, floppy disks, nuclear medicine cameras)
- Safety zones must be established around the MRI magnet to protect personnel (e.g., housekeeping staff and security) and the public from the effects of strong magnetic fields and RF radiation
- MRI units and associated instrumentation are extremely expensive

Even with these limitations, the uses of MRI in medicine have just begun to be explored.

Principles of Magnetic Resonance Imaging

During the 1940s, it was observed that certain atomic nuclei such as hydrogen behave like tiny magnets. When these nuclei are placed in a strong magnetic field and are bombarded by radiowaves of the right frequency, they absorb the radiowaves and almost immediately re-emit this energy, also in the form of radiowaves, like tiny radio transmitters.

Since a major portion of the body is composed of water, there is a more than an adequate supply of hydrogen atoms, which can act as receivers and transmitters of the RF radiation. In the magnetic resonance imaging unit, the patient is positioned inside a large magnet in which the magnetic field strength may be as much as 30,000 times stronger than the Earth's magnetic field. The patient is then bombarded by the appropriate RF radiation. Sensitive radio receivers surrounding the patient's body detect the weak radio signals re-emitted by the hydrogen nuclei within the patient's body.

The signals that are returned from the patient's body are extremely complex and contain a variety of information concerning the tissues from which they originate. The signals generally contain information regarding two tissue parameters referred to as the spin-lattice relaxation time (T_1) and the spin-spin relaxation time (T_2) as well as hydrogen concentration information and flow information. Each of these parameters can individually be affected by disease states to such a degree that if an image could be generated based solely upon a particular parameter, pathologies could possibly be visualized. With MRI the individual contributions of each of these parameters to the output signal cannot totally be separated. However, using certain well-defined series of RF pulses (known as *pulsing sequences*), images in which the contrast is more dependent on T_1, T_2, or hydrogen concentration can be generated. These are referred to as T_1-weighted, T_2-weighted, and proton density–weighted images.

It happens that T_1 and T_2 are more sensitive to pathological changes, and as a result, T_1- and T_2-weighted images are more useful from a diagnostic standpoint.

In addition to image production, MRI units having large enough field strengths can be used to generate specific chemical profiles for tissues such as cardiac muscle. What is of primary interest to cardiologists is the relative quantity of phosphorous compounds (e.g., inorganic phosphates, phosphocreatine, and ATP) present in the cardiac muscle. The relative quantity of each of these compounds tends to change, depending on the condition of the heart muscle. This technique, referred to as NMR spectroscopy, holds great promise as a noninvasive technique in determining the extent of damage done to the cardiac muscle as a result of a heart attack (i.e., a myocardial infarction).

Magnetic Resonance Imaging Equipment

The heart of the magnetic resonance imaging unit is a magnet—one typically having a magnetic field strength some 50,000 times stronger than the Earth's magnetic field measured at sea level. This strong magnetic field is produced by current-carrying coils of wire. If the coils are constructed of ordinary metals

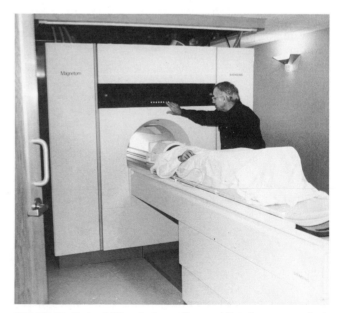

FIGURE 22–7. An MRI unit that utilizes a 1.5 tesla superconducting magnet.

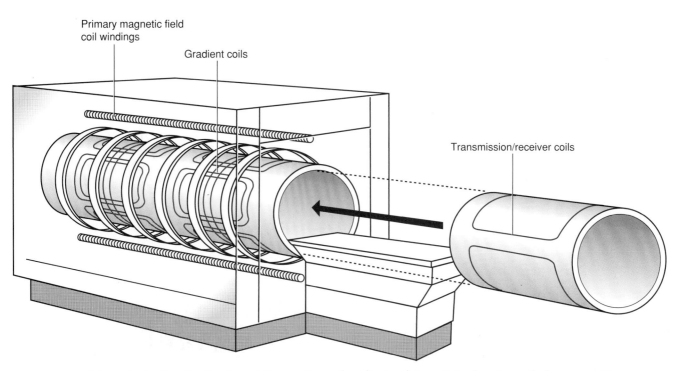

Primary magnetic field coil windings

Gradient coils

Transmission/receiver coils

FIGURE 22-8. Schematic drawing showing the relative positions of gradient and transmission/receiver coils for a magnetic resonance imaging (MRI) unit.

that have electrical resistance, they are termed *resistive magnets*. It is perhaps more common to find the coils made of niobium-titanium, which when cooled with liquid helium becomes *superconducting*. This term indicates that as long as the wires remain at these extremely low temperatures, electrical resistance in the wires essentially drops to zero, and the unit can operate for several weeks without being connected to a power source. Most imaging centers have opted for superconducting magnets such as that shown in Figure 22–7 because of their increased field strength, stability, uniformity, and relative inexpense of operation.

Arranged internally around the magnet's bore (i.e., the opening into which the patient is positioned) is a complex array of current-carrying coils known as gradient coils. The magnitude and direction of currents flowing through these coils are computer-controlled. By varying the currents, the magnetic field strength across the patient's body can be varied. This variation allows images to be produced in almost any body plane. This is an advantage not shared by any other imaging modality. Gradient coil design and positions around the cylindrical bore are illustrated in Figure 22–8.

RF transmitter and receiver coils are another important component of MR imaging units. These coils either surround the patient's body or may be placed directly on the body. In the latter case, they are known as surface coils. The coils are connected to RF transmitters, illustrated in Figure 22–9, and are responsible for sending the RF signals into the patient's body and receiving the signals re-emitted from the body tissues. These signals are extremely weak. To minimize the possibility of external radiofrequency interference, RF shielding is commonly used with MR imaging systems. It usually takes the form of a metal screen (known as a Faraday cage), which may be extended over the patient's body during the imaging process. Some MR facilities need to enclose the entire imaging room with metal screening to minimize external interference.

The complexity of generating images using magnetic resonance requires the use of computers. Computers are used not only to analyze the complex MR signal and produce the final digital image but computers also control RF transmission, the current flow through the gradient coils necessary for slice selection, and adjustments necessary for magnetic field uniformity.

DIAGNOSTIC MEDICAL SONOGRAPHY (ULTRASOUND)

The use of sound waves to locate objects submerged under water had its first major application during World War II. It was known as SONAR (an acronym for *so*und *na*vigation and *r*anging) and was used to locate submarines below the ocean surface. By the early 1960s, ultrasound has made the transition from war-time applications to its uses in medical diagnosis and therapy.

Principles of Ultrasonic Imaging

Sound waves carry energy but not in the same way as x-rays. Recall that x-rays and other forms of elec-

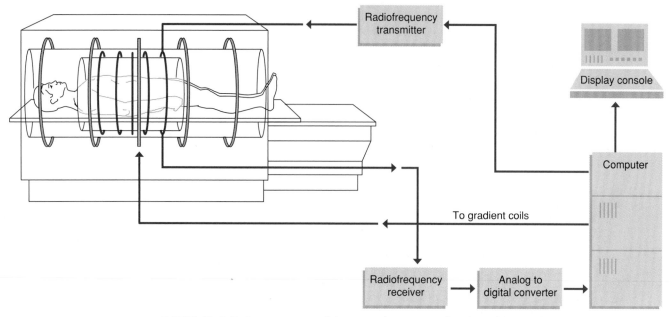

FIGURE 22-9. Basic components of the magnetic resonance imaging system.

tromagnetic radiation travel in the form of transverse waves; sound waves, however, travel in the form of pressure or longitudinal waves (Fig. 22–10). The sound waves used for medical diagnosis utilize frequencies above the audible hearing range, as indicated in Table 22–3, and is therefore referred to as ultrasound.

Diagnostic medical sonography, or ultrasonic imaging, is based on the principle that as sound waves are sent into the patient's body and strike structures such as bones and organs, a portion of the incident wave is transmitted through the structure and a portion is reflected (Fig. 22–11). How much of the incident sound energy is reflected depends on the acoustic properties of the tissues. For example, bone produces extremely strong *echoes* compared with soft tissue structures.

Ultrasound has found great acceptance in the medical community because of several factors. Ultrasound does not employ ionizing radiation as do radiography and nuclear medicine. This makes ultrasound the imaging modality of choice for obstetrics and gynecology. Another strong capability of ultrasound is its ability to distinguish between soft tissue and fluid-filled structures such as cysts. It is also easy to gauge size and depth of structures based on knowledge of the speed of sound in tissue and the length of time required for the echo to reach the surface.

Some features of body structure do pose significant problems for ultrasound. Air poses the first problem. Whenever a sound wave encounters air, there is a major reflection of the incident sound wave. This is first encountered at the skin surface as the sound wave is transmitted from the sound source (known as a *transducer*) into the body. For the sound wave to enter the body, the air layer between the transducer and the patient's body must be removed. This is accomplished by filling in the air space with a coupling gel or min-

eral oil on the skin surface before placement of the transducer on the patient's body. Air can still pose a significant problem—for example, in an abdominal study when the patient has abdominal gas. The gas may reflect such a major portion of the sound wave that deeper structures cannot be seen. In this situation, the patient is sent back to his or her room, and imaging may be attempted at a later time.

Bone poses the other major problem for ultrasound. Since bone also reflects a major portion of the incident sound waves, structures located behind bones can be missed. One example of this is in ultrasonic imaging of the heart (known as *echocardiography*). Because of the anatomical location of the heart, the ultrasonic beam must be carefully angled between the ribs in order to image the heart and its internal structures.

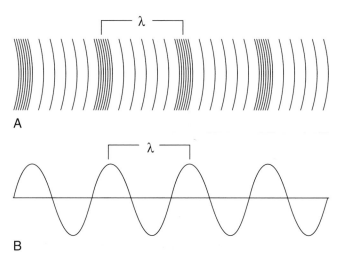

FIGURE 22-10. Sound travels in the form of a longitudinal wave (*A*), whereas x-rays travel in the form of transverse waves (*B*).

Table 22–3: CLASSIFICATION OF SOUND WAVES BY FREQUENCY

Frequency	Classification	Comments
$<\sim 20$ Hz	Infrasound	Seismic waves are of this type
20–20,000 Hz	Audible sound	Hearing range of average human
$>20,000$ Hz	Ultrasound	Cannot be heard by humans
1–20 MHz	Diagnostic ultrasound	Low intensities used for diagnostic imaging
1–10 MHz	Therapeutic ultrasound	High intensities are used to produce deep-heating effects

Hz = hertz; MHz = megahertz.

Ultrasonic Imaging Equipment

Ultrasonic sound waves are produced by the device known as a transducer, a general term used to describe any device that converts one form of energy to another. The heart of the transducer is a thin piezoelectric crystal, typically a ceramic material such as lead zirconate titanate (PZT). Electrical contacts attached to the crystal provide electrical voltage to the faces of the crystal. As the voltage polarity is rapidly changed (Fig. 22–12*A*), the crystal quickly expands and contracts. This expansion and contraction of the crystal produces ultrasonic pulses.

As the ultrasonic pulses enter the patient's body, they encounter different tissues and tissue structures. The greater the differences in the acoustic properties of the tissues encountered, the greater the reflections occurring at their surfaces. These echoes of various intensity travel back to the transducer. During the "receiving phase," the transducer does not send out sound pulses but "listens" for the returning echoes. As the returning echoes strike the transducer crystal at the surface of the patient's body, the pressure waves cause the crystal to expand and contract as the compressions and rarefactions of the reflected sound waves move across the crystal. This reaction generates voltage

pulses (i.e., electrical signals) of varying magnitudes, depending on the strength or intensity of the incoming echoes. This phase is illustrated in Figure 22–12*B*. This method of sending out sound pulses (transmission phase) when waiting for a period of time to receive the reflected waves (receiving phase) is referred to as *pulsed ultrasound*. Most common ultrasound procedures use this technique.

As the reflected sound waves are received and converted into electrical pulses, the pulses are converted into "echo" images, which are visualized on a CRT screen. The medical sonographer can generate numerous cross-sectional images of the patient and when the best view is obtained, the image can be transferred to film to obtain a hard copy. Such an echo image is shown in Figure 22–13. All images obtained with standard ultrasound are transverse slices. For this reason, sonographers must be familiar with transverse anatomy.

Typically, in imaging with ultrasound, sound frequencies ranging from 1 to 20 megahertz (MHz) have been used. In general, as the frequency is increased, image resolution improves. However, at the same time as the frequency is increased, the penetrating ability decreases. For this reason, abdominal studies, which need a greater depth of penetration, use frequencies from about 2 to 5 MHz. In examinations of smaller structures such as the eye, higher frequencies, from 10 to 20 MHz, can be employed. Frequencies are changed simply by physically interchanging transducers.

Motion can also be viewed with ultrasound using multicrystal transducers known as linear array transducers. With this type of transducer, each crystal element sends out its sound waves in sequence. As each echo returns in sequence and is converted to an image on the display screen, apparent movement of the structure is displayed. This is called *real-time ultrasound*. Many specialized transducers of this type have been designed to meet special types of imaging requirements. Such imaging techniques have been extremely useful in obstetrics and cardiology.

Advances in ultrasound technology also permit the measurement of blood flow rates through carotid arteries, which is useful in diagnosing potential stroke victims. Using sound waves to measure blood flow rates is known as *Doppler ultrasound*. This has also become an extremely useful tool in cardiology in the evaluation of blood flow through the chambers of the heart.

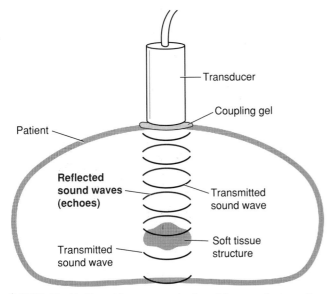

FIGURE 22–11. Sound images are produced by sound waves that are reflected (echoes) from internal body structures.

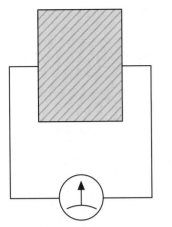
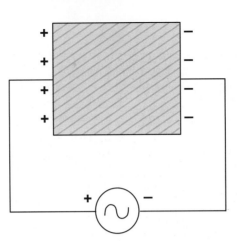
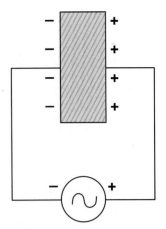

No voltage applied; no crystal deformation observed

Voltage applied; crystal expansion observed

Voltage of opposite polarity applied; crystal compression observed

A

Transmission phase

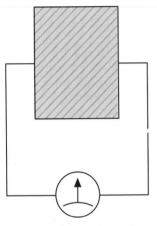
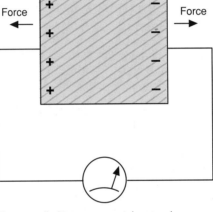
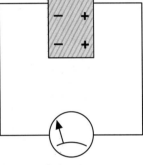

No pressure exerted; no voltage measured

Force applied to cause crystal expansion; voltage measured

Force applied to compress crystal; voltage of opposite polarity observed

B

Receiving phase

FIGURE 22–12. *A*, Transmission and *B*, receiving phases of the piezoelectric element of an ultrasonic transducer.

FIGURE 22–13. An ultrasonic image of the heart, showing both left (LV) and right ventricles (RV) and left (LA) and right atria (RA).

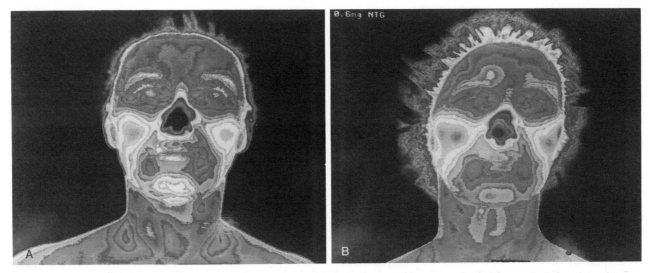

FIGURE 22-14. A, normal thermographic image, indicating symmetrical distribution of heat over the facial area. B, A thermographic image indicating an abnormal heat distribution over the patient's right eye. This was caused by dilated blood vessels as the patient experienced a migraine headache.

MEDICAL THERMOGRAPHY

Another mode of medical imaging which is gaining more acceptance in the American medical community is medical *thermography.* Thermography produces images based on variations in body surface temperature. Although this mode of imaging has been more widely accepted in Europe, improvements in infrared (IR) imaging cameras have revived an interest in this noninvasive modality.

Principles of Thermographic Imaging

Heat in measurable quantities is a by-product of many body metabolic processes. Heat generated from production sites deep within body structures is conducted to nearby cooler tissue. Heat is also transferred by the flowing blood and is brought to the body surface, where it is dissipated. As a result, body surface temperature can vary from one point on the body to another, depending on metabolic activity and circulatory processes just below the skin. Variations from these normal temperature distributions may then be symptomatic of pathology or circulatory problems. Thermographic images illustrating a flow defect are shown in Figure 22-14.

Thermographic Imaging Units

Skin having a surface temperature of 30°C typically emits electromagnetic radiation having wavelengths within the range of 4000 to 40,000 nm, most wavelengths being approximately 9500 nm. These wavelengths fall within the infrared portion of the electromagnetic energy spectrum. Although there are several

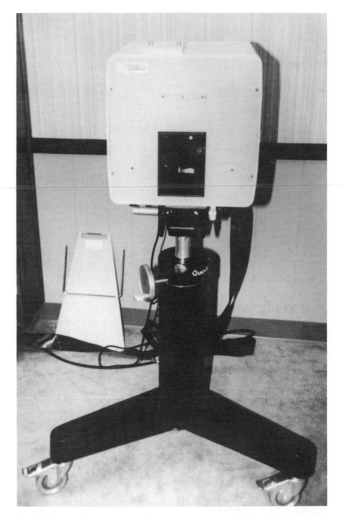

FIGURE 22-15. An infrared camera used to obtain medical thermographic images.

basic designs of infrared detectors, each basically consists of a device that converts infrared radiation emitted from the body surface into electrical signals. The magnitude of the signals may be made temperature-dependent as with thermal detectors. Another type produces electrical signals proportional to the wavelength of the IR radiation received by the detector. This is called a photon detector; it is sensitive to IR radiation within a narrow wavelength band and is usually cooled with liquid nitrogen to increase sensitivity. Such an infrared detector is shown in Figure 22–15.

Electrical signals from these units can be electronically sorted and displayed, using an appropriate color scale. Newer IR imaging systems allow studies to be stored electronically and hard copies to be produced, using color laser-jet printers.

Studies conducted with these units require some degree of patient preparation. Patients undergoing such studies must have clean, dry skin free of cosmetic creams, deodorants, or anything that can alter skin surface temperature. Clothing must also be removed and the body allowed to adapt to room temperature (~21°C for approximately 20 minutes). Doing this tends to enhance temperature differences and therefore affects thermographic image contrast.

Chapter Summary/ Important Concepts

Computed tomography (CT) is a specialized type of radiographic imaging utilizing an x-ray tube that rotates around the patient's body to produce tomographic, or slice, images. The primary difference between CT and conventional linear tomographic systems is that with CT the images are computer-generated. X-ray beam attenuation is measured at a large number of angles around the patient's body, and the data acquired are stored in the computer and then used to reconstruct a digital image of the body slice. Although primarily used to produce transverse images, the data acquired can be computer-manipulated to produce images in other body planes or three-dimensional images.

Nuclear medicine performs functional imaging with the use of small quantities of radioactive material attached to specific chemical compounds known as radiopharmaceuticals, which are injected into a patient's bloodstream. The body recognizes the compound only by its chemical identity, not by its radioactive tag. The radioactive tag most commonly used in nuclear medicine procedures is technetium-99m (^{99m}Tc), which emits a 140-keV gamma photon. The biodistribution of the radiopharmaceutical within the patient's body can then be monitored using an extremely sensitive gamma detector known as a scintillation camera positioned above the patient's body. The distribution of the radiopharmaceutical within the patient's body can then be used to determine whether a particular organ is functioning correctly or if disease is present. In some cases, some radioactive materials may be administered in higher doses to treat certain types of cancer. Since radioactive materials are used in solid, liquid, and gaseous form, great care must be taken to avoid radioactive contamination of facilities and personnel.

Magnetic resonance imaging (MRI) combines the use of strong magnetic fields, radiofrequency (RF) radiation, and the computer to produce its images. With MRI radiowaves of a specific frequency are transmitted into the patient's body. Hydrogen nuclei in the body absorb this radiation and then re-emit the radiation. The radiation that is re-emitted is detected by sensitive receiver coils placed around the anatomical part being imaged. The signals received are complex and contain information regarding MR tissue parameters known as relaxation times T_1 and T_2. Computer images that are T_1- or T_2-weighted can then be generated. Certain pathologies may be better visualized on a T_1- than on a T_2-weighted image and vice versa. MR can also be used to obtain flow information. Because of the strength of the magnetic fields employed, great care must be taken by personnel working in MRI. This imaging modality does not use ionizing radiation. It is the only imaging modality that can obtain tomographic slices in almost any body plane.

Diagnostic medical sonography (ultrasound) provides its images by sending sound waves (~1 MHZ–20 MHz) into the body and measuring the strength of the echoes produced. The sound waves are produced by an ultrasonic transducer that acts as both transmitter and receiver. When the transducer acts as both, the process is referred to as pulsed ultrasound. Ultrasound does not use ionizing radiation. One of the strengths of ultrasound is its ability to visualize cystic (fluid-filled) structures that can be missed by x-ray. Imaging problems can however occur when ultrasound strikes bone, air, or abdominal gas. Multi-element transducers can be used to produce motion images that are referred to as real-time ultrasound. Ultrasound also employs Doppler techniques to measure flow velocities. This has proved useful in measuring blood flow through carotid arteries and the chambers of the heart.

Medical thermography creates its images by mapping the temperature differences that exist over the skin surface. Images are usually produced using infrared cameras. Thermography is both a useful and noninvasive technique for localizing areas of inflammation and altered blood flow.

Important Terminology

Computed Tomography (CT). A specialized form of medical imaging utilizing a rotating x-ray tube and digital computer to generate cross-sectional images of the body, most commonly in the transverse plane

Contamination. The spread of radioactive materials to places where it should not be

Diagnostic Medical Sonography (ultrasound). A medical imaging modality that produces its images by measuring the intensity of echoes reflected from body structures when ultrasonic pulses are transmitted into the body; also referred to as sonar

Digital Image. A computer-generated image formed when individual picture elements (pixels) within an image matrix are assigned a specific shade of gray (or color) based on the numerical value of the individual pixel

Doppler ultrasound. An ultrasonic imaging technique used to measure flow velocities

Echocardiography. The imaging of the heart using diagnostic medical ultrasound

Echoes. The ultrasonic waves reflected from body structures when ultrasonic waves are transmitted into the body

Magnetic Resonance Imaging (MRI). A medical imaging modality that uses strong magnetic fields, radiowaves, and a digital computer to generate cross-sectional images in almost any plane of the body

PET. Positron emission tomography; a specialized nuclear medicine imaging technique that utilizes positron-emitting radionuclides

Pixel. A picture element; an individual element of a digital maxtrix

Pulsed Ultrasound. A technique employed in diagnostic ultrasound in which the transducer transmits ultrasonic pulses (transmitting phase) for a short period of time then waits to receive the reflected pulses (receiving phase) from body structures

Pulsing Sequences. A specific sequence of radiowaves transmitted into the patient's body during an MR imaging procedure and used to obtain images that are T_1-, T_2-, or proton-density–weighted

Radiopharmaceutical. The radioactive compound administered to the patient in order to perform a nuclear medicine study

Real-Time Ultrasound. Ultrasonic imaging technique using multi-element transducers to produce dynamic images

Resistive Magnet. A type of magnet whose magnetic field is produced by conventional current-carrying wires

Scintillation Camera. An extremely sensitive radiation detector used to produce an image in nuclear medicine

SPECT. Single photon emission computed tomography; a nuclear medicine technique for acquiring tomographic images with commonly used radioactive materials such as ^{99m}Tc

Superconducting Magnet. A type of magnet whose magnetic field is produced by current-carrying wires that when cooled to extremely low temperatures lose their electrical resistance

Technetium-99m (^{99m}Tc). The radioisotope used to label chemical compounds used most commonly in performing nuclear medicine studies; this radionuclide emits a 140-keV photon and has a physical half-life of six hours

Thermography. A medical imaging modality that generates images of the body based on skin surface temperature differences; such images can be used to localize sites of inflammation and blood flow abnormalities

Tomography. Any form of medical imaging in which slice images are produced

Transducer. Any device which converts one form of energy into another

Voxel. A volume element; the small volume of tissue represented by a pixel in a digital image

Bibliography

Bushong, S.C.; Archer, B.R. Diagnostic ultrasound: Physics, Biology and Instrumentation. St. Louis: Mosby-Year Book, 1991.

Chilton, H.M.; Witcofski, R.L. Nuclear Pharmacy: An Introduction to the Clinical Applications of Radiopharmaceuticals. Philadelphia: Lea & Febiger, 1986.

Coulam, C.M.; Erickson, J.J.; Rollo, F.D.; James, A.E. The Physical Basis of Medical Imaging. New York: Appleton-Century-Crofts, 1981.

Curry, T.S.; Dowdey, J.E.; Murry, R.C. Jr. Christenson's Physics of Diagnostic Radiology, 4th ed. Philadelphia: Lea & Febiger, 1990.

Kremkau, Frederick W. Diagnostic Ultrasound: Principles, Instruments and Exercises, 3rd ed. Philadelphia: W.B. Saunders, 1989.

Sprawls, P. Physical Principles of Medical Imaging. Rockville, MD: Aspen Publishers, 1987.

Wells, P.N.T. Scientific Basis of Medical Imaging. New York: Churchill Livingstone, 1982.

Williams, L.E. Nuclear Medical Physics, Vol 3. Boca Raton: CRC Press, 1987.

░░░ Review Questions

1. Indicate several basic differences between CT and conventional radiography.
2. Explain the type of images produced in nuclear medicine procedures in terms of what is represented in the images.
3. Compare the energies used in diagnostic radiography with that of ^{99m}Tc, commonly used in nuclear medicine studies.
4. What additional radiation protection precautions must be taken in nuclear medicine departments that are not required in radiology departments?
5. How does the radiation used in MRI compare with diagnostic energy x-rays?
6. List two advantages MRI has over conventional radiography and nuclear medicine.
7. Although MRI uses non-ionizing radiation, what aspects of MRI can cause concern for potential biological effects?
8. What type of radiation is detected and mapped in thermographic images.
9. What are the positive aspects of thermography as an imaging modality?

Index

Note: Page numbers in *italics* refer to illustrations; numbers followed by (t) indicate tables.

ISBN 0-7216-3428-1

90071

MOST COMMONLY USED GREEK PREFIXES

Prefix	Multiple	Symbol	Example
mega-	10^6	M	MeV
kilo-	10^3	k	keV, kV, kg
centi-	10^{-2}	c	cm
milli-	10^{-3}	m	mm, mg, ms
micro-	10^{-6}	μ, mc	μm, mcg
nano-	10^{-9}	n	nm

USEFUL CONSTANTS

Quantity	Symbol	Numerical Value
Speed of light	c	3×10^8 m/sec
Charge on electron	e	-1.6×10^{-19} coulomb
Electron mass	m_e	9.1×10^{-31} kg
Proton mass	m_p	1.673×10^{-27} kg
Neutron mass	m_n	1.675×10^{-27} kg
Gravitational constant	G	$6.67 \times 10^{-11} \dfrac{N\text{-}m^2}{kg^2}$
Electric constant	k	$9 \times 10^9 \dfrac{N\text{-}m^2}{coul^2}$
Planck's constant	h	6.63×10^{-34} J-sec $= 4.14 \times 10^{-15}$ eV-sec